Introducing Social Policy

Second Edition

Cliff Alcock
Guy Daly
Edwin Griggs

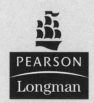

PEARSON

Longman

Harlow, England • London • New York • Boston • San Francisco • Toronto • Sydney • Singapore • Hong Kong
Tokyo • Seoul • Taipei • New Delhi • Cape Town • Madrid • Mexico City • Amsterdam • Munich • Paris • Milan

Pearson Education Limited
Edinburgh Gate
Harlow
Essex CM20 2JE
England

and Associated Companies throughout the world

Visit us on the World Wide Web at:
www.pearsoned.co.uk

First published 2000
Revised edition published 2004
Second edition published 2008

ISBN: 978-1-4058-5848-9

British Library Cataloguing-in-Publication Data
A catalogue record for this book is available from the British Library

Library of Congress Cataloging-in-Publication Data
Alcock, Cliff.
  Introducing social policy / Cliff Alcock, Guy Daly, Edwin Griggs.-- 2nd ed.
     p. cm.
  Includes bibliographical references and index.
  ISBN-13: 978-1-4058-5848-9 (alk. paper)
  1. Great Britain--Social policy. 2. Public welfare--Great Britain. 3. Public welfare administration--Great Britain. 4. Social service--Great Britain. I. Daly, Guy. II. Griggs, Edwin. III. Title.
  HV248.A43 2008
  320.60941--dc22

                          2008012618

10 9 8 7 6 5 4 3 2 1
12 11 10 09 08

Typeset in 10/12.5pt Sabon by 3
Printed by Ashford Colour Press Ltd., Gosport

The publisher's policy is to use paper manufactured from sustainable forests.

Introducing Social Policy

Visit the *Introducing Social Policy*, Second Edition Companion Website at
www.pearsoned.co.uk/alcock to find valuable **student** learning material
including:

- Updates and questions on the latest developments in social policy
- Updated links to relevant online resources

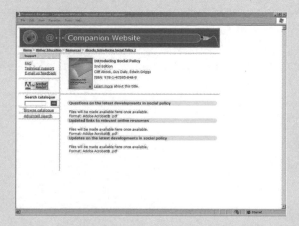

We work with leading authors to develop the strongest educational materials in social policy, bringing cutting-edge thinking and best learning practice to a global market.

Under a range of well-known imprints, including Longman, we craft high quality print and electronic publications which help readers to understand and apply their content, whether studying or at work.

To find out more about the complete range of our publishing, please visit us on the World Wide Web at: www.pearsoned.co.uk

Contents

Part IV Welfare themes   234

Authors and Contributors

Cliff Alcock was until recently Senior Lecturer in Social Policy at Coventry University.

Guy Daly is Associate Dean in the Faculty of Health and Life Sciences at Coventry University.

Edwin Griggs teaches Social Policy at the Universities of Birmingham and Wolverhampton.

Tony Colombo is Senior Lecturer in Criminology in the Department of Social and Community Studies, Coventry University.

Harry Cowen is Principal Lecturer in Social Policy and Sociology in the Department of Natural and Social Sciences at the University of Gloucestershire.

Mary Knyspel is Senior Lecturer in Sociology in the Department of International Studies and Social Science, Coventry University.

Helen Poole is Senior Lecturer in Criminology in the Department of Social and Community Studies, Coventry University.

Guided tour

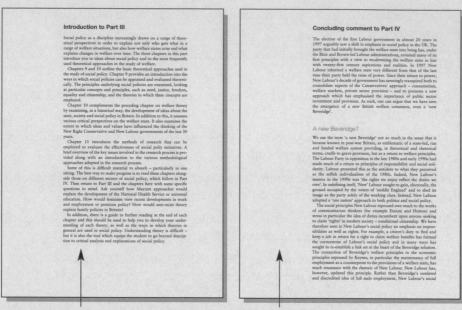

Introductions and **Conclusions** to Parts draw together the main themes of, and relationships between, the chapters in each Part.

Objectives and Introductions respectively provide a concise summary of the chapter aims plus a more general outline of the chapter in a wider context.

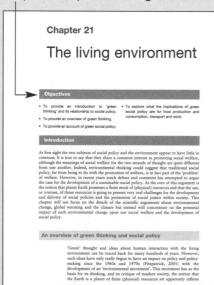

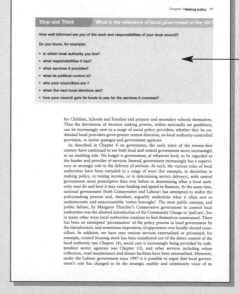

Stop and Think boxes present short, thought-provoking issues to reflect upon as you read.

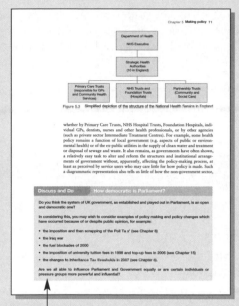

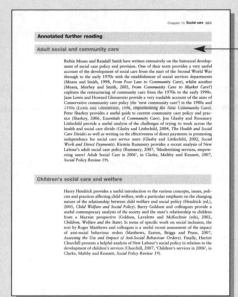

Annotated further reading provides avenues for further investigation into the key issues.

Discuss and Do boxes show deeper issues to discuss and reflect upon, useful for wider discussion or project work.

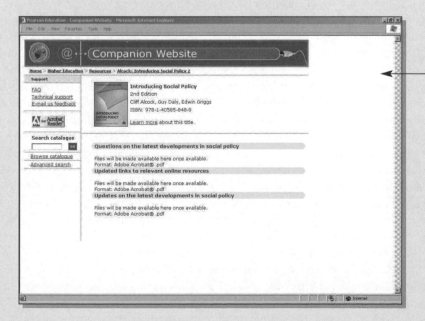

The **Companion Website** provides updates and extra links to keep the subject alive beyond the text.

Preface

Social policy is an academic field that most of us encounter in one way or other, even if we do not recognise it. Conversations at home, at work or with friends are frequently related, directly or indirectly, to the discipline. When we discuss or debate:

- whether education is being 'dumbed down';
- whether as a country we can afford to provide health care free to all at the point of delivery;
- whether too many people are going to university;
- whether university tuition fees will discourage the participation of people from poorer backgrounds;
- whether the state should provide more or less financial support to the unemployed;
- whether the state should fund free childcare;
- what role the individual, as opposed to the wider society, plays in tackling environmental concerns such as climate change;
- what provision should be made for those who cannot afford to buy their own home;
- whether older people and other groups should be provided with free long term care;
- whether any welfare service should be provided to people dependent upon their means ('means tested') or 'free' irrespective of one's own income and wealth (for example child benefit which is a universal benefit);

we are tackling questions directly related to the subject and practice of social policy.

As a discipline, social policy draws on a variety of academic subject areas including sociology, politics, economics, philosophy, history and social and public administration. It posits relevant questions and suggests appropriate solutions as to how social welfare should be formulated and provided. The discipline of social policy both analyses social issues and proposes new ways to tackle such issues.

This book therefore provides an introduction to social policy for undergraduate students in British universities, whether they are studying specifically for a social policy degree or are encountering the subject area as part of their studies – for example as part of a nursing, social work, social welfare, youth or community work qualification as well as those undertaking degrees in the other health professions. We hope that other students encountering social policy for the first time, whether at sub-degree level (for example A level, GNVQ or BTEC Awards) or even postgraduate students who need a gentle introduction into the subject, will also find this book a helpful introduction.

We have structured the second edition into four parts. First of all, we provide an historical overview of the development of the welfare state in Britain over the nineteenth and twentieth centuries. Next, we consider contemporary aspects of providing welfare. We also provide some of the theoretical background to understanding social policy and welfare provision – philosophically, ideologically and methodologically. Fourthly, we provide an overview and examination of the key areas of social policy and welfare services.

We would hope that the book is one that many students will choose to read 'from beginning to end', but we have also designed it to be a text that other students can call upon for particular chapters or sections dependent upon their interests or needs.

To help students to understand the subject matter being covered, we have included within each chapter a number of brief exercises – which we have called 'Stop and Think' activities – as well as more substantial topics for consideration – 'Discuss and Do' activities. We hope that these will help to bring the material alive and allow the reader to apply the content to 'real life' issues and situations. Each chapter is substantially referenced (with full references presented together at the end of the book) along with suggested further readings to which students can refer in order to develop their understanding to a greater depth and level of detail. There is also a glossary section at the end of the book which provides explanations of some of the key terms and abbreviations that are part and parcel of the language of social policy.

Overall, we hope that you find the book to be interesting and enjoyable since, in our view, social policy is and should be 'serious fun'.

Acknowledgements

Cliff Alcock would like to thank Lorraine, Faye, Leigh, Christopher and Eve for their encouragement and their laughter, and would especially like to thank Lorraine for her continued support and patience. Without them all the work on this volume would not have been possible.

Guy Daly would like to thank Michele, Isabella, Amelia and Marianne for their forbearance during the period of the production of the book. In addition, he would like to thank Timothy Cronick and Paul Hunter for their assistance in providing access to topical case study material. Lastly, he would like to thank his work colleagues, Julia Crisp, Claire Lovick and Linda Merriman for their support.

Edwin Griggs would like to thank Pam, Alex, Will and Lizzie for the enormous and beneficial difference they have made to his life in recent years. He would also like to thank his teachers at the Universities of Bristol and York many years ago, from whom he learnt so much, whose scholarship he can never hope to emulate, and for whom his contribution to this book is small and inadequate acknowledgement.

We would also like to express a heartfelt thanks to colleagues at Pearson Education who have provided us with assistance and encouragement during the production of the second edition. In particular, we are extremely grateful to Andrew Taylor, Sarah Busby and Emma Easy for their support. We would also like to thank the copy-editor, Patrick Bonham. In addition, we are grateful to Dr Binqin Li (London School of Economics), Dr Majella Kilkey (University of Hull) and Dr Hyun B. Shin (University of Leeds) who provided swift and insightful feedback to draft chapters.

Publisher's acknowledgements

We would like to express thanks to all contributing authors for their donation of their time, effort and expertise towards this new edition. Particular thanks are due to the principal authors – Guy Daly, Edwin Griggs and Cliff Alcock – for their substantial contribution towards such a major revision. Finally, to Guy Daly, without whose dedication and editorial management this edition would have never appeared, we extend our particular gratitude.

We are grateful to the following for permission to reproduce copyright material:

Figure 3.1 from The National Archives, http://www.nationalarchives.gov.uk; Figure 5.2 from *Politics UK*, *6th Edition*, Longman (Jones, B. *et al*. 2006); Figure 6.1 from *Modernising Governance: New Labour, Policy and Society*, Sage (Newman. J 2001); Figure 7.1 from Fury over Cameron Plan to Silence Scottish MPs in *Daily Mail* (Chapman, J. 29 October 2007); Figure 7.2 from *Health Policy Review*, Issue 2, Healthy Policy and Economic Research Unit, BMA (Smith, T. and Babbington, E. 2006); Tables 8.1, 8.2, 8.3 and 8.4 from *Public Expenditure Statistical Analyses Cm 6811*, The Stationary Office (H.M. Treasury 2006). Crown copyright material is reproduced with the permission of the Controller of HMSO and the Queen's

Printer for Scotland under the terms of the Click-Use Licence; Figures 12.1 and 12.3 and Tables 17.1, 17.2 and 17.3 from *Social Trends No. 36*, Office of National Statistics (ONS 2005). Crown copyright material is reproduced with the permission of the Controller of HMSO and the Queen's Printer for Scotland under the terms of the Click-Use Licence; Figure 12.2 and 14.4 from *Social Trends No. 35*, Office of National Statistics (ONS 2005). Crown copyright material is reproduced with the permission of the Controller of HMSO and the Queen's Printer for Scotland under the terms of the Click-Use Licence; Table 13.1 from *Children Looked After by Local Authorities Year Ending 31 March 2001*, Office of National Statistics (ONS 2005). Crown copyright material is reproduced with the permission of the Controller of HMSO and the Queen's Printer for Scotland under the terms of the Click-Use Licence: Figures 13.1, 13.2 and 13.3 from *Community Care Statistics 2006, Home Care Services for Adults, England*, The Information Centre, Adult Social Services Statistics (The Information Centre 2006). Crown copyright material is reproduced with the permission of the Controller of HMSO and the Queen's Printer for Scotland under the PSI Licence; Figures 14.1 and 14.2 and Table 14.1 from *Social Trends No. 34*, Office of National Statistics (ONS 2005). Crown copyright material is reproduced with the permission of the Controller of HMSO and the Queen's Printer for Scotland under the terms of the Click-Use Licence; Table 14.2 from *Housing Statistics*, ODPM/National Statistics (ODPM 2005). Crown copyright material is reproduced with the permission of the Controller of HMSO and the Queen's Printer for Scotland under the terms of the Click-Use Licence; Figure 14.3 from www.statistics.gov.uk. Crown copyright material is reproduced with the permission of the Controller of HMSO and the Queen's Printer for Scotland under the terms of the Click-Use Licence; Figure 15.1 taken from McNally, S. (2007) Centre For Economic Performance Policy Analysis, *Has Labour Delivered on the Policy Priorities of 'Education, Education, Education' – The Evidence on School Standards, Parental choice and staying on*, Centre for Economic Performance, London School of Economics. Available to download at http://cep.lse.ac.uk/pubs/download/pa008.pdf; Figures 16.1, 16.2 and 16.3 and Table 16.1 from *Labour Force Survey*, Office of National Statistics (ONS 2006). Crown copyright material is reproduced with the permission of the Controller of HMSO and the Queen's Printer for Scotland under the terms of the Click-Use Licence; Figures 18.1, 18.2 and Tables 18.1, 18.2, 18.3 and 18.4 from *Social Trends No. 37*, Office of National Statistics (ONS 2005). Crown copyright material is reproduced with the permission of the Controller of HMSO and the Queen's Printer for Scotland under the terms of the Click-Use Licence; Figure 19.1 from *Individual Income 1996/97 – 20003/04*, Women and Equality Unit (National Statistics: Department of Trade and Industry 2005). Crown copyright material is reproduced with the permission of the Controller of HMSO and the Queen's Printer for Scotland under the terms of the Click-Use Licence; Figure 19.2 from www.statistics.gov.uk. Crown copyright material is reproduced with the permission of the Controller of HMSO and the Queen's Printer for Scotland under the terms of the Click-Use Licence.

We are grateful to the following for permission to reproduce the following texts:

Box 5.1 from Wintour, P. and White, M., No fuel tax concessions says Brown. Chancellor rejects early move on prices as pickets lift blockades, *The Guardian*, 15 September 2000. Copyright Guardian News & Media Ltd 2006; Box 5.1 from

Pensioners and motorists gain from mini-Budget, *The Guardian*, 8 November 2000. Copyright Guardian News & Media Ltd 2006; Box 7.3 from Chapman, J., Fury over Cameron Plan to Silence Scottish MPs', *Daily Mail*, 29 October 2007; Box 11.1 from Ahthana, A., Bullying is exaggerated, says childhood expert, *The Observer*, 28 October 2007. Copyright Guardian News & Media Ltd 2006; Box 13.1 from Batty, D., Timeline for the Climbié case, *The Guardian*, 24 September 2001. Copyright Guardian News & Media Ltd 2006; Box 14.1 from Booth, R., ITN man once interviewed the influential, now he sleeps rough. Journalist homeless after losing job and going through divorce, *The Guardian*, 15 December 2007. Copyright Guardian News & Media Ltd 2007; Box 14.2 from Summers, D., Brown outlines legislative programme, *The Guardian*, 11 July 2007. Copyright Guardian News & Media Ltd 2007; Box 15.1 from Laville, S. and Smithers, R., War over school boundaries divides Brighton. Council brings in lottery for sought-after places; Parents in old catchment area threaten court action, *The Guardian*, 1 March 2007. Copyright Guardian News & Media Ltd 2007; Box 15.2 from Curtis, P., Test results for third of primary students wrong, says study, *The Guardian*, 2 November 2007. Copyright Guardian News & Media Ltd 2007; Box 15.3 from Meikle, J., Cameron faces Tory revolt after retreat on grammar schools, *The Guardian*, 17 May 2007. Copyright Guardian News & Media Ltd 2007; Box 19.1 from Curtis, P., Councils face £2.8bn bill for equal pay. Wage discrimination claims leave black hole in local authority finances, *The Guardian*, 2 January 2008. Copyright Guardian News & Media Ltd 2008; Box 19.2 from Teather, D., Glass ceiling still blocks women from executive floor, *The Guardian*, 2 October 2006. Copyright Guardian News & Media Ltd 2006; Box 19.3 from Atkinson, R., Everyone in Jodee Mundy's family is deaf – except for her, *The Guardian*, 29 December 2007. Copyright Guardian News & Media Ltd 2007.

In some instances we have been unable to trace the owners of copyright material and we would appreciate any information that would enable us to do so.

Chapter 1

Introduction – what is social policy?

Social policy as an academic field of study is one of those curious items, rather like an elephant, which we recognise when we see it but which is notoriously difficult to describe. It is, at one and the same time, the theoretical pursuit of norms about how we think society 'ought' to behave, but also the practical application and implementation of those policies that we consider to be 'social'. We could, of course, argue that all areas of policy inherently have implications for the well-being of society. Consider, for instance, the debate in the years since the onset of the Iraq War in 2003 and the realisation of the budgetary and political implications both for the armed forces and for those industries involved in their supply. Yet we do not automatically consider either defence or armed forces policy to be within the remit of 'social policy'. What, then, is social policy?

> Social policy is the study of the social services and the welfare state. The field of study has grown over time, and it stretches rather more widely than at might first appear, but the social services are where the subject began, and they are still at the core of what the subject is about. The social services are mainly understood to include social security, housing, health, social work and education – the 'Big Five' – along with others which are like social services, including employment, prisons, legal services or drains. (Spicker, 1995)
>
> The term social policy is not only used to refer to an academic discipline and its study, however, it is also used to refer to social action in the real world. Social policy is the term used to describe actions aimed at promoting well being; it is also the term used to denote the academic study of such actions. (Alcock, 1997)

The two quotations above provide us with fairly standard definitions of the term 'social policy'. Both suggest that, as an area of study, it is concerned with the welfare or well-being of society and its members. Furthermore, as an area of study, social policy is closely concerned with the activities of the 'welfare state', that is the range of government policies and social services used to enhance the welfare of citizens within a country. Some writers (Spicker, 1995; Hill, 2003) suggest that social policy is intimately concerned with the activities of the 'Big Five' which make up the classic welfare state. This classic welfare state (though the Big Five may not be universally agreed) will normally comprise policies of income maintenance and social security, health policy and services, the personal social services, education and training policy, and employment policy and housing policy. Some writers might consider that policies concerned with employment rightly belong to the field of economics and economic policy rather than social policy; similarly policies of criminal justice enjoy a transience between social policy and legal studies. Such an apparent confusion, however, does provide us with an insight into the difficulties in defining social policy. We can suggest that all government policy has a social element, but that is not to suggest that all government policy is social policy. We may also note here the multi-disciplinary nature of social policy: it is an academic subject which draws upon the academic techniques and skills of many other disciplines – sociology, economics, politics and policy making and history. This itself remains an unresolved debate among social policy academics between those who regard social policy as a 'field of study' which draws heavily upon other academic disciplines, and those who regard social policy as an academic discipline in its own right, drawing together those other academic elements (see the chapters by Alcock and Erskine in Alcock, Erskine and May, 1997).

> ... although it is on the one hand, an academic discipline – to be studied and developed in its own right – it is also an inter-disciplinary field – drawing on and developing links with other cognate disciplines at every stage and overlapping at times with these in terms of both empirical foci and methods of analysis ... the boundaries between social policy and other social science disciplines are porous and shifting.... (Alcock, 1997)
>
> While social policy cannot claim to be a science, it draws its legitimacy as a subject on its ability to draw upon the methods of a number of social sciences and apply these in a rigorous and disciplined way to understand the field in which we are interested.... social policy involves understanding a range of philosophical and political perspectives. (Erskine, 1997)

The scope of social policy

Although debates such as those indicated above may prove interesting to those academics employed within social policy departments, they do not necessarily hold the same interest for students of social policy. Instead, students of social policy may be (rightly) more concerned with the study of social phenomena, such as poverty, inequality and social justice, and policies that attempt to address such phenomena. Implicitly and following such a definition, the student of social policy is concerned to discover whether such policies may be said to be effective – that is whether the policies achieve the aims they set out to pursue and crucially whether social welfare can be said to have been improved as a result of the introduction of one or other policy. Here we can borrow, from policy studies, the notion of a cyclical policy process (Figure 1.1).

Although this might be described as a simplistic model of policy making, it does, nonetheless, provide us with a useful frame of reference for thinking about social policy (for a detailed exposition of policy making and its study, see Hill, 1997). Social policy, then, is not simply the study of society and its problems, but is intimately concerned with how to address and ameliorate social problems and with the

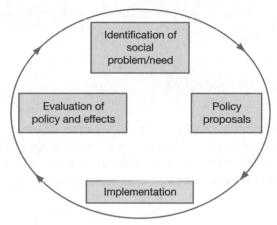

Figure 1.1 The policy cycle

analysis of the success or failure of policies designed to improve welfare and well-being. Implicitly, too, the study of social policy is concerned with the creation and appropriateness of structures and institutions designed to implement social policies.

Here we have introduced the term 'welfare' to our notion of social policy, and often the terms social policy and welfare, or welfare state, will be used interchangeably in texts about the subject (Ginsburg, 1992). This interchangeability has been and can continue to be the source of confusion, as we may be tempted to regard the activities of the welfare state as coterminous with social policy. Indeed for many years, under the guise of social administration, the distinction between welfare and the welfare state was not clear, and may still today be blurred. Yet social administration determined the content and direction of social policy and framed its debate for much of the post-war period.

> The discipline of social policy is relatively new, ... [T]he first department of social policy opened at the London School of Economics in 1950 headed by Richard Titmuss. This department ... [was] primarily concerned with the training of welfare professionals during a period of expansion in the welfare state ... The scope of the discipline in these early years was therefore strongly influenced by the institutional structures of the welfare state. Academic concern thus focused on the role of the state as the primary provider of welfare. (Ackers and Abbott, 1996)

Social policy was, by this definition, what the welfare state did, and no longer was it simply possible for the state to act; it became regarded as the 'natural' provider of welfare, apparently at the exclusion of others. During the 1960s and 1970s this view of social administration as social policy became somewhat discredited and since then a more holistic approach to social policy has developed. (For a more detailed discussion and appraisal of the transition from social administration to social policy, see Mishra, 1981.)

Broadly speaking, the study of social policy is the study of the role of the state in relation to the welfare of its citizens. This leads immediately to two questions. First, since the welfare of citizens is affected by their own actions and by the actions of others, including those of collective organisations of different kinds, what is it about the role of the state in relation to welfare that is different? Secondly, what are the kinds of actions that have an impact on welfare? (Hill, 1995).

The structure of the book

This volume is intended to be an introduction for students having their first experience of social policy, whether as undergraduates of social policy, or taking relevant A-levels, BTEC courses or access students. It is written on the assumption that students have little or no prior knowledge or experience of social policy but may have encountered social policy in other contexts. The text aims to provide an up-to-date yet accessible overview of the development of and the context for the provision of social welfare in the contemporary United Kingdom. Chapters are included that discuss the historical, ideological and political context within which social policy has developed and the changing contemporary context within which social policy is developing today.

The book is divided into four substantive parts. Part I explores the historical development of social policy through the nineteenth and twentieth centuries, with one chapter (Chapter 2) devoted to the development of welfare services following the introduction of the Poor Law Amendment Act of 1834, and a second chapter (Chapter 3) charting the changes from the Liberal welfare reforms through to the widespread adoption of the welfare principles laid down in the Beveridge Report in 1942. The distinction between the two centuries is somewhat arbitrary, but the chapters seek to explore the ideas and principles laid down during those years that we might say still guide the implementation and delivery of social policy in twenty-first-century Britain.*

Part II examines the policy and political context within which social policy is made. It begins by examining the changes to the political environment that the welfare state has experienced in the last three decades. The first chapter (Chapter 4) of this part considers the so-called 'crisis of welfare states' that heralded the end of the Beveridgean consensus in British politics generally but in social welfare in particular. The other chapters of this part consider, first, the policy-making process (Chapter 5), that is how policies come into being and are implemented. This is followed by a chapter on how the governance of welfare has changed since the establishment of the post-war welfare state (Chapter 6), followed by one that explores the changes that have occurred in the provision of welfare with the advent of devolutionary arrangements in Scotland, Wales and Northern Ireland over the last 10 years (Chapter 7). This section closes with a chapter (Chapter 8) that considers the financial environment of social policy making, that is, how we prioritise and allocate resources to welfare services and the mechanisms by which resources are collected and distributed.

Part III explores the ways in which different ideologies are used to explain social policy and how such theoretical concepts are necessary for an understanding of social policy. The first chapter (Chapter 9) considers the ways in which social poli-

*It should be noted that throughout this book, unless stated otherwise, the terms 'Britain' and 'British' are used as a convenient shorthand for the United Kingdom of Great Britain and Northern Ireland.

cies can be appraised and evaluated. This is done by examining the principles underlying social policies, looking at such concepts and principles as need, justice, freedom, equality and citizenship, and the theories within which these concepts are employed. This is followed by Chapter 10 which examines the development of ideas about the state, society and social policy in Britain. In addition to this, the chapter also assesses various critical perspectives on the welfare state. Lastly, the chapter examines the ideas and values of Thatcherism and New Labour, the key driving forces behind the changes to social policy and welfare over the last 30 years. The final chapter (Chapter 11) in this section considers the place of research in understanding social policy and welfare, not least by providing an overview of the processes involved in researching social policy.

Part IV looks at the 'policy areas' that form the backbone of the British welfare state and have traditionally been considered the very essence of social policy thinking and analysis. Therefore we have chapters considering developments in social welfare: health, social care, housing, education, employment and pensions. These chapters tend to present a brief historical overview of developments before and since the publication of the Beveridge Report and then to outline the development of our modern 'welfare services'. We also include in this part, however, chapters examining less traditional areas, including the development of 'family' policy, social divisions, the role of the criminal justice system and environmental policy which, although not typically regarded as social policy, have a considerable impact on social welfare. Although we do not go so far as to construct these as part of the so-called 'new' social policy (see Cahill, 1994), we do believe such areas are valid and worthy areas of social policy analysis. The book concludes with a final chapter on international social policy (Chapter 22), not least via the impact of both the pressures of globalisation and the development of a social policy agenda within the European Union.

The structure of the book is intended to provide the reader with a flexible and accessible introduction to social policy making in modern Britain. It is hoped that readers and students of social policy will be able to approach the text in a linear fashion but also to be selective and take a more random approach to their study of social policy.

Other features of the book

We believe that in order to understand social policy and all that it entails, one needs to engage in the debates, questions and issues that any consideration of social policy and social welfare throw up. Therefore, all of the subsequent chapters in the book have activities within them that aim to assist the student reader in particular with their understanding of the material being presented. To this end, we have included two types of pedagogical (teaching and learning) features. The first of these is what we have called '**stop and think**' activities, where the reader is asked to spend a little time thinking about a particular issue related to that part of the chapter. The second set of activities is what we have termed '**discuss and do**' activities, which are somewhat longer questions requiring the reader to consider in greater depth more general issues and questions related to the chapter.

Part I

Historical development of welfare

Introduction to Part I

This part examines the historical context within which social policy in Britain has developed over the nineteenth and twentieth centuries and seeks to establish the background behind much of contemporary social policies and welfare structures. An historical perspective helps us to understand better the present climate of social policy and may lead us to speculate about the future. We also may be able to trace the development of particular social policies over a considerable period of time and to understand what is often the apparently cyclical nature of policy developments.

Any historical approach to policy development inevitably involves an amount of arbitrariness, especially in deciding where to begin. Since this volume is intended to explore contemporary social policy issues and debates, these two historical chapters are brief and seek merely to explore context and environment. Inevitably, then, they may omit or deal only briefly with aspects that some readers may feel deserve more detailed consideration. Since our focus is to introduce social policy in the British 'welfare state' in the twenty-first century, we have chosen to begin in the year 1834.

Chapter 2 introduces the reader to a range of developments in welfare policy that were pioneered in the nineteenth century. The year 1834 is a landmark year since it marks the point at which government announced its own permanent presence on the welfare stage. The introduction of a New Poor Law, founded upon scientific principles, marked a fundamental turning point in social policy and heralded interventions in many other aspects of society. The chapter goes on to discuss legislative developments in public health, employment regulation and education, each of which experienced reform to a greater or lesser degree, though in each case developments were tentative and sporadic.

Chapter 3 discusses developments in the early decades of the twentieth century, beginning with the Liberal governments in power before the First World War. These governments, armed with new ideas and new thinking in social policy, established the roots of what was to become, after the Beveridge Report in 1942 and the legislative programme of the post-war Labour government, the welfare state. Successive governments adopted, usually in the face of deep-seated opposition, wider and more pervasive powers in the regulation of our social life. These governments also laid down welfare principles, such as insurance, that remain with us today.

The distinction between the developments of the nineteenth century and those of the twentieth is another arbitrary choice since, as many writers will indicate, many of the ideas adopted by the Liberal governments were the result of a process of debate that began in the late nineteenth century. Similarly the philosophical and ideological foundations of the Beveridge era have roots going back some decades. There are many other texts available that examine these and other developments of this era and to which readers are directed within both the chapters and the annotated readings.

Chapter 2

Welfare before the state

Objectives

- To provide a broad historical overview of the development of British social policy before the twentieth century.

- To explore the development of the principles of welfare and the foundations of contemporary social policy.

- To describe the development of welfare services, including public health, income maintenance, education and employment regulation.

Introduction

It is often tempting when examining the modern welfare state to trace its beginnings to the post-1945 expansion of welfare that followed the publication of the 1942 Beveridge Report. But such an approach runs the risk that we omit to consider some of the principles that have characterised the development of British social policy and the welfare state before Beveridge. Similarly it may be tempting to take a lengthy historical detour in order to provide the fullest possible background to the contemporary picture and contemporary developments. We may, for instance, wish to elaborate the feudal and religious foundations of welfare, which stressed both the religious duty of caring for those less fortunate and the duty of the feudal lord to protect those within one's own domain. We can also suggest, with some degree of accuracy, that many of the founding principles, for instance the distinction between the deserving and undeserving poor drawn in the Elizabethan Poor Law of 1598, remain with us today or that the parable of the good Samaritan is still apposite. Similarly we might argue that the residency qualification and the powers vested in parishes by the various Acts of Settlement, embodied in the Old Poor Law, which parishes used to limit the burden on their own funds by driving the 'travelling poor' from their boundaries, may be found in the modern-day treatment of both travellers and the single homeless. However, although such an approach may prove interesting for both reader and writer, it remains a detour from the contemporary scene that we wish to examine and, of course, there are numerous historical accounts already available to which we might usefully refer the reader (Fraser, 1976; Marshall, 1985; Slack, 1995).

We have chosen instead to begin our historical overview with the Poor Law Amendment Act of 1834, which, although not the first instance of the involvement of the state in the welfare of its citizens, represents a fundamental turning point. For it is with this Act that the state's role is consolidated in an attempt to redefine the Poor Law on the basis of universal laws and principles; it is here then that we can discern the foundations of the modern 'welfare state'. It is also from this point that the state begins to adopt ever greater responsibilities in the everyday lives of its citizens and gradually, over the next century or so, increases the number of activities for which it assumes responsibility or control. And, although we do not wish to characterise the expansion of state activity as linear or necessarily progressive, and about which there has been much debate, 1834 nonetheless represents a significant turning point in the history of social policy.

We then turn from the Poor Law Amendment Act to examine other areas of state involvement in the regulation of the social sphere, for example in the regulation of working hours and conditions, in the attempts to improve public health and the sanitary conditions of our major towns and cities of the nineteenth century, and in the beginnings of the development of state education. We also briefly examine popular reaction to an increasing state role in the provision of social policy and welfare services as compared to the range of provision already made by individuals and groups such as friendly societies and charities. Finally in this chapter we discuss what we call the 'winds of welfare change', by which we mean the period towards the end of the nineteenth century during which to continue a 'hands-off' approach with the minimum of state provision no longer seemed adequate or sufficient. We refer here to the ideological roots of what was to become a 'new liberalism' in which the state in Britain was to re-evaluate its own social role and was to conclude, along with other modern industrial nations, that a far greater level of intervention was right and proper. In Britain this provoked constitutional crisis which was itself to help redefine not only the course of social policy for the twentieth century but also the role and function of government and the balance of power within the British constitution.

Poor Law reform

Poor Law legislation can be dated back as far as 1388 when attempts were made both to fix wages and to limit the mobility of labour which may cause wages to rise. But the more systematic operation of a system of poor relief came in two Acts passed under Elizabeth I in 1598 and 1601. These Acts created three classifications of the poor together with appropriate treatment for each: the impotent poor (old, sick, lunatic) would be accommodated in poor houses or almshouses; the able-bodied poor would be set to work in the parish, and their children apprenticed to a trade; and finally the able-bodied poor who absconded would be punished in the 'house of correction'. The Poor Law would be administered by each parish, which would appoint overseers of the poor who were empowered to raise a poor rate to pay for poor relief (Fraser, 2003: 33–36).

The Elizabethan Poor Law made each parish responsible for its own paupers. This was the cause of many disputes between parishes about who was responsible for particular individuals. It led to especially harsh treatment of those deemed vagrants, and to expectant women whose child might be able to claim residency, and thus dependency on the parish, should she give birth within the parish boundary. The Act of Settlement of 1662 attempted to clarify the definition of those legally entitled to settle, but this did little to improve matters, since the costs associated with removing a stranger would often be greater than those incurred by allowing them to settle, particularly since they may not ever claim poor relief. What we can note, however, is that the Elizabethan Act enshrined in law, and as a principle for subsequent social policy, the notion that some of the poor were more worthy than others and would be categorised as either deserving or undeserving poor.

Over time the Poor Law came to be dominated by various means of 'outdoor relief' rather than the systematic use of workhouses to alternatively employ or punish the different categories of pauper. In many parts of the country outdoor relief took the form of wage subsidy, perhaps most prevalent in rural areas and in times of food shortages caused by poor harvests. The system of wage subsidy received much attention especially towards the end of the eighteenth century, after several years of poor harvests and the impact of war with France saw the costs of the Poor Law rising, peaking at around £8 million in 1817–19. Although annual costs did begin to fall again in the early years of the 1820s, by the end of that decade the cost was again creeping upwards to reach £7 million in 1831 (Fraser, 2003: 43–44). Critics suggested that the system of wage subsidy induced labourers to idleness, as they would sooner allow the parish to supplement their wages than work hard to improve their situation. Thomas Malthus went further and suggested that the Poor Law encouraged the poor to have more children in order to receive extra relief, and that this system would have catastrophic consequences since the country was able to supply only a limited amount of food. Population, on the other hand, would carry on increasing until the country could simply no longer feed itself (Harris, 2004). For critics of the Poor Law this provided ample evidence of the folly of allowing the state to interfere in the welfare of its people and the damage that state-sponsored charity could cause. The working poor would lose any motivation to improve their position while 'generous' relief was provided and might even adjust their behaviour to take advantage of poor relief.

The pressure to reform the Elizabethan Poor Law was founded on the many concerns and worries in the minds of officials and reformers. First was the often random nature and application of the existing Poor Law, which was administered by local parishes. The often cited, we may say famous, systems of parish relief, such as that of Speenhamland, were by no means universal and there remained great diversity and variation in the administration, availability and generosity of parish relief, so that it may be incorrect to refer to the 'Old Poor Law' as though it were a single entity.

Secondly, there was the concern outlined above that parish relief undermined principles of thrift and hard work that people and the economy depended upon. Parish relief was felt to be an expensive luxury which, instead of simply relieving the poor, was encouraging them to remain idle and burden the parish and its ratepayers. That burden fell disproportionately, they felt, on aristocratic landowners and new groups of middle-class entrepreneurs. We can go further to suggest that the existence of parish relief was itself a cause of poverty, not because it encouraged indolence in the poor but because it encouraged employers to reduce wages. Employers were able to maintain wages at low levels in the knowledge that the parish would 'top-up' the wages of their labourers. This was most keenly felt in rural areas as employers artificially reduced local levels of pay in the knowledge that the parish would supplement incomes. Those same employers, this time as ratepayers, also pressed for a reduction in the burden of their poor rates and thereby a reduction in payments of relief. This they regarded as a tax on employment which itself damaged the successful working of the economy. Such factors were themselves cited in the Swing riots of 1830 which witnessed in Hampshire the breaking of agricultural machinery and the destruction of local workhouses in some parishes (Hobsbawm and Rudé, 1969: 119–120).

Finally, there was the fear that the Poor Law of the previous two and a half centuries was no longer able to meet the demands of nineteenth-century Britain. The dual processes of industrialisation and urban development were attracting new populations to towns in search of work. In times of unemployment, existing residency qualifications, embodied in the various Acts of Settlement, would disqualify individuals from turning to the parish for help; indeed we may argue that the parish boundaries themselves had become outdated and meaningless as new towns and cities had grown. A Poor Law designed to meet the needs of a medieval, largely rural and agricultural population was self-evidently outdated by the early decades of the nineteenth century.

The 1834 Amendment Act

The combination, therefore, of the rising costs and inconsistent application and obsolescence of the existing system of the Poor Law together paved the way for its review and subsequent amendment. In 1832 the government established a Royal Commission to examine the operation of the Poor Law. The review was largely the work of Nassau Senior, a leading economist of the day, and Edwin Chadwick (see Box 2.1 overleaf). The intention behind the review was to found the New Poor Law on more rational and 'scientific' principles and in particular a principle of deterrence. Following this notion, the Poor Law would no longer simply provide relief for the poor, those subsisting on low wages who could improve their position by hard work, but only for the destitute, those who had nowhere else to turn. The establishment of a centralised administrative system, laying down the rules to be implemented at a local level, was a keystone in the new system. Similarly the random distinction between 'deserving' and 'undeserving' poor would be more systematically, and bureaucratically, defined, leading in time to the establishment of notions of 'rights to welfare'.

The Commission's Report, however, focused largely on the question of rural poverty and on the position of the able-bodied; other categories of pauper were mostly ignored as were the changing conditions of urban industrial areas. This is perhaps unsurprising, given the extent of rural unrest in the years preceding the foundation of the Royal Commission, but it meant that the New Poor Law changed little from the Elizabethan system in many parts of the country for years to come.

The 1834 Act removed the responsibility of the Poor Law from the parish and instead created a locally elected Board of Guardians who were to administer relief in 'unions' (groups of parishes) which were supervised at a central level by the Poor Law Board. (The Local Government Board replaced this in 1871.) Central supervision, which was advisory rather than directive in nature, was intended to ensure that the principles of the Poor Law were applied uniformly. These principles were, first, the ending of most 'outdoor relief' and the application of the workhouse test. Each Poor Law union was to establish a workhouse, the intention of which was to discourage all but the destitute from turning to the Poor Law for relief: '... it would

Box 2.1 **Sir Edwin Chadwick**

Edwin Chadwick was born in 1800 near Manchester. In 1818 he embarked on a legal career as an attorney, later changing to train as a barrister. Chadwick was influenced by the political philosophy of Jeremy Bentham and later served as his secretary. In 1832 he was invited to serve on the Royal Commission, examining ways in which the Poor Law might be improved, and he also reported on conditions for children in factories; this work resulted in the Factory Act of 1833. He then returned to the Poor Law Commission and is credited with that part of the report which enshrined the principle of less eligibility (see Box 2.2).

He later turned his attention to questions of public health and of whether poor sanitary conditions contributed to increases in the poor rate. Chadwick's Sanitary Report of 1842 led to the passing of the first Public Health Act in 1848 and his appointment as the first Secretary of the General Board of Health. Later in life he stood for Parliament, unsuccessfully, in both 1859 and 1868 and was knighted in 1889 shortly before his death at the age of 90.

Box 2.2 **Less eligibility**

The first and most essential of all conditions; a principle which we find universally admitted, even by those whose practice is at variance with it, is that his situation on the whole shall not be made really or apparently so eligible as the situation of the independent labourer of the lowest class. Throughout the evidence it is shown that in proportion as the condition of any pauper class is elevated above the condition of independent labourers, the condition of the independent class is depressed; their industry is impaired, their employment becomes unsteady, and its remuneration in wages is diminished. Such persons, therefore, are under the strongest inducements to quit the less eligible class of labourers and enter the more eligible class of paupers. (Taken from the Poor Law Report, 1832)

remove at once the "poor" (i.e. the labourer whose wages were being subsidised) from the Poor Law and cater only for the indigent (the truly destitute) as was its proper function' (Fraser, 2003: 49). Those granted relief would no longer receive subsidies to their wages (the former system of outdoor relief) but would enter the workhouse and engage in work in return for relief. It is true to say, however, that although this may have been the intention of the reformers of the day, much local variation continued in the administration and delivery of Poor Relief and in many areas outdoor relief continued to be available, though perhaps more stringently controlled.

Secondly, the notion of 'less eligibility' (Box 2.2) sought to determine that levels of relief would not be so generous as to discourage the poor from finding work. This in turn would mean that only the destitute would turn to the Poor Law for help and that those simply suffering lower wages would be encouraged to turn to other systems of support such as friendly societies or charities. Therefore the system of relief founded by the 1834 Act was one which, in theory, offered relief to those individuals whose poverty was not their own fault and whose behaviour was respectable (Thane, 1996). One purpose of the workhouse system embodied in the

New Poor Law was to put the poor to work in return for assistance and to discourage the (re)production of further mouths to feed. The notion that no one should receive something, in this case assistance, without a corresponding duty to work, is one we find resonant in some of the notions of 'workfare' and the 'New Deal' debated in contemporary political circles.

In theory, then, the able labouring poor would be provided for by the workhouse whilst other groups, the elderly, widows, sick and physically or mentally unfit, would continue to receive outdoor relief. In practice the workhouse came to dominate Poor Law provision in the later years of the nineteenth century as the deterrent principles of the Act were enforced most vigorously. The poor often instead refused to submit to the indignities of the Poor Law and the ultimate indignity of a pauper funeral. This might suggest that the poor of the nineteenth century had only the prospect of destitution and the Poor Law as some kind of safety net, cast so narrowly as to miss the bulk of the poor (Fraser, 1976). The workhouse system also garnered a reputation for harshness and brutality, particularly following the Andover scandal in 1845 when inspectors found workhouse inmates fighting over the bones they were crushing to make fertiliser.

Stop and Think

Are the principles embodied in the New Poor Law still relevant to the modern welfare state, for example in more modern 'welfare to work' approaches?

The above brief account of the Poor Law may leave one with the impression that the Act concerned itself primarily with the income maintenance of the poor and destitute. However, there was also the much wider consideration of the health and moral welfare of the poor. Local Boards of Guardians also sanctioned the creation of other forms of institutional welfare by way of infirmaries providing medical care and secure hospitals providing for the incarceration of the mentally ill. Such 'indoor relief' we might usefully suggest remained within the twentieth-century welfare system, in the provision for both the elderly and the mentally ill, until perhaps the practical development of ideas about community care in the decades following the Second World War.

The Poor Law was not, however, the sole form of provision available to the poor: savings, mutual aid funds, insurance schemes, friendly societies and trades unions all offered the working classes ways of providing for themselves and their families in bad times. Also during this period building societies, which often operated as local, short-term organisations to enable a small group of working people to borrow the funds to build their own homes, began to expand and develop as commercial organisations operating as long-term savings banks and mortgage lenders. Unemployment, sickness, old age and death could all be covered by the variety of schemes operating, often by the working people themselves and outside the realm of Poor Law Guardians, especially as the century progressed (Johnson, 1985a). Alongside the various forms of self-help that the Poor Law was keen to encourage, there also developed wide-ranging elements of charitable poor relief. Attempts to coordinate charitable relief under the auspices of the Charity Organisation Society (COS) and to deliver charitable relief according to 'universal and consistent principles' so that help was distributed systematically and to those 'deemed capable of becoming self-supporting' (Thane, 1996) proved largely unsuccessful. However, the 'casework' approach pioneered by the COS involving attempts to deal with the problems facing an individual or family has persisted in much charitable and, in the personal social services, state provision today.

Much of the available charitable provision was organised by religious organisations such as the Jewish Board of Guardians and later organisations such as the Salvation Army. Such organisations often regarded this kind of work as their duty towards humanity but also saw the opportunity to act as though urban missionaries with a quest to save the fallen or convert the heathen. Many such charities were locally based and many were short-lived, but estimates from the period suggest that in the late 1860s charitable expenditure in London was more than £5.5 million (Harris, 2004). Much of the work of the charity sector in the nineteenth century arose as a result of the perception of failure of the Poor Law system and paved the way for its piecemeal replacement and eventual abolition during the end of that century and the early decades of the twentieth century.

This brief foray into the world of the Victorian Poor Law, whilst not attempting to be a wholesale review of nineteenth-century attitudes towards the poor, does illustrate that many of the principles upon which state intervention in individual lives was predicated remain with us today. Distinctions between the deserving and undeserving, the discouragement of dependence and the targeting of help to the most needy are all the stuff of the welfare reform debate initiated by successive governments in the 1980s and 1990s. However, though crucial in the development of a welfare state, the Poor Law was by no means the only factor in the evolution of British social policy. The state also began to develop its responsibilities in public health, employment regulation and education, and it is these other areas of state intervention to which we now turn.

Public Health

If the need for change in the operation of the Poor Law can be attributed to the rapid growth of an industrial, urban population, then the pressure for action over public health was doubly felt as a result of rural migration. The population of Britain doubled in the first half of the nineteenth century, with a fourfold or even eightfold increase in the populations of some urban areas. In the first 50 years of the nineteenth century, for example, the population of Birmingham grew from 71,000 to 233,000, of Glasgow from 77,000 to 345,000, of Liverpool from 82,000 to 376,000, and of Manchester from 75,000 to 303,000 (Fraser, 2003). Such accelerated growth heralded the development of towns and cities in which housing was closely built, so as to be near places of work, and lacked amenities which we now take for granted, such as a clean water supply, sewerage systems and refuse disposal.

The development of public health as a legitimate concern of government, and indeed the development of systems of both a clean water supply and sewage disposal, are often credited to one man, Edwin Chadwick (see Box 2.1). Chadwick had been crucially involved in the collection of evidence for and the preparation of the Poor Law review which itself formed the basis of the 1834 Poor Law Amendment Act. It was in this capacity that Chadwick and his colleagues first began to perceive the link between sanitary conditions and the spread of illness and disease, and in its turn the contribution of disease (and death) to the prevalence of poverty and, of course, the costs of the Poor Law.

The acceptance by government for public health responsibilities was, however, faltering. Death rates, it was generally agreed, particularly in towns and cities, were rising and the increasing incidence of epidemic diseases such as cholera alarmed the middle classes. Even in the 1840s, these diseases were preventable. Chadwick, in preparing his report on sanitary conditions, was able to use the newly founded central machinery of the Poor Law to collect his evidence. Poor Law Assistant Commissioners, Boards of Guardians and Poor Law medical officers were all used to give testimony to the health and sanitary conditions endured by the 'labouring classes' (Fraser, 2003). His report, published in 1842, was not, however, widely and readily accepted and it was not until 1848 that legislation, in the form of the Public Health Act, saw the light of day. Political infighting and unwillingness to raise additional revenues – the costs involved in creating a water supply and sewage disposal systems would be considerable – resulted only in inaction. Also the whole debate was itself overshadowed by the debate surrounding the proper role for the state in regulating its people, again an issue frequently revisited since.

Provision for clean water and sewage disposal was initially a discretionary responsibility of municipal authorities who found themselves facing a host of vested interests in the form of the building industry, landlords, water companies and ratepayers. The Public Health Act made provision for setting up local boards of health and the appointment of Medical Officers of Health (MOH), although this was only permissory unless death rates were unusually high. Although some earlier legislation had provided, for example, for the creation of a municipally controlled water supply in Leeds and an MOH in Liverpool, the development of the state's role in public or environmental health was initially patchy. An overseeing role was ascribed to the General Board of Health, also established under the Act, although so ineffective was the legislation that the Board was replaced in 1854, with Chadwick himself being dismissed. Even after an epidemic of cholera in 1848–49 the General Board of Health found itself almost powerless in its attempts to improve sanitary conditions – they were able to report on local conditions and preventive actions but were unable to enforce action. Although the Board did appoint its first Medical Officer, Sir John Simon, in 1855, the Board itself was abolished in 1858. However, Simon's work did continue when he became Medical Officer to the Privy Council (1858–71) and later to the Local Government Board (1871–76) where he oversaw enquiries into infant mortality, diet and housing conditions (Finer, 1952; Harris, 2004). With the passing of the Sanitation Act of 1866 municipal local government began to derive compulsory powers to act in the interests of public health or for the prevention of 'nuisances'. Further change came in an Act of 1890 (the Housing of the Working Classes Act), which allowed local government to impose minimum standards in the construction of housing and to develop municipal (council) housing, adding to earlier powers, from 1878, to demolish insanitary dwellings.

Other developments in the provision of public standards of health derived from improvements in medical technology and knowledge. The increasingly widespread use of immunisation against disease, together with increasing knowledge about disinfection, made hospitals themselves safer places to be treated. Later still, the provision of public hospital services was distanced from the Poor Law. The provision of hospitals also gradually became a responsibility of local authorities, as it was they who from 1929 assumed control of Poor Law infirmaries. Further developments were to be noted in the passing of legislation designed to control the use of poisonous or hazardous materials and the safety of food and legislation to regulate working conditions in factories and other workplaces. Local doctors were also required from 1889 to notify the authorities of the outbreaks of certain infectious or communicable diseases.

Many of the public health provisions discussed here, like the Poor Law itself, have been retained as principles by which the modern welfare state continues to operate. Much responsibility for public health today remains with local authorities, and for those reforms pioneered by Chadwick and others, responsibility lies with Environmental Health Officers and the Health & Safety Executive as well as with the National Health Service. And, although the priorities of public health may have developed such that the provision of clean water, sewerage systems and refuse disposal are now taken for granted, new areas of responsibility, for example in food hygiene standards or noise pollution control, have been incorporated. Once again we are able to see how the contemporary welfare state owes a debt to an age long forgotten.

Stop and Think

Why was public health such an important issue in nineteenth-century Britain? How are public health issues dealt with in the modern welfare system?

Employment regulation

Looking back to the nineteenth century, it often appears that the pioneering spirit of *laissez-faire* capitalism, the industrial revolution and the creation of an empire were foremost in the minds of the government of the day. Yet within that century of revolution we can discern the seeds of latter-day social policy developments, tempered though they were by considerations of the moral virtue of the working classes and a strongly held principle that the state should only become involved when absolutely necessary. That meant a clear understanding that the free market had failed to provide and that any intervention should not itself be the cause of harm – sentiments clearly resonant of many debates today.

Employment regulation was, however, possibly one of the most sacrosanct areas of welfare, and as in the Poor Law and sanitation, change was slow to come. Government involvement in the control of employment and conditions in the workplace at a time when supply and demand determined the price and conditions of labour was, to say the least, a tentative venture. Many employers and politicians of the time continued to believe in the value of free trade, and thereby regular employment, as the most effective way of providing for the welfare of the working classes. At a time when trades unions, though legal, were effectively emasculated by the law, legislation to regulate hours and safety in the workplace was patchy and slow to develop. Many employers were able to do little more than comply with the minimum standards in the full knowledge that enforcement was lax and punishment light.

Box 2.3	Regulation of child labour

In recommending legislative restrictions of the labour of children, as not being free agents, and not being able to protect themselves, we have been careful not to lose sight of the practical limits . . .

The restrictions we venture to propose . . . are, that children under nine years of age shall not be employed in mills or factories . . . that until the . . . fourteenth year the hours of labour during any one day shall not in any case exceed eight . . . until the fourteenth year children shall not in any case be allowed to work at night; that is to say between the hours of ten at night and five in the morning.

Since the whole of our recommendations have for their object the care and benefit of children, we have been desirous of devising means for securing the occupation of a portion of the time abridged from their hours of labour to their own advantage. We think the best mode of accomplishing this object will be the occupation, supports of three (or four) hours of every day in education. (Taken from Report of the Commission of Enquiry into Factories, 1833)

Reformers initially focused their attentions on the employment of children in factories (see Box 2.3). Child labour itself was, of course, nothing new and children would be put to work in agricultural regions or cottage industries as soon as they were able. But the conditions in which children worked and lived in industrialising Britain proved an offence to the humanitarian sentiments of a country that came to regard itself as the most civilised in the world. The conditions endured by children, the long hours and the physical hazards they faced when operating machinery, were likened to slavery, since children in contrast to adults often had little choice over their labour. They could not trade their labour in the free market as *laissez-faire* economics predicted and gradually, though by no means easily, the case for government regulation was accepted. Employers constantly stressed the damage to their industry if child labour were banned and often sought to place the blame at the doors of parents who insisted that their children work as soon as they were able. Similarly they stressed the likely increase in poverty amongst the labouring classes, and therefore the increased Poor Law burden, if children were prevented from working.

Some employers, enlightened reformers such as Robert Owen, sought to show that they could continue to profit whilst maintaining a watchful eye on the welfare of their employees, but they were often the exception in the early industrial revolution. So it was that children, often as young as four, came to work in coal mines and factories across the country, often simply because their stature allowed them to work in places adults could not reach. Indeed in many districts workhouses and Boards of Guardians would 'apprentice' children to colliers or factory owners and so reduce the burden on their local rates (for a description of children's working conditions in the coal industry, see Pollard, 1984).

Restrictions on the hours that either children or women were able to work, or the industries in which they were able to work, were also beset with problems. An overall reduction in the income available to a family placed that family under greater pressure and strain and might lead them to the doors of the workhouse. Such proposals also raised in the minds of Victorians the prospect of social unrest as children, out of gainful employment and in families under increased social pressure, might turn to crime. Images such as this were reinforced in the popular conscience by stories such as those of Fagin and the Artful Dodger in Dickens' *Oliver Twist*. But reformers too were concerned with the moral and educational welfare of children, and accounts of long hours, beatings, sexual promiscuity, drunken and indolent parents and the physical injuries suffered by many children meant that the intervention of the state could be put off no longer.

As we might expect, however, the introduction of legislation to regulate the conditions and hours worked by children, and later by women and men too, was slow and hard fought. Credit for the ending of child labour is often given to Lord Shaftesbury and his parliamentary campaigning but, as Fraser notes, his work was the climax to that started by others before the passage of the 1844 Factory Act (Fraser, 2003). Indeed, the previous decade and a half had heralded vigorous efforts in the pursuit of a legally enforceable 10-hour day. Incremental legislative change throughout the middle decades of the nineteenth century gradually introduced protection first for children, for instance prohibiting their employment in textile mills at ages younger than nine years and limiting their daily hours of work to eight, rising to 12 hours at age 13. Legislation also introduced the factory inspectors who had powers to enforce rules governing the employment of children.

The legislation, however, remained weak and difficult to enforce – only one mines inspector was appointed by the 1842 Mines Act – and this itself indicated the difficulty of and opposition to something as fundamental as control of the 'free market'. Indeed, the 10-hour day was not achieved until the 1874 Factory Act by which time pressure from workers themselves was growing, as indicated by the growth of the 'new unionism' (the TUC had been formed in 1868) and gradual reforms in the franchise giving more working men the right to vote.

Education

Education and its provision during the nineteenth century remained very much a minority undertaking. Formal and structured education remained, as it had done for previous centuries, largely a privilege for the aristocracy and the emerging middle classes who could afford the costs of private tuition, fee-paying grammar schools and eventually perhaps Oxford or Cambridge. But, for the mass of the population, education, where it existed at all, remained basic, often little more than basic literacy and numeracy. There was, of course, much between these two extremes, for example church-run schools, industrial schools, dame schools or those provided by charitable funds; for the mass of the population, however, education was both scarce and patchy.

Indeed there remained for much of the century deep-seated opposition to mass educational provision, with those arguing variously that anything more than a basic education would upset the given social order. Similarly, the state had no business in deciding the education of individuals, and compulsion in education would pauperise the labouring classes whose children would no longer be able to work and learn their trade. Much of the opposition had its roots in the religious divisions of the time and successive governments had to tread very carefully between the various churches and their dogmas. These factors in their turn guaranteed that formal state involvement in the provision of learning was delayed until the final quarter of the nineteenth century. So difficult did it prove for governments to agree on the nature and extent of their role in education that early interventions were confined to the regulation of teacher training, which was felt could help overcome often bitter conflict over the teaching of religion (Fraser, 1976; Henriques, 1979).

There existed some state support for schooling in that provided for children under the care of the workhouse. However, Poor Law education was not considered to be of very high status, offering low pay and low status to teachers. Efforts towards education for pauper children continued to attract voluntary and charitable effort, notably in the form of the Ragged Schools from the 1840s, but government support for such schools was rejected. Other provision came in the form of the Factory School that proved attractive to some owners as a method of disciplining and improving the standards of their workforce. But herein lay the roots of a conflict, since working children were expected to contribute to their family income, and schooling, albeit free, could deny the family one source of extra income. Similarly, factory owners were often unwilling to subsidise such projects, since they would interfere with their production. Indeed, many would refuse to allow time out of the factory for schooling and instead insisted that it be undertaken in the free time of the child, little though that may have been. Legislation in this area was usually ineffective. The provisions of the Health and Morals of Apprentices Act (1802) which 'laid down that the mill owner was to provide schoolroom and paid teacher', or the 1833 Factory Act which placed a responsibility for the education of non-apprenticed children on mill owners, proved difficult to enforce or were simply ignored (Henriques, 1979).

The most significant step taken by the nineteenth-century state in the establishment of a national system of education was that embodied in the Education Act of 1870. As a result of this Act, local School Boards were to be established 'where there was clear educational need' to provide 'non-denominational elementary schools financed out of the rates in addition to Government grants' (Fraser, 1976). The aim of the Act was to permit local authorities to act to improve the attendance of working-class children in some form of schooling and to try to overcome the religious bickering that had engulfed the education debate for the previous half-century. Although the Act did not establish a national education system, it did lay down a more systematic role for the state in the provision of education, the culmination of which was a national education system based upon free and compulsory education up to age 14.

Stop and Think

Why were children considered so important in the welfare reform campaigns, and how did the state respond to the needs of children?

Reaction to the welfare of the state

Whilst it has been popular to view the development of a welfare state as necessary, desirable and inevitable, a view reflected in the writings upon which we have relied in the preceding section, other writers point out the level of discord which greeted successive attempts to secure state involvement in the provision of welfare services. It is by no means certain that such changes, which preceded the more comprehensive pattern of state welfare that developed in the first half of the twentieth century, received universal or even popular acclaim. There was, as many writers indicate, a strong ethos among the working poor of self-help and self-reliance and often a deep and bitter distrust of what the state tried to do (Johnson, 1985a; Finlayson, 1994; Thane, 1996).

Mistrust of the motives of the state in extending its welfare role stems from the punitive and often brutal experiences of working people at the hand of local Poor Law Guardians. Family and community resources would usually be available to a family falling on hard times and returned to others in better times. If such resources either were not available or had been exhausted, the mercy of charity was to be preferred to the workhouse (Thane, 1996). Alongside the mass of frequently undocumented charitable activity was the broad range of working-class self-help, ranging from informal insurance and savings clubs to the more formal insurance schemes provided by friendly societies and trades unions. Membership of such societies was widespread, though often the vagaries of employment would mean that individuals would enter and leave such societies as they were alternately in and out of work. But such schemes proved popular in providing insurance to cover illness, death or, less frequently, unemployment. Membership of such societies has been estimated at around a million by the end of the nineteenth century (Thane, 1996).

Also increasingly common as a form of self-help during this period were cooperative arrangements for the purchase or construction of homes – the building society. Many of the building societies would be short-lived and terminate their activities when each of their members had built or bought their own home. From the middle of the century the move towards permanent building societies was underway. This would provide longer-term opportunities for members to borrow and invest but also marked a move 'away from working-class participation ... the movement also became commercial' (Finlayson, 1994).

There is therefore evidence of widespread working-class self-help across the range of social policies for which the government was beginning to take responsibility. Such self-help sat well with an economic and social doctrine of *laissez-faire* which dominated political thought in Victorian Britain and which preached that the proper role of the state was residual. However, there was at the same time a mood of change. Most of the self-help provision was attractive to, and in many ways restricted to, the better-off working class and those for whom steady and regular employment was available. Large numbers of unskilled workers either found themselves unable to take advantage of mutual society membership or found that their benefits were as temporary as their work. With organised self-help apparently the preserve of a labour aristocracy, it appeared as though numbers of working people would, however diligently they may try, continue to be unable to provide for themselves. To a growing number of 'Benthamites', followers of the utilitarian thinking of Jeremy Bentham, such a situation was inefficient and wasteful of human resources. Herein lay the ideological justification for an expanded state role that allowed the market its free hand but would temper its worst effects by (collective) state action (Pearson and Williams, 1984).

Towards the end of the nineteenth century, concern grew for the position of working people who, though not indolent or lazy, suffered from the effects of poverty for reasons that were perceptibly outside their control. Concern most frequently fell on the elderly who were poor by virtue of their inability to continue to work, often caused by their ill health. After a lifetime of work the elderly appeared to be able to rely only on charity or the workhouse in circumstances for which they appeared free of blame. Pressure grew, particularly following the studies conducted by Charles Booth, to do something about the aged poor for whom reliance on the Poor Law appeared as a final indignity at the end of a life of privation. The political mood then was in the process of change, partly motivated by a change in ideas away from *laissez-faire* towards a 'new liberalism' and by a realisation that the effects of state intervention might not be as damaging as first thought. Such acceptance of a wider role for the state in social policy was to lead, at the end of the century, to a view that the state 'should be used as a vehicle for social reform, to improve the condition of the weakest and the poorest' (Clarke *et al.*, 1992). This change in mood was to receive legislative elaboration in the Liberal reforms of the first decade of the twentieth century.

Our brief examination of an expanding state welfare role in nineteenth-century Britain indicates a polity itself unwilling to commit the state to widespread activity and cautious of the opposition such concerted action might bring. The government in each of these areas of poor relief – sanitation, employment regulation and education – took, at each stage, unsteady and faltering steps towards welfare reform. But what these tentative steps did do was to provide the justification to build upon and engage in further activities in the future. Slowly, then, the state adopted and accepted, though never unequivocally, an ever wider role in the regulation and provision of social welfare.

The winds of welfare change

The final decades of the nineteenth century proved to be something of a political watershed in the development of the role of the British state in welfare provision. The economic doctrine of *laissez-faire* was gradually giving way to a collective ideal embodied in what was termed 'New Liberalism' which envisaged 'a positive role for the state in the amelioration of social problems' (Pearson and Williams, 1984). The legislative development of New Liberalism is something to which we turn in the next chapter; however, it is useful here to review the political and social environment within which New Liberalism developed.

One factor often cited in the creation of a new 'social' ethos for the Liberals was their changing political fortune. More and more working men were obtaining the electoral franchise which, in turn, facilitated the development of a working-class politics. The establishment first of a 'new unionism' and later the Labour Party posed a not inconsiderable electoral threat to the Liberal Party which had to be addressed. There were also concerns expressed that conditions of poverty and illness at home might threaten the dominance of Britain over her global empire. Military defeats in the Boer war led some to suggest that Britain's young men may not be up to the physical challenges of fighting for and defending their country, and that social conditions at home might be in part to blame for this state of affairs, particularly in regard to the health of children. Similarly there was a change in attitudes towards social issues. The studies by Booth in London and Rowntree in York indicated that poverty might not be simply down to laziness within the labouring classes. Instead the economic operation of society, the unfettered free market might, it was suggested, be the cause of some poverty, which in turn 'could be the cause of people being unable to live freely' (Clarke *et al.*, 1992).

The studies by Booth and Rowntree contributed to a debate about how society might attempt to measure poverty objectively and how minimum social standards might be defined and achieved. Rowntree's study talked of a minimum necessary to maintain physical efficiency, whilst Booth spoke of a 'line of poverty' below which were grouped classes of people who had only casual, intermittent or small but regular earnings. 'By the word "poor" I mean to describe those who have a sufficiently regular though bare income, such as 18s to 21s per week for a moderate family, and by "very poor" those who from any cause fall much below this standard' (Booth, 1892). Rowntree refined this in his attempt to define conditions of primary and secondary poverty wherein those suffering primary poverty were 'families whose total earnings were insufficient ... for the maintenance of merely physical efficiency' (Rowntree, 1901). The conclusions reached by these two surveys, though not universally accepted, were that around 30% of the population were living in poverty (Booth suggested 30% and Rowntree 28%). Rowntree went further in his analysis by suggesting that there existed a cycle of poverty throughout the lives of the labouring poor. The years of childhood, early marriage and old age were those in which poverty was highly likely, often for reasons that were beyond the control of the individual concerned, but as a result of 'complex economic and social factors' (Fraser, 2003).

Such surveys, themselves groundbreaking in the development of social research, together with a changing and turbulent political climate, altered fundamentally the basis of debate about social policies and the proper role of the state in providing welfare. We will go on to see that the first two decades of the twentieth century, rooted as they were in the changes of the nineteenth, laid the foundations of a formally organised welfare state which would not become a reality for another half-century.

Discuss and Do

The emerging welfare services in the early twentieth century were not universally welcomed, even by those they were designed to help.

Reflecting on some of the ideas and explanations presented in this chapter, for example:

- eligibility
- deserving and undeserving poor
- pride and self-reliance
- *laissez-faire* economics
- state welfare efficiency and effectiveness
- increased power of the working class

describe some of the various reasons that might be put forward to explain:

- the reluctance to support state welfare
- the acceptance of state-provided welfare.

Conclusion

What we have concerned ourselves with in this chapter has been the foundations of our twenty-first-century welfare state. Clearly the welfare state was not established by, nor did it develop from the publication of the Beveridge Report. Many of the principles of welfare, ideological, political and philosophical, have been with us for many centuries. The changes in state welfare introduced and developed in the nineteenth century that we have discussed in this chapter represent an attempt to place those principles in a legislative and structural framework. Similarly, many of those principles remain with us today, in the rules and policies adopted by our modern welfare state.

Web resources

A number of websites now exist that will supplement any study of social policy and open up many interesting new areas for debate and discussion. A number of general history websites exist, one of the more accessible being Spartacus (www.spartacus.schoolnet.co.uk). While this site is primarily for schools, it does provide a wide-ranging historical background, and access to historical documents, to many of the social policy changes we discuss here. For example, it explores the growth of towns and cities, political changes in the nineteenth century, public health and general social conditions – see, for example, its resources on child labour and changes to the regulation of work (www.spartacus.schoolnet.co.uk/Irchild).

Another interesting site pertinent to the development of nineteenth-century welfare services is Peter Higginbotham's website dedicated to the role and operation of the workhouse in Britain, which can be found at www.users.ox.ac.uk/~peter/workhouse. The detailed poverty studies undertaken by Charles Booth in the East End of London are also now available online and can be found at www.booth.lse.ac.uk.

Annotated further reading

One of the most comprehensive and accessible accounts of legislative change across the range of social policy, particularly in the nineteenth century, remains Derek Fraser's *The Evolution of the British Welfare State* (2003), and a further useful source is Henriques' *Before the Welfare State* (1979). An important and very accessible addition to the range of literature exploring the foundations and development of the welfare state in Britain is Bernard Harris's *The Origins of the British Welfare State* (2004). As well as providing a comprehensive analysis of welfare state developments, this text also explores the various historical approaches to studying welfare (its historiography). The most accessible account of the later nineteenth century and the Liberal welfare reforms before the First World War can be found in Thane's *Foundations of the Welfare State* (1996).

Discussion and analysis of the area we might usefully refer to as non-state welfare has been growing in recent years. Johnson's *Saving and Spending* (1985a) gives perhaps the fullest account of the working-class economy during the industrial revolution, whilst Finlayson's *Citizen, State and Social Welfare in Britain 1830–1990* (1994) explores the development of self-help and mutual aid as alternatives to the 'state-led' notion of welfare reform.

For an exposition of the ideas and ideals and the political debates behind the welfare reforms of the day and the controversy over the right role for the state in promoting public welfare, see Pearson and Williams's *Political Thought and Public Policy in the Nineteenth Century* (1984). Clarke, Cochrane and Smart's *Ideologies of Welfare* (1987) explores similar territory, whilst an interesting biographical detour may be found in Barker's *Founders of the Welfare State* (1984).

Chapter 3

The welfare state years: consensus and conflict

Objectives

- To describe the institutional development of the British welfare state through the first half of the twentieth century.

- To explore the existence of consensus in British social policy.

- To introduce and examine the idea of a crisis of the welfare state.

Introduction

As we indicated in the preceding chapter, it may be tempting to lay the foundation of the British welfare state with the publication of the Beveridge Report in 1942. However, as we have seen, many of the principles embodied within the welfare state have their roots in the often pioneering work of social reformers in the nineteenth century. Similarly we can identify, in the structures of the contemporary welfare state, an earlier ancestry. In particular, we can suggest that the modern structures of British welfare are those laid down in the reforms introduced under the Liberal government in the first decade of the twentieth century.

We begin by examining these reforms and go on to suggest that the introduction of measures such as school meals, old-age pensions and later the principle of insurance-based social security were the basis of many, if not most, of the welfare principles upon which we rely today. The impact of Fabianism, as a coherent set of ideas, together with the impact of war combined to lend legitimacy to the idea of widespread and formalised state action across a wide range of social and economic activities. Such was the effect of this new state activity that the notion of a welfare consensus, a broad acceptance of the role of the state in many areas of public and private life, developed in the post-war decades. This notion of consensus on social policy we explore in the latter part of this chapter; we discuss whether such a term is itself meaningful and what the nature of that consensus might be.

Liberal social policy

In January 1906 the Liberals under Campbell-Bannerman won a landslide general election victory, ending almost 20 years of Conservative rule, and, though social reform was not high on their list of priorities, it did benefit from the victory. The presence of 53 Labour MPs was more than anything else a symbolic and powerful symbol of the aspirations of working-class men and women and of the failure of the two-party system (Sullivan, 1992; Thane, 1996). Britain had also undergone something of a demographic transformation, witnessing the relative decline of agriculture and rural depopulation and a corresponding rise in industrial manufacturing and a concentration of population in the developing towns and cities (Harris, 2004). The twin processes of urbanisation and industrialisation had political consequences in the growth of the 'new unionism' and the development of workers' political representation in the form of the Labour Representation Committee. There had been a Labour presence in the Commons for five years, though small, and many of those Labour MPs elected had taken the Liberal whip in Parliament. But their presence in Parliament was growing and as one contemporary report put it:

> The emergence of a strong Labour element in the House of Commons has been generally welcomed as the most significant outcome of the present election. It lifts the occasion out of the ordinary groove of domestic politics and will have far wider influence than any mere turnover of party voters. (*The Times,* 30 January 1906)

The General Election of 1906, which saw a landslide Liberal victory, returned 53 Labour MPs, 29 of whom were sponsored by the Labour Representation Committee (Fraser, 2003). In some ways this Labour presence in the House acted as a social conscience for the Liberal majority and prompted the first stirrings of 'welfarism'.

The embryonic welfare state

As we have suggested in Chapter 2, what have come to be known as the Liberal Welfare Reforms had their origins in a changing social consciousness in the final years of the nineteenth century. In particular concerns had been expressed about the physical condition of the young, the persistence of widespread poverty, particularly following the publication of the reports by Booth and Rowntree, and the continued reliance of many elderly and infirm individuals on the provisions of the Poor Law and the workhouse. The first reforms introduced by the new Liberal government therefore appealed to public sentiment by concentrating on measures to improve the welfare of children and the elderly. By the time of the outbreak of war in Europe in 1914, the government had endured constitutional crisis and had sought to introduce welfare provision for the ordinary working man.

The Liberal government's first moves were to focus on the welfare of children in the provision of free school meals. Some measures for the provision of school meals for the children of families receiving poor relief had been introduced by the Conservatives in 1905, and followed the deliberations of The Interdepartmental Committee on Physical Deterioration to 'investigate claims that the health of the population was indeed deteriorating' (Harris, 2004: 156). The Liberal measure – the Education (Provision of Meals) Act – passed by Parliament in 1906 placed the responsibility for such provision in the hands of the local education authority. The implication was clearly that meals could be provided for children of all poor families rather than those considered destitute enough to receive poor relief. The government then went further the following year by introducing a Bill requiring local education authorities to provide for the medical examination of children in elementary schools and for the promotion of the health of such children. What both provisions marked was a point at which Government began to gradually remove responsibility for welfare from the institutions of the Poor Law and, since both services continue to operate 100 years later, to establish what we have come to regard as a 'welfare state'.

The next significant development, in 1908, was the introduction by the government of the first old-age pensions, again outside the operation of the Poor Law, but not before being prodded into action by the back benches and activities outside the House. Although the government were wary of the Conservative opposition in the House of Lords, further prompting by Labour members of the House, as well as further Labour electoral gains in by-elections, encouraged the government to act. The introduction of old-age pensions was significant for a number of reasons, as it marked the development of (central) state welfare funded out of general taxation and subject to a national system of regulation rather than being left to local Boards of Guardians or local authorities.

Herbert Asquith, who had taken over as Prime Minister, and David Lloyd-George, the Chancellor of the Exchequer, were to be powerful movers in the introduction of new pension legislation. Lloyd-George felt that a large number of older people would rather endure poverty than submit themselves to their local Poor Law Board of Guardians; there was, he said, 'a mass of poverty and destitution which is too proud to wear the badge of pauperism' (Fraser, 2003: 167). The Bill proposed that old-age pensions be non-contributory and that they be introduced to offer relief to aged paupers and relieve the strain on the Poor Law, which was itself under consideration by a Royal Commission. Lloyd-George proposed the introduction of a means-tested pension for those aged 70 years or over, and so it was, with the successful passage of the legislation, that pensions were introduced from 1 January 1909. The new pension was paid as a right, and collected by recipients from their local post office, and by this measure reformers hoped to remove the stigma that had been associated with the Poor Law, though it was restricted to exclude those who had recently been in receipt of poor relief. The government was apparently concerned that local Boards of Guardians may simply try to offload the financial burden of their pensioners on to the Treasury (Harris, 2004).

Lloyd-George was to ensure his name in welfare history by his next intervention into the realm of social reform. As Chancellor in 1909 he was faced with a projected budget deficit of £16 million and he decided that the solution to his financial dilemma was to be by the introduction of his 'people's budget'. He intended to raise revenue by increasing duty on alcohol and tobacco, but also on petrol and the use of motor vehicles, a levy that fell in greater part on the wealthy. He also introduced a progressive form of income tax which Lloyd-George described as:

A War Budget. It is for raising money to wage implacable warfare against poverty and squalidness. I cannot help hoping that before this generation has passed away we shall have advanced a great step towards that good time when poverty and wretchedness and human degradation which always follow in its camp will be as remote to the people of this country as the wolves which once infested the forests. (*Hansard*, 29 April 1909)

So radical were these proposals for their day that the House of Lords rejected them and brought the two Houses of Parliament directly into conflict with one another. Lloyd-George warned that the Lords 'five hundred men chosen accidentally from among the unemployed' would not frustrate the will of the democratically elected government. The conflict prompted a constitutional crisis over which two general elections were fought in 1910; the first confirmed the 'people's budget' and the second caused the reform of the constitutional powers of the House of Lords who from then on would no longer be able to thwart the will of the Commons. Lloyd-George proposed the Parliament Bill and threatened to create enough Liberal peers to force the Bill through the Lords, and the outcome was that the House of Lords had to concede defeat. Since that time the House of Lords has been limited in the extent to which it is able to reject, or delay, legislation agreed by the Commons, particularly when considering the Finance Bill (budget) of a sitting government.

Following the constitutional crisis surrounding the adoption of the 'people's budget', the government was able to press ahead with further welfare reform. One of the most important structural principles of the British welfare state, which remains an important pillar today, was the introduction of social insurance to cover the interruption of earnings, by either ill-health or unemployment (see Figure 3.1).

Stop and Think

How far is it possible to suggest that the Liberal government's radical welfare reforms of the early part of the twentieth century were principally a result of the growth of the trades unions and a Labour presence in Parliament?

Lloyd-George proposed the introduction of a tripartite scheme into which contributions would be paid by employee, employer and the government itself. The contributions would insure the worker against the 'accidents of life', such as ill-health or death of the breadwinner, which had been recognised as major causes of poverty and destitution, and which would bring destitution onto whole families. The Act was in two parts. The first provided for free medical treatment for insured workers and treatment for family members who were suffering from tuberculosis, together with cash benefits. Workers could receive 26 weeks' benefit for a period of sickness, followed by a disablement benefit if they were unable to work after 26 weeks. The Act also provided for maternity benefits for insured women and wives of insured men (Harris, 2004). Part Two of the Act provided for benefits to be paid during periods of unemployment, for up to 15 weeks in a 52-week period, and paid lower rates of benefit than under the scheme of health insurance. However, the Act was limited to workers in certain industries; for example, it was not extended to agricultural workers until 1934. The Insurance Act was thus placed alongside an earlier piece of legislation, the Labour Exchanges Act 1909, which had established a national system of labour exchanges (Jobcentre Plus) to assist the unemployed

THE DAWN OF HOPE.

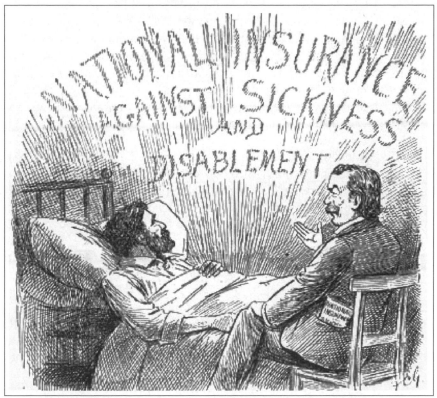

Mr. LLOYD GEORGE'S National Health Insurance Bill provides for the insurance of the Worker in case of Sickness.

Support the Liberal Government
in their policy of
SOCIAL REFORM.

Figure 3.1 'The Dawn of Hope' – poster produced by the Liberal Party to promote the 1911 National Insurance Act
Source: The National Archives, www.nationalarchives.gov.uk, ref. PRO: PIN 900/42. Reprinted with permission.

to find work, and we can see this same principle still in operation today within the programmes of the New Deal and welfare to work. The principle of insurance against periods of interruption to employment was extended during and after the years of the First World War to include periods of casual unemployment due to temporary recession, a cornerstone of the proposals contained in the Beveridge Report three decades later.

The impact of war and the inter-war years

The impact of the First World War was felt right across British society and at all levels. The men killed and injured during the fighting itself amounted to some 2.5 million, from around 6 million men who volunteered or were called up to fight. This 'total war' also forced society, and government, to address the effect of the fighting on those who returned, albeit slowly and in a piecemeal fashion. The injuries sustained, both physical and mental, were on a scale never before witnessed and demanded new responses from the medical profession. What we have now come to call Post Traumatic Stress (shell shock as it had been termed) had been grounds, on the front line, for charges of cowardice in the face of the enemy and dereliction of duty for which some had been executed. But both the physical and mental scars endured by soldiers demanded that new approaches and techniques be developed in health care, such as prosthetic limbs or psychological treatments. The effect of these changing attitudes to war can be seen in the Liberal government's election campaign at the end of the conflict, arguing that it wanted to build a land fit for heroes and in some way reward those men, and their families, who had sacrificed so much for their country. This, says Fraser (2003), marked a new attitude towards welfare, with the growth in the post-war years of a strong 'collectivist urge' (p. 193) and the notion that people may have a 'right' to demand support from the state.

The war also had a profound impact on society at home. The rates of taxation levied by the government in pursuance of the war increased dramatically over previous levels but had become accepted and came to be tolerated at higher peacetime levels after the conflict was over. The numbers of women who were brought into industry to maintain war production, over 1.5 million, marked the beginnings of a fundamental shift in the role of women in society, and many of the previous certainties of Edwardian and Victorian society were swept away by the social impact of the war. Class distinctions became blurred as men of all social ranks died together, and rationing and price controls on food were introduced at home, both of which imposed a sense of greater equality.

The years of the First World War and the decades up to the outbreak of the Second World War witnessed profound social change that in turn had its impact on the political and welfare landscapes. Economically Britain, which had been and still regarded itself as the powerhouse of the industrial revolution, was in a much weaker position. Although the economy did continue to grow, Britain had entered a period of economic decline relative to other economies and was overtaken by the new American powerhouse. The growth was underlined by the development of new industries in new industrial areas, such as the chemical industry, electronics and the automotive industry, but areas of 'traditional' industry were weak and declining. Thus for some parts of the country the inter-war years were characterised by high and persistent unemployment, continued industrial unrest and the highly emotive hunger marches, all of which were exacerbated by the advent of the 'Depression' of the early 1930s. Average incomes in the period did rise, in part due to the development of the new industries and in part due to the development of what might be considered more 'middle-class' (white collar) occupations, but the enduring picture of those decades is one of economic uncertainty and increasing militancy.

However, despite the image of economic depression, the picture varied considerably. Overall poverty levels continued to fall and there were general improvements in housing conditions and the provision of social security benefits and pensions. Significantly there were dramatic improvements in Britain's health as mortality rates fell, life expectancy rose by an average of 15 years, to 66 for men and 71 for women, and infant mortality fell equally dramatically, halving to 50 infant deaths per 1,000 live births. Gone now were the days of mass epidemics of infectious diseases such as typhus, cholera and smallpox that had characterised the nineteenth century and, though some infections did dominate with persistent outbreaks of diseases such as meningitis and tuberculosis, they too were coming under the control of the health professionals. Despite the public spending cutbacks of the 1920s, overall levels of spending continued to rise from 12% of GDP up to 25% and the period witnessed a large-scale expansion in public sector employment (Harris, 2004). In part, of course, the rise in public sector spending is explained by the increasing cost of benefits to cover the large-scale and persistent unemployment of the period which, despite cutbacks in the 'doles' of the early 1930s, was more than countered by the extension of entitlements to other industries and the widening of the allowances net to provide cover to family members rather than simply the 'breadwinner'.

Unemployment between 1921 and 1940 averaged around 1.5 million (mainly men) which represented around 10% of the insured workforce. Indeed the figure was never below one million and in 1932 peaked at just below 3 million. It is worth remembering in this regard, however, that this was the 'official' unemployment figure and, since many workers were not eligible or simply did not register, the actual figure must have been considerably higher. The problem of unemployment was also exacerbated by its concentration both regionally and industrially, though this was frequently one and the same thing. Unemployment was concentrated in certain, what came to be regarded as traditional, industries such as coal mining, shipbuilding, iron and steel working and textiles. But these industries were also concentrated geographically and dominated the north-east and north-west of England, South Wales, Scotland and Northern Ireland.

One thing we can say is that this level of unemployment undoubtedly damaged the juvenile welfare system. The system of National Insurance had been extended in 1920 to include some new areas of industry and to cover a wider range of dependents. As a result the costs of the system rose rapidly, which in turn undermined the insurance principle underlying the scheme. Rising costs in particular brought the government into conflict with local Poor Law Boards of Guardians in the East End of London (Poplar and West Ham), who still had a role in the relief of poverty at this time and who were accused of paying excessive relief. The government's response was largely ad hoc, however, as they sought to balance the insurance budget and introduced reductions of 10% in spending on Unemployment Benefit. They did, however, also finally remove the responsibility for poor relief completely from the local Poor Law by the abolition of Boards of Guardians and the introduction of Public Assistance Committees in the Local Government Act of 1929. This was of particular importance as it established a pattern of centrally controlled and managed dual relief in the form of insurance and assistance that was to become the model of British social security after 1945.

One area of welfare change that was significant in the inter-war years was that of housing. Lloyd-George's promise to build 'homes for heroes' had started a seemingly unstoppable change. Local government was given greater power to construct housing of good quality for working people to be able to rent. The building industry too was encouraged, by way of subsidy, to engage in a building programme of homes for sale. Between both local government and private industry around one million homes were built between 1919 and 1930 of which some 200,000 were subsidised by government and built by local authorities in the years 1919–22, though this programme was curtailed by reductions in public spending under the Geddes Axe of 1923. During the 1930s the programme of house building continued with greater urgency as local authorities acquired powers to designate areas for slum clearance and re-housing under the Housing Act of 1930 and later powers to address overcrowding in the Housing Act of 1935. In this decade some 3 million houses were built, most of which were for private sale, but the two decades together saw a significant increase in the state provision of housing with over one million council houses built.

By contrast the area of education saw almost no government activity during these two decades and it was not until 1944 that significant change in education policy came about. There were some changes in schooling during this time, however. A school-building programme was begun which focused on attempts to reduce the use of unsuitable buildings as schools and to reduce class sizes to more acceptable levels, as classes of 50–60 were not uncommon. There was also some expansion of nursery provision, the division between primary and secondary education became established, and there was some small change in university education with the establishment of three new universities and the introduction of scholarships for students of working families.

Politically too the era was one of great change. The 1920s saw the election of the first (minority) Labour governments under Ramsay MacDonald in 1922 and 1929, and then the first majority government headed by a Labour prime minister as MacDonald led the first coalition government of the 1930s. But the period was one dominated by coalition governments of various hues, as the country attempted to respond to national economic emergency and later the outbreak of war. Politically, however, the inter-war years, particularly the 1930s, were dominated by debates on foreign policy rather than domestic or social policy. The rise of fascism and communism in continental Europe polarised opinion in Britain as politicians attempted to respond to the rise of Hitler in Germany and the pending threat of another war.

The years between the two world wars, during which time the Labour Party gradually replaced the Liberals as the 'natural party of opposition', were also years during which Britain itself moved from welfare scepticism to welfare collectivism. Early attempts at state intervention in individual welfare had often been viewed with suspicion, as a threat to the attempts of working-class people to better their lives (Pelling, 1984; Sullivan, 1996; Thane, 1996). Early Labour response was to oppose the extension of state power implicit in the Liberal welfare reforms; it was the state, after all, whose welfare of the Poor Law was the most hated. Working-class experience of the welfare 'state' had been unequivocally oppressive, and it is unsurprising therefore that the working classes viewed Lloyd-George's reforms as some attempt to extend the workhouse solution to poverty (Pelling, 1968).

It was not only in the attempts at the relief of poverty, however, that there was suspicion. Experience in both education and housing policies suggested that welfarism would be nothing more than another burden. The construction of homes for working people, in the aftermath of slum clearance at the end of the nineteenth century, by charitable organisations was frequently the cause of resentment. Large well-ventilated rooms might be congenial to the health of large working-class families, but were also impossibly expensive to heat, and the rules and regulation of behaviour that went with such charitable tenancies were felt to be an unwelcome incursion into people's liberty and lifestyle. The Labour movement itself sought to redress the balance by the construction of 'model' working-class housing in the inter-war years, such as those of the Co-operative movement or the Tolpuddle Martyrs Memorial Cottages, and such a move might indicate a guarded welcome for municipal housing projects.

Interventions into the field of education raised similar worries and feelings of hostility amongst working people. One of the most ardent objections was the potential loss of earnings for a working-class family that compulsory education implied. Many families were in fact dependent for their very survival on the earnings from their children's employment. The progression of education reforms, which has continually increased the element of compulsion, alongside moves to restrict the hours worked by children, remained substantially unsupported by ordinary working people in the late nineteenth and early twentieth centuries. Their fears were grounded in an anti-statist philosophy which regarded the state as something that worked for and protected the interests of the wealthy (see Pelling, 1968). Likewise, the welfarism of the state, as expressed by the Liberal welfare reforms of the first decade of the twentieth century, was viewed as something antithetical to the alternative forms of working-class welfare provision already in place (Johnson, 1985a; Finlayson, 1994; Thane, 1996). The clearest statement of an alternative form of welfare was the widespread existence of the Friendly Society whose central concern was mutual insurance against sickness and unemployment. Strong within such societies was the belief that mutual self-help was socially and morally preferable to redistributive provision implemented by state functionaries, whose activities would inevitably involve intrusion into the private lives of citizens (Thane, 1996).

Stop and Think

How far would you agree that welfare reformers during the years between the First and Second World Wars were motivated by a feeling of 'never again', and saw the welfare state as a way to prevent future wars as well as the misery of mass unemployment?

The foundations of the social administration

The reasons for the gradual acceptance of welfarism within the Labour movement and the wider working classes has much to do with the development of the ideas of Fabianism. The Fabian Society, led by the indomitable Sidney and Beatrice Webb who themselves played a crucial role in the production of the Minority Royal Commission Report into the Poor Law, held that socialism in Britain was entirely compatible with the institutions of the state and could, and should, be realised through a parliamentary route. The state itself, they held, could be harnessed to promote the collective good and act as a neutral umpire between the demands of different interests. This view of the state, and its role in the promotion of welfare and the collective good, was to form the backbone of 'social administration', the forefather of today's 'social policy' (see Chapter 1). Put simply, the election of a Labour government would give the working class control of the state machinery of Westminster and Whitehall.

Social democracy in Fabian eyes, then, required not the 'withering away' of the state, but that it be fashioned into an instrument of social change and that the *expert administrator*, the civil servant, under the guiding hand of the elected parliament, become the tool for the implementation of (gradual) social change.

Inherent in the notion of gradual social change was the concept of ethical socialism apparent in the writings of theorists such as Tawney and Marshall. Within their writings was a notion of equality which emphasised self-esteem and dignity. Unevenness was acceptable but not the grotesque and blatant exploitation that they said characterised British capitalism; equality was to be a concept consistent with both individual difference and economic growth – ideas resonant of modern Labour thinking. Social policy within this ethical socialism would be used to diminish artificially created differences (Tawney, 1952).

Wartime welfare

It is of course also right to view the collective experience of the Second World War as a seed bed for the post-war welfare state. The nationalisation of hospital services and the development of an education policy that would make secondary education a right for all children played their part in creating a political climate in which post-war welfare measures would flourish. Several factors came together to create the climate of collective suffering; personal income was taxed at a high level, wage rates overtook inflation and unemployment was virtually abolished as both men and women joined either the armed forces or the home front services working in munitions or the Land Army (Jones, 1991; Addison, 1992). The social and economic planning of the war years led to a real and apparent redistribution of resources and may then be viewed as a 'dry-run' or prototype of post-war welfare state planning (Titmuss, 1950).

Thus it might be claimed that these factors, together with the shared danger of wartime, created a greater sense of social solidarity in British society than had hitherto been the case. Conscripts from different walks of life and social classes were thrown together and formed close bonds of comradeship. Dockers and doctors shared the security of air-raid shelters in the major cities, and rural, often middle-class, families provided homes for evacuees, which for one commentator was the nearest British society came to socialism (Foot, 1983).

By 1945 and the landslide general election, the hostility of the labour movement to state social welfare appears to have evaporated. The experience of crushing poverty and privation in the depressions of the 1920s and 1930s left many with the feeling that something had to be done and that the state may, after all, be the obvious solution. The experience of the war years, of collective deprivation and a collective, state, response, reinforced that feeling. The calls by Keynes and Beveridge for a twin pillar approach of full employment and a welfare state looked increasingly attractive and the Labour Party became identified with the crucial social issues of the day. All of these factors then, we might say, set the seal on the post-war orthodoxy of social reform and welfare statism.

Stop and Think

To what extend did the Beveridge Report represent a 'revolution' in the development of a welfare state?

Or, is it more appropriate to think of the Beveridge Report as part of a process of evolution?

Welfare consensus?

One important outcome of the collectivism of the war years was the creation of what was to become described as the 'post-war consensus' on welfare and the welfare state. Much of the post-war period is said to have been characterised by broad agreement in political debate about the role of the state in civil society. There was, it seemed, a continuity between the domestic politics of the Labour and Conservative parties and a substantial degree of agreement, in principle, about the need for government intervention to ensure economic growth, full employment and the provision of more or less comprehensive welfare services (Middlemass, 1979, 1986; Greenleaf, 1983).

The assumed nature of the welfare state was summed up in the oft-quoted phrase 'from cradle to grave', or 'womb to grave', in which 'life ... is monitored by, or is dependent upon, a vast network of state social legislation and provision' (Jones and Novak, 1980). The welfare state itself became regarded as a creature of consensus politics which, irrespective of their objective success or failure in meeting social need, was to be fostered, defended and extended as the mark of a civilised society. We shall, in the rest of this chapter, aim to untangle the conflicting arguments about the existence, nature and scope of the post-war British consensus.

The consensus, so it was said, evolved from the aping, by the Conservative Chancellor of the Exchequer, Butler, of the economic policies of his Labour predecessor, Hugh Gaitskell. So clear was the belief in the consensus that it acquired its own identity in the phrase 'Butskellism'. That the consensus existed appears to be in little doubt, since we are told that from the early 1970s it came under increasing strain in the austere economic climate of the day. Indeed we are further told that the consensus was responsible for many of the social problems visible in Britain in the 1970s and early 1980s.

But the roots of this apparent consensus can be traced back to the inter-war years. The privations, at least for working people, of the 1920s and 1930s and the clearly polarised, along class lines, response of the government to that period of economic crisis, which sought to protect the owners of finance capital, were still clear in the post-war memory. In addition, the minority Labour governments of 1923 and 1929 appeared powerless to break free from the drive for profit of British capitalism. It was in this environment that the idea of a negotiated settlement between labour and capital, which would ensure steady economic growth but also alleviate the suffering of many, gained currency (Addison, 1975; Sked and Cook, 1979; Briggs, 1983).

The range of policies which made up the post-war consensus are those stemming from the economic philosophy of John Maynard Keynes and the social philosophy of Sir William Beveridge in what has come to be called the Keynesian Welfare State (KWS) (Burrows and Loader, 1994). Keynesian policies were ones which assumed, or were consistent with, the intervention of government through fiscal and monetary techniques to regulate demand and encourage full employment. Beveridgian social policies were intended to contribute to the development of comprehensive welfare services, access to which would confer a sort of social citizenship. Accordingly, Keynes plus Beveridge were seen to equal Keynesian social democracy, or welfare capitalism or consensus.

The elements of that consensus can be conceptualised in the following way. In the first place the settlement represented a political turnabout. The inter-war years had been dominated by one political party at the helm of government. Although Labour formed two short-lived administrations, the Conservative Party, on its own or in coalition with the rump of the other parties, monopolised the politics of policy making in government. The formation of a genuine coalition government, a political expedient for Churchill as wartime Prime Minister, was the first step in this turn-around. The landslide of the 1945 general election completed the transformation. A new two-party system emerged in which both parties, now Conservative and Labour rather than Liberal, enjoyed relatively stable and relatively equal support (see Butler and Stokes, 1974, for an analysis of post-war 'consensus' voting patterns).

The second element of the new political consensus was that the policies said to characterise the years of consensus could be clearly distinguished from those of the inter-war years. The post-war settlement which included the social security plans of the Beveridge Report, the establishment of the National Health Service, the introduction of compulsory free secondary education and the pursuit of full employment as a policy goal, represented to many the creation of new 'rights' of citizenship (Parker, 1972; Gamble, 1987; Sullivan, 1989), indeed as a 'sustained attempt to reduce inequality through public action' (Gamble, 1987).

The third element of the post-war settlement is often seen as foreshadowing what was to happen in later years in both the politics of industrial relations and the politics of social policy making. That is, in accepting the trades unions, which had fought through the inter-war years for their right to be consulted and even incorporated into the decision-making processes of government, powerful state and private interests were embarking on a momentous change in direction from inter-war practices and principles. Of special significance is the legitimation of a tripartite structure of decision making in industry (and wider economic planning), in the form of the National Economic Development Council, and in social policy making. The introduction of this 'corporatist' format of decision making reached its zenith with the negotiation of the Social Contract between the Labour administration and trades unions in the mid-1970s. It is this policy-making change which is said to most epitomise the years of consensus in which successive Labour and Conservative administrations showed themselves willing to continue the policies of their predecessors. One of the clearest examples of policy consensus may be said to be the advent of comprehensive education in the 1960s, continued and consolidated under Margaret Thatcher's tenure as Education Secretary (Weeks, 1986; Reynolds and Sullivan, 1987; Sullivan, 1992).

Some commentaries point to the issue of nationalisation, and the apparent disagreement over the state's role in the direct management of industry, to suggest a lack of consensus. The post-war Labour government had established a mixed economy in which public and private corporations would coexist. In pursuit of this strategy the Attlee government had nationalised a number of major industries, including coal and steel. The following Conservative administration, from 1951, returned steel to private control but retained most of the others under state control, though arguably remained lukewarm towards them. Those industries that remained in public control were encouraged to operate as though they were private enterprises and brought in private sector businessmen to senior positions (Greenleaf, 1983; Blake, 1985). The Conservatives then appeared to accept major elements of Labour's post-war settlement, such as full employment and the welfare state, as both evolutionary and desirable.

There are, of course, as we indicate above, differences in emphasis between the parties, but much of the evidence seems to attest to the existence, over almost 30 post-war years, of a *de facto* political consensus on a mixed economy, full employment and a welfare state. The notion of consensus appears stronger when contrasted to the politics of conflict which characterised the inter-war years, rather than agreement at the level of individual policy in the post-war years. Whether or not we accept the existence of a consensus in British post-war politics, what does seem clear is that the ideas embodied in Keynesianism about economic management and in Beveridge's social philosophy acted as midwives to a relatively durable form of welfare capitalism.

The nature of that welfare capitalism is perhaps nowhere better analysed than in Marshall's seminal essay 'Citizenship and social class' (Marshall, 1963), which identifies the foundations of consensus not so much in the pursuit of particular policies or the formation of particular political structures, but in the establishment of wider and deeper social rights for citizens. These rights, including access to welfare in the famous phrase 'free at the point of delivery' and full employment, are important elements of the post-war consensus. They were viewed as the culmination of a process which delivered a wider package of social rights, which included the civil and legal rights already won. According to Marshall, these rights were important to the development of capitalism, since although they promised greater access to material wealth they also attempted to incorporate potentially disruptive individuals or groups into the value structure of capitalism (Marshall, 1963). The significance of the consensus, which Marshall believes to have been created by the addition of social rights, was that it altered the emphasis of twentieth-century British capitalism without altering its organisation and power.

Other commentators, whose views were held to be peripheral and minority views, took a rather different approach. This group, latterly referred to as neo-liberals or the radical right, acknowledged the creation and operation of a post-war political consensus, yet perceived it not as a boon but as a back-door tyranny. Their views, which over the past 20 years gained the status of political orthodoxy, suggested that:

• the development of state intervention in the advanced nations of the twentieth century represented an embryonic state socialism and is one step on the 'road to serfdom' (Hayek, 1944) and the loss of individual freedom;

• the development of welfare states and protective legislation removed the responsibility for behaviour from individuals. Welfare states, as a consequence, have created irresponsible societies (Boyson, 1971) in which individuals and families and communities look to the state for the provision of resources, cash and services which they ought to provide for themselves.

The welfare consensus, or so it is believed, was the creation of misguided, though possibly genuine, political reformers. They legitimated wide-ranging interventionist activities for the state in areas of the economy, in industry and in issues of personal welfare. As a result they distorted the true and historic independent status of the individual and the role of the 'natural' operation of the market in the allocation of resources. Instead of engaging in unregulated exchange relationships with employers, sellers of goods and other individuals, citizens were made the servants of the state. Instead of promoting social rights, consensus politics conferred the status of serfdom on citizens whose actions were circumscribed by the all-pervasive regulatory actions of the state. One of the consequences was to place the state in the role of family head or *pater familias*. (The New Right's views on the consensus and the need for its destruction are explored in greater depth in Chapter 10 of this volume.)

What neo-liberalism is in no doubt about is that the development of the post-war consensus led to a transformation in the nature of and relations between the state and the market. The state changed from its minimal predecessor, with residual economic and social functions, to a collectivist state exhibiting extensive central planning functions in the economy and in welfare (Hayek, 1960).

The orthodox understanding of post-war British politics is one that seldom doubts the reality of consensus as a guiding political principle and practice in which the bipartisan administration of a shared set of policy frameworks was a political reality. However, one dissenting voice is apparent in the works of historian Ben Pimlott who seeks to dissect what he regards as the 'myth of consensus'. His scepticism is founded in the overtly conflictual politics of the Thatcher era against which earlier politics indeed appear consensual in nature. He further argues that if consensus existed it remained a well-kept secret from the political actors of the day. Indeed, he regards the Beveridge Report, which provided the rationale for the welfare settlement, as less than unanimously accepted. The Conservative wartime leadership felt the proposals to be expensive and potentially divisive. He also cites a widespread lack of enthusiasm from amongst Labour ministers, especially Ernest Bevan, who felt that Beveridge's proposals would not allow a future Labour government sufficient flexibility in the introduction of social welfare and social security policy. Bevan also clearly believed that the proposals would weaken the ability of trades unions to secure adequate wage settlements because of the implicit adoption of a 'social wage' (see also Bullock, 1967; Harris, 1981; Morgan, 1990).

Pimlott also cites the clear hostility of the medical profession to the introduction of a National Health Service (NHS) which implied limitations to the professional power of doctors. The Conservatives also opposed the introduction of the NHS, and Bevan's concessions to the doctors might be seen as further evidence of conflict – 'I choked the doctors' throats with gold' – rather than as a manifestation of political consensus. Similarly there was continued hostility towards comprehensive schooling, before and after its introduction, until a Labour government forced the issue with the passage of the 1976 Education Act (repealed by the Conservatives within five years).

Discuss and Do

The phrase 'welfare consensus' is frequently used to describe the developing welfare state between the end of the Second World War and the early 1970s.

Thinking about the discussion in the closing section of this chapter, not least regarding ideas of:

- a political consensus between Labour and Conservative governments

- a shared belief that the state could and should provide welfare

- a social contract between labour and capital or welfare-capitalism

- all citizens having social rights, that is rights to state welfare support

- the neo-liberals, not least in relation to individual freedoms and responsibilities

discuss the extent to which you think the phrase 'welfare consensus' is an accurate and useful description of the socio-political period of 1945 to the early 1970s.

Conclusion

Whether or not we accept the advent of consensus between the governments of post-war Britain as a broad agreement over elements of policy, or a broad agreement within which there was room for diverse political opinion (Kavanagh, 1987), or indeed we reject the notion of consensus as a more hopeful than realistic analysis, one thing we can be sure of is the upheavals in British politics and policy which came to be known as the end of consensus. It is to this that we shall turn in our next chapter.

Annotated further reading

The volume by Bernard Harris, *The Origins of the British Welfare State* (2004), is a particularly useful and very readable account of the establishment and development of the welfare state in the nineteenth and early twentieth centuries, while the works by Finlayson, *Citizen, State and Social Welfare in Britain 1830–1990* (1994), and Johnson, *Saving and Spending: The working class economy in Britain 1870–1939* (1985a), give very detailed and accessible accounts of the attitude and response to the growth of state welfare provision. There are also a number of useful historical descriptions and analyses of the development of the post-war welfare state in Britain. Readers may find those by Lowe (1993), *The Welfare State in Britain since 1945*, Hill (1993a), *The Welfare State in Britain: A political history since 1945*, and Glennerster (1995), *British Social Policy since 1945*, particularly informative.

For discussions of the changing political economy, the welfare consensus and its demise, Sullivan's (1992) *The Politics of Social Policy* and Deakin's (1994) *The Politics of Welfare: Continuities and change* are both thorough and insightful, while the rise of Thatcherism may be explored in Gamble's (1988) *The Free Economy and the Strong State* and Kavanagh's (1987) *Thatcherism and British Politics*.

Concluding comment to Part I

In this part we have introduced and explored some of the background to and historical development of social policy in Britain over the nineteenth and twentieth centuries. From within such an historical overview we can point to a number of features that remain important to the development of modern social policy.

The distinction between the deserving and the undeserving, first drawn in Elizabethan legislation, between those who suffer poverty as a result of external factors, perhaps beyond the control of an individual, and the lazy or indolent poor who would rather beg than work, is one we still make today. The debate over the last 20 or so years of the existence, or persistence, of an underclass trapped in poverty and following different, and therefore anti-social, codes of conduct is clearly resonant of an earlier age. Similarly the revulsion and panic induced by the pitching of travellers' caravans on vacant land across the nation reminds us of the fortress mentality adopted by many parishes under the old Poor Law system.

The New Poor Law, as we have seen, brought to us a new vocabulary and new ideas, again which inform the course of policy today. The deterrent effect introduced by the doctrine of less eligibility and the workhouse system of duty to those who provided for one's welfare have survived through successive generations of welfare policy. The twin notions of duty and responsibility, mirroring the language of rights that has grown up in social policy, have been revived under New Labour and its mantra that 'the rights we enjoy reflect the duties we owe'.

Developments begun in the nineteenth century in the creation of environmental, as opposed to medically based, health services, and of non-denominational state-funded education again remain with us today, essentially unchanged. Both services when created were rooted in a tradition of local government which itself dates back to the Elizabethan Poor Law and is jealously guarded and frequently the source of conflict.

The later years of our historical overview witnessed the development of a welfare state built upon principles of insurance, introduced by the Liberal legislation of the first decade of the twentieth century, and later upon the twin pillars of steady economic growth and full employment. The building blocks of the welfare state added in the Beveridge era, that government and the welfare state were vital to successful economic management, themselves created the foundations of a welfare and economic crisis that were to be part of British political culture until the dark days of economic recession in the 1970s and 1980s. These years of development also built into the welfare state an institutionalised gender and ethnic imbalance that is still being addressed in the twenty-first century.

Part II

Contemporary welfare

Introduction to Part II

In this part we turn to the contemporary social policy environment and to five aspects in particular. The climate for much government activity, and more especially social policy, since the mid-1970s has been one of great turmoil. The welfare state in Britain has undergone a crisis of confidence, brought about largely by external factors. This led in the 1980s and 1990s to a reassessment of its own position within the British polity, including revision of the role of government itself and a re-evaluation of how governments finance, structure and deliver public services.

The first chapter in this part explores the idea of the crisis of the welfare state and the end of the golden years of welfare consensus that were thought to have developed in the decades following the Second World War. The upshot of this crisis has been a rethinking of the proper role of the state in providing welfare and in particular of its role in financing welfare.

These two themes are taken up in the following three chapters which go on to examine, firstly in Chapter 5, the policy process, that is how policy is made and who is responsible for the initiation, implementation and evaluation of policy generally and of welfare policy more particularly. Chapter 6 explores how government has changed the manner in which social policy is developed, structured and delivered. It does this by exploring the idea of 'governance' to explain the approach of the Conservative New Right governments of the 1980s and 1990s, and their emphasis on markets, as well as that of New Labour since 1997 which has tended to utilise a discourse of partnership to construct its approach to the governing of social policy and welfare. Chapter 7 then goes on to explore the restructuring of the British welfare state with the implementation of devolved structures in Scotland, Wales and Northern Ireland. The chapter suggests that this is leading to the emergence of differing social policy regimes in each of the countries of the UK.

The final chapter of this part examines two interrelated questions: how we pay for our welfare services and how we spend such funds. Included within this are discussions of recent trends in welfare spending, particularly under New Labour since 1997, and the developing relationship between public and private sectors in the financing and provision of welfare services.

Chapter 4

A 'crisis' of the welfare state

Objectives

- To examine and explore the meaning, implications and usefulness of a widely-discussed social scientific concept: 'crisis'.

- To consider recent trends in the growth and development of welfare states.

- To explore theories and arguments – Marxist, neo-liberal and other – of institutional and social change, with particular relevance to welfare systems.

- To highlight the interconnectedness of economics, politics, social policy and broader social changes.

- To demonstrate the contested nature of the modern state's role in relation to welfare.

- To complement material and argument within other chapters, particularly those on public spending, governance, comparative analysis and globalisation.

Introduction

In this chapter we explore the concept of a 'crisis' in the welfare state, which has allegedly overtaken it in the course of the last 30 years, and which has given rise to a mountain of commentary, analysis and prescription. There are a number of reasons why the subject is an interesting one and worth exploring. It provides us with an opportunity for looking at issues of policy change and development from a novel perspective. It draws our attention to the linkages between social policy, politics and the economy. Consideration of the subject complements chapters on the historical evolution of the welfare state; in this sense 'the crisis' may be regarded as a (recent) phase of welfare state history. It also complements other chapters on the topics of governance (see Chapter 6), globalisation, and comparative and international perspectives (see Chapter 22). The concept of crisis also usefully reminds us of the interconnectedness of different areas of social life – society, the economy, politics and welfare. It draws our attention to issues of policy evaluation – of what counts as 'success' and 'failure' in social policy. Finally, it enables us to consider some general theoretical issues and problems of explanation, and to assess the utility of various models and paradigms which purport to explain social and institutional change.

The concept of 'crisis'

The premise of this chapter is that the concept of crisis is a useful way of organising discussion about welfare state developments in recent decades. Welfare states have since the 1970s been confronted by a series of challenges, pressures, constraints and limits. The source of these challenges and constraints has varied, over time, between countries and among analysts. Official, in some sense, acknowledgement of the arrival of a welfare state crisis was marked by a conference in 1980 organised by the Organisation for Economic Cooperation and Development (OECD), a body which represents the advanced liberal capitalist countries, and the publication of its proceedings the following year (OECD, 1981). Since the 1990s the source of the challenge has been subtly reconceptualised and identified with *globalisation*, one of the most fashionable social science concepts of the 1990s and beyond. Since the topic of globalisation is the subject of Chapter 22, it will not be dealt with here.

There is in fact a remarkable amount of disagreement in the vast literature which the subject has generated about the nature, dimensions and seriousness of the issues which the concept of crisis is supposed to identify. The concept of 'crisis' is one whose usefulness is far from generally accepted, and many analysts and commentators have questioned its reality and applicability to social policy and the welfare state.

There is indeed no single meaning of the term 'crisis' in the social scientific literature on the subject. 'Crisis' is in origin a medical term. In that context it refers to a turning-point in the progress of an acute illness; after it, the patient either dies or recovers. The term has been employed in the social sciences, applied to whole societies, political systems and economies, as well as welfare states. A number of different senses of the term have been identified in contemporary discussions: crisis as *turning point*; crisis as *external shock*; crisis as *long-standing contradiction*; and crisis as any *large-scale or long-standing problem* (Smith, 1989: 9; Pierson, 1998: 138). It follows therefore that there is disagreement at a conceptual level about what is being discussed, and writers with differing ideological persuasions and differing points on the political spectrum offer differing interpretations of the significance of particular states of affairs.

A disputable concept

One of the difficulties with the subject stems from its open-ended and ramifying character, and the need to keep any discussion of it relatively brief. It is hard or impossible to separate the supposed welfare or welfare state crisis from crises of the economy, the state and politics, and what some people might regard as crises of personal and private life – changing family forms, and changing gender and sexual relations. In principle, 'crisis' could invite a consideration of virtually everything that has happened to the British and other welfare states in the last 30 years.

The list of associated issues is a very long one: economic problems of low growth, inflation and macro-economic instability; the return of mass unemployment; economic and industrial 'restructuring'; 'post-Fordist' economic transition; supposed negative impacts of social policy on the economy; demographic change and the demographic 'time bomb'; trends in public spending and taxation; tax and public expenditure constraints and 'retrenchment' ('cuts'); issues of 'legitimation', public opinion and popular support for the welfare state; supposed failures of egalitarian redistributive strategies; the persistence of poverty and other social divisions; the rise of 'new social movements' associated with gender, race, ecology, sexuality and disability; globalisation and its impacts; changes in the governing socio-political consensus; the crisis of social democracy; the advent and impact of Thatcherism; the 'postmodern turn' in social science and culture; the 'hollowing-out' of the British state, changes in 'governance' and the rise of 'New Public Management'. Some of these issues are dealt with in other chapters, so we can conveniently limit ourselves in this one to a consideration of just a few of these topics.

'Crisis of the welfare state' or 'crisis of state welfare'?

A 'welfare crisis' might be supposed to mean one of (at least) two things. It might mean a crisis of a *particular type of society, social order* or political system – the liberal-democratic capitalist state typical of developed Western countries since the Second World War – what is sometimes referred to as 'welfare capitalism'. We might label this a 'crisis of the welfare state'. This would be a systemic crisis in the Marxist sense (if not necessarily open to interpretation in Marxist terms, or only in such terms). On the other hand, it might mean something narrower and more limited than this – a *crisis in or of* one or more particular *welfare services or programmes*, such as a crisis of the NHS or NHS funding, or the 'old age crisis', what we might label a 'crisis of state welfare'.

Stop and Think	Crisis of welfare or crisis in welfare?

What do you think is meant by a 'crisis *of* the welfare state'? What do you think is meant by a 'crisis *in* the welfare state'?

'Crisis' as persuasive rhetoric or 'moral panic'

The term 'crisis' has been employed by a variety of commentators on the welfare state, of varying backgrounds and ideological and political persuasions – academic commentators and researchers, think-tank publicists, journalists, politicians and, not least, welfare bureaucrats, professionals and practitioners – those who work in social service agencies and bureaucracies. It is a term which various groups and individuals, left and right, have found highly serviceable. This ought to put us on our guard. In a sense, 'crisis' may be a construct (or 'social construction'), a rhetorical device, a persuasive rather than descriptive or analytical concept, designed to serve particular interests. The American political scientist Robert Alford called attention to this feature of crisis rhetoric a long time ago in his comment on health care 'crises' in the USA: '"Crises" are usually creations of specific interest groups seeking to make political capital out of a situation that has existed for many years and will continue to exist after the "crisis" has disappeared from public view' (Alford, 1975: xi). In this sense, the term 'crisis' may come into the category of 'moral panic', that well-known tool of radical social critique, with the difference that the originators of this particular rhetoric of moral panic are as likely to be left as right in terms of political and ideological affiliation.

At the present time, for example, there are a number of ongoing 'crises' in the area of welfare, some of them of possibly dubious legitimacy. An 'old age crisis' has, for example, been identified by one international agency. In the UK there is a pensions 'crisis', an astonishing change in perception in the space of a few years; not so long ago the British were being encouraged to congratulate themselves on a retirement income regime that represented an ideal balance of principles and avoided the errors and dysfunctions of foreign systems (see Chapter 17). There is also, we are told constantly, an NHS financial crisis (see Chapter 12).

In America there are related crises – a Medicare funding 'crisis' (Medicare is the US public health care programme for the retired), as well as a 'crisis' of social security (meaning, in the American context, retirement pensions). In the case of the NHS, most of the talk of crisis emanates, as it always has, from within the Service itself, from professionals and managers, bearing out Alford's argument. The NHS financial 'crisis' of 2006 is a replay of an old tune which periodically comes back into favour; it has often been noted that such 'crises' in the NHS are endemic and semi-permanent.

Historical context: the growth and development of post-war welfare states

Before looking in any detail at welfare state 'crisis' itself, real or imagined, we need to begin by looking at its historical background – the growth and development of welfare states, mainly since the Second World War. The second half of the twentieth century was the age of the welfare state in the advanced capitalist and OECD countries. In the Continental and Scandinavian countries of Western Europe, Canada, and Australasia, as well as the UK, Poor Law-type welfare systems were superseded, welfare provision was broadly universalised, and entitlements to a range of benefits and services were extended to most sections of the population on the basis of some notion of citizenship, continuing and in some respects completing processes which, varying from country to country, had begun towards the end of the nineteenth century and beginning of the twentieth (Pierson, 1998: Ch. 4). Welfare state growth and consolidation was marked by expanded entitlement to a range of benefits, improvements in their quality, and rising expenditure levels. Improvements took place even in the United States, generally regarded as a welfare state 'laggard' by comparison with European states. (Of course, there were exclusions and limitations to the realisation of citizenship-based welfare entitlements, relating to, for example, women and disabled persons, which subsequently became apparent.)

The three decades from 1945 to the mid-1970s were the so-called 'golden age' of the welfare state. This over-simplifies a complex story to some extent and it is probably the last half of the period, from 1960 to 1975, which more truly exhibits 'golden age' characteristics (Pierson, 1998: 131–135). Other writers periodise developments slightly differently (Heclo, 1981; Mishra, 1990; Glennerster, 1995).

Mishra, for example, divides post-war welfare state development into three phases: the period of the so-called 'Keynesian Welfare State' (1950–75); the phase of 'crisis' (1975–80); and a post-crisis phase involving a break with the earlier Keynesian welfare state consensus after 1980 (Mishra, 1990: 96). 'Crisis' is, in Mishra's view, therefore, a qualitatively different but temporary phase of welfare state development.

Stop and Think	Consensus and crisis?

How meaningful is it to talk of a post-war consensus period followed by a period of welfare crisis?

A key aspect of welfare state growth is public spending on welfare (see Chapter 8). Public spending is the necessary condition for the provision of social welfare benefits, services and programmes. Government spending on welfare services increased inexorably and apparently unstoppably, although discontinuously, after the Second World War, however measured – in monetary terms, in 'real' terms (deflated by some index to reflect 'constant' prices) and as a share of national income or GDP.

Welfare spending has in fact not merely kept pace with the growth of national income but has outstripped it (Glennerster, 1995: 97, Fig. 5.1). This explains why welfare spending has increased as a proportion of GDP. By way of example: in 1950, health care spending in the UK amounted to around 4% of GDP; by the 1980s this share had increased by around 50% to about 6% of GDP and it is now close to 9% of GDP.

There are a number of explanations for the long-term growth of welfare spending, including the role of social movements associated with labour and trade unions, the rise of democracy, population growth, the 'relative price effect' (see Chapter 8), the expansion and maturing over time of welfare state entitlements, the ageing of populations and the development of new medical technology (Pierson, 1998: 135).

Economic growth and welfare spending

The underpinning for welfare spending and welfare state growth during this period was, of course, economic growth. The 'golden age' was characterised by policies in most Western countries designed to maintain high rates of economic growth, as well as high and stable levels of employment (so-called 'full' employment), low inflation and a stable balance of payments (Marquand, 1988; Glennerster, 1995). Whether or not these policies were really successful in achieving it, economic performance was certainly good.

The astounding success of the global capitalist economy was all the more remarkable in the context of capitalism's apparent failure during the inter-war years. Capitalism's success was a global phenomenon. The economic success of individual countries, including the UK, was buoyed up by the growth of world trade, supported by global financial arrangements – the so-called 'Bretton Woods' system of fixed exchange rates and the International Monetary Fund (IMF), effectively an international bank – created at the end of the Second World War to ensure exchange-rate stability and the reduction of global financial imbalances. Economic growth created new demands for labour, and in many countries of the OECD group unemployment of the kind that had existed in the inter-war period disappeared. At the same time, strong demand for labour created opportunities for immigration and the employment of groups hitherto excluded from the labour market, such as women.

An increment of economic growth was available to be appropriated by governments via taxation to spend on public programmes, including social services. This is the point of Rudolf Klein's remark in 1980 that 'the Welfare State is the residual beneficiary of the growth state' (Klein, 1980a, 1996a). Klein also commented in the same year in relation to welfare cutbacks that 'the resumption of economic growth is the most effective social policy that we have got' (Klein, 1980b, 1996b: 291).

Welfare spending as a positive-sum game

Spending on the welfare state was therefore a '*positive-sum*', as opposed to a '*zero-sum*', game (Pierson, 1998: 126). Hard distributive decisions – who gains, who loses – could be glossed over and obscured in a context in which everyone is doing better. There was no need for struggle between interest groups and social classes over the distribution of the product of growth. Where there is no growth, one interest group can only gain at the expense of another. A positive-sum, growth strategy had to some extent been advocated by the Labour politician and theorist of post-war social democracy Anthony Crosland in 1956 (Crosland, 1956). The growth of welfare spending in this period was also facilitated by reductions in other public programmes, notably defence, which has taken a steadily reducing share of public spending since the 1950s.

Figure 4.1 overleaf shows trends in social expenditure in the OECD group of countries in the period 1960–81. The vertical axis refers to annual percentage changes in social spending. There are two pairs of lines. The upper pair show the 'nominal', i.e. actual cash, expenditure trend. The lower pair show cash expenditure 'deflated' to take account of price changes, or adjusted for inflation. The solid line refers to the seven major (at the time) OECD economies, which included the UK; the dashed line refers to the average for all OECD countries (19 countries at the time). Although both sets of lines are jagged and discontinuous, it will be seen that there is a clear difference between the periods before and after 1975. Between 1960 and 1975 the average growth of spending is between 5% and 10% per year; after 1975 there is a steep fall, and the average is 5% or less. The very large increases in nominal spending during the 1970s alert us to the very high rates of inflation then prevailing. Note that throughout this period these rates of real welfare spending growth mean that welfare spending increases outstripped average economic growth rates, and welfare spending continued to grow as a share of GDP.

The UK's *relatively* poor economic growth performance, by comparison with European and OECD countries, began to be a cause of concern among commentators and policy makers in the 1960s and later; there was talk of 'the British disease' and of Britain as 'the sick man of Europe'. The UK was certainly one of the slower-growing economies in the OECD group, by comparison with Germany, Japan or France. In fact the UK's growth rate was well below the average for the seven major OECD economies between the 1950s and the 1980s. For the decade 1950–60 the UK's rate was at an

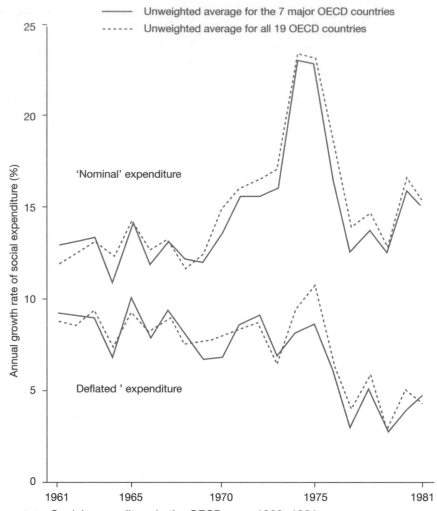

Figure 4.1   Social expenditure in the OECD area, 1960–1981
Source: OECD (1985) *Social Expenditure 1960–1990*, Chart 4, p. 19, Paris: OECD.

annual average of 2.3% (OECD 7 average 4.4%); for the period 1960–73 the UK's rate was 3.1% (OECD 7 average 5.5%) (OECD, 1985: 13, Chart 2; Pierson, 1998: 126). The UK's performance over this period was, nevertheless, by comparison with its own past performance, if not that of other countries, quite respectable, and was such as to facilitate increases in social welfare spending, particularly during the 1960s and early 1970s.

Economic performance for OECD countries after 1973 was very different from what had apparently become the post-war norm. For the period 1973–81 the OECD 7 average economic growth rate was 2.3% (the UK's was 0.5%). The decline in growth rates in the 1970s which characterised the OECD group in general was considerably worse for the UK economy (OECD, 1985: 13, Chart 2; Pierson, 1998: 126). The 1970s was a period in which growth declined, inflation rose, and unemployment also rose, something which, according to orthodox 'Keynesian' analysis of the economy, could not happen. By 1975, a year in which nine OECD economies did not merely not grow, but actually shrank, unemployment in the OECD group of countries had risen to 15 million (Pierson, 1998: 139). At the same time, inflation rates were very high – the UK rate in 1975 touched 25%. This state of affairs was referred to as 'stagflation' (stagnation plus inflation) or 'slumpflation' (slump plus inflation). Levels of investment and profitability also fell. This was a picture of economic policy failure.

For the UK, this eventually coincided in 1976 with a period of exchange-rate instability, requiring a loan from the IMF, which in turn ushered in a period of severe public spending cuts. For many observers, perhaps particularly those on the left, working in the social welfare industry and the universities, the era of 'the cuts' was the real welfare state crisis (Pierson, 1998: 153–154).

When was the 'crisis'?

Use of the term 'crisis' in welfare contexts is nothing new, and long predates the supposed crisis of the 1970s. Leaving aside the experience of the inter-war period in the UK, when economic crisis seemed to be endemic and arguably most welfare services were in a state of financial crisis for much of the time (the 'Geddes Axe' of 1922 and the benefit cuts of 1931 associated with the exchange-rate crisis and the election defeat of the Labour government of that year are simply the most high-profile examples) (Thane, 1996: Ch. 6; Fraser, 2003: Ch. 8), it is interesting to come across the following comment, published in 1961: '... the ideals which inspired the achievement of a "welfare state" are now no longer universally shared ... Against a background of recurring fiscal crises, "paying for services" has replaced "fair shares for all" as a current political slogan' (Briggs, 1961). It is the period of the supposed 'golden age' which is being described here. Talk of 'crisis' in relation to welfare and social programmes was not in fact uncommon in the 1960s (Robson and Crick, 1970).

If crisis is something, from a UK perspective, that has already happened, or is happening, it is also something that lies in the future. Talk of an 'old age crisis' or of a demographic time-bomb adverts to something that is looming, but has not yet necessarily arrived. The major economies of the EU, with their sluggish growth, high levels of unemployment and associated tax and regulatory burdens on industry, may be said to be facing a crisis – of economic performance and of welfare state affordability, and in this case it looks as if economy and welfare are in conflict.

An intellectual crisis? Ideological challenges to the welfare state

As we have already suggested, employment of the term 'crisis' might be as much a persuasive or rhetorical use of language as a descriptive or analytical one, as much a matter of perceptions as reality. 'Crisis' may be identified with intellectual critique, loss of confidence, ideological shifts, or an end of 'consensus', or be the product of a more detailed, dispassionate and rigorous evaluation of welfare state performance, resulting in disillusion and scepticism about the whole project and its apparent failure to overcome such problems as poverty, economic inequality, social divisions, educational under-achievement and health inequalities. As more is known, arguably, about the workings and outcomes of welfare state activities, with the greatly increased volume of welfare-related social research in the past few decades, the greater is the opportunity for disappointment and disillusion, in comparison with what obtained in the 1940s and 1950s. The last 30 years have seen the development of a variety of ideological and intellectual challenges to the welfare state. 'Crisis' has been employed to call attention to changes in elite and popular opinion. We explore these changes further in the section below on 'crisis containment: an end to consensus?'.

What crisis? The crisis debate

In this section we turn to consider some competing views and theories about the nature and dimensions of the welfare state crisis. First there is the view of crisis as a 'contingent' or 'sporadic' crisis, or as an 'external shock' to the system. In other words, the crisis is essentially accidental, a hiccup in the otherwise smooth upward progression of post-war liberal or social democratic capitalist states, caused by external shocks such as oil price rises. The implication is that crisis is likely to be temporary and that business as usual will eventually be resumed. Secondly, there is the view, partially a criticism of the first one, that the crisis was one of 'systemic contradiction' – this is the Marxist and neo-liberal view. This view implies that crisis is more fundamental, arising out of the particular, 'contradictory', relationships between the economy and politics in liberal capitalist democratic states, and further implies that crisis will be harder to escape. Thirdly, and finally, there are theories that may be called 'crisis containment' theories. These involve such ideas as an 'end of consensus', a decline in popular support for state welfare, and moves towards 'restructuring' the welfare state (Taylor-Gooby, 1985: 14).

An economic crisis? Crisis as 'external shock'

The concept of an economic crisis of welfare can be construed in various ways and as existing at various levels. At one level there was clearly an economic crisis of sorts in the UK and other countries in the 1970s, in which unprecedentedly high rates of inflation coincided with high and rising levels of unemployment and economic recession, involving actual reductions in national income, after 25 years in which advanced capitalist countries had grown continuously. 'Stagflation', or 'slumpflation', as this state of affairs was called, was provoked by, firstly, a quadrupling of oil prices in 1973 (there was another dramatic price increase in 1979, with similar effects), and secondly the policy responses pursued by governments in reaction to this. There were consequences for welfare spending and social policies and programmes.

The crisis in the sense just described, however, is not necessarily a 'crisis *of* the welfare state' so much as a 'crisis *for* the welfare state'. It is an economic crisis which had consequences for welfare. It was not something intrinsic to the welfare state – a 'systemic' crisis – but an 'external shock' to the system, a non-systemic, 'contingent' or 'sporadic' (to use Offe's term) crisis (Pierson, 1998: 140). The view that this is all the welfare state crisis really amounted to was the dominant mainstream view of most policy makers and policy analysts.

In the UK, for example, it was believed by many people in the mid-1970s, of all political parties, that public spending growth had got out of control and had to be limited. A statement of this view was the comment by Roy Jenkins, the then Labour Home Secretary, that a public expenditure ratio of 60% of GDP was a threat to freedom. Another was Anthony Crosland's remark, in 1975, to local authority leaders that 'the party's over' – in other words that the public expenditure feast that had hitherto prevailed had turned to famine, in relation to local authority spending (Crosland was Secretary of State for the Environment at the time, with responsibility for local government). This was highly significant for welfare because of local government's major role in providing so much of it (education, housing, personal social services).

There was some evidence, in the mid-1970s, of reduced willingness to fund higher levels of public spending in the UK. The period 1973–75 saw the most severe economic recession since the Second World War, and national income (GDP) actually fell, as did average take-home pay. As a result, both the Wilson and Callaghan governments and their successor under Margaret Thatcher sought to reduce both public spending and taxation (Glennerster, 1995: 172). People at that time were prepared, it was believed, not least among politicians, to support higher public spending and improved services only if their own private consumption was improving as well, which was not the case between 1974 and 1977 (Glennerster, 1995: 173). In other words, from being a positive-sum game, which it had been in the 1950s and 1960s, welfare growth became a zero-sum game and therefore much harder (Klein, 1980a, 1996a: 283). Economic crisis increased pressures on the welfare state, for example by increasing demands for unemployment benefits, at the same time that it reduced the capacity of the welfare state to respond (Klein, 1980b: 290).

This view of events still held, nevertheless, that the crisis, if it can be called such, was contingent rather than necessary.

A fiscal crisis of the state?

The 'contingent', 'economic shock' view was criticised by those who argued that the crisis could be construed as a systemic *'fiscal' crisis* or crisis of *affordability*. 'Fiscal' refers to public finances – taxes and spending (see Chapter 8). This has probably been the most general meaning and interpretation of welfare state crisis, implying a mismatch between needed and available financial resources. This usually implies that in some way the present or future costs of welfare programmes cannot be met either by taxation or by borrowing. In some way the limits of taxable capacity have been reached; taxpayers are unwilling to go on footing the bills for welfare expenditure. Analyses of fiscal crisis have been provided by both Marxist left and neo-liberal right, and in some respects they are similar.

Crisis as systemic contradiction I: Marxist accounts

The concept of socio-economic crisis was, of course, famously developed and used by Karl Marx. Marxist political economy may be regarded as a theory of crisis; in the Marxist view, capitalism is a socio-economic 'formation' prone to destabilising and perhaps fatal crises, presaging its transformation into something else – socialism or communism. For many Marxists, therefore, the economic experience of the 1970s was no surprise; it was what they had been expecting all along. In the same way, 'declinist' analyses of British economic weakness in the 1960s and 1970s were something with which Marxists could engage and agree. Eric Hobsbawm's classic economic and social history of modern Britain, *Industry and Empire*, is, for example, in its final chapters, a 'declinist' narrative, congruent with other accounts of poor British economic performance from the same era (Hobsbawm, 1968).

A sophisticated theory of capitalist state fiscal crisis from a Marxist perspective was developed by the American Marxist James O'Connor (O'Connor, 1973). Very similar analysis was provided by the German sociologist Claus Offe (Offe, 1984). This is a 'political economy' approach, since it treats society, economy, politics and the state together in an integrated way, as interrelated. This was an issue that had been ignored by Marx and most later Marxists, and has become a fruitful area for debate and criticism by both Marxists and non-Marxists (Gough, 1979; Judge, 1982: 32–35; Heald, 1983: Ch. 11; Klein, 1993; Bell, 1996: Ch. 5).

O'Connor's discussion represents a genuinely original contribution to a Marxist theory of the state. He held that the fiscal crisis of the state is a systemic and endogenous problem for capitalist states, reflecting basic 'contradictions' in the capitalist mode of production and its relationship to the capitalist state. It is therefore not something accidental, such as an external 'shock to the system', deriving from quadrupled oil prices after 1973, and resulting in macro-economic instability, which is how many mainstream analysts construed the welfare state crisis of the 1970s – it is an endemic problem for such states.

O'Connor's theory drew attention to what he called the 'legitimation' and 'reproduction' roles of the state, suggesting that these two aspects of the state's role are in fundamental conflict. Legitimation requires state spending on welfare to win support for the system on the part of workers. (This is, in other words, a 'social control' theory of welfare.) On the other hand, taxing capitalists and the rich destroys the motor of the system – accumulation – by undermining incentives to work, save and invest. In this sense, capitalism is seen to be self-defeating and is therefore bound to be crisis-prone. Traditional Marxist theory, of course, also saw capitalism as crisis-prone, but not quite in this way. Bearing in mind that O'Connor's analysis was published in 1973, so he was not providing an interpretation of what has subsequently come to be known as *the* 'welfare crisis' of the 1970s, because that was yet to break, his interpretation of the events of the mid-1970s, therefore, might be that 'stagflation' – the coexistence of economic stagnation, unemployment and inflation – something unamenable to analysis in terms of the dominant Keynesian paradigm – was a manifestation of inherent, systemic crisis, the only solution to which was some sort of transition, revolutionary or otherwise, to some kind of socialist regime.

Crisis as systemic contradiction II: Neo-liberal accounts

Neo-liberal diagnoses of the state of British capitalism and the welfare state became fashionable and influential during the course of the 1970s and 1980s. Neo-liberal analyses, often referred to as exemplifying a 'New Right' perspective, would seem to be at the opposite pole to a Marxist analysis, but in some respects they are rather similar (for discussion and elucidation of the terms 'neo-liberal' and 'New Right', see Chapter 10). There are different versions of what may be regarded as a neo-liberal critique.

Some neo-liberal analyses, by contrast with the Marxist approaches of O'Connor and Offe described above, generally employed the 'rational choice' models of behaviour and motivation which underpin mainstream economic theory, applying this to the state and public sector, the behaviour of bureaucrats, politicians and welfare professionals, and voting and electoral behaviour and choice. More or less formalised, this is known as 'public choice' theory (Judge, 1982: 36–39; Heald, 1983: Chs 1 and 2; Foster and Plowden, 1996).

The theory possesses a number of elements. It employs the concept of a political marketplace, in which politicians and parties compete to supply 'product' – policies – in return for the votes of electors. It has also developed a theory of state bureaucracy which views bureaucrats as 'rational maximisers' who have an interest in stimulating the growth of public budgets (over which they preside and from which they benefit).

In part the neo-liberal argument is a critique of liberal democratic representative government (Brittan, 1976). The theory is a theory of 'contradictions', rather like that of the Marxist argument of O'Connor. Brittan summarises the 'contradictions' of liberal representative democracy as follows: (1) the generation of 'excessive expectations', and (2) the disruptive effects of the pursuit of group self-interest in the marketplace (Brittan, 1976: 97). Brittan goes on to observe that 'an excessive burden is placed on the "sharing out" function of government'.

Neo-liberals would predict the existence of semi-permanent 'crisis' within organisations such as the NHS, operating both through the political 'marketplace' constituted by voters' choices and in terms of the organisation's own internal dynamics and incentive structures. In the first case voters are 'rational maximisers' who want more of what the NHS provides and will vote for it; on the other hand, there is a 'disconnect' between demanding the service and paying for it (unlike privately provided services). NHS services are mostly free at the point of use; users, who are also voters, have no incentive not to demand more, but are unwilling (so the argument goes) to pay for it through higher taxes.

In addition to this, the organisation's internal incentives operate to manufacture perceptions of crisis. The NHS workforce constitutes a lobby for higher spending, not only because of its perceptions of unmet patient need but because its own rewards and promotion prospects depend on it. As workers in a tax-financed public bureaucracy, decision makers and resource users face no cost or competitive constraints (unlike private sector health care providers). However, as a tax-financed public bureaucracy, financial resources for the NHS are subject to high-level political decision making by politicians faced with multiple and competing demands for public spending. The result is 'crisis', or at any rate a perception of one.

It cannot be said that this analysis is wholly unpersuasive. The first aspect is largely unpersuasive, because it does appear that taxpayers have a highly favourable view of NHS spending and are willing to fund more of it. The second has, perhaps, more plausibility.

These interpretations of 'crisis' are not purely economic; they may be regarded as 'political-economic' in character, in that crisis is seen as arising out of the relation between state, society and the economy.

The analysis of Bacon and Eltis

Another, perhaps even more influential, neo-liberal-type analysis of the British crisis of the 1970s was offered by two Oxford economists, Robert Bacon and Walter Eltis (Bacon and Eltis, 1996). This offered a more 'structural' explanation of Britain's economic difficulties than the neo-liberal explanations discussed above.

Bacon and Eltis drew attention to the way in which public sector employment 'crowded out' private or market sector employment. Growing public sector employment, in welfare-related or other activities, drove up public spending, helped by the 'relative price effect' (faster growth of relative costs in the public sector compared with the private sector, because productivity in the public sector, which is labour-intensive, grows more slowly than that in the private sector, whereas public sector wages increase at a similar rate). Higher public spending must be paid for through higher taxes on the private sector. Higher taxes are resisted by workers, who demand higher wages to compensate for their loss of earnings. This threatens company profitability, in turn threatening and bringing about reductions in company investment in new plant and machinery, leading ultimately to loss of competitiveness, company failures and redundancies. Government attempts to 'mop up' rising unemployment in line with orthodox Keynesian prescriptions by creating public sector jobs only have the effect af administering another twist to a vicious spiral of 'slowing growth, rising unemployment, accelerating inflation and deteriorating external balance' which, so the authors claimed, could only end in total economic breakdown (Bacon and Eltis, 1996: Ch. 4). The thesis does make a connection between welfare state growth and economic crisis, inasmuch as it is growth in welfare-related public employment that causes difficulties, via the effect of rising taxes to pay for this, creating profitability problems for private businesses.

The popularity of the Bacon–Eltis thesis was assisted by its prior publication as articles in the *Sunday Times* in 1975. The thesis perhaps 'caught a temporary anti-statist fashion', to quote Robert Skidelsky, although he went on to remark that the authors 'helped arrest the muddled British creep towards collectivism and create an intellectual climate favourable to Thatcherism' and initiate policies of 'market-promoting "structural adjustment"' which became later orthodoxy (Bacon and Eltis, 1996: xii, xiv). The authors themselves claimed some influence for their ideas on the policies of the Wilson and Callaghan Labour governments of the period (Bacon and Eltis, 1996: 117–119).

The Bacon–Eltis thesis would seem to have been refuted by subsequent events. The period of the Thatcher and Major governments, for example, did not witness any reduction in public spending, and the tax burden grew slightly in the 1980s. These governments tackled the underlying weaknesses of the British economy, indirectly through attempts to reduce inflation by monetary control, and directly by reducing the power of trade unions and introducing a range of policies to enhance productivity and competitiveness (see Chapter 16). Although it is true that private sector manufacturing employment fell continuously throughout this period, and unemployment grew, with some of the slack thus generated being taken up by service employment in the public sector, there was no direct transfer of employment from one to the other, since it was mostly men in the one sector who lost jobs and women in the other who gained them. Furthermore, it was not company profits and investment that suffered from the impact of higher taxes, but personal incomes and market sector consumption. There was no 'crowding-out' of private sector investment by tax-financed consumption (Bacon and Eltis, 1996: xi–xii).

Although the thesis was thus wrong in part, critics have suggested that some of the argument can be salvaged, in particular the claims about tax resistance on the part of workers. The Thatcher government dealt with workers' tax resistance by refusing to create sufficient new public sector jobs to mop up high levels of unemployment and was thus able to cap taxes to some extent, allowing workers to enjoy higher real levels of take-home pay. (The contrast with the present Labour government's policies is notable, as is the contrast with European countries during the 1980s.) The Labour governments of 1974–79 had promoted the concept of the 'social wage' – roughly, the cashed-out value of all social benefits, including health care and education, paid for by taxes – as something that could be sold to workers as an equivalent to foregone take-home pay, thereby buying agreement to the government's *de facto* incomes policy, the 'Social Contract', a policy which, of course, failed in the end. The Conservative approach, on the other hand, was premised on the idea that the 'social wage' is a myth, which workers would not be fooled into buying (Bacon and Eltis, 1996: xiii, xv, Ch. 4).

Discuss and Do	The social wage

The '*social wage*' is arguably a concept whose time has come round again. Labour governments of the 1970s thought that the 'social wage' concept could be used, at a time when disposable incomes were stagnant or falling, to buy workers' support for higher taxes (to pay for improved social services) and the government's anti-inflation incomes policy. The present Labour government, although not using the term, is effectively doing the same thing. Disposable (as opposed to gross) incomes – money in the pocket – for people on average and above-average incomes have hardly grown at all since the early 2000s, while the tax burden and spending on social services has risen. The present government's calculation is that people (i.e. voters) will buy this because they will make the connection between higher taxes and improved health, education and other social services and will not mind having less money in their pockets.

How plausible do you think this is?

'Crisis containment': an end to 'consensus'?

We turn now to consider some alternatives to the 'systemic' theories we have looked at above, which focus on the idea of 'crisis containment'. These views take it for granted that the crisis has in fact been overcome or resolved – there is no longer an overt crisis. The 'contradictions' have been overcome. One of these viewpoints makes use of the idea that there has been an 'end of consensus', or at any rate that the consensus has been reshaped. The crisis of the 1970s and 1980s has been associated with the end of the post-war welfare state consensus in the Anglophone countries.

The ruling political ideology – 'Keynesian social democracy' – which accompanied and underpinned the 'golden age' of the Keynesian welfare state has dissipated and been replaced by something else, usually construed as 'neo-liberalism', 'neo-conservatism' or the 'New Right'. This might take various forms, including 'Thatcherism' and what are sometimes regarded as derivatives of Thatcherism, such as the 'Third Way' or 'Blairism' (see Chapter 10).

'Thatcherism'

Analysts have drawn particular attention, in the British context, to 'Thatcherism' and the election of a supposedly consensus-busting, radical right government in 1979 (for fuller discussion of Thatcherite ideology, see Chapter 10). Thatcherism has been interpreted, for example, as representing the construction of a new, radical, right-wing hegemony based on the ideas of the 'free economy and the strong state' (Gamble, 1988). The 'full employment' consensus apparently vanished, as did the maintenance of harmonious relations with the trade union movement, and, with extensive privatisations, the commitment to the 'mixed economy'. It is, however, possible to exaggerate the impact of Thatcherism in relation to the welfare state.

First, the consensus started to break up before the advent of the Thatcher governments. Consensus 'break-up' can be dated to the period of Labour governments in the 1970s, especially after 1976. A further, related, point, looking at this issue in an international context, is that even left-wing governments, such as that of France, started pursuing 'right-wing' policies in the 1980s; New Zealand after 1984 was a particularly notable example.

Second, the story on welfare is more complicated than a simple 'end of consensus' account suggests. The first two Thatcher governments from 1979 to 1987 arguably had little or no policy for the welfare state. Large-scale privatisation, of either funding or provision, was effectively ruled out early on. What the Thatcher governments had was a policy for public spending, namely, to control it rigorously and limit increases as far as possible, which obviously had implications for welfare. This was not entirely successful, and public spending on welfare actually increased during the 1980s as a share of GDP, due, of course, in part, to much higher levels of unemployment and slower economic growth (Taylor-Gooby, 1985: 72, Table 9).

Thatcherism and welfare state 'restructuring'

After 1987 the agenda changed, and the Conservative government engaged in a programme of what looked like wholesale 'restructuring' of the major social services, attempting to decentralise, make services more 'responsive', increase efficiency, and introduce elements of competition and choice via the creation of 'quasi-markets' or 'internal markets', but within a public ownership and public funding model. This was not a classic neo-liberal strategy for the public sector, since it eschewed complete privatisation (Pierson, 1998: 157). Neo-liberals had always argued for genuine privatisation, of either funding or provision or both. The Conservative strategy was really more about management and managerialism than about markets; it was an attempt to develop and promote efficient management of public sector welfare institutions (Foster and Plowden, 1996). This was certainly a change in a consensus about how state welfare institutions should be managed and welfare delivered. It is, of course, a consensus that is still with us, since it has been broadly accepted by Labour governments since 1997.

Left critiques of the welfare state: a new consensus?

In the light of a supposed Thatcherite/neo-liberal dominated 'end of consensus' we have just considered, it should be borne in mind that the welfare state has been criticised from the left as well as the right. There has been long-standing criticism from both left and right of welfare state effectiveness, efficiency and lack of responsiveness. The view that welfare state provision is now poorly matched to a changing pattern of needs is widely accepted, providing justification for various 'restructuring' or 'new public management' reforms, such as those of the Thatcher governments just described. This could be interpreted in terms of some conception of 'crisis', in a narrower sense of delivery or organisation or values, rather than the wider sense of 'systemic' crisis.

From the left, for example, the Danish sociologist Gøsta Esping-Andersen has argued that there is a 'growing discrepancy between existing programme design and social demands' and that the contemporary welfare state 'addresses a past social order' (Esping-Andersen, 1996: 8–9). Esping-Andersen was particularly concerned in this critique with changing patterns of work, the changing position of women and changing family forms. This theme is continued in a later publication significantly entitled *Why We Need a New Welfare State* (Esping-Andersen, 2002). In this it is noted that 'The continuing viability of the existing welfare state edifice is being questioned across all of Europe' and that 'The status quo will be difficult to sustain given adverse demographic or financial conditions . . . the same status quo appears increasingly out of date' (Esping-Andersen, 2002). Another kind of left critique, couched in similar terms, comes from the proponents of 'basic income' or 'citizen's income' schemes (Van Parijs, 1992, 1995), who have argued for something to replace the 'second marriage of justice and efficiency' that the post-war welfare state represented.

Welfare state legitimacy and popular support

A 'welfare crisis' may be interpreted in terms of the idea of *legitimacy*, by which is meant public support or popularity. Welfare crisis may be construed as loss of legitimacy in relation to the welfare state or welfare services among the citizenry. This may be the result of various social and cultural changes which result in growing and changing public expectations about cost, volume, responsiveness and quality. The welfare state might be viewed as inflexible, unresponsive, monolithic, bureaucratic, no longer meeting a changing set of needs on the part of a population, who may, for example, have become much more diverse culturally, or in terms of family forms, or who simply expect and demand more choice or higher quality.

On the other hand, loss of legitimacy may take the form of tax 'backlash' – a belief on the part of people that they are over-taxed in relation to what they receive. Symptoms of such backlash may take the form of tax evasion and avoidance and the growth of the 'black' economy, or they might take the form of 'voice', exercised by voters choosing to vote for lower-tax parties in elections. Evidence of tax backlash in the UK is limited, but a belief in the possibility of such backlash, and of a predilection for lower taxes on the part of the electorate, is entrenched among politicians and political parties. New Labour's current muffled politics of 'tax and spend' – essentially pursuing tax and spend policies while pretending not to – have been strongly influenced by the experience of the 1992 election, in which the Labour party was defeated on an allegedly high-tax programme.

More recently the experience of the fuel protests of autumn 2000 has reminded parties and governments of what appears to be tax-resistance on the part of the population, as has the recent spectacle of a pensioner being jailed for refusing to pay greatly increased council tax bills. The marked reluctance of the government to deal with the long-standing issue of local taxation – it has recently postponed consideration of the issue, because reform is widely expected to result in increased council tax bills – is another reminder of élite sensitivities (see Chapters 5 and 8). In terms of the distinctions introduced above, a 'legitimacy crisis' might be viewed as a 'crisis of state welfare'.

Researchers have sought to answer questions about welfare state legitimacy via the medium of public opinion surveys, and such surveys of opinion in relation to welfare have now become a minor industry.

In fact evidence for tax backlash in the UK at this time is remarkably meagre. There were more overt tax backlashes in other countries at the time – in the USA, in California, with the celebrated tax-reducing Proposition 13 in the State elections in 1976, and in elections in Denmark. Although British workers may have been sceptical about the idea of the 'social wage' (see above), there is little evidence that Labour's defeat in the 1979 General Election had anything to do with popular perceptions of excessive tax burdens. Britain's tax and spending burden then as now was in any case considerably lower than that of most Continental European and Scandinavian welfare states.

Although there has been, since the 1970s, a pervasive belief in the existence of tax resistance among the public on the part of politicians and parties, it is not the case that the public have an unselective hostility to public spending. The public are quite discriminating and have consistently favoured higher spending on particular programmes and services, such as education, health and pensions, according to opinion survey evidence (Taylor-Gooby, 1991: Ch. 5, 111–119). These are services from which a majority of the population will expect to benefit, unlike 'minority' services such as council housing, unemployment benefit and means-tested assistance for the unemployed and single mothers. In fact, public support for the welfare state strengthened among all social groups during the course of the 1980s.

Pierson concluded his review of public opinion on state welfare by remarking that 'Overall, the pattern of popular attitudes to state welfare is complex but stable ... There is little evidence of large-scale popular backlash against the welfare state' (Pierson, 1998: 160–161).

An assessment: critiques of crisis

We now turn to some of the sceptics who have questioned the whole idea of the unaffordability and unsustainability of the welfare state. If the 1970s and 1980s were the decades of radical questioning of the welfare state, the 1990s and subsequently have been the period in which its intellectual and political defenders have fought back, generally successfully. That is why 'crisis' debates have a somewhat musty historical flavour to them. Whatever current problems of the welfare state there may be, talk of a systemic general welfare state crisis is now rare, although the label continues to be attached to particular issues, such as the pensions 'crisis' (see Chapter 17).

Left and right, as well as professional and occupational interest groups, made use of the rhetoric of crisis for their own purposes. Marxist and neo-liberal analyses of systemic fiscal crisis were, needless to say, rejected by those of a mainstream social democratic political and ideological persuasion, who dismissed the idea of a general crisis arising out of the particular economic and political dynamics of liberal representative democratic capitalism (Davies and Piachaud, 1985; Klein, 1993; Bell, 1996). These critics consistently denied its applicability to the situation of the UK, arguing that the welfare state is not 'unaffordable', and that there is no inherent conflict or trade-off between economic performance and extensive state welfare provision (Davies and Piachaud, 1985; Deakin, 1987: 3). The growth of welfare spending is not necessarily a problem, nor should it, by itself, be associated with fiscal crisis. If the rest of society is happy to support a growing welfare sector through increased taxes, well and good. If, however, there is a 'tax backlash', or tax resistance on the part of the citizenry, then there may be a problem.

The thesis that there was a systemic fiscal crisis appeared to be swiftly refuted by experience after 1979, in the UK and USA, by the election of governments committed to tax reductions and expenditure restraint, even though these goals were only imperfectly and partially realised. The success of the Conservatives in the UK, winning four general elections under Margaret Thatcher and then John Major, suggests that there are no inherent flaws or 'contradictions' in liberal democracy, nor that the 'legitimacy' and 'reproductive' functions of the modern state cannot be reconciled. From this perspective, such claims about welfare as those made by Conservative governments of the 1980s come into the category of 'crisis as moral panic'.

Some Marxist writers also dismissed the idea that the welfare state was threatened in the sense of being seriously cut or dismantled, arguing that the welfare state was now (i.e. by the 1980s) 'irreversible', because of its universalism and the fact that the middle classes were effectively incorporated as a major interest favouring welfare state maintenance, if not expansion (Therborn and Roebroek, 1986).

A careful summary of evidence, international as well as British, on various aspects of welfare state 'affordability' and achievement was provided by John Hills, who concluded by giving a negative answer to the question 'Is the welfare state in crisis?' (Hills, 1997). The level of welfare spending in the UK, as about a quarter of GDP, had been roughly stable from the 1970s to the 1990s and was below the level of most European countries. There was no 'demographic time bomb'; the upward pressures exerted by an ageing population feeding demands for increased pension provision and health care spending on the elderly were easily containable, resulting by the 2040s in no more than the addition of another 5% of GDP. This is the case for the UK, although some other countries face greater difficulties in these respects (Hills, 1997: Ch. 1).

The other main question reviewed in Hills's report, that of how successfully the welfare state, British and other, 'works' in achieving its objectives, is also given a largely positive, although not uncritical, answer. The welfare state does redistribute from rich to poor, from men to women and over people's lifecycles; the tax and benefit systems together operate to reduce the overall degree of inequality in society. The welfare state has had to work harder in the 1980s and 1990s in these respects because the overall degree of socio-economic inequality has increased in all advanced capitalist countries in this period, due to greater inequality in earnings (Hills, 1997: Ch. 2).

The 'crisis of affordability' or 'fiscal crisis' of the welfare state in general may therefore be dismissed as basically unsound. Levels of public spending and taxation were not, and are not, incompatible with the survival of the capitalist system, whether this is considered from a neo-liberal or a Marxist standpoint. It was observed in 1985 that 'since the roots of the current critique of the welfare state are ideological, the way in which the system operates and its measurable economic and social effects are largely irrelevant to the critics' (Johnson, 1985b: 37–38, cited in Deakin, 1987: 3).

This is a reference to the then Conservative government's critique of welfare. The sense in which it was 'ideological' is that this critique reflected political choices, not inexorable economic constraints. Two observers concluded at the time that 'the case for zero growth in public expenditure is not based on economic constraints but rather on a political desire to give absolute priority to tax cuts' (Davies and Piachaud, 1985: 110). In fact, the definitive answer to the 'affordability' thesis has been provided by the tax and spend policies of the present 'New' Labour government, first elected in 1997, which has pursued an expansionist policy in both these areas since 1999, in the context of steadily rising national income.

The context of the UK debate: British national 'decline'

We may observe that, in practice, much of the British debate about 'the crisis' refers to a specific historical situation – that of the 1970s and 1980s, when the British economy and welfare state faced particular difficulties. An interesting point about discussions of crisis in this period, in the UK, is the way they connected with a long-standing theme of commentary on post-war British politics and society – the theme of national 'decline', one of the most potent narratives in twentieth-century political and economic commentary (Smith, 1989: 11; English and Kenny, 2000). The 'crisis' of the 1970s and 1980s was, in this light, simply the most recent instalment of a long-running saga. Since 1992, of course, the economic picture has changed substantially and the British economy seems to have been set on a qualitatively new and vigorous growth path, unemployment has fallen steadily and inflation appears to have been conquered.

The future of the welfare state: globalisation challenges

Finally, and very briefly, consideration of the current state of welfare naturally invites consideration of the future. The 'crisis' of welfare provides an invitation to look forward as well as back. To begin with, the terms of the debate about the future of state welfare have changed in the past decade. Discussions of challenges to the welfare state are now much more likely to refer to the phenomenon of *globalisation* and its impacts (Mishra, 1999; Yeates, 2001). A debate has raged since the mid-1990s about whether the effects of globalisation are positive, negative or neutral for welfare states. Globalisation and its effects will not be discussed here, since it is a subject for Chapter 22.

Discuss and Do   Crisis, what crisis?

To what extent do you think the rhetoric or discourse of a crisis in the welfare state is:

- an episode in the development of the British welfare state arrangements?
- a recognition of the limits of a nation state's activity in welfare support when faced with opposing pressures, for example of globalisation and individualism?

Conclusion

In this chapter we have sought to explore various dimensions of 'crisis' in relation to welfare. In part, we have been exploring some aspects of welfare state development and welfare expenditure growth in the latter half of the twentieth century; in part we have been examining some of the problems of paying for welfare; and in part we have been considering some of the issues and problems confronting any mature welfare system. We have sought to analyse the many meanings of the term 'crisis', suggesting that its use may be rhetorical and persuasive as much as analytical, serving the varied political agendas of left and right.

In this chapter, we have

- examined the concept of crisis;
- explored post-war trends in the development of welfare states;
- assessed some theories and arguments – Marxist, neo-liberal and other – about the nature of crisis;
- located these issues and debates in the context of other chapters on public spending, governance, comparative analysis and globalisation.

Annotated further reading

The debate about welfare state 'crisis' is partly historical. A reading of welfare state history is a good way of putting much of the UK 'crisis' debate into context. There are excellent histories of the post-war UK welfare state by Rodney Lowe and Howard Glennerster (Glennerster, 1995; Lowe, 2005) and of earlier UK twentieth century social policy by Derek Fraser, Pat Thane and Bentley Gilbert (Gilbert, 1970; Thane, 1996; Fraser, 2003).

The best general book on the sociology and politics of the welfare state, with a chapter which puts 'crisis' in broad comparative historical and sociological context, is Chris Pierson's *Beyond the Welfare State?* (Pierson, 1998: Ch. 5). Older texts which are still useful, and give a flavour of the kind of debates that were taking place in the early 1980s, include Taylor-Gooby's *Public Opinion, Ideology and State Welfare* (Taylor-Gooby, 1985) and Mishra's *The Welfare State in Crisis* (Mishra, 1984). Mishra's follow-up book, *The Welfare State in Capitalist Society*, is also useful (Mishra, 1990).

Two classics of the 'crisis' genre, representing varieties of Marxist left, are James O'Connor's *The Fiscal Crisis of the State* (O'Connor, 1973) and Claus Offe's *Contradictions of the Welfare State* (Offe, 1984). Offe's prose style is somewhat forbidding. An accessible text in this tradition, which interprets crisis in terms of welfare state 'restructuring', is Gough's *The Political Economy of Welfare* (Gough, 1979). Brief treatments of O'Connor's theory are provided by Gough and by Judge (Judge, 1982: 32–35) and Heald (Heald, 1983: Ch. 11). Their theories are accessibly presented and discussed by Pierson (Pierson, 1998: Chs 2 and 5). An amusing and trenchant critique of this literature is Rudolf Klein's 1993 article 'O'Goffe's tale', reprinted in his *Only Dissect* (Klein, 1993, 1996c).

A classic statement of the neo-liberal welfare state 'unsustainability' thesis is the article 'The economic contradictions of democracy' by the economic journalist and *Financial Times* correspondent Samuel Brittan (Brittan, 1975, 1976). The edited book in which a version of Brittan's article appeared contains a number of useful articles, from left and right, on the British crisis of the 1970s (King, 1976). Another influential economic journalist, the *Times* correspondent Peter Jay, presented a version of the Brittan argument in an IEA pamphlet, *Employment, Inflation and Politics* (Jay, 1976); Jay was the son-in-law of James Callaghan, the Labour Prime Minister from 1976 to 1979. The most celebrated statement of the idea that there is a fundamental conflict between economic performance and the growth of the public sector is the book by two Oxford economists, Robert Bacon and Walter Eltis, *Britain's Economic Problem: Too few producers* (2nd edition, 1978), reissued in a revised third edition in 1996 as *Britain's Economic Problem Revisited* with a useful critical foreword by Robert Skidelsky (Bacon and Eltis, 1996). A more recent sceptical view of the welfare state from a neo-liberal perspective is Skidelsky's *Beyond the Welfare State* (Skidelsky, 1997). For brief accounts of 'public choice' theory, see the books by Judge and Heald cited above (Judge, 1982: 36–39; Heald, 1983: Chs 1 and 2) and also *The State Under Stress* by Foster and Plowden (Foster and Plowden, 1996). Neo-liberal/'New Right' theories are examined by Pierson (Pierson, 1998: Chs. 2 and 5).

Excellent critiques of the idea of welfare state crisis have been offered by Paul Pierson and Francis Castles among others (Pierson, 1994; Castles, 2004). In fact Castles' book is probably the best single treatment, at an advanced level, of the whole crisis phenomenon. Further correctives to doom-laden scenarios have been provided, for the UK, by the LSE researchers in the past two decades. Particularly valuable are *The State of Welfare* (2nd edition) edited by Howard Glennerster and others (Glennerster and Hills, 1998) and the brief compilation of data and analysis, *The Future of Welfare* (2nd edition), by John Hills (Hills, 1997). The latter makes superb use of visual means of presenting quantitative data – in fact it is a model in this respect.

Welfare state futurology is interestingly and valuably discussed in books by Francis Castles, Gøsta Esping-Andersen and Nick Ellison (Esping-Andersen, 2002; Castles, 2004; Ellison, 2006). The final chapter of Chris Pierson's text is also useful (Pierson, 1998: Ch. 6). The future of welfare is also in part the theme of reports such as that of the Labour Party's Commission on Social Justice (Commission on Social Justice, 1994), as it is of discussions of 'Third Way' politics by sociologists such as Anthony Giddens (Giddens, 1998, 2000) and of texts on globalisation by Giddens and other writers such as Nicola Yeates (Giddens, 1999; Yeates, 2001). The final section of Chris Pierson's and Francis Castles' *The Welfare State Reader* contains useful articles on the future of welfare (Pierson and Castles, 2000).

Chapter 5

Making policy

Objectives

- To outline the political and policy environment within which social policy is developed and implemented.

- To explore the roles of central and local government in the development of social policy.

- To outline recent changes in the social policy making environment.

Introduction

This chapter explores the context within which social policy is created and implemented. This includes an explanation of the roles of central and local government as well as outlining recent changes in the policy making environment.

As can be seen from Box 5.1, on the fuel protests in 2000, government-based policy making can lead to 'unintended consequences' such as protest and political backlash which can ultimately lead to governments having to make significant policy changes. This chapter looks at the context within which social policy is made and implemented.

The political and policy environment

At its most basic level the policy process has been described as a 'black box' into which are entered 'inputs' and from which emerge 'outcomes'. Thus a typical input would be represented by the policies of an elected government and outcomes would be those policies as received by a population. Diagrammatically this might appear as depicted by David Easton (Easton, 1965; see Ham and Hill, 1993) some 40 years ago and shown in Figure 5.1 on page 68. This is the policy process at both its most simple and its most uninformative. Such a description merely tells us that there are demands made upon governments who respond with policies and tells us nothing of what is going on inside the 'black box'. In such a model the policy process is assumed to be a neutral and impartial arbiter of policies devised by a government, whatever the political shade of the party in

Box 5.1	The fuel protests of autumn 2000

No fuel tax concession, says Brown

Chancellor rejects early move on prices as pickets lift blockades

Patrick Wintour and Michael White, *The Guardian*, Friday 15 September 2000

As petrol stations across Britain struggled to get back to normal today, chancellor Gordon Brown dug in his heels against any early tax concessions on fuel prices before next March, despite a 60-day deadline for action imposed by pickets when they lifted their crippling blockades.

With Tony Blair's full support, Mr Brown let it be known that he will not be deflected by what ministers insist are 'illegal blockades and intimidation' in reaching his budget judgment as usual in March. Downing Street believes its firm stance will win round public opinion as tempers cool. A senior No. 10 official said: 'These people have got to take on board the facts of the budget process. You cannot make budget decisions as a response to protests. There is a budget process and a parallel democratic process. They can make representations if they wish.'

However, the government's strategy is high risk given the scale of action and strength of feeling shown this week. Protesters – who include farmers, hauliers and fishermen, already aggrieved at what they see as unfair treatment by the government – have threatened to reimpose blockades of oil refineries and depots if there is no move to cut fuel taxes.

Pensioners and motorists gain from mini-Budget

The Guardian, Wednesday 8 November 2000

The Chancellor Gordon Brown delivered his 'mini-Budget' today which, as anticipated, gave extra cash to pensioners and motorists .... Mr Brown announced a freeze in fuel duty and a cut of 3p per litre in 'green' (ULSP) petrol ... and diesel .... Mr Brown told MPs in his pre-budget statement in the Commons: 'I recognise and I understand the very genuine concerns of motorists and hauliers.' The chancellor said 1.5p per litre would normally have been added to petrol and diesel from Budget day next year, raising £560m – which he would now forgo by cancelling the planned increase.... Mr Brown stressed this was part of the government meeting its environmental obligations, as well as addressing motorists' concerns. He said he now expected ULSP to make up 100% of the market next year, and after announcing other changes to excise duties said his total package of help to motorists was equivalent to 4p a litre off fuel duty and for hauliers was worth 8p per litre off diesel.

The chancellor's gamble was that his announcements would be enough to head off another fuel blockade like the one in September which crippled fuel supplies. He said that overall his changes on fuel and excise duty for cars and lorries would cost £1bn.

Reprinted with permission.

power. Such a model therefore tells us little or nothing of the values and ideas which help to shape and form policies and the direction they take once implemented (see Ham and Hill, 1993).

Within the parameters of the British state, the central state may be considered to be crucial, since it is within the centrally based 'corridors of power' that many decisions are made. Constitutionally, Britain operates a tripartite division of powers

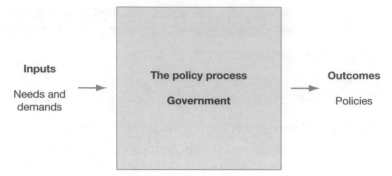

Figure 5.1 The 'black box' approach to policy making
Source: Based on data from D. Easton (1965) *A Framework for Political Analysis*, Englewood Cliffs, NJ: Prentice-Hall; and C. Ham (1992) *Health Policy in Britain* (3rd edn), London: Macmillan.

Discuss and Do   Critiquing Easton's model

What strengths or weaknesses can you identify in this model of making policy?

Weaknesses might include:

- over-simplification and too mechanistic

- no differentiation between outputs and outcomes

- no recognition of self-generating demands

- a naivety in thinking that the policy making process is equally open to all groups and individuals

- no recognition of the different levels of policy making (national, local, supra-national)

- no recognition of discretion of policy implementers (street-level bureaucrats) at the implementation stage and level.

Strengths might include:

- a straightforward depiction of the process for making policy

- a model that depicts a dynamic world

- a model that depicts a system open to a plurality of influences.

(see Figure 5.2) between the legislature (Parliament), the judiciary (judges, courts and tribunals) and the executive (the Civil Service and departments wherein they work). This remains something of a constitutional fiction, however, since there is a great deal of interplay between the three arms of the constitution. Crucial to this interplay is the role of the Prime Minister and the Cabinet which has developed over the past two centuries and is today pivotal in the making of policy. On re-election to government in 1997, Labour under Tony Blair's prime ministership signalled the importance of the Cabinet, for example by establishing within it the Social Exclusion Unit and with it the central planks of that government's programme.

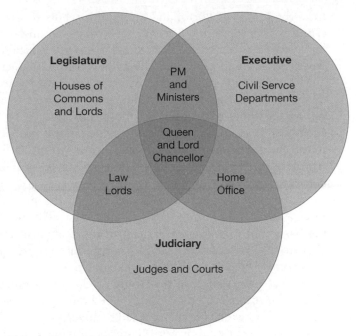

Figure 5.2 The making of policy
Source: Adapted from B. Jones *et al*. (2006) *Politics UK* (6th edn), Harlow: Longman. Reprinted with permission.

Indeed, the Prime Minister's Office specifically is regarded as having increased its powers during the period of the New Labour government.

This type of representation between the three realms of Parliament, the judiciary and the Civil Service illustrates the different constitutional functions of the various arms of the separation of powers.

Parliament

Thus the job of the legislature is to debate and consider the introduction of new laws, to consider the effective operation of existing policy and to oversee the efficient running of government departments. Members of Parliament exercise this power through the system of parliamentary committees (both Standing and Select Committees) where they are able to question ministers and senior civil servants. MPs are also able to inter-rogate ministers, including the Prime Minister, via the system of MPs' questions and a weekly 30-minute Question Time with the Prime Minister. Private individuals may also be summoned to give evidence to Select Committees, notably in recent years at the hearings to consider the Mirror Group pensions case, the selling of arms to Iraq and the collapse of the Matrix Churchill company (which led to the Scott Enquiry), and more recently the directors of the Northern Rock bank following the bank's 'financial crisis' due to difficulties in raising funds in the money markets.

New legislation passes through the apparently laborious process of First, Second and Third Readings in the House of Commons interspersed with detailed discussion of a Bill's content at the committee stage. A Bill will then also receive consideration from the House of Lords, and during this whole process MPs and lords from government and opposition have the opportunity to question and debate the principles and provisions of new legislation and to suggest amendments. Finally a Bill receives Royal Assent and passes into law as an Act of Parliament.

Most legislation today is that which is brought forward as part of the programme of the governing party in the Commons, and there is usually little time to debate opposition-sponsored Bills or those introduced by individual MPs (Private Members' Bills, the most famous of which is still probably the 1967 Abortion Act) unless the government agrees to make room within Parliament's schedule. In recent decades, as the business of government has become more time consuming and detailed, governments have resorted more to the introduction of Statutory Instruments (SIs) which amend and change the provisions of legislation but are rarely fully debated on the floor of the House. This technique has been pursued on the basis that it will make Parliament more efficient but has also brought with it charges that governments use SIs to introduce controversial new laws without the opportunity for proper debate and scrutiny.

Because most debate in the House of Commons concerns government business, and this is a tendency that mushroomed during the last century, increased significance and power has been accorded to government ministers, and most notably to those ministers (Secretaries of State) occupying seats within the Cabinet, and, of course, most importantly to the Prime Minister. This has led to charges that Britain is becoming a nation of executive government and is therefore losing its democratic legitimacy. (Lord Hailsham coined the term 'elective dictatorship' in the 1970s as a means of describing the undemocratic nature of Parliament.) Ministers, as MPs, participate in the legislative process outlined above, but occupy a special position as senior, and often longserving and experienced members. But Secretaries of State also occupy an executive role as titular heads of a government department and are so charged to fight for the interests of their own department within both Cabinet and Parliament. This creates a potential conflict of interest as one agenda for action within the executive comes into conflict with the policy agenda of government.

The Executive – the Civil Service and central government departments

We turn next to examining where policy is made and describe the structure and functions of central government departments, such as the Department of Health or the Department for Children, Schools and Families (previously the Department for Education and Skills). This is followed by a description of the structure of government at a local level. Such an approach provides us with a picture or plan of government and from this we might be able to discern which individuals, government ministers, civil servants or local government officials are responsible for making policy at different levels of government.

Here we face additional questions regarding the policy process. Figure 5.3 shows a simplified structure of the National Health Service in England, from which one can see that much of the delivery of health policy is conducted at a local level,

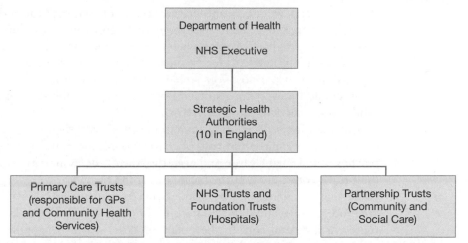

Figure 5.3 Simplified depiction of the structure of the National Health Service in England

whether by Primary Care Trusts, NHS Hospital Trusts, Foundation Hospitals, individual GPs, dentists, nurses and other health professionals, or by other agencies (such as private sector Intermediate Treatment Centres). For example, some health policy remains a function of local government (e.g. aspects of public or environmental health) or of the ex-public utilities in the supply of clean water and treatment or disposal of sewage and waste. It also remains, as governments have often shown, a relatively easy task to alter and reform the structures and institutional arrangements of government without, apparently, affecting the policy-making process, at least as perceived by service users who may care little for how policy is made. Such a diagrammatic representation also tells us little of how the non-government sector,

Discuss and Do   How democratic is Parliament?

Do you think the system of UK government, as established and played out in Parliament, is an open and democratic one?

In considering this, you may wish to consider examples of policy making and policy changes which have occurred because of or despite public opinion, for example:

- the imposition and then scrapping of the 'Poll Tax' (see Chapter 8)

- the Iraq war

- the fuel blockades of 2000

- the imposition of university tuition fees in 1998 and top-up fees in 2006 (see Chapter 15)

- the changes to Inheritance Tax thresholds in 2007 (see Chapter 8).

Are we all able to influence Parliament and Government equally or are certain individuals or pressure groups more powerful and influential?

the commercial, voluntary and private sectors of welfare, fit into the policy process. We might therefore be led to believe, by such representations, that social policy only involves the activities of government or a particular department of government. Indeed, as Tony Butcher clearly illustrates, many of the assumptions behind the establishment of the post-war welfare state evolved from the notion that government should do everything in terms of welfare provision, that is both provide and fund welfare services (Butcher, 1995).

A further, more detailed, examination of the executive role of government might then go on to explore the role of the Prime Minister and the Cabinet, the upper reaches of the Civil Service and even the role of the monarchy. Any examination of the British constitution at the beginning of the twenty-first century must surely conclude that the joint roles of Prime Minister and their Cabinet are pivotal in the creation, passage and implementation of policy. The PM and Cabinet (see Box 5.2) represent a central core in the policy process, which is supported by an array of Cabinet committees and a small army of (theoretically) 'neutral' civil servants and politically appointed advisors, the most celebrated of whom in recent times have been Mrs Thatcher's economics advisor Sir Alan Walters and her press officer Sir Bernard Ingham and, more recently, Tony Blair's press officer Alastair Campbell. Or, more formally, we might point to the role of the Bank of England Monetary Policy Committee (MPC), a non-elected committee of 'wise persons' appointed to advise the Treasury over the conduct of economic policy and, specifically, to decide on the national interest rate. The MPC does not represent a formal, constitutional part of the government machine but is nonetheless of vital importance in the creation of policy.

The civil servants of the Cabinet Office and political advisors exist to support the roles performed by Cabinet ministers. Even a cursory reading of the diaries of any of our recent political luminaries will illustrate the volume of work they faced as individuals whilst in office – a volume of work impossible to maintain without the aid of advisors who work on policy papers, prepare departmental briefings or press releases (see, for example, the various diaries of Richard Crossman (Crossman, 1979), Barbara Castle, Tony Benn, Margaret Thatcher, Nigel Lawson, Bernard Ingham, John Major, Clare Short, Robin Cooke and David Blunkett). Constitutionally, at least (see Bagehout, 2001; Hennessy, 1988, 1996), Britain employs a doctrine of ministerial responsibility by which a minister is held to be responsible for all the actions of their department and its civil servants, and although little can be done to enforce such a doctrine, which we may suggest in any case is outdated and in need of replacement, much of a minister's time in the House of Commons is spent answering questions about the activities of their department. In practice a minister will seldom resign over what might be considered the minor misdemeanour of a junior civil servant and over the last 10 to 20 years there has been the tendency to devolve departmental functions to agencies whereby some organisation other than a central government department delivers a service but is responsible to its manager rather than a minister (for example, the Benefits Agency, the Child Support Agency and the Environment Agency). We might argue that the creation, for example, of the Benefits Agency to deliver income maintenance benefits under the control of a chief officer or senior manager, more along the pattern adopted by a privately constituted company, damages the process of democratic responsibility to the House of Commons.

Box 5.2	The government in Cabinet

Prime Minister	Gordon Brown
Chancellor of the Exchequer	Alistair Darling
Secretary of State for Justice	Jack Straw
Home Secretary	Jacqui Smith
Foreign Secretary	David Miliband
Secretary of State for Business, Enterprise and Regulatory Reform	John Hutton
Secretary of State for Children, Schools and Families	Ed Balls
Secretary of State for Communities and Local Government	Hazel Blears
Secretary of State for Culture, Media and Sport	James Purnell
Secretary of State for Defence	Des Browne
Secretary of State for Environment, Food and Rural Affairs	Hilary Benn
Secretary of State for Transport	Ruth Kelly
Secretary of State for Work and Pensions	James Purnell
Minister for Housing	Yvette Cooper
Minister for Children, Young People and Families	Beverley Hughes

These are the main offices of state. Other members of a government's Cabinet would include Ministers for Scotland, Wales and Northern Ireland, and other junior ministerial positions which may at times be included in the Cabinet, or even non-government posts such as chairperson of a political party.

The judiciary

The final arm of the tripartite division of state power is collectively referred to as the judiciary. It comprises the system of courts and the role of the judges in interpreting policy and arbitrating in disputes over the principles or implementation of an Act of Parliament. The judges, of course, also play a role in the creation of policy, since they sit in the House of Lords as Law Lords. So too we can count here the vast array of semi judicial tribunals, which sit within the executive arm of government, such as Industrial Tribunals or Social Security Appeal Tribunals. Judgments made in courts, and those of higher level tribunals, such as the Social Security Commissioners, are said to set legal precedent and to bind lower courts and tribunals. In this sense the judiciary may also be said to make policy and not simply to interpret legislation, since their decisions may change the way in which policy is delivered by departments and may even operate counter to the intentions of the original legislation. Since 1973 an additional court has appeared in the hierarchy of the judiciary, the Court of the European Union, which is able to make decisions over the interpretation of EU legislation or the breaching of such legislation by member governments. Such decisions, in their turn, are binding on governments and the legal systems of the European Union.

The very brief sketch presented above gives us only a snapshot of the constitutional arrangements of government at the centre. However, how much does this really tell us about the making of policy in Britain today? For example, following the implementation of the Next Steps Report (*Improving Public Management in Government: The Next Steps*) the then Department of Social Security (more recently entitled the Department of Work and Pensions) had a core staff of a mere 2,000 based in Whitehall (Ling, 1994). The bulk of department staff are now employed by agencies (the Benefits, Contributions and Child Support Agencies are the largest) and not directly by the DWP, and these staff are employed in local offices where policy can be said to be 'delivered'. An important part of the making of policy, therefore, is the process of implementation locally. Ministers and senior civil servants often have little control over how staff choose to deliver a policy on the ground. These 'street level bureaucrats' (Lipsky, 1980) may be able to exercise a good deal of discretion over how a policy is implemented. A similar pattern may be discerned in all government departments with the majority of staff employed at a local level, whether in Strategic Health Authorities, Primary Care Trusts, NHS Hospital Trusts and Foundation Hospitals in the health service, or by local authorities or schools, colleges and universities in the education service. It is for this reason that we now turn to the local dimension of policy making.

Discuss and Do　　**Policy making and implementation at the periphery – street-level bureaucrats**

Can you think of examples of policy making or implementation where social welfare professionals and other staff are able to use their own discretion in the implementation of a particular policy?

Examples you may think of might include:

* how a head teacher in a school chooses to implement 'SATs' tests or the national literacy or numeracy strategies

* how a member of staff working for the Benefits Agency chooses to allocate (or not) benefits entitlements

* how a police officer chooses to deal with a motorist driving at 78 mph on a motorway where the speed limit is 70 mph.

Policy making at the periphery

The most obvious place to begin looking at the local dimension of policy, particularly social policy making, is to examine the role of the local authority or council (Daly and Davis, 2008). Local authorities are charged with responsibility, either mandatory or discretionary, for implementing a range of centrally determined policies. Specifically they may be responsible for overseeing and directing (though less and less actually delivering) education, adults' and children's social care and housing in the field of social policy, and for a range of other services, such as environmental and leisure services, as well as for making contributions in the delivery of local health, police and transport policies. Often, however, local authorities have little or no independent function in determining policy and may be limited to enacting the provisions of an Act of Parliament. Increasingly commonly, local authorities exercise a strategic role in the planning of services for their particular areas; services which are then provided by other agencies, such as schools or bus companies; or they may hold a supervisory role in overseeing the working of policy implemented through private or voluntary agencies, such as has happened in the delivery of community care policy.

In organisational terms many local authorities traditionally mirror the structures found in Whitehall, whereby specific service departments have an elected councillor playing the role of 'minister' and serving with other key councillors on the local authority's 'cabinet'. Alongside this, scrutiny committees (similar to Select Committees at a national level in Parliament), comprising councillors and serviced by local government officials (the 'civil service' of local authorities), examine the possible impact of new policy measures and the effectiveness of on-going delivery. However, there exists far greater variation in local policy making. First, there are different tiers of local authority with different functions (see Figure 5.4 overleaf). Second, there is far greater variation in the political make up of local authorities in that the Labour and Conservative parties do not dominate totally, with Liberal Democrats often ruling local councils and significant numbers of 'independent' councillors serving as individuals rather than following a party line. Many councils are recorded as 'hung' with no party having overall control, and although these factors may possibly be witnessed in Parliament they are far more common at a local level. Third, local authority political structures are now typically either a cabinet-style structure with a political leader (as described above) or with an elected mayor running things. Yet variation in policy has been far less common across authorities in recent years as central government, which after all controls the vast majority of purse-strings of local government finance, has sought to exercise its authority and to ensure that nationally standards in the delivery of services are comparable. Thus in education, the pursuit of national standards in literacy and numeracy, and the perceived need for Britain to catch up in the education of its children, has led to the introduction of a national curriculum and nationally established standards to be monitored by attainment tests.

However, local authorities are not the only local arm of the policy structure. In 1998, following referenda in Scotland and Wales and a vote in favour of the Good Friday Agreement in Northern Ireland, the Westminster Parliament agreed some degree of political devolution. We have since seen the establishment of a Scottish Parliament, with limited policy making and tax raising powers, a Welsh Assembly that has largely taken over the powers of the Secretary of State for Wales, and a Northern Ireland Assembly, again with limited powers and partly controlled by cross border agreements with the Irish Republic. This has led to some interesting changes, particularly in Scotland. (The impacts of 'variegated' devolution on the nations of Scotland, Wales and Northern Ireland are explained in detail in Chapter 7.) In addition, as we have already indicated, much central government business is conducted not by departments based in Whitehall but in the local offices of those departments, their agencies or semi-autonomous organisations (sometimes

Unitary Authorities	Shire County and District Authorities	London Borough Councils (LBCs) and Greater London Authority (GLA)
Local authorities that tend to oversee the delivery of all local authority services in their area, e.g. • Metropolitan Districts • Certain city councils	Local authorities in which there tends to be a split in the areas of responsibility between a county council and a more local district council	LBCs are similar to Metropolitan Districts in their scope The GLA does not provide services but oversees service provision
Example: • Birmingham City Council	**Example:** • Gloucestershire County Council and Cheltenham Borough Council	**Examples:** • Greater London Authority • Westminster City Council, Hackney LBC, Kensington and Chelsea
Responsibilities: • Children s education and social care • Adult education and social care • Housing • Leisure • Refuse collection and disposal • Environmental and public health • Planning and development control • Economic development • Overseeing local strategic partnerships	**Responsibilities:** *County Council –* • Children's education and social care • Adult education and social care • Refuse disposal • Environmental and public health • Overseeing local strategic partnerships *District Council –* • Housing • Leisure • Refuse collection • Planning and development control • Economic development	**Responsibilities:** *GLA – oversees* • Transport • Police • Fire and emergency planning • Planning and economic development *LBCs –* • Children's education and social care • Adult education and social care • Housing • Leisure • Refuse collection and disposal • Environmental and public health • Planning and development control • Economic development

Figure 5.4   Local authority structures and functions in England

described as 'quangos', quasi autonomous non/national government organisations). For example, in health, we would need to consider the roles of the regional and subregional arms of central government's Department of Health such as Strategic Health Authorities (SHAs) and the more local Primary Care Trusts, NHS Hospital Trusts and Foundation Hospitals. In education, the Department for Children, Schools and Families works with a variety of agencies. For example, under Labour one has seen the emergence of a type of school that is independent of local authority provision, that is city academies. These city academies have a greater degree of autonomy than that granted to local authority-controlled schools. At the same time, in education one has witnessed a more direct relationship between the Department

Stop and Think   **What is the relevance of local government in the UK?**

How well informed are you of the work and responsibilities of your local council?

Do you know, for example:

- in which local authority you live?
- what responsibilities it has?
- what services it provides?
- what its political control is?
- who your councillors are ?
- when the next local elections are?
- how your council gets its funds to pay for the services it oversees?

for Children, Schools and Families and primary and secondary schools themselves. Thus the devolution of decision making powers, within nationally set guidelines, can be increasingly seen in a range of social policy providers, whether they be traditional local providers given greater central direction, ex-local authority-controlled provision, or newer quangos and government agencies.

As described in Chapter 6 on governance, the early years of the twenty-first century have continued to see both local and central government move increasingly to an enabling role. No longer is government, at whatever level, to be regarded as the funder and provider of services. Instead, government increasingly has a supervisory or strategic role in the delivery of services. As such, the various roles of local authorities have been curtailed in a range of ways (for example, in discretion in making policy, in raising income, or in determining service delivery), with central government more prescriptive than ever before in determining what a local authority may do and how it may raise funding and spend its finances. At the same time, national government (both Conservative and Labour) has attempted to widen the policymaking process and, therefore, arguably undermine what it often saw as undemocratic and unaccountable 'rotten boroughs'. The most public attempt, and public failure, by Margaret Thatcher's Conservative government to control local authorities was the aborted introduction of the Community Charge or 'poll tax', but in many other ways local authorities continue to find themselves constrained. There has been an attempted 'privatisation' of the policy process in local government by the introduction, and sometimes imposition, of appointees over locally elected councillors. In addition, we have seen various services externalised or privatised; for example, council housing stock has been transferred out of the direct control of the local authority (see Chapter 14), social care is increasingly being provided by independent sector agencies (see Chapter 13), and other services including refuse collection, road maintenance and leisure facilities have been externalised. However, under the Labour government since 1997 it is possible to argue that local government's role has changed to be the strategic enabler and community voice of its citizens (Daly and Davis, 2004, 2008). This can be seen particularly in its responsi-bility for overseeing the 'Local Strategic Partnership' between itself and other local public services (see Box 5.3).

Box 5.3	An example of a Local Strategic Partnership

The Birmingham Strategic Partnership

The Birmingham Strategic Partnership (BSP) is the LSP for Birmingham and was established in 2001. The BSP brings together, at a citywide and district level, key public agencies and representatives of the business, community and voluntary sectors to achieve more effective joined-up action, particularly in relation to neighbourhood renewal and tackling deprivation.

The BSP is committed to:

- leading the coordination, planning, implementation and updating of the Community Strategy, Local Public Service Agreement, Local Area Agreement and other such government initiatives that may arise that help to deliver the vision and strategy for Birmingham;
- being a strong advocate for the vision and strategy within which individuals, organisations and key public, business, community and voluntary sector service providers can develop their strategies and re-align and improve their services;
- providing a mechanism for any agency, individual, organisation or group to both influence the vision and strategy for Birmingham and contribute to bringing it about;
- seeking to engage the people who live and work in Birmingham, and other stakeholders, in devel-oping and delivering the vision for the city;
- increasing opportunities to explore how services can be improved, particularly for groups and areas with the lowest outcomes, and providing a unified and challenging voice to rally change.

Organisations represented on the BSP board include:

- Advantage West Midlands [Regional Development Agency]
- Birmingham Association of Neighbourhood Forums
- Birmingham Chamber of Commerce and Industry
- Birmingham City Council
- Birmingham Community Empowerment Network
- Birmingham Environmental Partnership
- Birmingham Race Action Partnership
- Birmingham Strategic Housing Partnership
- Birmingham Voluntary Services Council
- Centro [West Midlands Passenger Transport Executive]
- Learning and Skills Council, Birmingham and Solihull
- Primary Care (on behalf of the four PCTs in Birmingham)
- West Midlands Police
- West Midlands Fire Service

Source: www.bhamsp.org.uk/index.php (2007).

The debate about such changes and their contribution to democracy continues to rage as the government argues for less direct political control of many of our local social services and an increased say for users and the local community more widely (as will be explored in the next chapter on 'Governance'). The government believes such changes make those services closer and more responsive to service users. Opponents of these changes argue that the proper forum for local democracy is a locally elected authority. Labour has, since 1997, set about an ambitious programme of 'democratic renewal' (Leach and Wingfield, 1999; Pratchett, 1999). Labour's 2001 General Election manifesto expressed a vision of local government that is 'active, in touch ... [and] serving the people' (The Labour Party, 2001: 34). The government's agenda (DTLR, 2001) has therefore been seeking to introduce measures to ensure that local government has a new democratic legitimacy and develops new ways of working to provide clearer, more efficient decision making and accountability. It is clear that such reforms are bringing fundamental change to the formulation and implementation of policy.

However, the type of policy-making model set out above describes a set of constitutional arrangements and, whilst it may tell us the layout of the policy map, gives us little information about how policy is made or implemented and what influences the creation and success or failure of social policy. We need now to turn to the vexed question of 'who makes policy?'.

Who makes policy?

As we have already indicated, the formal passage of legislation, that is the making of laws and Acts of Parliament, takes place within the confines of the Houses of Commons and Lords and the system of Select and Parliamentary Committees (as well as increasingly in the 'governments' of Scotland, Wales and Northern Ireland). We may therefore choose to examine the passage of legislation through the Houses of Parliament and seek to explore the importance of debates or of Second Readings and the committee stage for a particular piece of legislation. We would then have built up a reasonably detailed picture of one part of the institutional arrangements for the creation, passage and implementation of new policy. However, we have already indicated that much, possibly as much as 95%, of the business of Parliament is taken up in the debate of government-sponsored legislation and government policy.

We might next turn to the government, as chief initiator of policy, to ask again, who makes policy? We have stated above that the Cabinet and Prime Minister occupy a crucial position in the policy machine since they are, technically at least, responsible for the initiation and implementation of policy; thus we could turn to the operation of Cabinet and its committees. But again, as we have already noted, Cabinet ministers rely heavily upon their civil servants for information and advice; an individual would, after all, be unable to retain the sum of information relating to all the work of a department. The Cabinet meets once or twice per week for a morning and clearly would be unable, even as a group of 20 senior government members, to consider the breadth and depth of policies within its remit.

The role of civil servants may in turn suggest to us that it is they who, in controlling the flow of information between a minister and his or her department, are able to set and maybe even to manipulate the policy agenda. They may, for instance, if it is not too conspiratorial, present to a minister a set of 'preferred' policy options and thereby exclude more radical solutions to policy problems, so leading politicians to amend, and perhaps abandon, their ideologically motivated plans. Such a scenario would suggest that the policy process is inherently conservative and restricts itself to slow and incremental change (Ham and Hill, 1993).

But such a description of institutions and the way in which they operate does not seem to be sufficient for our needs. Such a study does not explain to us 'why' a particular piece of legislation is created, 'how' that policy is being implemented or its impact on the well-being of citizens. Thus we might go further than the descriptive study outlined above and seek to examine some of the factors that influence the creation and formulation of new policy. We could, for instance, look at the role of political parties in promoting policy as part of their electoral manifesto, which when in government they seek to implement. We need to know how, for instance, parties arrive at their manifesto, how proposals are discussed internally, and for example the role of the party conference (less and less influential, admittedly). In turn we can consider the role of the media in examining those policy proposals and the impact of the various pressure groups that pursue their own agenda and add their comments to party political manifestos. We can by this means create, as Mullard (1995) suggests, a policy hierarchy which has at its head an élite represented by Westminster and Whitehall, the so-called corridors of powers, followed by the political parties and range of interest and pressure groups whose role it is to engage in political debate and dialogue or ideological principles. That debate is said to resolve itself within the electoral process, with the victor claiming a mandate from the people for their principles and policies. The next stratum in this hierarchy is that of the grassroots (party or pressure group) activist whose perspective and interpretation of policy will often differ from that of their leadership, followed by the public or electorate who remain often the least well informed about policy and the policy process.

However, public debate over policy rarely considers the detail of policy and often seems to consist purely of the 'media soundbite'. Additionally, what public debate there may be over policy may often not concern social policy but any of the other areas with which government may be involved; most frequently it revolves around questions of the economy, which often dominates a domestic political agenda. The end point for such an analysis is to examine the role of the electoral process in the making of policy and the pursuit of power by political parties. Democratic theory would suggest, at its most ideal, that what we have is a system of government by the people for the people, and that our MPs are nothing more than our representatives in Parliament. But clearly MPs have a number of different pressures which affect the way in which they vote. They are representatives of their constituents. But they are also representatives of their party, which is enforced with party whips whose job it is to ensure that MPs are present and vote the 'right way'. And yet MPs are more than just constituency and party representatives; each swears allegiance to the monarch and thus also serves the 'national interest', however that may be defined. And, finally, an MP always has to consider his or her conscience in voting in the Commons.

What we are suggesting here is that we cannot, with any degree of credibility, identify which actor within the policy system is responsible for making policy. There is, in reality, no fixed hierarchy of decision making by which policy can be made at central government and passed down into implementation by the bureaucracy. Policy is more of a web of different interests, influences and actors all interlinked to one another in such a way that those linkages change over time and with different issues. This might suggest that a pluralist policy structure exists, but we may also be able to identify policy élites which are capable of exerting greater pressure or influence than other groups and occasionally disproportionate pressure or influence. We would therefore suggest that Rhodes's notion of a model of 'policy communities' or 'policy networks' provides a useful way of examining policy making in the British context (Rhodes, 1988). Again, for further elaboration of policy networks, refer to the next chapter.

Discuss and Do   Policy networks

Think of a particular policy issue, for example:

- increasing or scrapping prescription charges
- the effectiveness of GCSE exams
- the desire to increase the numbers of new houses being built per year

and try to map out the various policy players and interests that may be involved and influential in shaping and implementing a change in policy direction.

The overriding problem with the institutional method of analysis has been that the process itself has often remained at best hidden and at worst assumed obvious. More recent, institutional, changes, such as the development of links at a European level following the Single European Act (1986), the Maastricht Treaty (1992), the incorporation of the Human Rights Act into British law, and constitutional reform in Scotland, Wales and Northern Ireland, along with the shifting pattern of relationships between ministers and their departments (or agencies of a department), have appeared to change at a more fundamental level the process of making policy.

Conclusion

The policy process, as we have seen, is more than simply the sum of its parts. There is clearly more to making policy than we can determine by outlining and describing the nuts and bolts of the policy machine. An example might illustrate this point. If asked to talk about motor racing, we could draw an accurate picture of a racing car, its engine, aerodynamics or design. But that would not tell us how to drive such a machine or about the psychological thrill we might derive from driving it. Similarly, to describe the policy process in terms of its mechanics is insufficient, as it tells us little of how to make policy or why some people are attracted to become policy makers, that is, what makes the machine, and its driver, tick?

Spicker (1995) argues that social policy making in particular and the policy process in general are very much to do with power and the values of those engaged within the policy process (see Chapters 9 and 10). We could equally well suggest that the community or environment within which policy is made is of crucial importance and, in the era of globalisation, those factors external to and beyond the control of our domestic policy environment assume ever greater importance (see Chapter 22).

We have already suggested above that the institutional structures are in a continuous process of flux and change and that the relationship between central policy making and what goes on at the local level, including the delivery of policy, informs the way in which policy is made and implemented. Thus we have a number of interesting and useful avenues to explore which might give us greater insight into the making of social policy.

Annotated further reading

For an expanded and up-to-date description and discussion of the institutions and structures of the British policy machinery, readers should consult Bill Jones *et al.*, *Politics UK* (6th edition, 2006). For lively and lighter introductions to UK policy and politics, the following are very accessible: Jeremy Paxman's *The Political Animal* (2003), Andrew Marr's *Ruling Britannia* (1996), and Simon Jenkins, *Accountable to None* (1995). For a wider examination of the policy process within the structural framework, Simon James's *British Government: A reader in policy making* (1997) illustrates a number of useful points; similarly Maurice Mullard's *Policy-Making in Britain: An introduction* (1995) offers some useful case studies of different aspects of the policy process. The most comprehensive thematic approach is provided by Ham and Hill's, *The Policy Process in the Modern Capitalist State* (1993) along with its accompanying set of key readings in Hill's *The Policy Process: A reader* (1993). Peter Hennessy's *Whitehall* (1988) provides an accessible account of the operation of politics and policy making at national level, whilst his *The Hidden Wiring* (1996) presents an equally readable explanation of how the machine of governing works without a written constitution. There have been various ministerial diaries, but the first of note and arguably the most illuminating is Richard Crossman's diaries (*The Crossman Diaries*, 1979). Description and analysis of local policy-making institutions and procedures may be found in Howard Elcock's *Local Government* (1994), whilst recent developments in social services in particular are examined in Tony Butcher's, *Delivering Welfare: The governance of the social services in the 1990s* (1995). More specific analysis of policy making for social policy may be found in Peter Levin's *Making Social Policy: The mechanisms of government and politics and how to investigate them* (1997) which gives an interesting case study approach to different social policies pursued during the 1980s and 1990s, whilst a more detailed analysis in the management of social policies and their departments is offered by John Clarke *et al.* in *Managing Social Policy* (1994).

Chapter 6

The governance of social policy

Objectives

- To describe the hierarchical government structures within traditional public administration.

- To review the reasons for the break-up of the post-war social policy and welfare consensus.

- To explain the nature of the changes in governance under the governments of the New Right.

- To explain how New Labour's partnership approach to the governance and management of welfare contains both similarities to and differences from the approach of the New Right.

- To evaluate the various governance models and the usefulness of governance as an analytical tool in social policy analysis.

Introduction

Governance is an area of theoretical analysis not typically considered by general introductory social policy texts. And yet, the significant changes in social policy over the last 25 years under the governments of the New Right (with Prime Ministers Margaret Thatcher and John Major) and, latterly, New Labour have created a new set of (governance) arrangements through which we, as citizens, receive social welfare.

What do we mean by 'governance'? Although the term was used as far back as the fourteenth century (Weller, 2000), over the last 10 to 15 years governance has (re)appeared as a term to replace 'government' as a means of explaining how society is governed (Rhodes, 1997). A fairly straightforward definition, focusing directly on policy making, is provided by Richards and Smith (2003: 15):

> 'Governance' is a descriptive label that is used to highlight the changing nature of the policy process in recent decades. In particular, it sensitizes us to the ever-increasing variety of terrains and actors involved in the making of policy. Thus, governance demands that we consider all the actors and locations beyond the 'core executive' involved in the policy making process.

In contrast, Newman provides a more multi-dimensional definition, drawing together the work of various academics in suggesting that governance is concerned with power and authority, rights and duties, as well as changes to the nature and patterns of governing.

Governance has become a shorthand term used to describe a *particular* set of changes. It signifies a set of elusive but potentially deeply significant shifts in the way in which government seeks to govern (Pierre and Peters, 2000). It denotes the development of ways of coordinating economic activity that transcends the limitations of both hierarchy and markets (Rhodes, 1997; Smith, 1999). It highlights the role of the state in 'steering' action within complex social systems (Kooiman, 1993, 2000). It denotes the reshaping of the role of local government away from service delivery towards 'community governance' (Clarke and Stewart, 1999; Stewart and Stoker, 1988; Stoker, 1999). (Newman, 2001: 11, emphasis in original)

As such, governance is concerned with *government*, the *state*, *economic activity and systems*, and *local government*. Governments, it is argued, govern differently from in the past. Interrelatedly, the state 'steers' and influences rather than directly controls and delivers. Economic activity is no longer either controlled by the state (state planning) or determined solely by the market. Local government, which very much used to be concerned with service delivery (that is, directly providing services), is less and less responsible for such things and is increasingly seen as being responsible for 'community leadership', that is the coordinator and voice for local priorities and concerns. Essentially, governance is concerned with the economic, the political and the social.

As such, 'governance' attempts to explain how it is no longer 'the government from the centre' that controls the production and consumption of (public) goods and services. Rather, it is argued, governments have ceded control on the one hand to supra-national organisations, corporations, non-governmental organisations (NGOs) and quasi-autonomous non-governmental organisations (QUANGOs), and on the other hand to civil society at the local level: communities, voluntary organisations and individual citizens. Therefore, whilst in the past government could plan the production and consumption of social welfare and other goods, this is no longer the case.

This chapter maps out the changes that have occurred to the governance arrangements in Britain. It is possible to suggest that these changes relate to four governance arrangements that have existed: *hierarchies*, *markets*, *networks* and *partnerships* (Newman, 2001; Richards and Smith, 2003). This chapter explores the evolution from *government* to *governance* by describing the four models of governance:

- *Hierarchies* – the governance structures within traditional public administration.
- *Markets* – the break-up of the post-war consensus which preceded the shift in the management and governance of social policy, the changes to the governance and management of welfare services under the New Right.
- *Networks* – the rise of governance networks.
- *Partnerships* – New Labour's approach to the governance and management of social welfare.

Finally, an evaluation of whether we have really moved in any significant sense from hierarchical governance, and the worth of governance as an analytical tool, is explored.

Models of governance

Newman (2001) has suggested that there have historically been four types of governance arrangements – hierarchies, markets, networks and partnerships:

- Traditional public administration – the hierarchical model.
- Markets – the rational goal model.
- Networks – the open systems model.
- Partnerships – the self-governance model.

Newman suggested that these four models can be distinguished by reference to two 'dimensions of difference':

- Power – centralised or decentralised.
- Disposition to change – stability or innovation.

She mapped the four models of governance against these two axes (see Figure 6.1).

The following sections of the chapter will examine these different governance models. However, before doing that, it is important to note that it would be too simple to depict or overlay particular epochs, ideologies or governments with particular governance models. As Richards and Smith (2003: 9) have observed:

> In reality there is no distinct temporal breach between each [model of governance]. The reality is there is a great deal of fuzziness and overlap.

However, for the purposes of simplification, we will use Newman's four models of governance to structure the developments in the governance of welfare: 'from hierarchies to markets to networks to partnerships'.

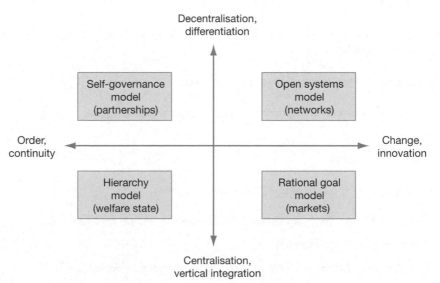

Figure 6.1 Newman's models of governance

Source: J. Newman (2001) *Modernising Governance: New Labour, Policy and Society*, Figure 2.1, p. 34, London: Sage. Reprinted with permission.

Traditional governance structures – hierarchies

The period of the last 20 to 30 years has seen a shift away from the traditional, centralised (at either national or local government level), hierarchical structures of government. It was said of Aneurin Bevan after the inception of the National Health Service in 1948 that, as the Minister for Health, he expected to be able 'to hear the sound of a bedpan dropping in a hospital ward in South Wales' and be involved in the subsequent action. Certainly with the advent of the post-war welfare state, there was a belief in state planning and delivery of a uniform and universal social welfare provision. The British people had come through the experience of the Second World War in which the state had taken on the responsibility for managing both the supply and demand of many goods. State responsibility had not simply extended to the control of the *production* of many goods and services, such as health services, housing, child care and food production. In addition, government had taken on the responsibility for managing *demand*, for example for food and fuel. In many respects, the Warfare State had become the Welfare State.

Discuss and Do   Food rationing

During the Second World War and then with the creation of the post-war welfare state, it was felt that the state could and should manage both supply and demand of many essential goods. When one looks at the production and consumption of food, for example, it is believed that with the need to produce more fresh food locally or nationally, and the impact of food rationing where consumption of particular foods was controlled through rationing, the nation's health was better during the war period than it had been prior to the outset of hostilities or was to be when rationing was lifted in the 1950s.

Do you think food should be rationed? Give three reasons why it should and three reasons why it should not be rationed.

Reasons for the rationing of food may include:

- It is fairer – food is an important resource (public good).
- It is more efficient.
- It is more effective.

Reasons against the rationing of food may include:

- People are free agents and should be allowed to decide for themselves.
- The market is more efficient.
- The market will more effectively respond to changes in demand.

In the 'era of government' (Richards and Smith, 2003) the state (directly) controlled the production of a variety of goods:

- Welfare services – education, health care, housing, welfare benefits, social services.

- Utilities – electricity, gas, water, coal, transport, telephone and postal communications, broadcasting.
- Manufacturing – steel, shipbuilding, motor vehicle manufacturing.

The state managed supply and demand more generally. There was a general belief, informed by Keynesian economic theory, that the state could control both demand and supply rather than leave it to the market to balance supply to individual demand.

At the core of hierarchical government was the sovereignty of government at Westminster. Government governed its citizens in a hierarchical, top-down manner (see Box 6.1).

Box 6.1	The Westminster model

- Parliamentary sovereignty
- Accountability through fair and free elections
- The party with the majority of seats has control
- Government is via a strong Cabinet (the Executive)
- Doctrine of ministerial responsibility
- Central government dominance
- Non-political civil servants

Source: Richards and Smith (2003: 4).

Public administration and bureaucracy

The 'warfare state' and the post-war welfare state were predicated, however, not just on Keynesian economic theory and hierarchical government from the centre but also on Weberian-like hierarchical, bureaucratic organisations. In exercising control, the post-war state can be regarded as epitomising the essentials of Weber's *bureaucracy* in that it, and its subordinate departments, agencies and organisations, typified bureaucratic arrangements (see Box 6.2 overleaf).

Working alongside the public administrators were a burgeoning number and variety of welfare professionals. In nearly all of the welfare services, those responsible for the direct provision are members of professional groups: doctors and nurses, teachers and lecturers, social workers, housing officers, architects and town planners. It is perhaps not surprising that Klein (1973: 4) remarked: 'The Welfare State is, in many respects, also the Professional State'. Whilst the bureaucrats are employed to exercise rationality and neutrality in the application of the rules of the system, professionals are empowered to exercise their expert judgement, informed by education and service or vocation (see Box 6.3 overleaf).

Hierarchical government and public accountability

In 'the era of government' the bureaucratic modern state was organised such that the citizen was able to apportion responsibility and hold to account those

Box 6.2 — The hierarchical state – Weber's bureaucratic organisation

- A hierarchy of relationships
- Rule-bound decision making
- Clear lines of responsibility
- Hierarchical discipline
- Responsibility gravitates upwards
- A culture of control and procedure/process
- Organisational structures are linear, rigid and impermeable
- Organisational structures are relatively stable
- Predictability and uniformity
- Stable and enduring with only gradual changes over time
- Underpinned by a strong set of public service values or ethos
- Public servants are impartial, incorruptible, permanent, anonymous, professional/expert
- Elected representatives are temporary, amateur/non-expert, ultimately responsible

Box 6.3 — The essentials of a profession

- Control over entrance into its membership
- Self-regulation of members
- Distinct knowledge base
- Authority that cannot easily be challenged by an 'uninformed' public
- State-licensed monopoly of provision
- Regulatory code of ethics
- Professional culture

responsible. For the citizen, it was their elected representatives who were ultimately responsible and held to account (with the Executive responsible to the elected representatives as a whole); they, in turn, held accountable their senior bureaucrats who then held to account their junior colleagues and so forth down the lines of the bureaucratic modern state. Therefore, in the traditional, hierarchical, bureaucratic state:

> Governing was basically regarded as one-way traffic from those governing to those governed. (Kooiman, 2000: 142)

Therefore, government in the modern state during 'the era of government' had the following features:

- an elected representative set of institutions whose ultimate responsibility it is to govern;
- a set of administrative bureaucratic institutions that are there to support the political representatives in the development of policy and its implementation;
- a territorial locale within which these institutions of the state operate;
- levels of government and administration with that at the national level being supreme or primary;

- the state developing social policies that aim to improve the lot of its citizens, promote the development of the nation or polity, and secure social inclusion and therefore legitimacy;
- control of the national and local economy, not least through influencing the supply and demand of goods;
- the promotion of the involvement of citizens in terms of both their rights and duties. (After Richards and Smith, 2003: 46)

Governance in the epoch of hierarchical government meant that:

> In the UK the post-war welfare settlement was based on the conception of the state as a direct service provider, with large, bureaucratic state organisations forming a public sector predominantly based on governing through hierarchy. (Newman, 2001: 13)

However, as we will see in the next section, by the mid-1970s these arrangements were seen to be no longer appropriate, and were criticised for promulgating monolithic, inefficient, unresponsive, supplier-dominant welfare services. A period of reform under the governments of the New Right and New Labour has since ensued with the intention of tackling these perceived problems.

The break up of the post-war consensus and the demise of hierarchical governance

Part of the drive for change in social policy over the last 25 years has been related to how services are delivered, the aim being to provide more effective social and public services, including arrangements to allow the citizen to shape and influence the nature of those services. The drive for change in the governance and management of public services from both the New Right governments of Margaret Thatcher and John Mayor and, latterly, New Labour has been in part to ensure that social and other public services cease to be: monolithic, inefficient, unresponsive and supplier dominant.

First, public services were regarded as *monolithic* or uniform. That is, there was a notion that the state would provide the same type and level of service to each user, patient, tenant, pupil or student without acknowledging the diversity of needs. This was characterised by the criticism that state provision meant 'one size fits all'. Irrespective of whom you were or what your particular needs were, you would get the same service as your neighbour and fellow citizens throughout the United Kingdom.

Second, public services were depicted, perhaps unfairly, as *inefficient*. Local government in particular was generally thought to be wasteful of public money, whilst the NHS was believed to be over-managed by inefficient 'state bureaucrats'. Indeed, it was argued by some that public services tended to expand their budgets to maximise their own interests rather than to improve or increase services.

Discuss and Do   **Problems with hierarchical governance**

What criticisms could you make and what examples can you give of the traditional, hierarchical welfare state? Think of a particular service, for example housing, the NHS or education, and relate the service to criticisms of the traditional welfare state in terms of the service being:

- Monolithic – 'one size fits all'.

- Inefficient – slow, costly, bureaucratic.

- Unresponsive – no choice, long queues.

- Supplier dominant – serving the interests of providers, e.g. welfare professionals.

> ... [B]ureaucrats benefited in direct proportion to the size of the budget they held .... [C]laims for improved spending on public services [were seen] as a reflection of public servants' and professionals' desire to earn more and run larger organisations. (Glennerster, 2003: 27)

When budgets were tight, rather than becoming more efficient it was argued that professionals simply reduced their workload or output.

Perhaps unsurprisingly, both local government and the NHS have been subjected to virtually continuous reorganisation over the last 25 to 30 years. And yet, if one explores the use of resources in the NHS, for example, one sees first that the UK has traditionally spent less of its GDP than comparable OECD countries on health care and, second, when it comes to expenditure on administrative costs, the UK is relatively efficient (see Chapter 12 for a fuller discussion).

Related to the perceptions of inefficiency was the belief that public welfare services were also *unresponsive*. Hospital waiting lists and council housing queues are two examples of state provision perceived to be slow in responding to the needs of citizens. Part of the argument here is that, unlike in a pure market where supply responds to demand by an increase in supply and/or an increase in price, with public services an increase in demand was often managed by extending the waiting time or the length of the queue.

> ... [T]he tendency of firms in a non-competitive situation [is] to be less than wholly efficient in the way they produce their product. Working practices may be slack, *responses* to consumers slow .... The 'monopoly profit' may not be reaped by the shareholders but by the workers and managers not being as *responsive* and effective as they could be. (Glennerster, 2003: 28, emphasis added)

The final criticism made against public services was that, again unlike in a pure market where the customer is depicted as sovereign, with public services it was argued that it was the *suppliers* of services, not least the public service professionals, who were *dominant*. The user, whether he or she was a patient, a housing tenant, a pupil or a student, remained subservient to the provider or supplier: hospital consultants and family GPs, local authority housing officers, school teachers and university lecturers. William Waldegrave, a Conservative Secretary of State in the 1990s, articulated the perceived problem thus:

> [We have] designed public services where the interests of the providers systematically outweighed those of the users .... (Waldegrave, 1993: 9–10)

Overall, there was a view that welfare users were unable to exercise either voice or choice. Hirschman (1970) had argued that consumers can influence providers in two ways, by exercising 'exit' and/or voice. However, by the late 1970s it was felt that the consumers of the welfare state could neither exit from existing providers by taking their custom elsewhere nor voice their dissatisfaction satisfactorily.

These criticisms were levelled at the set of arrangements that epitomised the British post-war welfare state from its inception in 1945 up until the break-up of the post-war consensus encapsulated in the election of the Thatcher Conservative government in 1979. However, it should be remembered that the New Right governments of Margaret Thatcher and John Major were not the first post-war governments to 'attack' state welfare and public expenditure. It was, after all, Anthony Crosland, a Labour government minister, who advocated that 'the party was over' and it was his Labour government which oversaw, in 1977–78, the 'largest' post-war cuts to public expenditure (see Sullivan, 1992; Clarke *et al.*, 2000). Even so, the New Right was overtly anti-welfarist and anti-statist (Clarke and Newman, 1997; Hughes and Lewis, 1998; Jones and Novak, 1999; Clarke *et al.*, 2000).

Having set the context for governance arrangements, this chapter now explores the changing nature of the governance and management of social welfare in which it has been argued that we have moved from hierarchies to markets, to networks and, latterly, to partnerships. We will start by examining the nature of the New Right's reforms, where attempts were made to incorporate the values of the market in the provision of social welfare, and hence the move to market governance.

New Right solutions – the market, new managerialism and user empowerment

The New Right sought to redefine the nature of welfare provision and public services more generally. Among their aims were to reform public services through attacking those perceived problems of state welfare mapped out earlier: uniformity, inefficiency, unresponsiveness and supplier dominance. All of these were regarded as failures inherent in public provision. The solution was to be found in the promotion (interrelatedly) of privatisation, new managerialism and user empowerment.

The New Right's strategy to reform the provision of welfare, and its governance, took three approaches: privatisation, managerialism and user empowerment. How do you think each of these approaches might be seen to be able to improve the provision and governance of welfare services? Choose a particular service area and consider the impact of each of these approaches:

- Privatisation – in order to make provision more efficient and responsive.

- Managerialisation – which challenges the power of suppliers (professionals and technocrats).

- User involvement – whereby users get what they want, when they want it, and are able to influence the nature of provision more generally.

Privatisation – the role of markets and the family

The New Right was anti-statist (and, particularly, anti-welfare statist) in terms of its proponents' belief in the primacy of the 'free market' and that state provision interfered with the 'natural' and 'efficient' manner in which markets distributed goods, services and resources. The New Right argued that the state provision of welfare had left citizens with limited choices and diminished responsibilities (see Nozick, 1974; Hayek, 1976).

Part of the New Right's response, therefore, was to 'privatise' welfare in two respects (Clarke *et al.*, 2000). First, it proposed to privatise services, or to use 'quasi-markets' (Le Grand and Bartlett, 1993) where it was not appropriate for the private sector to take over. Indeed, throughout the 1980s and into the mid-1990s, one witnessed the privatisation of many industries and services which had been nationalised during the 1940s (Swann, 1988):

- Public utilities – electricity, gas, water, coal, transport, telecommunications.
- Manufacturing – steel, shipbuilding, motor manufacturing.

In addition, local authorities, the NHS and other public services had to 'contract out' many of their services, including cleaning, catering, grounds maintenance and refuse collection. Other services were either taken out of the direct control of central government by being set up as agencies or made independent of local authorities, often being recast as local quangos:

- Government agencies – Benefits Agency, Passport Authority, DVLA.
- Ex-local authorities – polytechnics, further education colleges, grant-maintained schools, careers services, economic development, social housing, residential care.

Those welfare services that remained the direct responsibility of central or local government were reconfigured through the creation of 'quasi-markets' (Le Grand and Bartlett, 1993). Quasi-markets are markets in which there is a split between the supplier and the purchaser. However, unlike in a pure market, the purchaser is not the direct consumer or user. Quasi-markets were introduced in the delivery of a number of services. For example, the NHS and Community Care Act 1990 created in the NHS a 'purchaser-provider' split between GP fundholders and NHS Hospital Trust providers, whilst in social care Social Services departments increasingly became enablers rather than direct providers of community care. This was all done with the aim of reconstructing ('re-imagining') welfare users as welfare *customers*.

Second, the New Right sought to privatise welfare in terms of repositioning parts of it back in the private realm, that is back with individuals, families and communities. Therefore, responsibility was privatised, by making individuals, families and communities responsible for meeting their own welfare needs. This can be seen particularly in the changes that were made in the provision of health and social care.

> [I]n the fields of health and social care ... the family or the community has been expected to take on a greater role in the provision of care .... In these changes it is now well established that the community-as-carer has primarily meant the family, and within the family the gendered division of labour has meant that caring work has primarily fallen on women as mothers, daughters and wives. (Clarke and Newman, 1997: 28)

However, the marketisation of welfare and other public services led to greater fragmentation of control mechanisms. The state, and government more specifically, could not control or command the provision of social welfare in the way that it had in the past. As Newman observed,

> The introduction of market mechanisms led to a more fragmented and dispersed pattern of service delivery and regulation ... that required new forms of coordination. Privatisation, contracting out, quasi-markets, the removal of functions from local authorities and the proliferation of quangos, the separation between policy and delivery functions in the civil service with the setting up of Executive Agencies all meant that governments had to develop new forms of control. (Newman, 2001: 13)

The rise of new managerialism – combating supplier dominance

In addition to the privatisation of welfare, the New Right wished to exert greater control on social welfare and other public service providers by bringing in stronger management. New managerialism was an approach that imported the dominant ideology of management from the private sector to run public services. Welfare and other public services were to be reconstructed via this 'managerialist' *paradigm* (Clarke *et al.*, 1994; Clarke and Newman, 1997). Managerialisation is 'the process of subjecting the control of public services to the principles, powers and practices of managerial co-ordination' (Clarke *et al.*, 2000: 5). As such, the new managerialism (Pollitt, 1993; Dunleavy and Hood, 1994; Flynn, 1997; Clarke *et al.*, 2000) reoriented the way that welfare and public services were to be administered and provided, away from hierarchical governance, explored earlier in this chapter, into a new managerialist one which contained:

> ... a new set of practices and values, based upon a new language of welfare delivery which emphasises efficiency and value for money, competition and markets, consumerism and customer care. (Butcher, 1995: 161)

The new mangerialism typically featured 'attention to outputs and performance rather than inputs and personal authority to line managers' (Clarke *et al.*, 2000: 6).

In reality, the New Right's emphasis was to be on controlling all three of economy, efficiency and effectiveness – the three 'Es' (see Carter, 1989; Carter *et al.*, 1992; Power, 1993, 1997; Flynn, 1997):

- inputs such as costs (economy);
- outputs (efficiency);
- outcomes (effectiveness).

Therefore, throughout the 1980s and up to 1997 there was a great emphasis on reducing budgets, 'getting more for less', and freeing up managers to manage and deliver outputs and outcomes (to 'get results'), almost irrespective of how this was to be achieved. Some have suggested that this was at least a two-stage process. The first stage was a 'neo-Taylorist' (after Frederick Taylor) form of managerialism (see Clarke *et al.*, 1994; Newman and Clarke, 1994; Clarke and Newman, 1997), focusing on importing a culture of strong management, and controlling costs and the behaviour of service providers:

> The central thrust, endlessly reiterated in official documents, is to set clear targets, to develop performance indicators to measure the achievement of those targets, and to single out, by means of merit awards, those individuals who get 'results'. The strengthening of and incentivising of line management is a constant theme .... In official terms, what seems to be required is a culture shift of a kind that will facilitate a more thoroughgoing functional/neo-Taylorist management process. (Pollitt, 1993: 56)

The second stage built on this by introducing quasi-markets, decentralisation, a concentration on quality, and a customer focus (see Clarke and Newman, 1997). Therefore, by the mid-1990s, the new public management paradigm had replaced that of the old public administration and was epitomised by the changes listed in Box 6.4 (after Dunleavy and Hood, 1994: 9; Clarke and Newman, 1997: 21). In so doing, new managerialism sought to manage the welfare professionals and public administrators and did this partly by promoting a greater customer focus (Clarke and Newman, 1997; Newman and Clarke, 1994; Stoker and Mossberger, 1995).

User involvement – empowering the citizen-consumer

The third dimension to the New Right's 'market governance' was their advocacy of consumerism. There had been a growing critique of welfare statism from both left and right leading up to the mid-1970s. The left and new social movements of the 1960s and 1970s (disability, mental health, 'race', gender movements) had all begun to challenge the monolithic, top-down state welfare provision that had become established in the post-war welfare state settlement. These movements had started to question the principles underpinning the post-war welfare state with its presumptions of:

- full male employment;
- a particular notion of family centred on women providing the majority of care and welfare;
- a particular notion of British citizenship based on the predominant ethnic group;
- able-bodiedness and age.

Box 6.4	New public management

- Transparent budgets
- Devolved budgets and services
- Costs attributed to outputs, not inputs
- Greater emphasis on quality
- Outputs measured by quantitative performance indicators
- Introduction of quasi-markets through separating purchasers from providers
- Encouragement of other agencies to take on the provider roles (public, private and voluntary/not-for-profit)
- Facilitation of users to 'exit' from one provider and switch to another instead of having to rely on 'voice' options in order to make changes

This, it was argued, had led to a welfare state that supported a particular set of social arrangements in relation to 'race', gender, age, able-bodiedness and sexuality.

> The 'universalism' of citizenship is ... deeply circumscribed – a highly conditional universalism which presumes a family-based social and economic structure. It addresses an indigenous population at whose heart are wage earning males supported by families surrounded by a set of dependent populations positioned by age (both young and old), by gender (the 'anomaly of the married woman'), by infirmity and by 'race' (the 'alien' non-citizen). (Langan and Clarke, 1993: 28, in Clarke and Newman, 1997: 4)

It certain ways the New Right was able to seize on these criticisms and incorporate them alongside their own arguments when presenting their case for a greater focus on users as customers. For the New Right, state welfare was an unproductive drain on the 'real economy' (Nozick, 1974; Hayek, 1976) and socially damaging through creating a 'dependency culture' (see Joseph, 1977; Mead, 1986). The New Right's remedy was to seek to decrease the powers of the state, reduce the individual citizen's tax burden, and thus return power and responsibility to the individual.

The New Right duly implemented changes in social policy, with the avowed intention of empowering individuals – for example, as parents, school governors, tenants, patients and clients. The 1980s and early 1990s saw, for example, the creation of the local management of schools and the option of grant-maintained status free from local authority control, the purchaser/provider split in the health service, and the advent of GP fundholders, compulsory competitive tendering of local authority services and the creation of housing action trusts. The political right's argument was that these moves empowered citizens as sovereign consumers, for example through the self-government of schools and hospitals, coupled with the emphasis on consumer choice (as opposed to supplier control) and a mixed economy of welfare provision, consequently leading to increased responsiveness from welfare providers (Hill, 1994).

The New Right's attempts to privatise welfare and public services more generally, to bring in a new managerialist approach, and to empower users as customers, can be seen as part of the process of shifting governance arrangements from hierarchies to markets. They certainly went some way to break up the post-war welfare state settlement and its governance structures based on hierarchy. No longer were public administrators necessarily directly responsible, whilst welfare professionals were being increasingly directed and managed rather than allowed to use their professional discretion, markets and quasi-markets were being brought in, and users reconstructed as customers.

Governance through networks

As stated nearer the beginning of the chapter, it would be too simple to overlay particular epochs, ideologies or governments with particular governance models. Similarly, the development of governance arrangements is not a straightforward linear development, from hierarchies to markets and from markets to networks. Even so, a consequence of the New Right's changes to the nature of welfare provision was that the hierarchical bureaucratic post-war welfare state had indeed been refashioned or distorted, if not totally replaced.

Various forces, some internal to Britain and others exerted from outside the British state, had led to the reduction of hierarchical government. Government could no longer adequately respond by itself to the challenges of globalisation, internationalisation and supra-state organisations, decentralisation, fragmentation, dynamism, diversity and complexity. Yet this had not led straightforwardly to the rise of governance through markets. Rather, the New Right's changes had arguably resulted not in market governance but instead in a fragmented or 'differentiated polity'.

> [P]ower is ... dispersed: the once unified state is fragmented and *networks have replaced hierarchy*. The policy process has become much more complex: rather than being a linear process with decisions being made in the centre, it has become one where a range of actors are involved .... [P]olicy decisions now involve public and private sector actors, agencies, privatised industries, regulators, officials, and ministers. The process of policy-making and policy delivery has become more complex. (Richards and Smith, 2003: 276)

The authority, autonomy and power of the nation state's government was being 'hollowed out' or dispersed *outwards* (via privatisation and quasi-markets), *downwards* (via the creation of quangos and government agencies) and *upwards* (to the supranational level, for example the EU). Therefore, whilst in many respects the attempts of the New Right to refashion governance arrangements along market lines provide a coherent explanation, some commentators (notably Rhodes) argued that the New Right's reforms had resulted in a fragmenting of the hierarchical welfare state, the 'hollowing out of the state', in which the traditional hierarchical governance arrangements were replaced not so much or solely by market governance as by governance through networks (see Box 6.5):

> The phrase 'the hollowing out of the state' summarises many of the changes which have taken place, and are taking place, in British government. (Rhodes, 1997: 17)

As such, the 'hollowed out state' had led to a 'differentiated polity'. The main features of this were:

- an emphasis on governance, rather than government;
- power dependence, and thus exchange relationships;
- policy networks;
- a segmented executive;
- intergovernmental relationships;
- a hollowed out state. (Richards and Smith, 2003: 276)

Government could no longer 'govern from the centre', controlling both demand and supply. Paradoxically, sovereignty had not been simply or solely passed to the sovereign consumer in the marketplace. Instead, government was 'managing from a distance' through:

- performance indicators and performance management regimes;
- targets;
- contracts;
- charters;
- external scrutiny, via audit and inspection;
- self-regulation, for example through internal quality assurance regimes;
- sanctions and threats.

At the same time as exercising such command and control from a distance, government was becoming increasingly reliant on a range of actors and organisations from the independent as well as the public sector. These agents were difficult to control. Increasingly such agents became self-controlling and governing, through networking and linking with each other.

Governance through networks was epitomised by the thinking of Osbourne and Gaebler. For them, government could no longer 'row and steer' and was now able only to control or steer. They argued that government needed to withdraw from government (!) and concentrate on governance. Osbourne and Gaebler's (1992) influential text, *Reinventing Government*, argued that governments were living with outdated public systems that needed replacing with decentralised, entrepreneurial, responsive public organisations. Their key themes for government were to:

- empower communities instead of delivering services;
- decentralise authority;
- fund outcomes, not inputs;
- encourage competition rather than monopoly;
- meet the needs of the customer, not the bureaucracy;
- invest in prevention instead of cure;
- put the *polis* back into urban policy.

Government had to relinquish command over service delivery, steer through policy networks and act as an enabler within networks. As Rhodes said:

Interorganisational linkages are a defining characteristic of service delivery and I use the term to describe the several interdependent actors involved in delivering services. These networks are made up of organisations which need to exchange resources (for example, money, information, expertise) to achieve their objectives .... As British government creates agencies, bypasses local government, uses special purpose bodies to deliver services, and encourages public–private partnerships, so networks become increasingly prominent among British governing structures. (Rhodes, 1996: 658)

Box 6.5	Governance through networks

- The body politic is fragmented and complex rather than hierarchical.
- The state steers rather than exerts direct control.
- Policy is formulated via policy networks.
- Service providers are brought in.
- Users are brought in.
- There is a multiplicity of providers.
- Relationships are neither hierarchical nor contractual but are based on trust.
- Quality in service delivery is key.
- Long-term relational contracting rather than short-term gains.

Governance and New Labour – Partnership

Similarly to the overlap between markets and networks, the shift from networks to partnership is not a clearly defined one. Even so, as Driver (2005: 265) has observed:

> Labour entered government in 1997 not simply to defend key public services such as health and education but to reform them. Indeed, it promised forms of governance that would offer a 'third way' between traditional forms of public and social administration *and* the reliance on markets as mechanisms to reform the delivery of public services. (Emphasis in the original)

This *third way*, neither hierarchical nor market-based, was to be governance through partnerships. As Newman has said:

> ... a more distinctive feature of Labour's approach was a more explicit focus on partnership as a way of governing. This focus was evident in the strengthening of the partnership rhetoric and in the [Labour] government's approach to the delivery of public policy. (Newman, 2001: 105)

Richards and Smith (2003) have encapsulated New Labour's approach as being one focused on 'joined up-ness' whereby New Labour attempted to resolve one of the key challenges presented by governance, that is the inability of elected governments to control and coordinate policy. In New Labour's view, neither the state (hierarchies) nor markets nor networks had adequately tackled the social, political or economic challenges of governance. Therefore, the response of New Labour has been to try to 'wire the system back up' (see Newman, 2001). This section now looks at New Labour's approach to governance in the provision of welfare.

The reform of welfare and public services has been part of New Labour's 'modernisation agenda' since its election in 1997. This agenda included reform to the National Health Service (see Chapter 12), whereby the purchaser–provider split has been retained but reformed and the greater use of the private health sector encouraged. Education has seen the promotion of specialist schools and city academies (see Chapter 15). Education and social services have been reformed with the strengthening of performance management, the dismantling of separate LEAs and education and social services departments and their replacement by distinct Adult Services and Children's Services Directorates (see Chapter 13), and encouragement more generally for education and particularly social services to work more closely with primary health care trusts. Social housing has witnessed the continued encouragement of local authorities to transfer their council housing stock to housing associations or 'self managed tenant organisations' (see Chapter 14). The involvement of the private sector has been encouraged, whether through the continuation of the Private Finance Initiative for capital projects or by bringing in external (that is, private sector) expertise to the public sector, for example in education management.

There are arguably three aspects to New Labour's approach to governance. First, New Labour has pursued the agenda of *new managerialism* with added vigour. Accordingly, New Labour has continued to challenge the perceived 'supplier dominance' in public service provision. As the White Paper *Modernising Government* (Cabinet Office, 1999: para. 20) stated, public services 'need to meet the needs of citizens, not the convenience of service providers'. Related to this, the emphasis on quasi-markets remains in place under New Labour. Second, New Labour has placed an even greater emphasis on *choice*. The third and, arguably, the overriding aspect of New Labour's approach to governance has been its espousal of *partnership* (Glendinning *et al.*, 2002). In examining New Labour's approach to governance, this section will examine these three facets of new managerialism, choice and partnership.

New Labour and new managerialism

By the time Labour returned to power in 1997 it had jettisoned much of the basis of the 'Old Labour' ideology, not least a perhaps over-stated faith in traditional governance through public administration hierarchies as the mechanism for ensuring public accountability. New Labour has accepted much of the New Right's approach, in particular the new managerialism paradigm.

> New Labour has pushed marketisation and privatisation forward, at least as zealously as the Conservatives did, narrowing the frontiers of the public domain in the process .... Ministerial rhetoric is saturated with the language of consumerism. The public services are to be 'customer focused'; schools and colleges are to ensure that 'what is on offer responds to the needs of consumers'; the 'progressive project' is to be subjected to 'rebranding'. (Marquand, 2004: 118, in Clarke *et al.*, 2005: 169)

Accordingly, New Labour has continued to pursue new managerialist approaches, including:

- promoting markets and quasi-markets;
- using audit, inspection and performance management;
- challenging welfare professionals and their perceived supplier dominance;
- promoting user involvement and empowerment.

As far as markets and quasi-markets are concerned, New Labour has defined public services as publicly *funded* services which may be subject to 'externalisation' (privatisation), for example in health care, prison services, and various local authority services – such as housing, social care and leisure. It is true to say that many of these providers are within the 'not-for-profit' voluntary or independent sector. As Driver has said:

> New Labour has embraced the managerial reforms introduced by the Conservatives across the civil service, local government and the wider public sector. The [Labour] government expects the new public management to deliver better results by more effective and efficient use of resources by public sector managers. As long as public providers can show 'best value' (or just plain 'value for money'), government and auditors are happy. (Driver, 2005: 267)

Choice

As part of its attempts to challenge the supplier dominance of welfare professionals and promote user involvement and empowerment, New Labour has also placed a great emphasis on user choice in welfare provision:

> In simple terms, we are completing the recasting of the 1945 welfare state to end entirely the era of 'one size fits all' services .... We are proposing to put an entirely different dynamic in place to drive our public services: one where the service will be driven not by the managers but by the user – the patient, the parent, the public and the law-abiding citizen .... I believe that the vast majority ... now believe in the new personalised concept of public services .... In reality I believe people do want choice, in public services as in other services .... The next vital stage of public [services] reform [is] to design and provide truly personalised services .... (Blair, 2004)

Therefore, we have witnessed a number of social policy initiatives under New Labour with the stated aim of increasing user choice. For example, in health care we have seen the promotion of 'choose and book' for hospital admissions, council housing has seen the introduction of 'choice based lettings', education has seen the establishment of city academies and foundation schools and faith-based schools with the intention of widening parental choice, and in social care the expansion of direct payments is a stated aim of recent policy pronouncements.

However, choice remains as problematic under New Labour as it did under the governments of the New Right. As Clarke *et al.* (2005: 167–168, 267) have pointed out, there are a number of questions that arise from the promotion of choice and consumerism, including:

- How do we institutionalise choice?
- Can or should choice be the main coordinating mechanism for the provision of welfare services?
- What does choice mean in terms of the relationship between citizens, users, welfare professionals, managers and politicians?
- What is the relationship between choice and inequality?

For proponents within New Labour (such as Alan Milburn and John Reid), choice is democratic and egalitarian since everyone, rather than just the few, will be offered choice, for example, in the provision of health care and schooling. However, Clarke *et al.* (2005) have suggested that rather than reducing such inequalities, choice may exacerbate them – not least because access to welfare services is shaped by economic and social capital and social inequalities more generally.

Indeed, welfare users may not be concerned about choice but, instead, are more likely to be occupied by issues to do with quality, access and responsiveness (Schwartz, 2004; Clarke *et al.*, 2005).

> British citizens ... care a good deal less about choice than they do about being treated with dignity, being treated by competent and compassionate physicians rather than indifferent bureaucrats, being treated in a timely fashion, being informed of their condition, and being involved in medical decisions. In my opinion, British citizens care about the right things, and they are appropriately dubious that greater choice will make any of these things happen. (Schwartz, 2004)

Partnership

New Labour's third and, some might say, overarching strand within its approach to governance is partnership. New Labour's *Third Way* espoused attempts to distance itself from the neo-liberalist market governance of the New Right and also the traditional hierarchical governance arrangements that preceded the New Right. Therefore, whilst New Labour has continued with various aspects of the New Right's new managerialism and has promoted choice, it has also sought to articulate a model of governance based on partnership. One month after its election to government in 1997, Labour was seen to be articulating its emphasis on partnership:

> We are not just a new Government, we are a new type of Government. Our decisions will not be handed down from on high ... we do not have a monopoly of wisdom and ideas. We want to hear your ideas and want you to tell us what you think of ours. (Armstrong, 1997: 18–19)

As such, New Labour proposed to work in partnership:

- horizontally – for example, across government departments;
- vertically – for example between central and local government;
- with all stakeholders – users, citizens, business, communities.

> The election of a Labour government in May 1997 saw some evidence of a shift from market competition towards a reassertion of (new) public services values ...

[P]ublic agencies are being enjoined ... to develop partnerships .... (Barnes, 1999: 87)

Only by working in partnership did New Labour believe it would be possible to tackle the problems and complexities within modern society. Newman (2001) has identified a number of objectives that partnership working may meet in the governance and delivery of social welfare:

- *Synergetic solutions* – to develop new, innovative approaches to policy development or service provision by bringing together the contributions and expertise of different partners.
- *Joined-up solutions* – to ensure integrated and coordinated approaches to policy making as well as in welfare provision.
- *Breaking down 'silos'* – to ensure government departments work together rather than against each other.
- *Greater and more widespread involvement* – to ensure that the best solutions are pursued; therefore, all stakeholders need to be involved, at an individual and a community level as well as those operating at local, regional and national levels of governance.
- *Funding/resourcing* – to increase the financial resources available for investment by developing partnerships and joint ventures between the public, private and not-for-profit sectors.

New Labour has therefore promoted partnership working across a variety of social welfare areas:

- Education – for example, Education Action Zones, Education Business Partnerships.
- Health – for example, Health Action Zones, Health Improvement Partnerships.
- Between local government and other agencies and sectors – for example, Local Strategic Partnerships, New Deal for Communities.
- Criminal justice – for example, with the establishment of Youth Offending Teams.
- Financing – Private Finance Initiative, Public–Private Partnerships.

According to the Audit Commission (1998: 5–7) in *A Fruitful Partnership,*

... partnership working is difficult to do well and making partnerships work effectively is one of the toughest challenges facing public sector managers.

The report identified a number of difficulties, including:

- getting partners to agree on priorities for action;
- keeping partners actively involved;
- preventing the partnership from becoming simply a talking shop;
- making decisions that all partners endorse;
- deciding who will provide the resources needed to achieve the partnership's objectives;
- linking the partnership's work with partners' mainstream activities and budgets;
- monitoring the partnership's effectiveness;
- working out whether what is achieved justifies the costs involved;

Discuss and Do   **Difficulties of partnership working**

What difficulties can you envisage in partnership working? You can refer to your own experiences in terms of partnerships you may have – domestic, work or study-related. More specifically, what difficulties might the following have where there is an emphasis on partnership working:

- politicians (local or national)?

- welfare providers?

- users?

- citizens?

What advantages can you identify with 'governance through partnership' as compared with the other models of governance explored in this chapter:

- advantages over hierarchical governance?

- advantages over market governance?

- advantages over network governance?

What factors need to be in place to ensure effective 'partnership governance'?

- avoiding 'partnership overload', particularly where agencies are involved in large numbers of partnerships. (See Ling, 2000)

Critics of New Labour's promotion of governance through partnerships have argued that its achievements are over-stated and that there are a number of concerns. Such criticisms include the following:

- The promotion of partnership working has not led to real partnerships, as government still plays a centralising and controlling role.

- Partnership working is not egalitarian or democratic in that some partners are more equal than others.

- Partnership working makes demands only on some (poorer) citizens to participate.

- There are difficulties if and when certain partners choose not to get involved or choose to withdraw their support.

These misgivings will be touched on briefly below and then more fully later in this chapter in the discussion of whether the new models of governance have really led to a new set of arrangements.

Partnership or centralisation?

It is arguable that New Labour's rhetoric of governance through partnership has been matched by reality. Some have argued that the actual effect has been a tendency to adhere to centralised state command and control rather than decentralised partnerships. For Driver (2005: 25), at least:

In practice, there has been a tension between the setting of objectives and targets by central government and the devolutionary tendencies of the other aspects of the government's public sector reform programme. The centripetal forces in British government and politics are well established: the Whitehall-centred culture of public administration; the dominance of the treasury in that centralist culture, the desire for governments (Labour no less) to 'get things done'; the 'control freak' tendency of New Labour brought from opposition into government.

Therefore, whilst New Labour has espoused the rhetoric of partnership and community engagement, and matched this in certain respects in its policy making and implementation, one can also still see examples of 'government by the centre'.

Discuss and Do   New Labour – steering or rowing?

In what respects is it possible to argue that New Labour has tended to centralise or, conversely, to devolve its governance arrangements?

What explanations can you offer for why New Labour might have taken each of these approaches?

In thinking about these two questions, refer to real social policy examples.

Some of the reasons why New Labour has wrestled with the tension between centralisation (hierarchical governance) and devolution (partnership governance) are that the benefits of centralisation include universalism, uniformity, shared risk and hands-on control, while the benefits of devolution include diversity of provision and providers, regional and local variations, choice, autonomy and greater local control.

In some respects, the question of whether New Labour's rhetoric of partnership governance is matched by action depends on whether or not any of the governance arrangements (markets, networks, partnership) that have purportedly replaced hierarchical governance have actually shifted the balance away from the nation state and central government. The chapter will now briefly look at this question, followed by a discussion of the usefulness of the concept of governance for understanding social policy.

Taking stock of governance

Has big (hierarchical) government necessarily disappeared?

Have we really moved away from hierarchical governance? As you will see from Box 6.6, the four models of governance explored in this chapter make particular claims in terms of the basis of the relationship, degree of dependence, medium of exchange, economic model, means of conflict resolution, culture and accountability mechanisms.

And yet the question remains as to whether any of the alternative models (markets, networks, partnerships) have really superseded hierarchical governance.

Box 6.6	Comparing hierarchies, markets, networks and partnerships

	Hierarchies	Markets	Networks	Partnerships
Basis of relationships	Employment relationship	Contract and property rights	Resource exchange	Sum greater than the individual parts
Degree of dependence	Dependent	Independent	Interdependent	Co-dependent
Medium of exchange	Authority	Prices	Trust	Negotiation
Economic model	Markets are inefficient and prone to failure. Need public control of public/merit goods	Individuals are utility maximisers, to which the market responds	Enable service development locally, backroom steering	Mixed economy, 'what works is what counts'
Means of conflict resolution and coordination	Rules and commands	Haggling and the courts	Diplomacy	Deliberation
Culture	Subordination	Competition	Reciprocity	Synergetic enlightened self-interest
Accountability	To the centre via the ballot box	Via the market and contracts	Self-referring	Upwards, downwards, outwards to all its constituent parts

Source: Adapted and amended from Rhodes (1999) and Kjaer (2004).

While we have seen changes to how government and the state both command (steer) and control (row), it is still government and the state that is controlling, notwithstanding the pressures upwards (supra-nationally), outwards (to other state and non-state actors) and downwards (to regions, localities, communities and individuals). Therefore, social policy is increasingly delivered via market, network and partnership mechanisms. Even so, the relationship between government and other organisations remains uneven or asymmetrical. Whether government chooses to promote policy development and delivery through markets, networks or partnerships, the power remains at the centre; that is, within government. As Richards and Smith (2003: 279–281) observe:

> It is extremely difficult to think of any human activity that is not in some way regulated by the state .... The failure of one form of governance is the establishment of a higher level of regulation .... [W]hilst there have clearly been changes in the policy arena, the state [hierarchical government] remains the most dominant political actor within the British political system. It has the most resources in terms of income (taxation), personnel, information, and force. Whilst there are more actors involved in the policy process and the relationship between them have changed, the relationship continues to be asymmetrical in that the central state continues to dominate when it chooses.

Government essentially sanctions the creation of public service markets and quasi-markets, the development of social policy networks and the promotion of partnerships to develop and deliver social welfare. It is arguably still the hierarchical state which determines whether market, network or partnership governance approaches are pursued.

How useful for social policy is the notion of governance?

While governance is a quite recent phenomenon within social policy writing, it has managed to attract some analysis regarding its usefulness. Daly (2003) and Fitzpatrick (2005), for example, have expressed concerns with the governance paradigm. Their three main concerns are:

- 'the literature is replete with wishful thinking in which a particular version of governance is proposed as the only version in order to advance the very changes the proposer wishes to see' (Fitzpatrick),
- 'governance shies away from identifying the main origins of change' (Fitzpatrick);
- 'governance is situated in the political rather than the social' (Daly).

Even so, both Daly and Fitzpatrick acknowledge that the focus on governance has provided insights into the developments in the administration of social welfare. Daly (2003) has provided a thorough account of the strengths of the governance paradigm, including the following:

- It provides an overarching framework within which to describe New Labour's approach to social/public policy making and provision.
- It concentrates specifically on policy making.
- It is useful in analysing the impact of policy changes in terms of the power of government at the centre as against that devolved. Governance helps to explain how the state now exercises loose-tight control – or more control over less (Rhodes, 2000).
- It helps to identify and explain the different levels at which policy is made and implemented – supra-national, national, regional, local, and community-based.
- It helps us understand how social policy develops and how welfare is reformed, along with an explanation of the reasons why.
- It concentrates on the role of the state in policy making and delivery.

Conclusion

This chapter has sought to explore the development from government to governance in the provision of social welfare. In so doing, it has suggested the following:

- The development of governance regimes is fuzzy and non-linear.
- The post-war welfare state was a hierarchical bureaucratic regime.
- The governments of the New Right sought to replace hierarchical governance with a market model by promoting privatisation, new managerialism and user involvement.

- New Labour sought to replace previous governance models with that of partnerships, incorporating aspects of new managerialism and choice within their approach.
- The notion of governance has its own weaknesses but is useful in providing a framework to explain New Labour's social policy and in explaining more generally how government now exercises power in the realm of social policy.
- The reality of governance may still be one based on hierarchy.

Annotated further reading

Though quite a recent phenomenon in social policy and welfare textbooks, there have been a number of useful writings on governance in a general sense, including Kjaer's *Governance* (2004), Newman's *Modernising Governance* (2001), Rhodes's *Understanding Governance* (1997) and Richards and Smith's *Governance and Public Policy in the UK* (2003). More general considerations of the task of managing in the public sector and/or public services include Butcher's *Delivering Welfare: The governance of the social services in the 1990s* (1995), Flynn's *Public Sector Management* (1997) and Pollitt's *Managerialism and Public Services* (1993). Critiques of the rise of management – or 'new managerialism' – include Clarke, Cochrane and McLaughlin in *Managing Social Policy* (1994), Clarke, Gewirtz and McLaughlin in *New Managerialism, New Welfare?* (2000), and Clarke and Newman in *The Managerialist State* (1997). A useful text that explores the complexities of partnership working is Glendinning, Powell and Rummery's *Partnerships: A Third Way approach to delivering welfare* (2002), while Ling presents a useful chapter on 'Unpacking partnership: health care' in Clarke *et al.*'s *New Managerialism New Welfare?* (2000). In terms of considerations of quasi-markets, the seminal work here remains Le Grand and Bartlett's *Quasi-Markets and Social Policy* (1993).

Chapter 7

Welfare within a fragmented state – devolved social policy

Objectives

- To describe the nature of devolved social policy arrangements in each of the three countries of Scotland, Wales and Northern Ireland.

- To explain why these arrangements are different for each of these countries.

- To explore the dilemmas posed by the development of devolved social policy arrangements.

- To describe how these social policy developments are leading to a divergence within British social policy and the directions of that divergence in relation to the four countries of the UK.

Introduction

> ... the full effect of [devolutionary] changes has yet to be seen, but there is clear potential for a significant and long lasting impact on the future shape of social policy. (Sykes *et al.*, 2001a: 3, in Chaney and Drakeford, 2004: 121)

The aim of this chapter is to explain the nature of the devolved arrangements for social policy across the countries of Scotland, Wales and Northern Ireland (Parry, 2008). The reason why the chapter does not also consider the situation in England is twofold. First, in many respects the focus of much of the rest of this book is United Kingdom and English social policy (similar though not synonymous with each other). Second, attempts at devolution within England, for example elected regional assemblies, have yet to bear fruit.

Whilst proposals for devolution of powers and responsibilities to the separate countries of the United Kingdom (England, Scotland, Wales and Northern Ireland) have been part of political debate in the UK arguably ever since the 'Act of Union' between England and Scotland of 1707, more contemporaneously it is arguably with the election of New Labour in 1997 that one has seen significant developments.

Attempts had been made to set up devolved structures in Scotland and Wales in the 1960s and 1970s under two previous periods of Labour governments, that of 1964–70

Box 7.1	Social policy under devolution ·

The very sad news in November 2006 that Fraser, the youngest child of Gordon Brown and his wife, Sarah, has cystic fibrosis highlighted in stark terms the possible impact of devolved social policy across the four countries of the United Kingdom. As the media reported at the time, the child was diagnosed because screening for the disease has taken place in Scotland since 2002 while similar screening was not due to be available in all parts of England until mid-2007:

'The baby was diagnosed as a result of a routine screening programme for all new borns in Scotland which is expected to be extended to England next year.

Screening is important because the sooner treatment begins the more successful it is likely to be. But there is no cure for cystic fibrosis.' (Sandra Laville and Alex Kumi, *The Guardian*, 30 November 2006)

Devolution, as one would expect, results in differing social policies for each of the four countries of the United Kingdom.

Stop and Think	Devolutionary pressures

What do you think might be some of the pressures or reasons for the people of Scotland, Wales and Northern Ireland to support moves towards devolution?

and 1974–79. In 1969, 'the Crowther (later Kilbrandon) Commission was appointed by the Labour government to consider devolution in Scotland and Wales' (Department for Constitutional Affairs website, www.dca.gov.uk, 2006). However, by the time its recommendations were published in 1973 and then formulated into the White Paper 'Democracy and Devolution: proposals for Scotland and Wales' in 1974, the Conservatives were back in government. Even so, the subject was re-addressed near to the end of the 1974–79 Labour government when, in 1978, the Scotland Act and the Wales Act were passed. These pieces of legislation required positive endorsements by the people of Scotland and Wales in respective referenda. For Scotland there was the added proviso that the demand for devolution had to be supported by 40% of the electorate (that is eligible to vote). Referenda were held in each of the two countries on 1 March 1979. The results were that neither country voted sufficiently to support the implementation of devolution. In Wales there was a resounding rejection, with 80% voting against devolution. In Scotland there was a majority vote (52%) for devolution but, with a 63% turnout, this amounted to only 33% of the electorate and was not sufficient to meet the 40% threshold (Department for Constitutional Affairs website, 2006).

In Northern Ireland there is a very different history and context to devolution compared with the other countries of the UK (see McLaughlin, 2005). It can be argued that Northern Ireland had already experienced a form of devolution or local rule when it came into existence in 1922, in that from 1922 to 1972 the province was partly governed directly by the Northern Ireland Parliament. However, this was put on hold in the early 1970s with the escalation of the 'Troubles' in the province. There was a brief return to devolved government in 1974, but this was very short-lived due to the opposition of the Ulster Workers' Council. In the early 1980s there was another period of limited self-rule, but this period was curtailed by the opposition of the nationalists. It was not then until the talks between Westminster and Dublin that ensued in the mid- to late 1990s that a return to devolved government became a prospect once more.

However, it was as part of New Labour's *Modernisation Agenda* in the late 1990s that we saw significant developments in devolutionary structures. What resulted was different proposals or arrangements for each of the four countries of the UK:

- England – regional assemblies.
- Scotland – elected Parliament and Executive.
- Wales – elected Assembly and Executive/Assembly Government.
- Northern Ireland – elected Assembly and Executive.

Whilst no real progress has been made in establishing regional assemblies in England – there was a referendum in the North East of England in November 2004 where the electorate rejected the chance to establish a regional assembly – all of the other countries have established devolved structures of one shape or form.

Stop and Think   An English Parliament?

Why do you think there has been little support up until now for devolution in England, either with the establishment of English Regional Assemblies or an English Parliament?

In both Scotland and Wales referenda took place in 1997. The Scots were asked an additional question of whether they supported their Parliament having tax-raising powers. The Scottish referendum took place on 11 September 1997 and the Welsh referendum one week later. The results of the referenda were as follows:

- In Scotland (with a turnout of 60.4%), 74.3% voted for a Scottish Parliament with 63.5% supporting the Parliament having tax-raising powers.
- In Wales (with a turnout of 50.1%), 50.3% voted for the establishment of the Welsh Assembly.

The development of the arrangements in Northern Ireland did not include the putting of a proposal to the people of Northern Ireland. Instead, it was left to the political representatives of the main political parties to decide on whether or not to move to devolved government. Extremely protracted negotiations did eventually culminate in the Good Friday/Belfast/Northern Ireland Agreement in April 1998 which, amongst other things, allowed for the establishment of the Northern Ireland Assembly.

Scotland

Scottish context

The Scottish Parliament came into being in 1999 following elections to the Parliament of its 129 members. These members serve a four-year period of office and are elected on the Additional Member System of proportional representation. The Parliament is similar to the Westminster model in that it elects a First Minister who then governs with the assistance of an Executive. The 1998 Scotland Act listed all those matters which were 'reserved' to the Westminster UK government and, by implication, declared that all matters not listed would be within the jurisdiction of the Scottish Parliament and Executive. In the main, the Scottish expenditure is funded by a block grant allocated by Westminster but, unlike in Wales and Northern Ireland, included among the Scottish Parliament's powers is the authority to vary income tax levels set by Westminster by up to 3%. (The matter of funding is dealt with below.) The Scottish Nationalist Party's position has long been for Scotland to have full independence from Westminster.

In 1999 Scotland duly saw its first directly elected government in and by Scotland for nearly 300 years. Because the elections to the Scottish Parliament are contested on a form of proportional representation, this led to the first two terms of the Parliament and Executive (1999–2003 and 2003–07) being controlled by a Labour and Liberal Democrat coalition. This was superseded in May 2007 with the election of a minority Scottish Nationalist Party (SNP) administration. Perhaps of equal significance is that, unlike for the UK Parliament in Westminster, the main opposition party during those first two terms was the (arguably left-of-centre) Scottish Nationalist Party, not the Conservatives. However, Hassan and Warhurst (2001: 214) have argued that a myth has developed over ideological differences between Scotland and England:

> ... the discourse of difference and uniqueness in the Scottish home rule debate is an important totem in the Scottish home rule debate, and is a key mobilising 'myth'. The degree to which Scotland is different has long been exaggerated: the fact that 80 per cent of Scots vote for centre-left parties does not mean they are centre-left voters, because parties mean different things in different places ... [and] most of the difference between Scotland and England could be accounted for by social class ....

Even so, as mentioned above, the 2007 elections to the Scottish Parliament resulted in a change in political control. The SNP became the largest single party (with 47 out of a total of 129 seats and one more than Labour) and, as such, were able to form a minority administration.

The Scottish devolution system is such that, under the 1998 Scotland Act, the UK Parliament retains responsibility for:

- foreign affairs;
- defence and national security;
- macro-economic and fiscal matters;
- employment and social security;

while the Scottish Parliament and Executive do have devolved powers for domestic economic and social policy, particularly in relation to:

- education and training;
- health and social care;
- housing;
- environment;
- law and home affairs;

- local government;
- police and fire services;
- agriculture, forestry and fishing;
- sport and the arts;
- transport;
- tourism and economic development.

However, even in these devolved areas, the UK Parliament remains sovereign in that it is able to override the Scottish Parliament. As such, the Scottish devolution system has been described by Parry (Parry, 2002: 315, in Stewart, 2004: 102) as one of 'incomplete responsibilities'. Even so, Keating (2005) has argued that 'the formal divisions of powers gives Scotland possibly the widest range of competences of any devolved or federated government in Europe'.

Funding of social welfare in Scotland

As with Wales and Northern Ireland, Scotland's public expenditure is mainly funded via the UK Treasury. It is calculated using something called the Barnett formula, a system devised in the late 1970s. Under this system, Scottish service areas are allocated funds on an historical basis, that is based on funding levels of the previous year plus or minus an increase for that year based in proportion to the allocations given to the equivalent departments and spending areas in England. The funding allocation is not, therefore, a needs-based assessment of expenditure. Nor is it based on the Scottish Executive or its predecessor, the Scottish Office, having to negotiate with the Treasury. Rather, that surrogate negotiation is done by all the UK spending departments and once their allocations have been agreed, the Scottish Executive receives a per capita equivalent (but can vire between budget heads, that is, move money from one area of spending to a different area). Other points to note are that 'Scotland has historically spent more per capita on public services than England ... particularly in health and in education' (Stewart, 2004: 103). Because of the way that the Barnett formula works, this greater level of expenditure remains part of the system. However, the difference in expenditure levels between England and Scotland, Wales and Northern Ireland has diminished over the last few years. This is illustrated by using the two examples of health and education expenditure. Between 1999/2000 and 2004/05, spending in both of these policy areas in the four countries converged:

- Between 1999/2000 and 2004/05 *education and training* spending grew in the UK as follows:
  - by 56% in England, from £695 per head to £1,086 per head
  - by 38% in Scotland, from £852 per head to £1,179 per head
  - by 47% in Wales, from £755 per head to £1,107 per head
  - by 43% in Northern Ireland, from £1004 per head to £1,435 per head.
- Between 1999/2000 and 2004/05 *health* spending grew in the UK as follows:
  - by 65% in England, from £818 per head to £1,350 per head
  - by 57% in Scotland, from £997 per head to £1,563 per head

– by 55% in Wales, from £917 per head to £1,421 per head
– by 57% in Northern Ireland, from £940 per head to £1,476 per head. (Adams and Schmuecker, 2006)

A difference that Scotland does enjoy from Wales and Northern Ireland is its ability under devolution to vary income tax by up to 3% from UK rates. However, it has yet to exercise this power. It may need to do so in the future, though, or to enact some of the policy changes in England such as moves away from universalism and marketisation, because if it does not it may find that the levels of funding afforded to Scotland from Westminster are insufficient for its purposes. As Keating (2005) has noted:

> to the degree that England moves away from universal services and towards differentiation and fees, the Barnett transfers to Scotland will be reduced. At that point welfare state divergences will require fiscal autonomy, so re-opening an important part of the settlement.

Policy divergence in Scotland

Prior to the establishment of devolution in 1999, Scotland had enjoyed policy differences since the Act of Union in 1707, particularly in areas of education, local government, law and religion. Education and health care remained distinctive even with the creation of the post-war welfare state. And, throughout the period of the Thatcher and Major reforms, Scotland generally continued to support the Labour Party at both UK general elections and local elections, such that, unlike in England, Scotland generally declined to implement the marketisation and privatisation agendas of the New Right governments of the 1980s and early 1990s. This has led Parry to conclude (Parry, 1998: 213, in Stewart, 2004: 104) that 'Scotland's welfare state remained more old-fashioned, better resourced and less privatised than England's'. Therefore, in some respects one can argue that Scotland already had a diverging social policy even prior to the vote for devolution in 1998, though some writers have questioned the degree of divergence post-devolution (Mooney and Scott, 2005).

According to Stewart (2004), Scotland's social policy has a greater emphasis on social justice and inclusion than England's and a greater belief in the traditional post-war welfare state. Even so, post-devolution, there is a belief in Scotland that it has unique problems which it now has the power to tackle: 'Scottish solutions to Scottish problems' (see Box 7.2 overleaf). One of the main areas where the Scottish Parliament and Executive are able to exercise power is in education. Here Scotland has witnessed an emphasis on raising standards, on guaranteed pre-school education (and not just care) for all three- and four-year-old children, the abolition of the right of schools to opt out of local authority control, and the abolition of testing for primary and secondary pupils at Key Stages 1, 2 and 3 and therefore the consequent production of school league tables. At secondary level, there is broad support for a comprehensive schools system as opposed to selection or centres of excellence. City colleges have not manifested themselves. More generally, private education only makes up less than 5% of provision (as against 10% in England). In higher education, up-front tuition fees were abolished by the Scottish Executive in 2000.

Box 7.2   **Divergence in public policies in Scotland since devolution**

- Pre-school education for all 3- and 4-year-old children
- Abolition of local authority opt-out of schools
- Abolition of school tests and school league tables
- Abolition of up-front tuition fees and the earlier introduction of means-tested bursaries in higher education
- Early implementation of smoking ban
- 'Free' personal social care for older people
- No pursuit of foundation hospitals or more general concordat with the private health sector

Source: Adapted from information in Stewart (2004).

Alongside this, financial support was provided for students from low-income families. Together these measures helped in the achievement of the 50% higher education participation rate target before their English counterparts. Since the May 2007 elections, the SNP minority administration has promised to implement plans to abolish the tax levied on university graduates in order that they pay back university fees along with plans to pilot free school meals for all children in their first two years of primary school.

In health policy, in 1999 the Scottish Parliament and Executive were faced with tackling some of the poorest health and greatest health inequalities in the UK and the European Union. Certainly Scotland as a whole has the poorest health of the four countries of the UK and some of the starkest health inequalities. Many analysts see this as being a consequence of poverty and inequality as well as the prevalence of poor diet and relatively high levels of smoking. The Scottish Executive's health policy agenda has, therefore, included an emphasis on public health and partnership working between agencies (not least across health and social care generally) and professionals rather than internal competition or the promotion of foundation hospitals or more general working with the private sector. PFI has not been pursued overtly in Scotland, unlike in England, by any of the Scottish Parliament administrations. Indeed, rather than contracting with the private hospital sector, one has seen examples in Scotland where the NHS has bought out private providers. In addition, the Scottish Executive decided to support calls for 'free' personal social care for older people. Following the May 2007 elections, the SNP minority administration has promised to implement its plans to abolish NHS prescription charges by 2011 and has overturned proposals to close a number of hospital A&E departments.

In housing, Scotland has been seen to follow the Westminster policy line, at least as far as the stock transfer of council housing. Large cities such as Glasgow have seen their council housing stock transferred to other housing organisations. The Scottish Executive, for its part, has encouraged this to as great an extent as has been the case in England (see Daly *et al.*, 2005). However, others, such as Edinburgh, have seen their tenants reject the option to transfer.

Generally, policy development in Scotland was seen to be conducted within a consensorial context for the first two terms of the devolved Parliament. Political consensus was necessary across the political parties, or at least within the Labour and Liberal Democrat coalition Executive between 1998 and 2007. Since May 2007, the SNP administration has had to take great care in trying to get its policies through the Parliament.

However, there was seen to be consensus within policy networks more generally in that professionals and academics, instead of being regarded as having vested interests, were included in discussions on policy matters during 1999–2007. As Greer (2006) has observed in relation to Scottish health policy (though it can be applied to Scottish social policy as a whole):

> Since devolution, a coherent Scottish policy direction has been developed . . . . Its broad tone was professionalism [and partnership]: trust in the professions who run the system, and lack of trust in, or even antipathy towards, the markets and managers . . . .

Whether this will continue under the SNP's administration will be interesting to observe.

Box 7.3	Cameron threatens to strip Scottish MPs of voting rights

Fury over Cameron plan to silence Scottish MPs

James Chapman, *Daily Mail*, Monday 29 October 2007

David Cameron has been accused of risking the break-up of the UK over his plans to stop Gordon Brown and other Scottish MPs voting on legislation that applies only to England. The Tory leader is pressing ahead with a radical constitutional overhaul – first revealed by the Daily Mail – to end the unfairness caused by the creation of the Scottish Parliament. Scottish MPs in the Commons can vote on issues that affect only England, but English MPs have no say on Scots issues decided in Edinburgh.

A series of controversial measures – including foundation hospitals and university tuition fees – have become English law thanks to the votes of Labour's 'tartan army' of Scottish MPs. Neither applies to Scotland.

At the next election, Mr Cameron will propose a ban on Scottish MPs having a say on laws relating to English schools, hospitals and a range of policy areas. The decision will make the constitutional dilemma – known as the 'West Lothian Question' – a key election battleground.

Labour deputy leader Harriet Harman called Mr Cameron's plans 'a very dangerous line of argument' . . . .

But polls suggest there is [a] growing concern in England over the way Scots are enjoying benefits and perks funded by taxpayers throughout the UK but not available south of the border. Scots do not pay tuition fees, and they get free personal care for the elderly and quicker access to new NHS medicines. One survey yesterday said one in three English voters favoured breaking the Union.

Reprinted with permission.

Scotland: conclusion

Scotland may be construed post-devolution as presiding over 'Scottish solutions to Scottish problems' but this needs to be tempered by the reality that constitutionally, financially and politically, it is still in many respects beholden to Westminster:

Discuss and Do   The West Lothian question

The question refers to the constitutional anomaly by which Members representing Scottish con-
stituencies (and on occasion from Welsh and Northern Irish seats) may vote on legislation which
extends to England, but neither they nor Members representing English seats can vote on subjects
which have been devolved to the Scottish Parliament. (http://www.parliament.uk/
commons/lib/research/notes/snpc-02586.pdf)

In other words, Scottish MPs are able to vote with all other MPs on pieces of legislation which
relate only to England. Similar legislation for Scotland would be decided upon by the Scottish
Parliament and, therefore, neither English nor Scottish MPs are able to vote on legislation that is
the responsibility of the Scottish Parliament. Hence, some commentators think this is constitutionally unfair.

We have already seen that:

• Scotland still enjoys higher levels of expenditure on social services than England;

• Scotland has diverged from England in various policy areas, such as over higher education tuition
  fees, school tests and league tables, and foundation hospitals.

What do you think of the situation? Is it a 'constitutional anomaly'? Should Scottish MPs be permitted to vote for the implementation of tuition fees, etc., in England even though the Scottish
Parliament and its MSPs will not impose it on the Scottish people?

• Constitutionally Westminster is still sovereign.
• Financially, Westminster allocates resources.
• Politically, the Scottish Labour (and Liberal)-run Scottish Executive were
  beholden to the British Labour Party – often referred to as an exemplification of
  the 'West Lothian question'.
• The election of the SNP administration in 2007 may lead to the emergence of a
  more obviously Scottish social policy.

Even so, Stewart (2004: 115–116) has observed a number of points of note in
relation to Scotland and devolution:

• Scotland already had a degree of devolution pre-1999 and this had led to a degree
  of policy divergence pre-1999.
• Scotland has traditionally spent more on social policy than England.
• Scotland generally has a consensus of support for public services and welfare provision and an antipathy to marketisation and privatisation to a greater degree
  than England.
• Divergence has been on the part of England, therefore, rather than Scotland [and
  Wales].
• Scotland's welfare provision has historically been financially advantaged (and
  would be even more so if it used its discretionary 3% income tax raising
  powers).

- Scotland has arguably been ruled by a centre-left administration with centre-left political opposition irrespective of which parties were in control.

However, there are others who have questioned the degree of divergence post-devolution (Mooney and Scott, 2005).

Wales

Welsh context

As seen in the introduction to this chapter, Wales voted only narrowly in favour of devolution in 1997. The Welsh devolutionary arrangements on offer, and subsequently implemented, were of a more limited nature than those proposed for and implemented in Scotland. Although the National Assembly of Wales (NAW) does not have primary legislative powers, it may make secondary legislation, that is orders and regulations relating to the implementation of primary legislation; and the Wales Act 2006 does allow for some national policy making, subject to referendum approval. The Assembly itself consists of 60 Assembly Members, elected via an Additional Member System of proportional representation.

Even though the Assembly enjoyed only limited powers at the outset, it has taken on responsibility for implementation of many of the major social policy areas. Those responsibilities that have remained with the UK Parliament and central government departments include:

- foreign affairs;
- defence and national security;
- macro-economic and fiscal matters;
- employment and social security;
- police and criminal justice system (unlike in Scotland).

Shared responsibility between the NAW and central government includes responsibility for crime and disorder partnerships and youth justice matters. Therefore, whilst its powers are not as wide as those of the Scottish Parliament, the NAW does have devolved powers for implementing domestic economic and social policy, particularly in relation to:

- education and training;
- health and social care;
- housing;
- environment;
- law and home affairs;
- local government;
- police and fire services;
- agriculture, fisheries and food;
- sport and the arts;

- transport;
- tourism and economic development.

Similarly to Scotland, the NAW is funded from Westminster via the Barnett formula but, unlike the Scottish Parliament, the Assembly does not have (income) tax varying discretion. This, along with the lack of primary legislative powers, amounts to a constitutional weakness in the view of a number of analysts (see Chaney and Drakeford, 2004). As such, it is argued that the NAW is beholden on the wishes of the UK Parliament:

> ... the settlement is precarious because it is completely dependent on the goodwill of the British government to find legislative time (always in short supply) and their willingness to accommodate Welsh concerns. (Hazell, 2003: 298)

However, as mentioned above, the Government of Wales Act 2006 has led to the Welsh Assembly having greater powers, including the separation of powers between the Executive (Welsh Assembly government) and the Parliament (the National Assembly for Wales).

Ideologically, the NAW has instilled a centre-left set of values, initially in the legislative framework underpinning the establishment of devolution in Wales and then, post-devolution, firstly by the Labour–Liberal coalition, then under Labour control in the second term, and most recently under the Labour–Plaid Cymru coalition since the May 2007 elections. Therefore, the ideological underpinnings are ones shaped, rhetorically at least, by Wales's socialist and libertarian past, and based on the principles of:

- universalism as opposed to means testing;
- equality rather than choice;
- public services rather than market-based provision;
- cooperation rather than competition;
- sustainability;
- social inclusion (see Chaney and Drakeford, 2004).

Despite the fact that the NAW has only limited discretion over the design and implementation of social policy in Wales, a distinctive and diverging set of social policy arrangements has emerged in the country post-devolution.

Policy divergence in Wales

One can identify a number of areas of social policy in which Wales, despite at the outset having only secondary legislative powers and no revenue-raising powers, has diverged from UK and English social policy direction (Box 7.4). This is evident across a variety of social policy areas including education, health, social care, housing and leisure. In health, one can see a distinctive Welsh approach, for example in its emphasis on primary care and public health, the establishment of 22 Local Health Boards which replaced the five Welsh Health Authorities, the rejection of Foundation Hospitals and PFI, the retention of Community Health Councils, free prescriptions and the abolition of all prescription charges in 2007, as well as the universal provision of free breakfasts in primary schools, and free school milk for infant school children.

In education, the NAW and Welsh Assembly government have piloted a post-16 Welsh Baccalaureate qualification, abolished SATs for Key Stage 1 (seven-year-old children), rejected specialist and faith schools, implemented (means-tested) Assembly Learning Grants for further and higher education students, and chosen not to implement higher education top-up fees, as well as introducing its own, distinctive, Welsh National Curriculum. In social care, Wales has seen the establishment of a Children's Commissioner and an Older People's Commissioner for Wales, and the introduction of free nursing home care for nursing home residents (but not free social care as yet, though this remains an aspiration). More general policy changes have included the implementation of free access to national museums and galleries, free local bus travel for pensioners and disabled people, and universal free use of leisure centre swimming pools for school children and older people.

Box 7.4	Divergence in public policies in Wales since devolution

- Education:
  - Piloting of post-16 Welsh Baccalaureate qualification
  - Abolition of SATs for Key Stage 1 (seven-year-old children)
  - Means-tested Assembly Learning Grants for further and higher education students
  - Non-implementation of higher education top-up fees
  - Introduction of its own Welsh National Curriculum
  - Rejection of specialist or faith schools
- Social care:
  - Establishment of a children's Commissioner for Wales
  - Establishment of an Older People's Commissioner for Wales
  - Free nursing home care for nursing home residents
- Health:
  - Emphasis on primary care and public health
  - Establishment of 22 Local Health Boards which replaced the five Welsh Health Authorities
  - Universal free breakfasts in primary schools
  - Free school milk for infant-aged children (not in England as well)
  - Rejection of Foundation Hospitals and PFI
  - Retention of Community Health Councils
  - Free prescriptions
  - Abolition of all prescription charges
- More general policy changes include:
  - Establishment of the Voluntary Sector Partnership Council and 21 interest networks
  - Free access to national museums and galleries
  - Free local bus travel for pensioners and disabled people
  - Universal free use of leisure centre swimming pools for children and older people

Source: Adapted from Chaney and Drakeford (2004).

Wales: conclusion

Despite the limited legislative discretion, a distinctive social policy agenda has emerged in Wales post-devolution. Chaney and Drakeford's (2004: 121) analysis of the first term of the NAW concluded that the Welsh Assembly is:

> if it is anything, a social policy body, ... that the Government of the assembly has gone about discharging its social policy responsibilities in a way that has an explicit set of articulated, ideological principles, which mark out that agenda as distinctive, ... [and] this distinctiveness has not been confined to policy formulation but has also been translated into the detail of policy implementation and regulation.

Adapting Stewart's (2004) concluding points in relation to Scotland and devolution, one can see, similarly to Scotland in many ways, that:

- Wales did not have a degree of devolution pre-1999.
- Wales has traditionally spent more on social policy than England.
- Wales generally has a consensus of support for public services and welfare provision and an antipathy to marketisation and privatisation to a greater degree than England.
- Divergence has been on the part of England, therefore, rather than Wales (and Scotland and Northern Ireland).
- Wales's welfare provision has historically been financially advantaged.
- Wales, similarly to Scotland, has been ruled by a centre-left administration with a significant degree of centre-left political opposition.

As we will see in the next section, some of these points also pertain to Northern Ireland.

Northern Ireland

Northern Irish context

Northern Ireland has a very different history and context to devolution to the other countries of the UK (see McLaughlin, 2005). It 'came into existence' as a small territory within the UK in 1922, as a result of the partition of Ireland, and comprises six of the nine counties of the old province of Ulster. It has a population of approximately 2 million. Many of its people and communities continue to have their lives defined and shaped by allegiances to either the Nationalist (in simple terms, mainly Catholic and proponents of a United Ireland traditionally) or Unionist (again in simple terms, Protestant and supporters of Northern Ireland remaining within the United Kingdom) cause. Unionist dominance has, arguably, played a part in determining a restricted citizenship for minority Catholic communities. Therefore, Catholic citizens have not traditionally enjoyed the same civil, political or social rights as their majority Unionist–Protestant counterparts.

In some respects the province has enjoyed devolution in one form or another for most of the time since its inception in 1922 (see Box 7.5). From 1922 to 1972, the territory was governed in part by the Northern Ireland Parliament, which had responsibility for all things with the exception of foreign policy, taxation and national security (McLaughlin, 2005). With the 'escalation of the Troubles' in the region in the late 1960s and early 1970s, a period of 'Direct Rule' from Westminster ensued which lasted for the period 1972–82. During this time there was a brief period of devolved government – the Power Sharing Executive – in 1974, but this was terminated by the strike action of the Ulster Workers' Council. During 1982–86 a further attempt at limited devolution was made, though the Nationalist political parties (SDLP and Sinn Fein) boycotted these arrangements. Direct Rule by Westminster returned for the next 13 years: 1986–99.

Box 7.5	An historical summary of governance in Northern Ireland
1922–72	The Northern Ireland Parliament
1972–82	Direct Rule from Westminster (see below)
1982–86	Northern Ireland Assembly
1986–99	Direct Rule from Westminster
1999–2002	Northern Ireland Assembly
2002–07	Direct Rule from Westminster
2007–	Northern Ireland Assembly

Note: the period of Direct Rule of 1972–82 was interrupted in 1974 for a short period by a period of devolved government – the Power Sharing Executive.

Source: Adapted from McLaughlin (2005: 109).

In April 1998 the Good Friday Agreement (also known as the Belfast Agreement or Northern Ireland Agreement) was reached between the various political parties in Northern Ireland as well as the UK and Republic of Ireland governments, to establish devolved government once again. This ruled for a period during 1999–2002. However, from 2002 up until May 2007, the Assembly was suspended and replaced by a period of Direct Rule from Westminster whilst attempts were made to gain agreement between the dominant Protestant (Democratic Unionist) and Nationalist (Sinn Fein) Assembly Members on a number of constitutional and policy matters. This was achieved in May 2007 and the Northern Ireland Assembly had its powers returned to it from Westminster.

Therefore, following the Good Friday Agreement in April 1998, the Northern Ireland Assembly (NIA) was established with the election of 108 members. The Northern Ireland Assembly (NIA) has a similar set of powers to that enjoyed by the Scottish Parliament. The Assembly has an Executive that is made up of a First Minister and a Deputy First Minister, along with a further 10 ministers. These Executive positions are allocated in proportion to the strength of the Assembly Members of each of the political parties. The Assembly's Executive has a number of committees in relation to each of the executive responsibilities and functions of the Northern Ireland Executive. Once again, the membership and chairperson of each of these committees is determined on party political proportionality grounds. The committees are responsible for developing, scrutinising and consulting on policy. However, as mentioned above, the NIA and Executive only ruled for a period from December 1999 until October 2002, with a number of periods of suspension in 2002, the most recent of which, on 14 October 2002, led to a significant period of Direct Rule by Westminster (see Department for Constitutional Affairs website, 2006). However, agreement between Ian Paisley's Protestant Democratic Unionist Party and the Nationalist Sinn Fein party led to the re-establishment of rule from the Northern Ireland Assembly at Stormont, with Ian Paisley as First Minister and Martin McGuinness of Sinn Fein as Deputy First Minister.

There are 10 spending departments within Northern Ireland, each of which is scrutinised by a committee of the NIA. The 10 departments are:

- employment;
- education and learning;
- social development;
- culture, arts and leisure;
- health, personal social services and public safety;
- finance and personnel;
- environment;
- enterprise, trade and investment;
- agriculture and rural development;
- Office of the First Minister and Deputy First Minister.

Policy divergence in Northern Ireland

The fact that Northern Ireland has had significant periods of self-rule since 1922 has shaped the area's social policy. In addition, the unique context of the 'Troubles' has obviously coloured all aspects of social policy in the region. This can be seen directly in two ways. First of all, it is arguable that because of the problems of sectarianism between nationalist and loyalist communities and groups, some of the cutbacks and changes in social welfare provision experienced elsewhere in the UK during the Thatcher and Major governments were experienced to a lesser extent in the province. Second, in the period when the Northern Ireland Assembly and Executive ruled during 1999–2002, because of the way that the Executive and Assembly are comprised on proportionality grounds and because the Nationalist and Unionist groups have very different perspectives politically, there has been a need to try to build consensus on social policy developments in order to get them through the legislature. As such, one can identify a number of areas of social policy where Northern Ireland, despite the limited period of self-rule in 1999–2002, can be seen to have diverged from UK and English social policy direction. This is apparent across a variety of social policy areas including education, health and social care, housing, social security and public transport.

In education Northern Ireland has a bifurcated system at secondary level (that is, the abolition of selective secondary schooling). In higher education, means-tested bursaries were introduced earlier than in England and Wales. In health and social services, Northern Ireland has had an integrated system for health and social care without local government involvement since the early 1970s. Instead there are four Area Health and Social Services Boards. In housing policy, social housing has been directed and overseen by the Northern Ireland Housing Executive since the early 1970s, again similarly to social care, outside the control of local government (unlike in the rest of the UK). Regarding social security, unlike for Scotland and Wales, the Northern Ireland Assembly does have powers in relation to social security, though any variance in expenditure would require Whitehall Exchequer approval and would have to be met from the existing block grant, since the NIA does not have revenue-raising powers. Therefore any proposed increases in social security expenditure would have to be at the expense of funding going to health, education, housing and so forth. The one significant piece of legislation that the NIA has passed relating to social security has been to permit the removal of driving licences from those parents who have defaulted on child support payments. Other social policy divergences have included the establishment of a Commissioner for Children and free public transport for pensioners. Keating (2002: 5, in McLaughlin, 2005: 117) summarised the key policy divergences, as set out in Box 7.6.

Box 7.6	Divergence in social policy in Northern Ireland since devolution

- Abolition of school league tables
- Establishment of a Commissioner for Children
- Decision to provide for a Single Equality Act, considering legislation on religion, sex, race and disability with the new provisions on sexual orientation and age
- Free public transport fares for older people
- Introduction of bursaries for students
- Decision to abolish the 11+ examination
- Loss of car licences for default on child support payments
- Distinctive public health strategy based strongly on social model of health
- Establishment of local health and social care commissioning groups

Source: McLaughlin (2005: 117).

Northern Ireland: conclusion

Northern Ireland's approach to social policy has been influenced by a number of factors, including self-rule for substantial periods between 1922 and 1999; the impact of the 'Troubles', not least in dampening the 'excesses' of the New Right Thatcher and Major reforms; and more recently the need within the Assembly and Executive for consensus in order to drive through social policy reforms. Indeed, McLaughlin (2005: 116) has argued that Northern Ireland has 'continually' been ruled by 'conservative' ideological administrations, firstly via Unionist 'governments' prior to 1998 and more recently via Unionist/Nationalist power sharing. Both of these have tended to gravitate to a lowest common denominator conservative agenda, for example with a focus on 'family values' and on the needs of the 'unambiguously deserving poor', that is, children and older people. This has been at the expense of a more overt social justice agenda to tackle poverty as a whole and social exclusion more generally. Again adapting Stewart's (2004: 115–116) analysis, Northern Ireland has exhibited a number of points of note in relation to devolution:

- Northern Ireland had a degree of devolution pre-1999 which in turn meant a degree of policy divergence pre-1999.
- Northern Ireland has traditionally enjoyed greater social policy expenditure than England.
- Northern Ireland, similarly to Scotland and Wales, generally has a consensus of support for public services and welfare provision and an antipathy to marketisation and privatisation to a greater degree than England.
- Divergence has been on the part of England, therefore, rather than Northern Ireland (and Scotland and Wales).
- Northern Ireland's welfare provision has historically been financially advantaged, though part of the 'peace dividend' has seen attempts to cut this.
- During its periods of 'self-rule' Northern Ireland has been ruled by 'conservative' ideological administrations, firstly via Unionist 'governments' prior to 1998 and more recently via Unionist/Nationalist power sharing, with a tendency to gravitate to a lowest common denominator conservative agenda.

Comparing the three devolved countries of the UK

In this chapter we have seen how each of the three countries of Scotland, Wales and Northern Ireland responds to the opportunities of devolution provided to its policy makers. Box 7.7 summarises these differing responses.

Some parts of the (particularly English-based) media have reported that the UK is very much becoming a tale of two differing sets of welfare regimes – see, for example, the article from the *Daily Mail* in Figure 7.1 on page 126.

Discuss and Do   A fragmented polity?

Having explored the contrasting social policy arrangements in the four countries of the United Kingdom, you may wish to think about the following questions:

- To what extent do we have a divergence of social policy across the four countries of the UK?
- Why do we have these different devolved arrangements?
- To what extent is it possible to argue that it is England that is forging a distinctive social policy whilst the other countries of the Union are defenders of the traditional principles and arrangements of the post-war welfare state?
- Should England, therefore, have its own devolved structures or has it already got them?

Box 7.7	Comparing the devolved arrangements in Scotland, Wales and Northern Ireland					
	Structural arrangements	Ideological underpinning	Areas of policy	Funding	Powers and responsibilities	Areas for which not responsible
Scotland (population 5 million)	Scottish Parliament with 129 members elected every four years on an Additional Member proportional representation system. First Minister and Scottish Executive govern the country	Centre-left (Labour–Liberal coalition) for first two terms followed by nationalist–leftist minority administration (SNP controlled)	Housing, education, health and social care	UK Parliament (via Barnett formula). Can use its power to increase or decrease income tax by up to 3% – yet to be exercised	Devolved powers for domestic economic and social policy, particularly for education and health, criminal law	Foreign affairs, defence and national security, macro-economic and fiscal matters, employ-ment, social security
Wales (population 3 million)	National Assembly of Wales with 60 members elected every four years on an Additional Member proportional representation system	Centre-left (Labour–Liberal coalition) for first term, followed by solely Labour controlled Executive in second term	Health, education, social services and social care, housing, as well as economic, agricultural and industrial development	UK Parliament (via Barnett formula); no powers to raise extra revenue	Does not have powers of primary legislation but can make secondary legislation. Does not have tax-varying powers	Defence, foreign affairs, taxation, employ-ment, financial and macro-economic matters, social security, criminal law, policing, immigration and asylum policy
Northern Ireland (population 1.6 million)	Assembly comprising 108 members and an Executive which includes a First Minister and Deputy First Minister	Lowest common denominator conservative consensus	Education, health and social care, social security, employment, trade and investment, environment, arts and leisure, agriculture	UK Parliament (via Barnett formula); no powers to raise extra revenue. Never had a system of Poll Tax or Council Tax, therefore even less income is raised locally than for rest of UK	Has powers to legislate in areas of transferred matters	Defence, foreign affairs, taxation, financial and macro-economic matters, policing, criminal justice, immigration and asylum policy

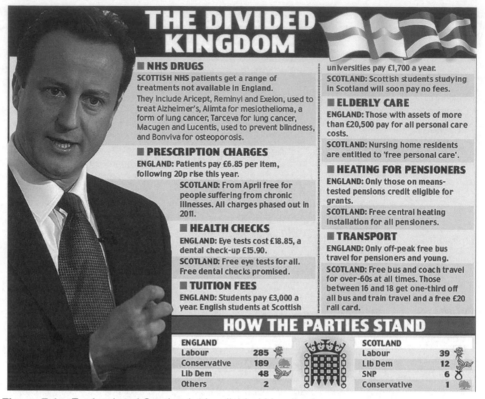

Figure 7.1 England and Scotland: 'the divided kingdom'
Source: J. Chapman (2007), 'Fury over Cameron plan to silence Scottish MPs', *Daily Mail*, 29 October 2007, p. 4. Reprinted with permission.

As such, all three devolved countries have to a greater or lesser extent shifted away from the Westminster (and therefore, by default, English) approach to social policy. Therefore, where there has been policy divergence, it is possible to argue that the devolved countries are defenders of the principles of the post-war welfare state from which England is diverging. For example, if one looks at health policy, Greer (2003: 213) has argued that 'England is the only country trying explicitly to reinvent its health services, and is certainly the only one that might reinvent the NHS out of existence . . . [and] this alone might strike people in Northern Ireland, Scotland and Wales as a reason for devolution'.

Among the implications of a set of devolved social policy arrangements is that UK citizens will experience a variegated citizenship, in which rights and duties are increasingly specific to the country of domicile:

> . . . a sign that Westminster, as a set of institutions and a political culture, may not be capable of creating or claiming for itself the oversight and guarantor of common standards of the citizenship role which . . . is required in the re-modelled 'looser' UK brought about by New Labour devolution and consequent policy divergence between the countries of the UK. (McLaughlin, 2005: 112)

However, as we have seen above, aspects of divergence between the four countries were apparent prior to New Labour's push for devolution. Even so, perhaps what we are starting to witness is a more marked divergence between England's social policy, still determined by Westminster, and those of the other countries of the

Union. Indeed, perhaps one needs to think of England as the one country among the four in the Union that is breaking away. On this point, Greer (2006) has argued that:

> The cardinal error of analysing devolved policies is to take England as a base-line. There is no reason to do so; different politics, debates and values and histories all conspire to mean that there is no reason to expect the four systems will line up neatly on some scale of achievement.

It is therefore possible to suggest that one is seeing a different focus and direction of travel for England as compared with the other three countries. We can generalise out of the depiction presented by Smith and Babbington (2006) of the differences in focus of the four countries in relation to health policy. They suggest a model with two dimensions, 'left–right' and 'unionist–nationalist' (see Figure 7.2). In this model, 'left' depicts a belief in the traditional values of the post-war welfare state such as universalism and equality, while 'right' represents a belief in the market, private financing, mixed economy of provision, and individual consumers; 'unionist' depicts a focus on policy being determined by the UK Parliament and government, as against 'nationalist' in which each of the Scottish Parliament and Northern Irish and Welsh Assemblies and their Executives determine policy and priorities. In this model, England is a country going in a particular direction all of its own, with policy shaped by the Parliament of the Union at Westminster informed by values of the right, while Scotland, Wales and, to a lesser extent, Northern Ireland are travelling in a very different direction based on traditional leftish-based values and national(ist) priorities (see Figure 7.1). The model is not unproblematic, however, particularly in the depiction and positioning of Northern Ireland as leftist and, therefore, universalist and championing of equality.

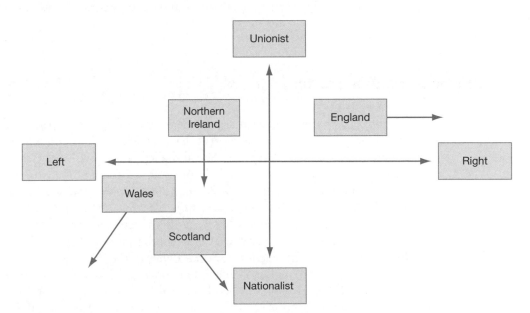

Figure 7.2 A left–right model of the four countries of the United Kingdom
Source: T. Smith and E. Babbington (2006) 'Devolution: a map of divergence in the NHS', in BMA, *Health Policy Review – Issue 2: Different Approaches to Reforming Health Services*, London: BMA. Reprinted with permission.

Conclusion

In conclusion, this chapter has set about explaining the nature of the devolved arrangements for social policy across the countries of Scotland, Wales and Northern Ireland. In so doing, we have looked at the context of devolution for each of the three countries, the financial arrangements, the nature of the devolved powers and what this has meant in terms of specific policy development and divergence in each of the three countries. This can all be summarised as follows:

• Scotland and Northern Ireland already had a degree of devolution pre-1999, leading to a degree of policy divergence pre-1999.

• Scotland, Wales and Northern Ireland, via the Barnett formula, have all traditionally spent more on social policy than England.

• Scotland, Wales and Northern Ireland generally have a consensus of support for public services and welfare provision and an antipathy to marketisation and privatisation to a greater degree than England.

• Scotland's welfare provision has historically been financially advantaged (and would be even more so if it used its discretionary 3% income tax raising powers).

• Scotland has been ruled by a centre-left administration with centre-left political opposition, while Northern Ireland has been ruled by conservative (and not necessarily pro-market) administrations both pre- and post-1999.

• Scotland, Wales and Northern Ireland have all started to develop their own specific social policy and welfare arrangements.

• If policy divergence is emerging between the countries of the UK, the fracture is between England and the three countries of Scotland, Wales and Northern Ireland.

Annotated further reading

Although there has not been a great deal written on the impact of devolution on social policy, some useful materials have emerged. A useful introduction is the chapter by Richard Parry on 'Social policy and devolution' in *The Student's Companion to Social Policy* (3rd edition, 2008). Comparative work includes Adams and Schmuecker's *Devolution in Practice 2006: Public policy differences within the UK* (2006) and Hazell's *The State of the Nations 2003: The third year of devolution in the United Kingdom* (2003). Works specifically on Scotland include a very useful text on the nature and level of devolution and policy divergence in Scotland by Mooney and Scott, *Exploring Social Policy in the 'New' Scotland* (2005); Greer's 'Policy divergence: will it change something in Greenock?' in Hazell (*op. cit.*); Hassan and Warhurst's 'New Scotland? Policy, parties and institutions', in *Political Quarterly*, vol. 72, no. 2 (2001); Keating's 'Devolution Briefings: Policy making and policy divergence in Scotland after devolution'(2005), published by the ESRC Research Programme on Devolution and Constitutional Change; and Stewart's '"Scottish solutions to Scottish problems"? Social welfare in Scotland since devolution' in Ellison *et al.* (eds), *Social Policy Review* 16 (2004). Works specifically on Wales include Chaney and Drakeford's 'The primacy of ideology: social policy and the first term of the National Assembly for Wales' in Ellison *et al.* (*op. cit.*). Works specifically on Northern Ireland include McLaughlin's 'Governance and social policy in Northern Ireland (1999–2004): the devolution years and postscript' in Powell *et al.* (eds), *Social Policy Review* 17 (2005).

Chapter 8

Paying for welfare

Objectives

- To introduce issues of taxing and spending on welfare programmes.

- To provide an understanding of the rationales for public financing and provision of welfare services.

- To provide an understanding of the developing relationship between public and private sectors in the financing and provision of welfare services.

- To explore recent trends in welfare spending, particularly under New Labour since 1997.

Introduction

This chapter looks at the financial underpinnings of many of the welfare state's social services and programmes.

> 'Capping "threat" limits council tax' ... 'Poorest households pay higher share of tax and get lower proportion of benefits, says study' ... 'Cameron firm on tax breaks for married couples' ... 'Tories to fight the next election without the promise of tax cuts' ... 'Chancellor rebuffs alcopop tax request rise'.

These are some recent headlines from a national newspaper. What all these stories have in common is that they refer to stories about taxes or public spending, or both – in other words, money. Another thing they have in common is that they suggest that these issues are political. These are issues which are close to the heart of political and public policy debate in Britain today. Political parties compete on their policies for taxes and public spending. Finally, most of the stories explicitly make a connection between spending, taxing and welfare in one way or another. (In this context the Conservative Party policy of encouraging marriage may be seen as welfare-affecting in some way in a broad sense, either welfare-enhancing or welfare-reducing, depending on your point of view.)

This chapter is concerned with money – the raising and spending of it for welfare purposes. Discussions of social policy sometimes give the impression that social policy is a 'free lunch', in which questions of resources for welfare purposes, how they are to be obtained and used, are ignored or played down. To a considerable extent, however, social policy is about money. It involves the mobilisation and deployment by governments of financial resources for welfare objectives. The cash, goods and services with whose distribution and redistribution welfare systems are concerned must be acquired and paid for somehow.

Although we might seem to be concerned in this chapter with economics and economic questions, economics being about such issues as the allocation of scarce resources among competing uses, 'opportunity cost' and so on, we are in fact concerned as much or more with politics as with economics. Taxation and public spending are essentially political, and the substance of contemporary politics is as much about taxation and public spending as about anything else. They are certainly economic issues, but not therefore issues which are best characterised in terms of the mainstream economic paradigm of the free market as a decision-making device for allocating resources or otherwise affecting their distribution. In fact they are about the use of political power to allocate resources, often, in the process, violating or overriding pure economic or free market criteria and values.

Some issues and questions

In the course of exploring the subject, we must consider a number of important issues. For example: What is the *justification* for public spending as opposed to private spending on welfare? A related issue is that of the economic *efficiency* of public and private spending on welfare. Is public superior to private spending, or vice versa? Another issue is that of *trends in welfare spending*, over time, and in comparison with other countries. Another is the *management and control of public spending* and the roles of such institutions as the Treasury, spending departments and Parliament in this. Innovations such as the Welfare to Work programme, the introduction of tax credits and the attempt to regulate social policy agencies through Public Service Agreements have made the Treasury a key social policy agency. We also examine different forms of revenue-raising – *income taxes*, *payroll taxes* such as *National Insurance*, and taxes on consumption. Finally, we consider, briefly, the taxing and spending policies of the Labour governments in office since 1997.

Stop and Think — Where does the money come from and where does it go?

List the various sources of funding that are available to society to assist in the funding of welfare.

What proportion of the UK's annual income do you think goes on welfare spending?

What welfare services do you think are the biggest spenders?

Public and private welfare spending

Our focus in this chapter is going to be on public, rather than private, spending, but we should recognise that not all welfare spending and provision in the UK is public.

It is both public and private. The term 'private' can mean a number of things. It can refer to welfare provided by commercial, 'for-profit', market-based organisations; it can refer to the *fees* and *charges* levied by public sector welfare providers for their services; it can refer to welfare provided by voluntary, 'not-for-profit' organisations or agencies; or it can refer to informal welfare provided by family, friends and neighbours. There is no area of public spending on welfare which is not also an area of private spending in some sense. In some cases private spending on a particular good or service is dominant, as in the case of housing. In others, such as health and education, public spending is dominant and the private sector residual. Some areas of income maintenance, such as the provision of income in unemployment, are dominated by public spending. Others, such as pensions, are, in the UK, heavily private. Social care is an area in which the private, informal, sector is dominant.

Private spending on welfare: commercial welfare provision

There is a great amount and variety of private, commercial, market-based welfare provision and financing in the UK, as in other countries. Education, health care, pensions, life assurance and long-term care are all examples. Individuals who choose to 'go private' rarely rely exclusively on the private sector. Private ('independent') schooling, for example, may be chosen by parents for secondary or sixth form education of their children but not for primary or tertiary level (there is as yet only one private university in the UK). For most users of private medical services, private provision supplements but does not displace public, NHS, provision. In some cases the State may subsidise, or partially subsidise, private provision. Independent schools, if able to claim charitable status, can take advantage of tax reliefs. Contributions to private pension schemes are eligible for income tax relief, as well as, in the case of company pension schemes, National Insurance rebates (see Chapter 17).

Private spending on welfare: fees and charges

Something which has been increasing in recent years is the raising of revenue for welfare spending through the imposition of *fees* or *charges* on users of public services. The introduction of university tuition fees, charges for eye tests, dentistry and means-tested support for long-term care are all examples of this. Charges – 'direct' or 'out-of-pocket' payments – are essentially private spending on welfare, even though the service is provided by a public agency most of whose funding is from public sources, such as taxes, National Insurance or the Council Tax. Fees or charges rarely or never cover the full cost of a service and are only a supplement to public spending. Charges for state-provided welfare are in fact nothing new. The charge for NHS prescriptions, for example, dates back to 1951, although removed for a short period by a Labour government in the 1960s. Charging for social services was widespread before the welfare state and continued to flourish subsequently, even under post-war Labour governments, despite the alleged incompatibility between universalist welfare state values and cash payment (Judge, 1980; Judge and Matthews, 1980: 1). Even 'model' welfare state countries, such as Sweden, make extensive use of charges for services such as primary health and hospital care (Ham *et al.*, 1990: 22; Rehnberg, 1997: 73).

Private spending on welfare: charity and the voluntary sector

Another area of private welfare spending is that of *charitable giving* and the *voluntary*, or *'not-for-profit'*, sector of service provision. The voluntary impulse has always been, and continues to be, important in welfare (Glennerster, 2003: 32–3). The total amount of charitable giving in the UK at around 1% of GDP – roughly £10 billion per year – is small by comparison with the amount raised by taxation and spent on social services, and also compared with that in other countries such as the USA, where it is around 2% of GDP, and of course not all of this is for what we would call 'welfare' – it includes donations to, for example, animal charities, the arts and religious organisations (Glennerster, 2003: 50–51). The voluntary sector is, nevertheless, valued as a dynamic and innovatory sector of the welfare industry.

Private spending on welfare: informal welfare

What we are going to discuss in this chapter is spending that is recorded as part of the *formal* economy and which will appear in national accounts statistics. We are completely ignoring the vast amount of *informal welfare* provision by the family in relation to social and health care and education. It must never be forgotten how important this is. Most of the welfare, in the broadest sense, produced in society is that produced by and within the family, not only by the nuclear family but by the extended family too, to some extent. We can also add to this welfare provided by friends and neighbours.

Why public spending?

Why do we typically have public spending on welfare? Why not leave it all to private markets and the private sector, commercial ('for-profit') or voluntary ('not-for-profit'), and the family? The argument that we explore in this section suggests that, in terms of the production and distribution of welfare, the market or commercial sector, the voluntary sector and the informal, family, sector 'fail'; that is, they do not ensure an amount and distribution of welfare that is 'ideal', or that we as citizens would like. This does not mean that they do not have a valuable role to play. It means that they must be supplemented, or even, in some areas of welfare, replaced, by the public sector – the state. We will begin by exploring some characteristics of the market.

In thinking about meeting our needs and wants for goods and services in a modern capitalist economy such as the UK, it is natural to begin by thinking of the *market* as an appropriate device for securing this. Many of our everyday wants are effectively met by private markets (as well as, of course, by the family). The market as a mechanism for supplying wants and allocating goods and services has been much studied by economists since the time of Adam Smith (1723–90) and his famous *The Wealth of Nations* (published 1776), who have identified many advantages and a number of disadvantages of the market mechanism. A basic feature of markets is the idea of *self-interested exchange between individuals for mutual advantage*. It is a system that is based on the profit motive, competition and choice, and, according to its defenders, possesses the characteristics of *dynamic efficiency*, *productive efficiency* and *consumer sovereignty* (Glennerster 2003: 17).

In their search for profit, individuals will establish businesses to meet consumers' wants; firms and businesses will innovate, creating new products and services; markets are thus said to be *dynamically efficient*. They will also attempt to organise production at the lowest possible cost – they are said to be *productively efficient*. At the same time they will be responsive to consumers' wants; in this sense there is said to be *consumer sovereignty*. Most productive activity in contemporary societies is apparently successfully carried on by markets, especially by comparison with the now virtually extinct 'planned' economies of the former communist states, such as the Soviet Union.

Given these supposed advantages, why can't social welfare be left entirely to the market? (As we have already seen, some welfare goods and services are supplied by the market.) Of course, there are a number of writers, of a liberal, free-market persuasion, who have favoured leaving most welfare to be provided by markets, the voluntary sector and the family (see Chapter 10). Milton Friedman's *Capitalism and Freedom* (Friedman, 1962) is a famous twentieth-century statement of the case for market provision of a range of social services, but on the whole, arguments of this type have never found general favour, at least in European countries.

There are two points to note about the description of the market given above. First, it is an idealised picture of the market and how it works. Few markets work perfectly in practice, and generations of economists have documented these failings in detail. Secondly, the market as depicted in this idealised way can be contrasted with the family, which is another major supplier of our wants and needs. The market embodies self-interested behaviour, whereas the family is supposed to embody altruism; it is about loving, caring, and taking care of others and their needs, rather than profiting from them. This too, of course, is an idealised picture. This is not, however, the place for a detailed examination of the family as a welfare agency (see Chapter 18).

'Market failure'

There are a number of explanations for public spending, in terms of economic *efficiency* as well as in terms of fairness or justice. The arguments against relying on private financing of welfare are therefore a mixture of economic arguments and ethical arguments.

A basic argument for some kind of public involvement in welfare provision is that, in relation to many aspects of welfare, there is, as we noted above, '*market failure*'. In other words, private markets for these goods sometimes or often do not work efficiently or fairly. (And private *insurance* markets for welfare, such as health insurance, also do not work efficiently or fairly.) Examples of market failure are the existence of what are called *public goods* and *externalities*. Another is that of *information failure*.

Public goods

Some welfare services possess some of the characteristics of *public goods*. A public good is a good which people cannot be excluded from consuming. They are not simply individual benefits which an individual can pay for and exclude others from consuming. Clean air is an example of a public good; defence is another. The existence of public goods provides arguments for public spending on some services, such as public or preventive health services. We all benefit from other people being healthy, in the sense of being free from infectious diseases. Disease control by public agencies via vaccination, screening and quarantine can therefore be justified. Not all aspects of health care have this public good character; much individual care and treatment provided by the NHS is presumably of benefit only to the individual and the individual's nearest and dearest (but see the remarks below on externalities and health care). Another example of an at least partial public good would be that of education. Education is not just a benefit to the individual who 'consumes' it, thereby acquiring skills and competences and enhancing their own earning power. We all benefit from other individuals being educated. There are collective or public benefits from living in an educated society, in which most people are literate.

Externalities

There is also a related problem of what are called *externalities*. These are the 'spill-over' effects of particular activities. Industrial pollution is a classic example of a 'negative externality'. (A public good might be viewed as a 'positive externality'.) A smoking factory chimney imposes a variety of costs, for example health costs and additional cleaning costs, on the surrounding area and its inhabitants, but from a pure free-market perspective, there is no way of dealing with these. The polluting factory owner imposes costs on others, but does not have to compensate affected people for these costs, nor is there any incentive for the owner to clean up the factory emissions. There is therefore a case for government to intervene to correct the externality, for example by regulation prohibiting smoke emissions. An example of this is the UK Clean Air Act of 1956 which limited smoke pollution in urban areas and is credited with significant improvements in the respiratory health of urban dwellers (Hall *et al.*, 1975: Ch. 13).

More recently, in the face of global, and not merely national, challenges such as climate change, the policy response to this kind of externality problem has shifted away from regulation and towards either taxation of the dangerous activity, as in 'carbon taxes', or 'carbon trading', which are schemes which effectively allow polluters to purchase the right to do so by buying 'carbon credits' from low- or non-carbon-emitting firms or businesses.

Traffic congestion in urban areas is an externality brought about by unrestricted, unpriced use of private transport. It has been dealt with by taxing or charging for the use of the externality-causing agent, as in the case of London's Congestion Charge, and by publicly subsidising the provision of public transport.

A further application of this approach to social issues is the idea of income redistribution as a way of overcoming the 'psychological' externality – distress to the non-poor who observe it – created by poverty and deprivation. One reaction to this particular externality, an individual one, is charitable giving, important in the nine-teenth century. The volume of charitable giving exceeded Poor Law budgets in this period, but much of it was haphazard and unregulated. Voluntary effort is thus inefficient and fails to overcome the externality. There is therefore a case for the state to take over and organise, via public systems of redistribution, involving taxation and cash benefits, the efficient correction of the externality (Glennerster, 2003: 20–21). It is also possible to view public health and education provision in the same way. We dislike, for example, the spectacle of untreated suffering produced by bad health and want to do something about it. (This is a point distinct from the one about public health as a way of correcting the externality imposed by infectious disease, referred to above.)

Information failure

Markets depend on information to work properly. As consumers, we need information about products – that they exist in the first place, for example, as well as something about their quality. No information, no market. Consider the vital role of advertising in a market economy. Advertising is information, but so is *Which?* magazine. This serves to remind us that information varies in terms of quality and accuracy. For many market-supplied products our knowledge is adequate, and there is a rough equality between supplier and consumer, a necessary condition for a market to work properly. For others, there may not be. Medical care is a well-known product about which consumers (i.e. patients) may be badly informed, relative to the supplier. This is an example of a service or product where the supplier – the doctor – knows more than the consumer about the latter's needs. There is information 'asymmetry'; consumers are vulnerable. It is hard to judge the quality of the 'product', and there is great uncertainty regarding outcomes of treatment (Glennerster, 2003: 22–25).

Private insurance and information failure

Another aspect of the information problem relates to insurance markets. Insurance is a way in which we attempt to deal with risks of various kinds and the costs that risks impose. Insurance is a way of sharing, or pooling, risks. Well-known examples of insurance are car insurance, house and home contents insurance, life insurance and health insurance. The insurance industry in a country like the UK is a dynamic one and is continually thinking up new risks for us to insure against. (It is now impossible, for example, to buy any piece of equipment of the 'white goods' or electronic variety from a large chain retailer of such goods without being offered an accompanying insurance policy; retailers in a highly competitive, low-margin business presumably now make more profit from selling the insurance than they do from selling the goods.) In relation to insurance, the imbalance between consumer and supplier can be the other way – the patient or insured person has more knowledge than the insurer about, for example, their health condition, and, further, has an incentive to conceal from the insurer the true state of their health and the seriousness of any condition they may be suffering from. This makes it difficult for the insurer to offer a premium to the insured person that is appropriately adjusted to the individual level of risk. The insurer will want to exclude 'bad' risks and will deny cover or will charge high premiums to customers perceived as bad risks, often people on low incomes. Public funding, through either taxation or social insurance, overcomes some of these inefficiencies of private insurance by expanding the size of the risk pool and preventing exclusions (Davis, 1998: 86–91).

These market failure and economic efficiency perspectives may seem an odd and unpersuasive way of presenting the case for state spending on welfare, and most people probably feel that such issues are better thought about directly in terms of some notion of justice, fairness or equality. It is nevertheless important to bear in mind that a useful defence of state provision can be constructed in terms of economic efficiency alone, without necessarily having to think about fairness, justice and equality. After all, people disagree about fairness, justice and equality, and what they require. These are challengeable, 'essentially contestable' concepts. 'Market failure' would seem, on the other hand, to be an empirical matter about which people could reach agreement. Social welfare economists such as Nick Barr are keen to stress the importance of constructing robust defences of state welfare provision in terms of such 'value-free' notions as economic efficiency and market failure (Barr, 2004).

Equity, fairness and justice

We turn now to consider some of the ethical objections to private spending and markets in welfare. An important deficiency of markets is that they are not necessarily 'fair'. Markets may respond to people's preferences – they may be 'consumer-responsive' – but only if these preferences are backed up by money, in other words, ability to pay. Services whose accessibility depends on ability to pay will discriminate against those on low incomes. This is a characteristic feature of free markets; they discriminate (another term is 'ration') by price. If equality is a social value and certain goods are held to be of great value to individuals, such that access to them should not be limited by inability to pay for them, then there is an argument for state funding of these services (see also Chapter 10, where these issues are discussed more fully). The context for this is, of course, that in a capitalist society, where incomes depend on market power and are unequal, access to goods and services is unequal (Davis, 1998: 47–50; Glennerster, 2003).

Discuss and Do Why have publicly funded welfare services?

Summarise and evaluate the reasons why the state may choose to fund welfare services.

The state and welfare

If the market 'fails', voluntary action 'fails' and the family 'fails' to provide for welfare needs to the extent that we would like, then we are, by elimination, apparently left with the state as an agency for overcoming these inadequacies. In other words, there is an argument for public spending and/or public provision of welfare services. It is possible to tell a story of the emergence of state welfare in the twentieth century in terms of the dawning recognition of the failure of non-state forms of welfare (see Chapters 1 and 2).

State 'failure'?

But the state itself can 'fail' too. 'State failure' has become an important issue in contemporary public policy making since the 1970s. A variety of failings of government have been identified. For example, public officials may be self-interested, rather than driven by concern for citizens' welfare. Professionals such as doctors and social workers may be similarly 'selfish' in their motivations. Voters, too, may be selfishly motivated rather than, as in the argument about externalities cited above, being sympathetically concerned about the welfare of the less well-off. Voting systems and political parties are imperfect means for representing citizen preferences (Glennerster, 2003: 25–30).

The alleged existence of state failure has been used by neo-liberal critics of state welfare as a rationale for privatisation and for the introduction of *quasi-markets* or 'internal' markets into hitherto publicly provided services, by, for example, the Thatcher and Major governments from 1979 to 1997, a policy continued to some extent by the Blair and Brown governments since 1997 (Le Grand and Bartlett, 1993; Glennerster, 2003: 25–32). This has been a highly controversial policy. It has also, on the other hand, led to attempts to manage the public services more rigorously, through targets, performance indicators, Public Service Agreements (see below) and payment and reward systems.

Public spending on welfare

Types of welfare spending: 'cash' and 'kind'

It is important to distinguish between benefits in *kind* – services such as health care, education, social care and housing – and benefits in *cash*. The latter are called '*transfer payments*' and include such things as Child Benefit, Income Support, Jobseekers' Allowance, state retirement pensions and the Pension Credit. These social security payments or cash benefits are *income transfers*, involving the transfer of purchasing power to individuals to meet their own needs. They have a variety of purposes including the relief of poverty, assisting individuals and families with the costs of child-rearing, and shifting income around over the life-cycles of individuals and families.

A vital distinction that we must introduce here is that between *financing* (or *funding*) of services on the one hand and *provision* or delivery of services on the other. These two things are separable. Governments may do both, or one or the other. (This is the theory – in practice no government anywhere provides a service without also funding that service.) The government may spend money on providing services directly, by employing front-line professionals – doctors, social workers, teachers – working in state-run agencies such as the NHS, local social services or schools. Public health care in Britain, for instance, is an example of a service funded publicly through taxes and National Insurance contributions which is also publicly provided via a public corporation called the National Health Service. Funding and provision are combined. Hospitals and health care producing assets are publicly owned, and health care personnel are public employees. State schooling in Britain is another example of combined funding and provision. Schools are owned by public authorities – local government in this case – and teachers are public employees.

Welfare services need not be directly provided by governments in publicly owned facilities using publicly employed workers. Governments may choose to provide the funding for services without engaging in direct provision. In fact, virtually all welfare states fund social services and programmes in some way or other, but service provision is often left to private providers. Most welfare systems are a mixture of public and private – the terms for this state of affairs are '*mixed economy of welfare*' or '*welfare pluralism*' – and this has long characterised systems such as those of the UK. Services may be provided by non-state organisations, either commercial (for-profit) or voluntary (non-profit).

In the Canadian health care system, for example, provincial governments pay for health care for their populations that is purchased from private providers – hospitals and physician practices. Financing of health care is mostly public, via federal and provincial taxes, but provision of hospital and physician services is mostly private. Coverage is universal and health care is available to all free of charge on the basis of need, as in the British NHS (Ham *et al.*, 1990: Ch. 6). Similar mixtures are found in many other health care systems, including those of Continental Europe, in which varying amounts of public and private in both funding and provision are combined (Freeman, 2000: Ch. 4).

In fact the public funding–private provision model is not unknown in Britain. Public money may be spent on goods and services purchased from the private sector, commercial or voluntary – for example, medical equipment and drugs bought by the NHS. A variation of this is the purchase of care services such as residential or nursing home care from private suppliers. Social care is often purchased from private-sector nursing and residential care homes by local authorities. These may be either commercial or voluntary organisations. Routine specialist surgical procedures, such as cataracts and hip replacements, have been purchased in bulk by the NHS from private suppliers – Independent Sector Treatment Centres (ISTCs) – since 2003 (see Chapter 12).

The question of public and private has been a hard-fought one in British social policy in recent years, since Conservative governments in the 1980s and 1990s sought to reform social services along more market-like lines, by means of competitive tendering, contracting-out and the attempt to devolve service provision via the creation of 'quasi' or 'internal' markets and semi-autonomous delivery agencies such as 'foundation' hospital trusts.

Private provision and fairness

It is important to realise that private provision of a service does not (necessarily) exclude equal provision for all on the basis of need and may be quite compatible with values of justice and fairness. Most developed-country health care systems provide universal coverage for their populations, while relying, often heavily, on private providers. It is public funding that is the key to ensuring universal access (Ham *et al.*, 1990: 107).

The growth of social welfare spending

In this section we look at some aspects of size and the growth of spending on welfare both over time and in comparison with other countries.

An important fact about welfare spending is its growth over time. From less than 5% of GDP or national income at the end of the nineteenth century, social welfare spending now accounts for around 25% of GDP. (Public spending as a whole now accounts for around 43% of GDP.) It is evident from these figures that social welfare spending therefore accounts for the greater part of public spending. In fact, the relative importance of welfare spending as a proportion of public spending has grown over time with the decline in such traditional areas of spending as defence and the payment of interest on the National Debt.

The picture throughout the twentieth century and into the twenty-first is one of seemingly relentless upward pressure to spend. If we look more closely at trends, however, we discern a pattern. Spending has not increased smoothly and continuously over the period but discontinuously, much faster in some periods than others. These are associated particularly with wars – the Boer War of 1899–1902, the First World War of 1914–18, and the Second World War of 1939–45. The period of the late 1960s and early 1970s also saw a period of faster than average growth. Since the mid-1970s, the picture has been one of greater stability and slower growth.

Explaining the growth of welfare budgets

How can we explain the inexorable growth of welfare spending? At a simple level, expansion in welfare budgets over time can be accounted for in terms of expanded coverage of the population and/or improved quality of benefits. If more people become entitled to benefits, and if benefit levels are raised and service quality improved, then quite obviously the cost of these benefits and services will increase. In education, for example, there has been an enormous expansion of higher education since the 1940s with the increase in the numbers of students and proportions of the population attending universities and other tertiary level educational institutions. (In this case some people might argue that increased coverage has not been accompanied by improved quality, at least during the most recent phase of expansion since the 1980s.) In the case of health care, the expansion of health care budgets since the creation of the NHS in 1948 is partly to be explained in terms of growth of the 'at risk' population, with the steady rise in the numbers of elderly resulting from increased life expectancy, and partly by expansion in the volume of what can be done for patients in the way of medical interventions due to improvements in medical technology.

Such explanations are true as far as they go, but do not provide a full explanation for spending growth. Various other explanations have been proposed.

War and welfare: the 'displacement effect'

Researchers in the 1960s drew attention to the importance of *war* as a promoter of higher public spending, and described the tendency of public spending to grow during wars, and then fall back afterwards, but not to the same level as pre-war, as a 'displacement effect' (Peacock and Wiseman, 1967). In other words, taxpayers became used to higher levels of tax during the war years and it was therefore easier for governments to maintain support for higher levels post-war. Wars of the twentieth century were different from earlier wars such as the Napoleonic wars when spending rose to relatively high levels, in that welfare spending increased. Social welfare programmes expanded during the First and Second World Wars, and in fact were part of the war effort. The two major wars of the twentieth century involved the mobilisation of the civilian population on an unprecedented scale, and improvements in social conditions in order to improve morale and the quality of 'human capital' were deemed essential.

Democracy

Another explanation for the growth of spending is provided by the growth of democracy since the late nineteenth century, which involved extensions of the vote to groups of the population hitherto excluded such as the working class and women (Pierson, 1998). These groups, it is argued, were more likely to favour government spending on welfare.

The 'relative price effect'

Another factor explaining the growth of welfare budgets is the so-called '*relative price effect*'. This refers to the relative increase in the price of publicly supplied services compared with privately produced ones, arising from the differing opportunities for productivity improvements in the two sectors. Productivity (output per worker) increases faster in the tradeable sector of the economy, which is mostly private and includes manufacturing industry. Pay in the private sector is linked to productivity. There is greater scope for productivity increases in the private sector, especially in manufacturing industry. Pay in the private sector ought therefore to increase faster than in the public sector. If the wages of workers in the public sector are, however, linked through comparability-based collective bargaining with those in the private sector, then the relative cost of providing a given volume of service will increase faster in the public than in the private sector. There will therefore be a rise in the GDP share of publicly provided services.

We can see, therefore, that the growth of welfare budgets is a complex, multi-causal phenomenon.

The composition of welfare spending

Official measures of public spending

Current official public expenditure documentation distinguishes between various aggregate measures for control and reporting purposes. *Departmental Expenditure Limits* (DELs) are firm three-year spending limits made up of departmental expenditures which can be planned and prioritised. These include, for example, NHS expenditure on hospital services. *Annual Managed Expenditure* (AME), on the other hand, is departmental expenditure which cannot be subject to such firm multi-year limits; it includes entitlement programmes like social security, which obviously cannot be capped, because spending fluctuates according to, for example, levels of unemployment, the numbers of people reaching retirement age, and levels of sickness and disability. It also includes NHS expenditure on primary health care. These two measures – DELs and AME – together make up *Total Managed Expenditure* (TME) (H.M. Treasury, 2006a: Ch. 1, Appendix D).

Another distinction is that between *current* spending and *capital* spending. Capital spending is basically investment – in new buildings and equipment, for example. Current spending is regular outgoings – for example, staff salaries and wages.

An important point to note is that in looking at trends over time, figures on public spending can be presented in various ways: for example, in terms of *cash*, unadjusted for inflation; in '*real*' terms, in which the figures are adjusted to take account of price changes – in other words, inflation – over the period under consideration and reduced to a common price basis; or in terms of a *percentage of GDP* or national income. The final measure gives a better idea of the change in relative importance of some particular item of spending over time as a component of the national economy.

Table 8.1 shows some trend data for selected years from the 1960s to the present for public spending as a whole, in cash, 'real' and GDP percentage figures, using both current expenditure and TME measures. The TME measure includes capital

Table 8.1 Public expenditure aggregates, 1967–68 to 2007–08

	Public sector current expenditure			Total Managed Expenditure		
	Cash (£ billion)	Real terms* (£ billion)	Percentage of GDP	Cash (£ billion)	Real terms* (£ billion)	Percentage of GDP
1967–68	13.7	165.0	33.6	18.2	218.2	44.5
1977–78	58.0	238.7	38.4	69.1	284.6	45.8
1987–88	166.4	301.7	38.6	181.5	329.1	42.1
1997–98	303.4	356.6	36.8	320.9	377.1	38.9
2004–05	455.4	455.4	38.7	491.0	491.0	41.7
2005–06	481.9	472.0	39.4	523.2	512.4	42.7
2006–07	506.7	484.5	39.6	552.3	528.1	43.1
2007–08	534.2	497.6	39.5	582.8	542.8	43.1

*Real terms figures are the cash figures adjusted to 2004–05 price levels using GDP deflators.
Source: H.M. Treasury (2006a) *Public Expenditure Statistical Analyses Cm 6811*, Table 3.1, p. 42, London: The Stationery Office. Crown copyright material is reproduced with the permission of the Controller of HMSO and the Queen's Printer for Scotland under the terms of the Click-Use Licence.

spending as well as current spending, which is why it is larger than the 'current' figures in the left three columns of the table. The figures for the last two years, 2006–07 and 2007–08, are planned figures, rather than actual spending ('outturn'). It will be noted that the 'real terms' figures take account of changes in the value of money and are expressed in terms of the 2004–05 price level.

Tables 8.2, 8.3 and 8.4 exhibit trends in public spending, focusing on welfare spending for three selected years, but also including defence expenditure and public order and safety, which is essentially expenditure on criminal justice or law and order (categories such as transport, agriculture, EU contributions and environmental protection have been omitted, but the totals including these excluded items

Table 8.2 Total expenditure on services by function, 1987–88 to 2005–06 (cash, £ billion)

	1987–88 outturn	1996–97 outturn	2005–06 estimated outturn
Defence	19.1	22.1	31.1
Public order and safety	8.0	16.3	30.1
Employment policies	3.0	3.0	3.9
Housing and community amenities	4.5	5.3	9.3
Health	20.4	42.9	89.4
Education and training	21.2	37.8	69.7
of which: Education	*20.4*	*36.4*	*67.9*
Social protection	55.1	112.1	170.3
Total expenditure on services	176.9	302.6	502.4
Total Managed Expenditure	181.5	313.9	523.2

Source: H.M. Treasury (2006a) *Public Expenditure Statistical Analyses Cm 6811*, Table 3.2, p. 43, London: The Stationery Office. Crown copyright material is reproduced with the permission of the Controller of HMSO and the Queen's Printer for Scotland under the terms of the Click-Use Licence.

Table 8.3 Total expenditure on services by function in real terms*, 1987–88 to 2005–06 (cash, £billion)

	1987–88 outturn	1996–97 outturn	2005–06 estimated outturn
Defence	34.6	26.7	30.5
Public order and safety	14.6	19.8	29.5
Employment policies	5.3	3.6	3.8
Housing and community amenities	8.2	6.4	9.1
Health	36.9	51.9	87.6
Education and training	38.5	45.7	68.3
of which: Education	*37.0*	*44.1*	*66.5*
Social protection	99.8	135.7	166.8
Total expenditure on services	320.7	366.2	492.1
Total Managed Expenditure	329.1	379.8	512.4

*Real terms figures are the cash figures adjusted to 2004–05 price levels using GDP deflators.
Source: H.M. Treasury (2006a) *Public Expenditure Statistical Analyses Cm 6811*, Table 3.3, p. 44, London: The Stationery Office. Crown copyright material is reproduced with the permission of the Controller of HMSO and the Queen's Printer for Scotland under the terms of the Click-Use Licence.

Table 8.4 Total expenditure on services by function as a percentage of GDP*, 1987–88 to 2005–06 (based on cash)

	1987–88 outturn	1996–97 outturn	2005–06 estimated outturn
Defence	4.4	2.9	2.5
Public order and safety	1.9	2.1	2.5
Employment policies	0.7	0.4	0.3
Housing and community amenities	1.0	0.7	0.8
Health	4.7	5.6	7.3
Education and training	4.9	4.9	5.7
of which: Education	4.7	4.7	5.5
Social protection	12.8	14.5	13.9
Total expenditure on services	41.0	39.1	41.0
Total Managed Expenditure	42.1	40.6	42.7

*For years 1987–88 to 2004–05 using GDP consistent with the latest figures from the Office for National Statistics (published 29 March 2006).
Source: H.M. Treasury (2006a) Public Expenditure Statistical Analyses Cm 6811, Table 3.4, p. 45, London: The Stationery Office. Crown copyright material is reproduced with the permission of the Controller of HMSO and the Queen's Printer for Scotland under the terms of the Click-Use Licence.

are shown in the bottom two rows of each table). Between them, they convey information about the composition of welfare spending in the same three ways as Table 8.1 – in cash terms, in 'real' terms, and as a percentage of GDP.

It will be noted that over the period 1987–88 to 2005–06 there have been some significant shifts in the volume and composition of welfare spending, with some interesting differences in trend between services. Thus defence shows a rise in cash spending over the period but a fall in spending in real terms, and an even more dramatic fall of around 40% as a percentage of GDP. Spending on 'public order and safety' has risen sharply according to all three measures, roughly quadrupling in cash terms, doubling in real terms and increasing by around a third as a percentage of GDP. We can see, from the three tables, that spending on 'social protection' – another name for social security – takes by far the largest share of the social spending budget. As a share of GDP it has fallen from its peak in the mid-1990s, although increasing in cash and real terms (it reached a peak of 15% of GDP in 1993–94). This is largely due to falls in unemployment since then, in a context of buoyant economic growth (i.e., rising GDP). Social protection is followed in scale by health care and education, with social care and housing trailing behind. Health has done especially well by comparison with other programmes, undergoing the most dramatic rise of all over the period of over 50% in terms of GDP share, while education has risen at a more modest rate of around one-sixth of GDP.

These programmes differ with regard to the influences on them and their degree of controllability. Thus social security is an almost entirely 'demand-led' programme. It is difficult to control in the short run because entitlements are difficult to eliminate or modify, although governments such as those of the Conservatives in the 1980s attempted to tighten eligibility criteria for some benefits (Atkinson and Micklewright, 1989). Spending is driven by factors which, in the short run, are beyond government control – unemployment, increasing life expectancy, divorce and family break-up. Other programmes, such as areas of health care and education, are easier to control. These differences are reflected in the differing spending control procedures operated by the Treasury.

These changes in the composition of spending and its division between the various programmes over the years are to some extent the product of deliberate political choices. The sharp rise in health spending, for example, is partly due to the fact that governments have responded to voters' perceived wants for more and better health care. It is also determined by factors specific to the health care industry, such as advances in medical technology and an ageing population. The rise in law and order spending reflects the increasing importance of such issues for voters and the public, and the belief of politicians of all parties that law and order is an election-winning (or losing) issue. Social spending has grown as a proportion of public spending, with declines in such areas as defence spending and, with Conservative privatisations of the 1980s, support for nationalised industries. In the 1950s, for example, defence spending accounted for 10% of GDP. With the disappearance of Empire and the decline in Britain's 'world role', and, since 1991, the ending of the Cold War, defence spending has declined in importance, permitting growth in other areas of spending.

Planning and controlling welfare spending: the role of the Treasury

Revenue-raising powers in the British system lie with central government, which has sole power to initiate taxing and spending proposals. Unlike the US Congress, the UK Parliament has little independent power to initiate or change taxes and spending, its role being largely confined to examining, approving and voting on Finance Bills and expenditure estimates introduced by the government. It does have, however, an important monitoring role (see below).

Local government, too, is weak in the UK. Unlike state- and provincial-level local governments in federal political systems such as those of the USA, Canada, Australia and Germany, it is subject to central control and has little financial independence. (A partial exception to this is the devolved governments for Scotland, Wales and Northern Ireland set up in the UK since 1998 – see below.)

The key agency in the planning and control of social spending is the *Treasury*, the most important department of British government, headed by the Chancellor of the Exchequer. The planning of individual departmental spending involves bilateral negotiations between the Treasury and departmental officials and politicians. The present system has evolved from the process established in the 1960s known as PESC, which was designed to place spending decisions on a more rational footing (Heclo and Wildavsky, 1981; Pliatzky, 1984; Glennerster, 2003: 183–185). Since 1998 the process has taken the form of two-yearly spending reviews, in which departments are given budgets for a three-year period beginning the year after the review (Glennerster, 2003: 186). The first of these reviews in 1998 was labelled a 'comprehensive' spending review, as is the latest one published, a year late, in October 2007. Spending reviews have subsequently taken place in 2000, 2002 and 2004.

In planning spending, the Treasury adheres to two rules – the so-called 'sustainable investment rule', which is the rule that public sector debt is limited to a maximum of 40% of GDP, and the 'golden rule', which is the rule that government borrowing takes place only to invest, that is, to spend on infrastructure (roads, hospitals, etc.)

rather than current spending, as on wages or benefits (Glennerster, 2003: 187–188). The purpose of these rules is to assist in creating a stable climate for economic activity and to promote confidence among business decision-makers and financial markets in the government's commitment to low inflation and economic growth. It should be noted that the Treasury has lost *direct* control over one key tool of economic management, with the Chancellor's decision to devolve power to set interest rates to the Bank of England and its Monetary Policy Committee in 1997 (Keegan, 2004). There is some flexibility in the interpretation of the two rules, however, and the Chancellor has some room for manoeuvre in determining when the rules have been conformed to.

Another important element in the system is Parliament, and particularly the House of Commons. Scrutiny of departmental spending and decision-making is one of its most important functions. Such scrutiny takes place via parliamentary agencies such as the National Audit Office, working especially in conjunction with the Public Accounts Committee of the House of Commons, and via a system of House of Commons Select Committees which shadow particular Departments of State. There is, for example, a Health Select Committee, which shadows the Department of Health in England, conducts inquiries and investigations of departmental policy, and publishes reports.

The basis of public expenditure planning at present is in terms of cash. The present system of cash planning has its origins in the spending control crises of the mid-1970s. Prior to that, spending was planned in 'volume' terms, that is, in specific amounts or levels of service 'inputs' – for example, numbers of teachers, doctors, nurses, social workers, and health and education infrastructure – regardless of the cash cost of these inputs. No regard was had to the effects of inflation on the costs of resources. With the high rates of inflation of the mid-1970s, this system became unworkable. A system of cash limits was established by the then Labour government and the cash planning system has been refined by successive governments.

In the 1990s the Treasury came to assume a more active role in relation to spending departments and programmes (Glennerster, 2003: 189) as a result of the Southgate Report on Treasury functions. This argued that the Treasury should have an active role in improving the supply side of the economy. Unemployment, for example, had come to be defined as a micro-economic rather than a macro-economic policy issue. The new view held that the Treasury had a role in encouraging improvements, perhaps through increased spending, or changed spending priorities, for example, relating to taxes and benefits. The Treasury's role in relation to claims

---

Box 8.1   **Public Service Agreements**

Public Service Agreements are a New Labour government innovation, particularly associated with the Chancellor from 1997 to 2007, Gordon Brown. They are essentially a device for central control over how money is used by service delivery agencies, national or local. All spending for particular functions detailed in the biennial comprehensive spending reviews that have taken place since 1998 comes with a Public Service Agreement attached, listing targets to be obtained in terms of specified outcomes to be brought about by the spending in question, usually with an associated timetable for implementation.

for new spending should not simply be negative or restrictive (Glennerster, 2003: 189). This approach has led to important changes in, for example, social security, with the introduction of tax credits, and the partial integration of the tax and benefit systems. We have also seen the introduction of Public Service Agreements (see Box 8.1).

Local expenditure, territorial devolution and formula funding

An important aspect of public expenditure planning and allocation is its distribution across the territorial area of the UK. With the exception of social security, which since the 1940s and the abolition of the Poor Law has been almost entirely a national service, with uniform benefit scales and entitlements across the whole country, welfare resources are spent and services delivered by local agencies – in the case of health by the NHS, and in the cases of education, housing and social care by local government. A further important aspect of this issue has been the administrative, and now political, devolution of power that has taken place in the UK since 1998 (see Chapter 7). There are now devolved governments for Scotland, Wales and Northern Ireland. Administrative devolution has a longer history, and the Scottish education system, for example, has always differed from the English one ever since the creation of the Union in 1707. This has meant that the four component countries of the UK have to some extent followed their own priorities for the delivery of such services as health, social care and education. Political devolution has given a further boost to this pursuit of sub-national priorities.

British governments have long employed systems of *formula funding* for sharing out resources across the territorial area of the UK. A formula in this context is simply a way of establishing a relationship between the needs of an area – which could be a local authority area, a health authority area, or a unit as large as the whole of Scotland – and the financial resources required to meet those needs. An obvious criterion of need is population size, and this is the basis of all funding formulas. Formula funding dates back to the 1890s, when a population-based formula for allocating Scottish expenditure was introduced. The allocation of resources by the Treasury to Scotland, Wales and Northern Ireland has been governed since the 1970s by a formula known, after its creator Joel Barnett, the Labour Chief Secretary to the Treasury from 1974 to 1979, as the Barnett formula. It is now commonly acknowledged that such social services as education and health in Scotland, Wales and Northern Ireland are more generously funded than those in England. These 'spending inequalities', though disputed, for example, by the Scottish Nationalist government in Scotland, have developed gradually over a long period, reflecting a variety of political pressures, and are not solely or even largely a principled response to, for example, higher levels of need in the other countries of the UK. The Barnett formula was supposed to regulate and gradually reduce these inequalities within the UK, but has not succeeded totally in this.

Within the territorial area of individual UK countries, such as England, formula funding is also used to allocate money from central departments to local agencies. Thus the Department of Health in England uses a formula to distribute money to agencies of the English NHS such as Primary Care Trusts, which commission health care for their resident populations. The present formula is a modified descendant of the so-called RAWP formula, introduced in the 1970s to fund English hospital services. These formulae are essentially based on population, weighted to reflect the particular needs of localities. Similar formulae are used in the other UK countries, and to fund the services provided by local government, which in the UK has only limited tax-raising powers of its own, and are in any case subject to stringent central control by the Treasury.

Taxation

Both taxing and spending need to be considered together in thinking about welfare. Government spending, to the extent that it is not funded by fees, charges or borrowing, must be paid for through taxes of some sort. Taxation can itself also have important effects on people's welfare, and a tax policy is in many respects also a welfare policy. Taxation policy will affect the distribution of income and wealth in a society, for example, and therefore its degree of inequality. In the 1970s the top rate of income tax on earned incomes was 83%; it is now 40%. At the same time, inequality, as measured by the distribution of income, has increased markedly in Britain, although reductions in tax rates are only part of the explanation for this phenomenon. Another reason for examining both taxation and spending is that they have become even more entwined since 1997 with the New Labour government's tax credit programme to assist the working poor.

The 'social division of welfare': taxation and fiscal welfare

The entwining of tax and spending policies goes back a long way, however, and the social scientist Richard Titmuss called attention in the 1950s to the connection between the two, and the welfare implications of taxation, in his famous article 'The social division of welfare' (Titmuss, 1958: Ch. 2). *Tax allowances* for earners with children, for example, were introduced in 1909, long predating the universal Family Allowance (now called Child Benefit) which was introduced in 1945 (Titmuss, 1958: 46; Hall *et al.*, 1975: 160). (A tax allowance is a band of income not subject to tax. In other words, it effectively raises the threshold – the starting-point – at which individuals start to pay tax on their income, with the result that they pay less tax.) This is an example of what Titmuss called *'fiscal' welfare* (Titmuss, 1958: 42); another example is described in Box 8.2. Tax allowances are effectively equivalent to a cash subsidy. Of course, at that time and for long after, only a small proportion of the employed population paid income tax, so this was essentially a form of welfare for the middle class. Other examples include tax allowances on contributions to private pension schemes, and, until recently, the tax relief allowed on mortgage interest payments (Glennerster, 2003: 51–52).

Box 8.2	**'Fiscal welfare'**

Another example of 'fiscal welfare' is tax reliefs for private education. Independent schools have traditionally enjoyed charitable status, which entitles them to reliefs from taxation (such as VAT), unlike commercial organisations. This is an implicit subsidy to the users of private education, generally, of course, the better-off. The Charity Commission, a public body which oversees all charitable organisations, has recently begun policing the independent school sector more rigorously. Such schools are now obliged to demonstrate that they provide 'public benefits' in order to justify their charitable status (Boone, 2007). 'Public benefits' could include providing scholarships for pupils from less well-off backgrounds and sharing facilities with local state schools.

Direct and indirect taxes

Taxes can be '*direct*' or '*indirect*'. Income tax is a well-known direct tax. Others include corporation tax (a tax on business profits) and inheritance tax (a tax on the assets – known as the 'estate' – left by those who have died; of course the tax is paid by the inheritors of the dead person's assets, not by the dead person). Taxes on economic activity such as Value Added Tax (VAT), and duties on tobacco and alcohol, are indirect taxes.

National Insurance

There are also so-called '*payroll' taxes* such as, in the UK, National Insurance contributions, paid by employers and employees, which are specifically linked to the financing of welfare programmes. Taxes raised for particular purposes are termed 'dedicated', 'earmarked' or 'hypothecated' taxes. National Insurance is not quite that, because it is used to finance a number of social security and health programmes, rather than a single one. (The TV licence might be regarded as an example of such a dedicated or earmarked tax.) National Insurance finances a range of social security benefits such as the state retirement pension, Jobseekers' Allowance, Invalidity Benefit and Widowed Mothers' Allowance, and also contributes in part to the financing of the National Health Service. Employers act as collection agencies on behalf of the government. Although employers, as well as employees, pay contributions, it is not clear that they really bear the cost of these contributions. Economists disagree about the real *incidence* of social insurance contributions, some arguing that employers merely pass the cost of contributions on to consumers in higher prices, others that they are a deduction from employees' wages. It should be noted that the *tax base* for National Insurance contributions is narrower than that for income in general, because it is levied only on earned income.

'Sin' taxes

Another important role for taxes is that of deliberately and intentionally modifying people's behaviour. A tax may be both revenue-raising and behaviour-regulating.

Thus taxes on harmful substances such as alcohol and tobacco – sometimes known as 'sin' taxes – are at least partially intended to discourage consumption of these substances, as well as raising revenue. In other words, they have a health-promoting function. Fuel taxes are similarly designed to encourage economy in vehicle use, the use of smaller cars and so on, and play a role in protecting the environment by reducing polluting emissions. Such effects may be numbered among the welfare aspects of taxes along with the more obvious redistributive effects of taxation.

Stop and Think

Do you think motorists should be taxed more heavily than they are currently?

It is interesting to reflect that governments in the UK and elsewhere are foregoing potentially useful sources of revenue by prohibiting and criminalising particular activities such as recreational drug distribution, sale and use, rather than permitting them and then imposing taxes such as VAT or special duties on them. The current drug control regime allows drug-dealing criminal entrepreneurs to amass superprofits on which they pay no tax, involving losses to the Treasury, in addition to the substantial losses foregone by failing to tax the sale and distribution of the product. At the same time, policing this regime involves costs.

Stop and Think

In the light of the discussion in an earlier section about 'externalities' and 'public goods', how do you think a British government might justify its drug control policy?

Of course, all taxes modify people's behaviour intentionally or unintentionally to some extent. Income tax may affect people's willingness to work, work harder or take higher-paying jobs. Economists, characteristically, disagree about the effects, some arguing that it may reduce people's willingness to work, others that it may have the opposite effect of encouraging people to work harder in order to earn a post-tax income that allows them to maintain a particular standard of living.

An important aspect of this question is the incentive or disincentive effects that taxes, in combination with loss of benefits as incomes rise, that people on low incomes may experience. It has been suggested that unemployed people, for example, may experience disincentives to take relatively low-paid work, if this results in loss of benefits as well as liability to pay income tax and National Insurance contributions. Concern about this issue has led to the present government's adoption of such policies as the Minimum Wage and Tax Credits (Glennerster, 2003: 46–49, 149–150).

An important development after 1979 and the election of the Conservative government in that year was the beginning of a shift away from direct taxes towards indirect taxes. Income tax rates were reduced and rates of VAT increased from 8.5% to 17.5%. This was to have significant distributive consequences, because income tax is a '*progressive*' tax, bearing more heavily on the better-off. Taxes such as VAT, on the other hand, are '*regressive*', in that they bear more heavily on those with lower incomes. The Conservatives reduced the top rate of income tax, initially from 83% to 60%, then a few years later to 40%, where it remains. The standard rate of income tax was also steadily reduced, from 33% to 30% and eventually, under New Labour, to 22%. The Conservatives sought from 1979 to 1997 to reduce the tax burden as far as possible, although they did not succeed in this. Historically high rates of unemployment in the 1980s and 1990s and other social and demographic changes ensured that the tax burden remained at above 40% of GDP for most of this period, falling to below 40% in the mid-1990s.

Taxation and political legitimacy

The level and kind of taxes we pay has continued to be a live issue since the election of New Labour in 1997. For politicians and governments it is an issue of great sensitivity. An inquiry into taxation established by the Fabian Society, a left-leaning think-tank close to the Labour Party, noted in the foreword to its report that 'Taxation is once again the central issue in British politics' (Commission on Taxation and Citizenship, 2000). The issue is one of whether people are willing to pay the taxes to finance the volume and quality of public services that they claim to want. In the 1990s it had appeared to some that the limits of people's willingness to pay taxes had been reached, and that either public spending on services must be cut, or alternative ways of paying for these services must be found, involving perhaps some degree of privatisation or the use of fees and charges. This was to some extent the basis of the Conservatives' policies on public spending and taxation.

Although it seems that since 1997 and the advent of New Labour this dilemma has been successfully and relatively uncontroversially resolved in favour of higher taxes and spending (see the following section), particular taxes and tax rises have generated controversy. A rise in fuel duties in 2000 precipitated a civil disobedience campaign. This has been successful in discouraging the Treasury from raising fuel duties. More recently rises in a local tax – the Council Tax – produced a backlash in which pensioners in some local authorities chose to go to jail rather than pay what were claimed to be unaffordable increases.

More recently still, the Inheritance Tax (IHT) seems to have become an object of public resentment, much aired in middle-market tabloid newspapers. Liability to pay Inheritance Tax has become much more common over the last few years, with rises in house prices pushing many estates above the tax threshold (which was still £300,000 in 2007). Although the tax threshold has been index-linked every year, the index has increased much less than average annual increases in house prices. This pressure from particular newspapers to abolish IHT or increase the threshold significantly, along with the promise from the Conservatives that they would increase the threshold so that IHT would only be paid on homes worth more than £1 million, resulted in Gordon Brown's Labour government's announcement in the autumn of 2007 that it would double the threshold to £600,000.

Stop and Think

Do you think that Inheritance Tax should be abolished, or the threshold for it increased, or do you think it is too generous and should be reduced?

The Fabian inquiry referred to above noted the sense of disconnection felt by many people from taxes paid and services received. People do not know where their tax money goes and are sceptical about government's ability to spend it appropriately. Re-establishing a connection was therefore a priority, and the inquiry recommended improvements in transparency and accountability and greater progressiveness in the tax system, and suggested that consideration be given to earmarking taxes for specific services such as the NHS (Commission on Taxation and Citizenship, 2000). Although not directly influential – the New Labour government has not accepted these specific proposals – the Fabian Report can be regarded as providing a general intellectual case for the value of taxes and spending and therefore an underpinning for the present government's tax and spend policies.

More recently, the Institute for Fiscal Studies, a public finance think-tank, has established a high-profile and wide-ranging review of the tax system to explore new challenges facing governments seeking to raise revenue, including those posed by globalisation, the increased mobility of capital and the impact of the EU (Houlder, 2006a). Taxation therefore continues to be a complex and difficult issue for governments and citizens alike.

Stop and Think

Do you think you ought to pay more tax, or less?

Do you think there are people who should pay more taxes and others who should pay less? What reasons would you give to support your argument?

New Labour's tax and spending policies

The 'New' Labour party under the leadership of Tony Blair, which won the 1997 General Election, inherited the Conservative commitment to low taxes and appeared to be committed to maintaining a low tax and spending stance. New Labour promised in the 1997 election to adhere to Conservative spending targets, and to maintain this commitment for two years (Labour Party, 1997: 13). Fiscal rectitude seemed to be the watchword of the then Chancellor, Gordon Brown. Labour were fearful of electoral backlash on the tax issue, mindful of the presumed effect of spending promises in the 1992 election on the result, the Labour Party's fourth successive election defeat.

'New' Labour – how new?

Is New Labour really 'new', however, as regards taxing and spending? Much of the enormous volume of mostly censorious commentary on New Labour politics in the last 10 years from the left has argued that New Labour is little different from its Conservative predecessors, owing most of its public philosophy, including, presumably, its attitude to public spending, to alien neo-liberal influences. This is the position taken by many left critics of New Labour such as David Marquand, Colin Leys and Colin Crouch, who argue that New Labour's approach to governance has eroded the values of the public sphere which prevailed in Britain during the twentieth century, and particularly since 1945 (Leys, 2001; Crouch, 2004; Marquand, 2004). Whatever the truth of these general propositions about the character of New Labour governance and public philosophy, they can be questioned insofar as they are supposed to apply to what is surely a core component of the public sphere, which is taxing and spending.

An alternative view about New Labour after 10 years in office is that it is more traditional than it appears. It may be regarded as, essentially, an old-fashioned social democratic 'tax and spend' government, not much different from its 'Old' Labour predecessors of earlier decades. Public spending, as a share of national income, has risen steadily since 1997 and has already reached 43% of GDP (it was 36% of GDP in 1996, the last full year of Conservative government). This is different from the experience of the Conservative years, because expansion under New Labour has occurred during a period of sustained economic growth and low unemployment. Although New Labour pledged in 1997, and thereafter, that top rates of income tax would not rise (Labour Party, 1997: 12), the tax burden has in fact steadily increased to match the increase in public spending. So-called 'stealth taxes' – taxes or tax rises that are invisible or unnoticeable – have worked to raise money for higher spending on public services, and have been more effective for this purpose than any increase in top rates of income tax could be. The phenomenon of 'fiscal drag' has reappeared to play a part in boosting tax revenues. Fiscal drag is an easy and painless way for governments to raise taxes while concealing the fact. As incomes from earnings rise, as they have done in a period of uninterrupted economic growth like that experienced since 1993, people pay more tax. They also move from lower to higher income tax bands. The tax thresholds between bands are indexed – increased – annually, but in line with prices, rather than average earnings (which have increased faster than prices over the period), ensuring that earners will therefore, over time, be dragged into higher tax bands. This has ensured that income tax yields have been buoyant. The increase in National Insurance contribution rates for both employers and employees in 2002 is another stealth tax. Yet another has been steep rises in Council Tax to pay for local authority-provided services (rather less successful as a stealth tax, since there has been some recent public backlash, particularly from pensioners).

It should be noted that the rising tax burden under New Labour does not constitute a 'soak the rich' strategy of a kind that was pursued to some extent in the 1970s. It is the tax burden on average incomes and a little above that has increased, not that on the highest incomes. Income inequality in the sense of the position of the richest 1% of the population relative to the rest has continued to widen, but the poorest have caught up to some extent with the average (Hills, 2004; Hills and Stewart, 2005; Stewart, 2005a).

Labour has clearly prioritised public spending, and been prepared to accept the fiscal consequences of doing so. In this respect there is 'clear blue water' between Labour and the Conservatives, at least until the advent of David Cameron as Conservative leader at the end of 2005, since when there appears to have been a shift in Conservative policy. The Conservatives consistently favoured tax cuts under Cameron's predecessors. Sustained economic growth and low unemployment would have been regarded by the Thatcher and Major governments as providing opportunities for tax reductions, not, as under New Labour, for tax and spending increases. Labour's tax policies appear to be in accord with the public's expressed desires for improved public services, and Labour in this respect has been closer to mainstream public opinion than the Conservatives. Just as the Blair-led Labour Party contesting the General Election in 1997 felt it necessary to adapt to what was, probably wrongly, perceived to be the prevailing policy climate on taxation and social welfare that had been created by the Conservatives, so a Conservative Party led by Cameron a decade later is apparently being forced to adapt to the climate of higher public spending, and associated public expectations, that have been shaped by a decade of Labour rule. What looks like recent Conservative repositioning under Cameron on taxing and spending issues suggests that New Labour's lack of openness about its stance on taxes may not be electorally necessary, and that the government could afford to be more honest with the public about its intentions and priorities.

This is not, however, the whole story as far as New Labour's tax policy is concerned. While increasing the tax burden for the better-off, the government has sought to reduce the tax burden on people with lower incomes. One of the key issues for poor and low-income people is the very high marginal rates of tax faced by people seeking to move off benefits, re-enter the labour market, or take higher-paid jobs, because of the effects of the combination of tax rates and benefit withdrawal as people's incomes increase. This is the so-called 'poverty trap'. The government has dealt with this in various ways. A new lower-rate tax band of 10% was introduced. (This was scrapped in the 2007 budget.) Various schemes of tax credits – Working Families Tax Credit, later replaced by Working Tax Credit and Child Tax Credit, and Child Care Tax Credit – have been introduced, which are designed to 'make work pay' by providing in-work financial support, mainly for people with family responsibilities. Tax Credits are administered by H.M. Revenue and Customs (the Pension Credit for the retired is an exception – it continues to be administered by the Department for Work and Pensions) and involve an integration of taxes and cash benefits which is supposed to result in a more coherent approach and a reduction of 'poverty trap'-type disincentives.

There are, however, flaws in the current management of the tax credit scheme which have come to light since 2005. Under- and over-payment have resulted from the difficulty of tracking changes in people's financial circumstances as their incomes fluctuate, and hardship has been caused to some families as H.M. Revenue and Customs has clawed back overpayments.

Whether New Labour's attempt to relieve the tax burden on low-income people has succeeded is a matter of controversy. A paper from the Centre for Policy Studies, a right-leaning think-tank, claimed that the tax take paid by the poorest fifth of households actually rose from 6.8% of the total in 1996–97 to 6.9% in 2004–05, while their share of benefits fell over the same period from 28.1% to 27.1%. The middle fifth of households appeared to be gainers on both the tax and benefit sides, according to the study. These findings were disputed by the Treasury, who argued that the tax paid by the bottom fifth of households had fallen by 1.4% since 1997–98, and that income inequality had also fallen over the period (Houlder, 2006b).

Stop and Think

Do you think that New Labour has been too timid in its approach to taxation? Should there, for example, be higher taxes on the better-off?

Conversely, why might New Labour have been reluctant to tax the better-off more than it has?

The private sector and public–private partnerships

A further, highly controversial issue, in England, is that of *public–private partnerships*. One area of public–private collaboration is that of the *Private Finance Initiative* (PFI), which involves the use of private capital investment in the building and equipping of infrastructure, such as NHS hospitals. The PFI programme was launched by the Conservatives in 1992, but the scheme failed to be implemented and no PFI deals were signed. The scheme was successfully relaunched after 1997 under New Labour. A large number of PFI deals have now been signed with private-sector consortia. There are advantages for governments in these arrangements, the main one being a reduction in public-sector capital costs, which henceforth no longer appear in the government's capital budget. Other claimed advantages include better project management – faster and more efficient building and commissioning of new schemes to time and on budget, things rarely achieved in the days of public-sector commissioning. PFI schemes have been bitterly attacked by the government's critics, mainly on the left, who argue that ostensible, up-front budgetary savings do not translate into overall lifetime savings on the projects. Public-sector agencies such as the NHS are essentially renting the assets from the private consortia for a fixed period, until they eventually revert to public ownership, and it is argued that the costs in the long run are higher (House of Commons Health Committee, 2002).

Conclusion

Welfare spending has enjoyed something of a golden age under New Labour, at least since 2000. The future is less certain, however, and the very high rates of increase enjoyed by such services as the NHS between 2000 and 2006 are ending. The next few years will see slower rates of increase. Despite these, by historical standards, very generous funding increases, problems of overspends and deficits have appeared in some public agencies, such as some NHS Primary Care Trusts, which suggests the existence of inadequacies either in financial control at a local level or in the broader financial framework of these services. There are questions about how far funding increases have actually brought about service improvements, as opposed to increasing staff remuneration and costs. New Labour has helped to reinvent the public sector, and re-establish public spending as a valid and worthwhile activity, after years when this was in doubt and the policy emphasis was on tax-cutting. Questions still remain, however, about acceptable levels of taxation, about how much the British population are willing to pay for improved services, and about the value for money and efficiency of public spending.

This chapter has introduced you to some issues in the financing of welfare and spending on social programmes. Having read the chapter, you should have some understanding of:

- why welfare services are publicly financed and provided;
- taxation and public spending issues as they relate to welfare programmes;
- the developing relationship between public and private sectors in the financing and provision of welfare services;
- recent trends in welfare spending, particularly under New Labour since 1997.

Annotated further reading

The best general introduction to issues of welfare spending, accessible and easy to read, is Howard Glennerster's *Understanding the Finance of Welfare: What welfare costs and how to pay for it* (2003), which adopts a mainly service-by-service approach. A straightforward introduction to some contemporary issues in public spending and the public sector in general is provided by the BBC economics correspondent Evan Davis in his book *Public Spending* (1998). A dated but still useful introductory book on public expenditure is Andrew Likierman's *Public Expenditure: The public spending process* (1988). A tougher, more advanced and comprehensive discussion of finance and expenditure issues is provided by Nicholas Barr's *The Economics of the Welfare State* (various editions, most recent edition 2004). Recent, fairly high-level discussions of public spending and social policy are presented in Deakin and Parry's *The Treasury and Social Policy: The contest for control of welfare strategy* (2000) and in Glennerster *et al.*'s *Paying for Health, Education and Housing* (2000). For a clear and balanced discussion of the problems of the present tax system and possible reforms, from a centre-left perspective, see the report of the Fabian Society's Commission on Taxation and Citizenship: *Paying for Progress: A new politics of tax for public spending* (2000).

For more argument on the 'state versus the market' controversy, in addition to the above, see some of the chapters in Wilson and Wilson (eds.), *The State and Social Welfare* (1991) and Helm (ed.), *The Economic Borders of the State* (1989), which discuss these issues at a fairly high level. On 'quasi-markets', see the collection edited by Le Grand and Bartlett (1993).

For analysis of public expenditure decision-making and the role of the Treasury, see the classic account by two American academics, Heclo and Wildavsky, in *The Private Government of Public Money* (1981). Howard Davies has edited an interesting collection of lectures delivered to an academic audience by former Chancellors from Healey to Clarke, with question and answer sessions (Davies, 2006). There are also valuable insider accounts of Treasury life by Leo Pliatzky, a former Treasury civil servant (Pliatzky, 1984), by Joel Barnett, a former Labour Chief Secretary to the Treasury (Barnett, 1982) and by the former Conservative Chancellor of the Exchequer Nigel Lawson (Lawson, 1992). A dated, but useful, short book by two journalists, essentially transcripts of BBC Radio 4 programmes involving interviews with Treasury officials and politicians, is Young and Sloman's *But, Chancellor* (1984).

It is well worth your while acquainting yourselves with official and parliamentary documentation on these issues. This can sometimes be more down-to-earth and revealing than many academic discussions. You could look at the Treasury's 2007 Comprehensive Spending Review itself, published in October, downloadable from the Treasury's website (H.M. Treasury, 2007). As well as a general statement on public spending priorities for the next three years, it contains separate annexes on spending plans for each government department. All the other spending reviews back to 1998 can also be downloaded. For a commentary on the issues underlying the 2007 Comprehensive Spending Review, which is also illuminating on public spending issues in general, see the report by the House of Commons Treasury Select Committee published in June 2007. The accompanying volume of verbal and written minutes of evidence is also interesting (House of Commons Treasury Committee, 2007). These are downloadable from the Treasury Committee's website. The Treasury Committee has also undertaken and reported on many other investigations into the work of the Treasury over the years, online versions of which are available from about 1997 onwards.

Concluding comment to Part II

This part has attempted to establish the contemporary environment within which social policy is currently developed and delivered. We have examined the political, structural and financial realms within which social policy is formulated and implemented and against which it may be evaluated.

As we have suggested, this is an environment in a process of continuing flux and change, not least because of the impact of devolved structures in Scotland, Wales and Northern Ireland. However, New Labour's approach has not only introduced devolved structures that have complicated the process of policy making but also developed an arguably distinctive approach to the governance of social policy. This has seen a shift from the New Right's emphasis on markets to one based on partnership, including the increased involvement of non-governmental bodies. The way that social welfare is financed and which areas of social welfare receive what levels of expenditure have also been explored, not least in relation to New Labour's approach, which has arguably resulted in significant increases to the funding of particular welfare services such as education and health.

Part III

Theorising and researching welfare

Introduction to Part III

Social policy as a discipline increasingly draws on a range of theoretical perspectives in order to explain not only who gets what in a range of welfare situations, but also how welfare states arise and what explains changes in welfare over time. The three chapters in this part introduce you to ideas about social policy and to the most frequently used theoretical approaches in the study of welfare.

Chapters 9 and 10 outline the basic theoretical approaches used in the study of social policy. Chapter 9 provides an introduction into the ways in which social policies can be appraised and evaluated theoretically. The principles underlying social policies are examined, looking at particular concepts and principles, such as need, justice, freedom, equality and citizenship, and the theories in which these concepts are employed.

Chapter 10 complements the preceding chapter on welfare theory by examining, in a historical way, the development of ideas about the state, society and social policy in Britain. In addition to this, it assesses various critical perspectives on the welfare state. It also examines the extent to which ideas and values have influenced the thinking of the New Right Conservative and New Labour governments of the last 30 years.

Chapter 11 introduces the methods of research that can be employed to evaluate the effectiveness of social poliy initiatives. A brief overview of the key issues involved in the research process is provided along with an introduction to the various methodological approaches adopted in the research process.

Some of this is difficult material to absorb – particularly in one sitting. The best way to make progress is to read these chapters alongside those on different sectors of social policy, which follow in Part IV. Then return to Part III and the chapters here with some specific questions in mind. Ask yourself how Marxist approaches would explain the development of the National Health Service or universal education. How would feminists view recent developments in work and employment or pensions policy? How would anti-racist theory explain family policies in Britain?

In addition, there is a guide to further reading at the end of each chapter and this should be used to help you to develop your understanding of each theory, as well as the ways in which theories in general are used in social policy. Understanding theory is difficult – but it is also the tool which equips the student to go beyond description to critical analysis and explanations of social policy.

Chapter 9

Political theory, the state and welfare

Objectives

- To introduce some concepts, principles and values used in welfare evaluation.

- To suggest that such concepts and principles are important.

- To show how these concepts have been employed in debates about social policy and the welfare state.

- To demonstrate the contested, controversial and disputable nature of these concepts and principles and that argument about them is necessary and ongoing.

Introduction

This chapter aims to introduce you to the ways in which social policies can be appraised and evaluated. We will examine the principles underlying social policies, looking at some concepts and principles, such as need, justice, freedom, equality and citizenship, and the theories in which these concepts are employed.

Facts and values

You may feel that, from a social science point of view, a discussion of values or principles like justice, equality and freedom is a waste of time. What is the relationship between social science on the one hand and values on the other in understanding what the welfare state is about? If the rise or development of the welfare state can be explained by social scientists, what need is there for any kind of understanding or justification in terms of values? Doesn't it constitute a return to discredited 'idealistic' interpretations of the welfare state as being about benevolence and altruism?

One possible reply to this question might be to say that sociological facts and values are connected in the realm of politics. The democratic politics of the kind that exists in most of the OECD countries implies the possibility of political and policy choice by an electorate that participates in politics, if only through a choice of representatives. The notion of a 'public interest' in politics seems to imply some kind of ethical or value orientation to political activity. The implication is that institutions, including welfare institutions, can be created and reshaped as a result of political choices. While it might be argued in response to this that democratic politics is simply the pursuit of private interests by other means, rather than the pursuit of any kind of public interest, it is arguable that in most countries it is more than this. Debate about policy typically involves argument, an attempt to persuade others, reference to values. An appeal to naked self-interest is rarely used on its own; it has at least to be cloaked by some reference to wider interests (Majone, 1989).

The twenty-first century state

The transformation of the lives of people in the developed countries in the twentieth century is a product not only of the phenomenal success of the capitalist economic system, but also of a transformation in the role and importance of the modern state compared with earlier centuries.

Since the beginning of the twentieth century it has come to be expected that the state will maintain and promote the well-being or quality of life of the population, not only through the regulation of private activities (such as economic activity), but through underwriting or guaranteeing people's access to a range of basic services and goods, such as housing, health and education. The welfare state is now an almost universal social institution among developed countries in the modern world.

Changing conceptions of 'the political'

One way of interpreting the events referred to above is in terms of changing ideas about what counts as 'politics' or a 'political issue'. In the past century what counts as 'political' has been progressively redefined and expanded. The distinction is between what are conventionally regarded as personal and private matters of concern only to the individual and the family, and what is public, political and therefore open to intervention and modification by the national government through legislation and regulation. Politics has come to embrace more and more realms of social and individual life (Habermas, 1976; Offe, 1984; Held, 1991: 5–8).

Welfare activities of various kinds, including health, education and housing, which in the nineteenth century would have been defined as non-political, that is, as private and personal matters for individuals and families, came to be defined as 'political' in the twentieth century and as matters of concern for governments. The nineteenth-century British state, by contrast, viewed the provision of welfare as something affecting a tiny minority of the population who were dependent; the state's attitude was one of fostering and encouraging self-reliance and independence as far as possible (Harris, 1990). Another way of describing this change is in terms of a shift from individualism to collectivism in the relations between state, individual and society (Marquand, 1996).

This process of expansion of 'the political' is of course far from over. The so-called 'new social movements' that have emerged in recent decades have been concerned with redefining the agenda of politics to include issues hitherto excluded. These include, for example, the interests and status of women, and of groups defined by ethnicity or culture, age, disability and sexuality. Feminists have been more explicit than most about this, with their slogan 'The personal is the political' (Habermas, 1976; Offe, 1984; Held, 1991: 6).

Stop and Think

To what extent is it possible to argue that 'everything' is political?

Conversely, do you think it is possible to de-politicise social welfare arrangements?

While it looks as if there has been, during the course of the twentieth century, a one-way process of change, from a restricted to an expanded conception of 'the political', or from individualism to collectivism, the last few decades of the century appear to have witnessed, at least in the Anglophone countries, something of a reversal of this process. There has been a reassertion and revival of individualism and allegedly a 'decline of the public' (Marquand, 2004). This is a trend particularly associated with the Thatcher and Major periods of government in Britain, from 1979 to 1997, but the trend, it is asserted, has continued undiminished under New Labour since 1997.

What is meant by this is an attempt to shift responsibilities for welfare away from governments back to the individual, the family and the private voluntary and commercial sectors. This has involved the privatisation and marketisation of some components of what were previously parts of the public sector, or at least the injection of market disciplines or market-type arrangements into formerly public organisations such as the NHS, local authority social care, state schooling, housing and even the BBC (Leys, 2001).

While these recent developments are significant, they do not affect the overall picture of the rise of the collectivist welfare sector painted above. In terms of size and importance, as measured by state spending and numbers employed, the welfare sector remains as significant as ever; and in terms of the state's interpenetration of society and everyday life, and of the expectations people place on the state, the state is arguably as significant as it was in the 1950s, even if the character of that significance has changed (the state no longer owns and controls one-fifth of British industry, for example, as it did before the 1980s).

An enabling or disabling state?

Most of us probably still take for granted the idea that contemporary government is on the whole a benevolent and beneficial institution which has effectively promoted the well-being of the population or of particular groups within it, and perhaps also that it has been effective in assuring stability and social harmony and in modifying and mitigating the status inequalities of capitalist market economies (Titmuss, 1958; Ringen, 1987; Hills, 1997). For three decades after the Second World War, comprehensive and universal state welfare was generally celebrated and admired as a major social achievement of democratic capitalist societies.

From a variety of points of view, these apparent achievements of the welfare state have been increasingly questioned since the 1970s. Critics of state welfare have argued that it is inefficient, self-defeating, oppressive, coercive and unjust or simply that it fails to achieve its objectives. Welfare states in such countries as Britain have been variously criticised as sexist, racist, undermining British economic performance, failing to promote equality and eliminate poverty, and creating a 'dependency culture'.

It has even been suggested that Western welfare states have been experiencing a 'crisis' in the past two decades, but even those sceptical about a crisis agree that welfare states are under pressure. The welfare state 'crisis', insofar as it exists, is probably more of an intellectual crisis than anything else, and results from the loss of certainty about the meaning and purposes of state welfare in the Anglophone countries that began during the 1980s.

Even if we reject these broad criticisms and decide that state welfare is acceptable, we still need to engage in evaluation and appraisal. Welfare systems in many countries are becoming increasingly sensitive to issues of appraisal and evaluation, to the impact of policies on individuals and communities and on a range of social issues such as poverty, inequality, social exclusion and social breakdown. Such issues as the quality, equity, efficiency and effectiveness of public services have become more important for policy makers. Such issues as freedom, paternalism, coercion, equality, justice and rights seem basic and essential to debates and disagreements about social policy.

Welfare principles and values

In the rest of this chapter we will examine a number of basic principles, or value concepts: well-being and need; freedom; justice and equality; and citizenship. These are not the only welfare concepts that we could look at, of course. Some might say that power is a highly relevant concept to look at in considering the politics and ideology of welfare. Another might be democracy. Those who are sceptical about the relevance of values or ethics in thinking about welfare would probably want to argue that the welfare state is about power, of classes, or social movements and groups, and the state, rather than about values. There are many more concepts that we could look at. 'Oppression', 'exploitation', 'identity', 'recognition', 'trust', 'community', 'professionalism', 'choice', 'consumerism' and 'social capital', amongst others, all deserve consideration, but limited space dictates a focus on those listed above. Anyone interested in power and democracy can turn to some excellent discussions of these more 'political' topics and their relationship to state welfare (Lukes, 2005; Pierson, 2006), and some of the others have been examined in recent texts on theory and welfare referred to in 'Annotated further reading' at the end of this chapter.

Need and well-being

There is a variety of ways of thinking about welfare or well-being in the social sciences (Marshall, 1950; Allardt, 1986: 118–121; Erikson and Åberg, 1987: 2–8;

Erikson, 1993). Social policy researchers tend to employ the concept of 'need'. Economists employ the concept of 'wants' or 'preferences' in their theories. In this view, human well-being consists in meeting and satisfying the wants, desires or preferences that people have, whatever these are.

From what point of view should we view a person's well-being? Should well-being be viewed in terms of the subjective feelings, wishes, choices or judgements of the individual, or is it to be viewed objectively, independently of the individual's subjective perceptions, by, for example, social researchers, expert professionals and policy-makers? Much social policy and social policy research has tended to take for granted that well-being should be viewed objectively. Poverty, for example, has always been defined objectively, since a subjective concept of poverty would be, it has been argued, impracticable (Ringen, 1987: 15). In relation to health and health care, health care professionals make judgements about a patient's health and the treatment, if any, that should be provided.

Stop and Think

Could we define and measure poverty by asking people whether they themselves felt poor? What problems might there be in doing this?

Private wants vs public needs?

Should social policy only be concerned with what are called needs, or should it be more broadly concerned with aspects of people's wants or preferences as well? It would be easy to assume that the public or non-market sector of social provision meets people's needs, while the private or market sector meets their wants. This would be an over-simplified view. The private sector clearly meets a large proportion of people's needs, perhaps most of them, informally, by supplying and providing for their wants and demands. People's involvements in the labour market and paid employment, consumer markets and family life underwrite a large proportion of their need-satisfaction (Allardt, 1986: 118).

The concept of need

The concept of need is constantly used in health care, education, housing, social security and social care as a criterion for distributing resources. Much welfare research is about the identification and measurement of a variety of needs and the evaluation of existing services and social provision in terms of how far such needs are successfully being met. The language of needs is typically employed by professionals – doctors, teachers, social workers – but also by managers, civil servants and politicians in relation to populations being served and in relation to individual clients, patients and service users. Needs, therefore, are determined by expert investigation, in relation to, for example, nutrition, housing and education. Appropriate degrees of purity in drinking water, the nutritional requirements of growing adolescents, the educational requirements of seven-year-old children, the area and number of rooms required by a four-person family in public housing – these are character-istic constituents of social policy debate and policy making.

The term 'need' seems to involve reference to requirements, prerequisites or con-ditions necessary for achieving some goal, objective or 'end-state'. Assertions that something is a 'need' may be completely factual and value-free, and the language of need is used in a wide variety of contexts which are entirely factual: 'I need a screw-driver to assemble this piece of furniture'; 'This car needs petrol in order to run' and so on.

A need is quite different from a want, a desire or a preference (Plant, 1991: 189–195). A person may need something without wanting it, or even knowing about it, because the existence of needs depends on reality, or 'the facts', independently of what people think or feel about it (Plant 1991: 192). 'What I need depends not on thought or the workings of my mind (or not only on those) *but on the way the world is*' (Wiggins 1985: 152). A human being's need for vitamin C has nothing to do with any subjective thoughts or feelings a person may have but is dependent on certain features of physical reality, in this case human physiology.

Are needs socially constructed?

An influential view among sociologists is that needs are 'constructed' through a variety of social processes. For example, the measurement of poverty, its extent and nature, involving amongst other things the construction of poverty indices by social researchers and policy makers, exemplifies these social processes of construction of poverty as a problem. What are the implications of this view? Does it undermine the account of needs given above? In fact, there is no incompatibility between asserting that poverty, for example, is a socially constructed concept, and that it is at the same time an objective phenomenon.

The social construction of poverty

An illustration is provided by the concept of poverty as 'relative deprivation'. This view of poverty acknowledges that poverty in a twenty-first-century Western society such as that of Britain can only be defined relative to a normal or average standard of living in that society, and is therefore socially defined and constructed. What con-stitutes a 'normal' or 'average' standard of living is, of course, constantly evolving and changing. What is regarded as an acceptable way of life changes as the average standard of living rises. But in fact there is not just one social construction of 'rela-tive' poverty; there are differing and competing constructions. British public policy, which has long acknowledged that poverty is relative, embodies one construction; radical critiques of official policy, such as Peter Townsend's, embody another (Townsend, 1979). (It should be noted that there is not and never has been an official 'poverty line' in Britain.)

Freedom and well-being

The concept of 'freedom' or 'liberty' appears to be another component of well-being. Is freedom something which social policy should be concerned about? One approach to this issue might be to say that social policy is concerned with the material preconditions of people's freedom, but not directly concerned with it. Constitutional law, for example through human rights legislation and bills of rights, and criminal justice, is concerned in part with freedom in a direct and obvious way, but surely this is not true of social policy? This would be too simple a view. In fact social policy is concerned in various ways with freedom, both promoting it and limiting it.

Concepts of freedom

Political theorists have distinguished between two concepts of freedom, 'negative' and 'positive' (Berlin, 1969). Proponents of the negative concept argue that freedom is the absence of intentional or deliberate interference or constraint by another. This is the classic liberal conception of freedom. On this view there is a difference between being able to do something and being free to do it; we may be free to do things that we are not able to do.

The positive concept of freedom (or tradition of thought) is more complex. It involves the idea of freedom as ability, power, opportunity or 'empowerment'; to be truly free to do something is to be able to do it. One interpretation of this 'positive' view is what has been called an 'idealist' conception, which views freedom as rational self-direction or self-command. Yet another 'positive' interpretation of freedom views it as collective self-determination or self-government, via democratic institutions. This has been described as a 'republican' conception (Miller, 1991: 2–5).

A classic statement of a positive view is that presented by the Victorian philosopher T.H. Green in a lecture in 1881. He defined freedom as 'a positive power or capacity of doing or enjoying something worth doing or enjoying, and that, too, something that we do or enjoy in common with others' (reprinted in Green, 1991). This embodies a view of freedom as empowerment, as well as containing an 'idealist' element in Green's reference to 'something worth doing or enjoying'. For Green, a person's freedom to get drunk for example, was not 'real' freedom, because this was an unworthy activity. A negative libertarian – a believer in negative freedom – would, on the contrary, say that a person choosing to get drunk was truly exercising their freedom, in this case the freedom to do as one likes. The negative libertarian might not necessarily approve of drunkenness, however, and would probably say that a person's getting drunk should not involve harm to others (Roberts, 1984; Green, 1991).

The distinction between negative and positive concepts was questioned by MacCallum, who put forward a 'triadic' concept of freedom. He argued that there is really only one concept of freedom, in terms of which both positive and negative freedom can be conceptualised. It can be stated as follows: 'X (an agent) is (un)free from Y (preventing condition) to do or become Z' (MacCallum, 1967, reprinted in

MacCallum, 1991). This might be an argument that there is really no difference between positive and negative conceptions, but that negative conceptions are incomplete, because they refer only to X and Y, ignoring Z – i.e., what it is valuable for people to be free to do. Lack of restraint as such has no value, unless it is specified what the agent is free to do (Taylor, 1979, 1991).

Negative and positive libertarians disagree about the constraints that limit people's freedom. What things or states of affairs constitute 'constraints'? The issue was posed starkly in a book by the late Conservative politician Keith Joseph and his co-author with their comment that 'poverty is not unfreedom' (Joseph and Sumption 1979: 47). This is a classic statement of the negative libertarian, or liberal, view. The fact that a person does not have the ability or the opportunity to do something because of lack of income or other resources does not limit their freedom. A person is free to dine at the Ritz, even if they do not have the money, and therefore the opportunity, to do so. The constraints that are relevant to freedom can only be identified with coercion or intentional actions by other human beings. If someone physically prevented you from entering the Ritz, or threatened you with violence if you attempted to do so, that would be coercion and a limiting of your freedom. A person cannot be coerced by a lack of resources or by poverty, if nobody intentionally willed or intended that that person be poor or lack resources or opportunities.

For the positive libertarian, on the other hand, lack of resources, lack of choice, lack of opportunities or abilities do constitute a lack of freedom. In short, providing people with material resources and opportunities can increase their freedom. To provide a person with education, for example, is to increase their freedom. It does this by increasing their range of choices and opportunities.

Stop and Think

Can we be free even if we are living in poverty, or do we need certain basic entitlements (and what would these be) in order to be able to exist freely in a modern society?

What are the implications of these views for social policy? The two views of freedom can be linked to two ideological perspectives about the morality of collective intervention and state action. One view, the classical liberal tradition, and its modern neo-liberal adherents, which holds to the negative view of freedom, says that state action to redistribute resources, promote equality and reduce poverty cannot be justified by the goal of increasing people's freedom. (It might theoretically allow the possibility that such activities could be justified in terms of some other value or values, such as justice.) The other view, associated with the positive tradition, asserts that freedom can be increased by state action, public spending and redistributive policies. It can be regarded as a socialist or social-democratic view of freedom.

Paternalism and social control

… one very simple principle … that the sole end for which mankind are warranted, individually or collectively, in interfering with the liberty of action of any of their number is self-protection. That the only purpose for which power can be rightfully exercised over any member of a civilised community, against his will, is to prevent harm to others ... Over himself, over his own body and mind, the individual is sovereign. (Mill, 1859, *On Liberty*)

It is basic to the liberal view that the individual is, with a few carefully specified exceptions, the best judge of his or her own welfare or interests. Nobody can know better than an individual what is in that individual's best interests. John Stuart Mill's principle, in the two quotations cited above, is a powerfully appealing one, particularly in an age like ours in which 'liberation' and 'empowerment' – the value of being able to 'do your own thing' – loom so large. Mill's principle is, however, controversial, and it is worth devoting a little attention to seeing why this is so.

Opposed to Mill's principle is the concept of 'paternalism'. 'Paternalism' refers to actions or a state of affairs in which an individual, or an organisation such as the state and its bureaucrats and politicians, substitute their own judgement about what individual(s) should do or how they should live for that of these individuals themselves. It assumes that individuals are not the best judges of their own welfare. Liberals regard paternalism as an ethically unacceptable degree of regulation or control of individual actions and behaviour, indeed as coercion.

The debate about paternalism is yet another aspect of the argument between liberals and socialists or social democrats about the limits of state action. Present-day neo-liberals typically claim that the welfare state is paternalist, a charge rebutted by socialists (Weale, 1978a).

According to its critics, the welfare state paternalistically reduces people's freedom in various ways – by taxing them, by directing and limiting their choices about goods and services, and by subjecting them to legal and bureaucratic regulation (Goodin, 1982, 1988: Ch. 11).

Paternalism is something that particularly worries some liberals, people ideologically on the political right. However, some people of an opposing ideological tendency on the political left, for example Marxists, have expressed what might seem to be rather similar concerns about state power and state action. Do left and right agree, therefore? The left employ the term 'social control' to refer to that which they dislike about the state's activities. Left-wing critics of welfare, who would claim not to be opposed to welfare itself but to welfare within the existing capitalist system, argue that welfare exists in such a society to pacify the working class and other subordinate groups. It is a way in which a basically unequal and unjust system can perpetuate itself by buying off opposition (Wedderburn, 1965; O'Connor, 1973; Gough, 1979; Offe, 1984).

Social control can, however, be given a more general and neutral meaning. Much social policy deliberately and intentionally sets out to regulate and modify the behaviour of private individuals and organisations. This is 'socially controlling', in one sense – it is regulation by another name. The ban on smoking in pubs and restaurants that came into force in England in 2007, earlier implemented in Scotland, is an example of this sort of thing. Virtually everything that government does involves social control.

Examples of collective interference with individual freedom include the following:

• legislation and regulations governing public, or preventive, health – clean water, sewerage, the collection and disposal of human wastes, communicable disease

control, environmental standards, regulations governing food standards and purity, and workplace health and safety;
- legislation which restricts maximum hours of work;
- housing standards;
- the minimum wage;
- regulations governing public house opening hours;
- the national curriculum;
- anti-discrimination legislation in relation to race, gender, age and disability;
- the law relating to the treatment of children;
- regulations governing the compulsory detention of the mentally ill.

Most people would say, on reflection, that social control is not only inescapable, it is very desirable. A society of any degree of size and complexity seems inconceivable without some kind of social control.

Mill's 'harm principle'

How far are these activities compatible with J.S. Mill's principle of freedom? In particular, Mill suggested that 'harm to others' was a justifiable basis for the state's regulating behaviour, and that such intervention would not be 'paternalist'. Mill thought it was possible to distinguish between actions that affected only the individual, what he called 'self-regarding' actions, and actions which affected other people, what he called 'other-regarding' actions. 'Self-regarding actions' were of no concern to the law or government, while 'other-regarding actions' could be, if they caused 'harm'.

Critics have pointed out how difficult it is in practice to distinguish self- from other-regarding actions, and how difficult it is to define harm. Mill's theory has been criticised as being either too restrictive of state action, or alternatively not restrictive enough.

Mill's principle appears to place severe limits on state action and the range of situations in which the state can intervene. It might seem to rule out a lot of what we take to be reasonable activities of the state, particularly in the realm of social policy. The individual must not be coerced in his or her own interest but only if the interests of others are threatened. But what is wrong with paternalism? Why not allow it? Much social control by the family, parents, state and society is justified on the grounds that this is in people's best interests. Children are subject to parental control. Much social policy is freedom-restricting and justified by reference to people's 'best interests'. It may be argued that, contrary to the basic liberal presumption, individuals may not know what is in their best interests. People's autonomy (freedom) may be reduced by advertising, public relations and propaganda. People may be insufficiently rational or lack foresight; they may fail to save or may under-invest for old age, sickness, unemployment and other contingencies. Even if only a minority are insufficiently rational, they risk becoming a burden to the rational majority. Economists such as Jones and Cullis have argued for the importance of what they call 'individual failure' (as opposed to 'market failure' or 'state failure') as providing a rationale for state intervention. The rational individual of economic theory, endowed with foresight and maximising individual utility, is a fiction (Weale, 1978b; Lee, 1986: 24; Jones and Cullis, 2000).

What conclusions can we draw from this discussion of Mill's principle? What it suggests is that we cannot rely on Mill's harm principle to do the work of defining the boundaries of state action and distinguishing between legitimate and illegitimate functions of the state. In other words, if we want to know what these are, we need to have recourse to other interpretations of the freedom principle, or to other principles or values altogether.

Freedom and Sen's theory of 'capabilities'

Freedom has been advocated as a welfare principle in recent years by the Indian economist and philosopher Amartya Sen, who has advanced an influential theory which connects freedom, poverty and material resources.

Sen identifies, and distinguishes between, three concepts: 'commodities', 'capabilities' and 'functionings'. Commodities (which are resources of various kinds, including income, health care and education) are the focus of most research on needs, poverty and social policy. The notion of a poverty line or subsistence, minimum income level is underpinned by a notion of a particular level of commodities. But a focus only on commodities is inadequate as a basis for poverty research. People vary in their ability to transform commodities into what Sen calls 'capabilities' and 'functionings', and these are what we should really be concerned with (Sen, 1980: 161).

'Capabilities' describe the necessary conditions human beings need to enable them to function fully. Examples of basic capabilities would include the ability to move about, the ability to meet our nutritional requirements, the wherewithal to be clothed and sheltered, and the ability to participate in the social life of the community. Capabilities are obviously close to the concept of 'needs'.

Capabilities are necessary conditions to achieve 'functionings'. Functionings involve the idea of activity, or of 'being and doing'. They relate directly to the kinds of lives that people are able to lead and the kinds of activities they can pursue, or 'being and doing' (which, Sen argues, is what our concern with the standard of living and poverty is all about). Commodities by themselves are 'opaque'; it is what people are able to do with them that matters. Social policy, therefore, should ensure a fair distribution of both commodities and capabilities in order to bring about a fair distribution of functionings.

Sen relates the capabilities concept to the idea of 'positive' freedom – freedom as 'empowerment' or as opportunity. Capabilities involve choice and the range of choice that individuals have. 'Capabilities . . . are notions of freedom, in the positive sense: what real opportunities you may have regarding the life you may lead.' In contrasting a capability and a functioning, the latter is an achievement, the former is 'the ability to achieve' (Sen, 1987: 36).

Stop and Think

On what grounds should government be allowed to regulate our behaviour? Try to think of some examples to illustrate your thoughts.

What arguments would you use to argue that government should not interfere with an individual's behaviour?

Justice

Justice has some relationship to the notion of equality, and a basic principle of justice implies equal or consistent treatment. This is referred to as the 'formal' or 'procedural' principle of justice (Weale, 1978b). If there is a set of rules governing or regulating some particular institution or set of social practices, then adherence to the rules in making decisions in relation to those practices constitutes justice of a kind, if the rules are applied impartially to all persons and situations. Public officials applying a set of rules in making decisions affecting the public, for example the rules governing social security entitlements, ought to apply the rules impartially and fairly to the persons and situations with which they deal. Not to do so would be unjust, and would be grounds for complaint and redress for affected members of the public.

The principle does not tell us in relation to what should people be treated equally. If we are concerned with health status and medical condition, for example, and the need for scarce life-saving medical treatment, most people would say that every individual has an equal right to have such treatment made available to them and to benefit from such treatment. On the other hand, each individual should be treated differently according to kind and degree of medical need. If we are concerned with people's liability to pay taxes, most would argue that the law should discriminate clearly between people in terms of treatment, and that a millionaire should pay more, a poor person little or nothing. In these cases the basic principle of equal treatment is 'defeated' by the application of some other norm, such as need (Weale, 1978b).

Social justice

John Rawls, one of the most notable modern theorists of justice, described justice as the 'first virtue of social institutions', in other words, as the most important social value. Rawls was referring to social justice – the justice of a society's basic institutions, laws, policies and practices, and also to the primacy of justice as a criterion of social evaluation (Rawls, 1972; Miller, 1976: 22).

Not all evaluations of social institutions and social policy employ the concept of justice, social or otherwise. Marx, and later Marxists, have had, notoriously, little use for the concept, although they certainly believed in human liberation, empowerment and freedom from exploitation (Lukes, 1985). Neo-liberal theorists such as Hayek rejected the concept of social justice as valueless (Hayek, 1982).

Social justice is not necessarily an ideologically left-wing, radical or socialist concept. There are many different conceptions or theories of social justice, ranging in ideological terms from left to right, from conservative to radical. In other words, there is no agreed view of what social justice is – it is the subject of fierce debate and disagreement. In the next two sections we look briefly at the 'contractarian' theory of the American philosopher John Rawls.

Rawls's theory of justice

The fullest presentation of Rawls's theory was in his book *A Theory of Justice* (Rawls, 1972). (All references are to this edition, rather than to the later, revised, edition.) Rawls's approach to justice is a so-called 'contractarian' one. People disagree about what justice is and what rules of justice there should be. The contractarian approach provides, so Rawls argued, a basis for reaching agreement about what justice is among individuals with conflicting views and interests. He suggested a 'thought experiment'. Imagine, he suggested, a group of individuals coming together to form a new society. They are required to agree on the principles that will govern their society. This choice situation Rawls refers to as the 'original position'. In this the participants in the choice process are ignorant of their likely future positions and roles in the society they are setting up. Rawls refers to this as the 'veil of ignorance'. Individuals in the original position reason behind this veil of ignorance to establish the principles they will live under (Rawls, 1972: Ch. 1, 11–22, Ch. 3).

They will choose those principles that will best secure their own future interests in the future society whose ground rules are here being chosen and agreed on. They do not know the roles and positions they will occupy in this future social order. They do not know whether they will turn out to be rich or poor, a captain of industry or a benefit claimant. Rawls argued that persons in a choice situation characterised by uncertainty adopt a particular form of reasoning and that the rational agent is pessimistic or risk-averse. In Rawls's view, the rational strategy to adopt in a situation of this kind is what is called a maximin strategy or decision-rule. Briefly, this strategy assumes that the rational agent is pessimistic about the future and will therefore choose an outcome which maximises the welfare of the worst-off position in the social order.

Three basic principles of justice will be chosen by rational contractors in the original position.

Rawls's theory prioritises freedom. His first, 'equal liberties', principle involves an equal distribution of certain basic resources such as rights and freedoms. Rawls has in mind here what we think of as basic civil and political rights (Rawls, 1972: Chs 2 and 4).

Rawls's equal opportunities principle is more radical than the usual liberal one, which is essentially the idea of a 'career open to talents'. Rawls stresses the importance of equalising starting points and ensuring that competition for jobs, promotion and educational opportunities is 'fair' – that all start from the same position and no individuals have undue privilege or advantage. This implies the possibility of policies of positive discrimination (not necessarily only in relation to familiar categories such as race, gender or disability) and therefore, by implication, of an extensive role for social policy in the areas of income and wealth redistribution, education, housing, health, labour market intervention and regulation and so on (Rawls, 1972: Ch. 2, 65–75, 83–90).

The 'maximin' or 'difference' principle concerns the distribution of resources such as income and wealth. It states that such resources should be redistributed in such a way as to maximise the position of the worst-off, or most deprived, group. It implies that resources should be transferred from the better-off to the worst-off until you cannot transfer any more without making the position of the worst-off worse in absolute terms (Rawls, 1972: Chs 2 and 5).

Many people would argue that a just society is one in which the distribution of goods and harms corresponds to the distribution of merit – moral merit, productive effort or creative ability, or capacity for entrepreneurial innovation. Thus the successful sportsman, entertainer or businessman is held to deserve the high fees, profits or remuneration they can command; similarly there is a popular belief that the 'punishment should fit the crime' in the treatment of criminals.

In Rawls's view nobody *deserves* anything, since nobody deserves the capacities, abilities or qualities that give rise to differential rewards. These are the product of genetic endowments and social environment. People's abilities, and the rewards to which they give rise, therefore, are the product of forces beyond their individual control. Rawls's theory allows little scope for individual responsibility and free choice in relation to, for example, choice of careers, occupational mobility or entrepreneurial success. Rawls regards the talents and abilities of those well endowed with these things as a societal resource, which it is appropriate to tax for the benefit of society. Rawls's theory is, therefore, sociologically determinist in character (Rawls, 1972: Ch. 5, 310–315).

Rawls's theory makes no reference to need, which might be thought to be a disadvantage from the point of view of social policy. Nor does it have any room for the idea of desert, that is, what each of us as individuals may deserve. Nevertheless, it contains elements that have interesting social policy implications. The 'difference' principle is a prescription for redistributing from those with high to those with low incomes. The principle of 'fair equality of opportunity' is quite a radical one, implying substantial state intervention to weaken the effects of family and inherited advantage. Rawls's theory embodies a strong emphasis on equality, which might make it attractive to those committed to an agenda of redistribution. The theory has been much discussed and much criticised, by free-market liberals, feminists (Rawls had little or nothing to say about the family) and Marxists. Some of these criticisms are presented and discussed in some of the 'Annotated further reading' at the end of the chapter.

Equality

The issue of equality is a major one for social policies and social services and welfare states. Equality as a goal poses major theoretical and practical questions. How can 'equality' be interpreted in relation to social policy? It is not immediately obvious. Equality is a complex value (Dworkin, 1981; Rae, 1981; Le Grand, 1982; Weale, 1985). What is equality about? What is it that is to be equalised? There are different

Discuss and Do

The founders of Google, Sergey Brin and Larry Page, are estimated to be worth around $10 billion (about £5 billion) apiece. At the same time, it is easy to identify large areas of deprivation and suffering in the United States among particular social groups and communities – some inner-city dwellers, some members of ethnic minorities, some people with no health care coverage, for example – quite apart from the rest of the world, which poses even larger issues about the scope and extent of social justice that we cannot, but ought to, address. It is very likely that Brin and Page do not 'need' all the money they have made, whereas deprived individuals could certainly use some of it.

How do you respond to this information? Are you (1) tempted by the view of Rawls, which is that it would be, presumably, appropriate to transfer a large (how much?) proportion of the Google founders' fortunes to the deprived? (It is presumably the case that Brin and Page have paid a lot of federal and state taxes already, to the extent that their fortunes are smaller than they would otherwise be.) Or are you (2) tempted by the view that the Google founders 'deserve' what they have made because they have created a highly successful product from which those of us (not everybody) with online computer access have benefited, and have in fact transformed the Web as a device for commerce as well as the general exchange of information, thereby assisting in a general creation of wealth? If you hold to (1), how far would your view be modified by an (unknown, unknowable) probability that Brin and Page were motivated to some degree by money in their creation of Google? If you hold to position (2), is it your view that the deservingness of Brin and Page outweighs the neediness of the deprived individuals? Would your view be modified by the extent to which you thought the deprived individuals did, or did not, 'deserve' (i.e. were responsible for) their deprived status?

concepts of equality and there is disagreement about whether and how far equality ought to be a goal of the welfare state. Thus the neo-liberal 'New Right' have opposed the goal of equalising material conditions among individuals. From another perspective, the 'postmodernist' perspective appears to undermine equality as a goal of government policy.

Miller, following the nineteenth century French sociologist Alexis de Tocqueville, suggests that equality is a progressive ideal: 'The history of egalitarianism is essentially a record of ideas that were at first visionary, then fiercely contested, then finally taken for granted as received wisdom' (Miller, 1990: 78). The wide acceptance of at least a minimal conception of equality was noted by the Commission on Social Justice: '... virtually everyone in the modern world believes in equality of *something*. All modern states are based on belief in some sort of equality and claim to treat their citizens equally. But what is involved in "treating people equally"?' (Commission on Social Justice, 1993: 7).

Some concepts of equality

We can distinguish between two concepts: social equality, and equality in and of social services and social programmes. Social equality is a broader concept that implies equalising people in some respect, which might include resources such as income and wealth but also, more importantly, rights, opportunities and social status. Equality in social services is a narrower concept and relates to the treatment of individuals by social programmes. Of course there is no hard and fast distinction between the two, and social policy in general is itself a way of promoting a broader conception of social equality. Social policy includes, for example, equal opportunities policies.

Equality in social service and programme provision cannot be conceptualised independently of the concept of need. Here, the principle is that of equal treatment, not literally, but in relation to need. This implies that, in relation to differing levels and kinds of need, equals should be treated equally, and unequals should be treated unequally. Equal levels and kinds of need should be treated equally, but greater needs should receive more in the way of resources. Standing behind this principle is the idea that the outcomes of social policy interventions should be greater equality in some respect.

'Social' equality

There are a number of versions of the idea of the social equality principle that might have some relevance to social policy. These include, for example, equality of opportunity, equality of material condition, and equality of outcome.

Equality of opportunity is the principle that all individuals should have equal opportunity to achieve whatever they are able to achieve. It applies chiefly to education and to employment. It can be interpreted in broader and narrower ways. Thus a liberal version of the principle would be the idea of the 'career open to talents'; individuals should not be discriminated against, in employment or education, on the basis of characteristics such as social class background, income, gender, race, religious background and so on. The hiring and promotion practices of firms, businesses and public bodies should be impartial; individuals should be hired or promoted on the basis of qualifications and ability. In relation to education, it implies that governments pursue education policies which do not exclude people on the basis of income and social class background, for example. The principle furnishes a case for universal school education, available to all, probably without fees or charges. This was a policy implemented, at least in part, by the 1944 Education Act in England.

Equality of material condition is the simple, if not crude, idea of equalising material conditions – income, wealth and other goods such as housing – between people. Resources should be transferred from those who have more to those with less until everybody is equal. It is not clear that any believer in equality has ever endorsed this view. Equality of resources need not imply equality of well-being, since people's ability to transform resources into well-being differs from person to person, as Sen has observed in relation to 'capabilities'.

What kind(s) of equality is or should social policy be concerned with promoting, and what is it reasonable to expect social policy to be able to achieve? A heated argument about this has taken place in recent years, one school of thought suggesting that the welfare state has failed to promote equality, others arguing that the issue has been misrepresented and that the welfare state has been accused of failing to do something which it was not designed to do and which it could never have succeeded in doing. This is the dispute about the so-called 'strategy of equality'.

The 'strategy of equality'

The 'strategy of equality' is a phrase (in fact a chapter heading) used by the social historian and socialist writer R.H. Tawney in his book *Equality*, first published in 1931 (Tawney, 1964), and later used as the title of a book by the economist Julian Le Grand. It embodies the idea of using welfare spending to equalise condition and status. The idea was promoted by a later socialist, the politician and writer Anthony Crosland in his 1956 book *The Future of Socialism* (Crosland, 1964).

A basic concept of the welfare state is that of subsidised consumption of a range of goods and services. This underlies the notion of 'specific egalitarianism' put forward by the American economist James Tobin in 1970: 'Certain specific commodities should be less unequally distributed than the ability to pay for them' (Tobin, 1970, reprinted in Phelps, 1973: 448). The welfare state redistributes income, wealth or purchasing power by ensuring the provision of services in kind; the consumption of these services is typically subsidised so that they are either free at the point of use or available at less than normal market prices. One point of Tobin's argument is that social policy is not simply about redistribution via taxation and cash benefits; it is also about in-kind redistribution, that is, redistribution of goods, such as health, education and housing, as opposed to cash. This view is opposed to those of neo-liberal writers such as Milton Friedman, for whom such in-kind transfers are paternalistic; if the state is allowed any redistributive role at all, it is the restricted one of cash transfers via, for example, the 'negative income tax' which Friedman proposed in the 1960s (Friedman, 1962). Tobin may also be making the point that our concern about equality is limited to a concern about people's consumption and use of specific commodities, goods and services, – education, health services, etc. – and whether there is a degree of equality of consumption in relation to these, rather than about overall or 'global' equality.

Le Grand attempted to give a more precise formulation of the idea of the 'strategy' in his book *The Strategy of Equality* (Le Grand, 1982). His conclusion was blunt: 'Almost all public expenditure on the social services in Britain benefits the better off to a greater extent than the poor' (Le Grand, 1982: 3). The welfare state did not significantly redistribute from rich to poor; the middle classes received more than their fair share of social provision, especially in relation to education. The strategy was largely a failure in securing equality of outcomes.

Universalism versus selectivism

One of the apparent implications of Le Grand's findings was the idea that universal social services failed to redistribute from rich to poor. If one wanted to achieve greater equality through the social services, then selective services, that is, services targeted on the poor or low-income groups, were more effective. In this, Le Grand seemed to be attacking one of the key principles of the welfare state as apparently established in the 1940s; that universal services, services equally available to all, were the key to promoting greater equality. It is interesting that the development of social policy since the early 1980s has seen a decline in the importance of some universal cash benefits – for example, the universal child benefit and the state retirement pension. The former has been supplemented by targeted child support in the form of various tax credits, the latter by expanded means-tested provision, the latest form of which is the Pension Credit. It is also interesting, however, that neither of these benefits featured in Le Grand's book, which ignored cash benefits.

In various ways, it can be argued, the British (perhaps more specifically the English, given intra-country differences within the UK) welfare state has become less universal in the past two decades. Private education and health and social care have grown in importance as a proportion of the 'welfare effort'. From the point of view of welfare state values this is important. Defenders of a universal welfare state, opposed to selectivity or targeting, have always argued that 'services for poor people are poor quality services' (Titmuss, 1968: 134). In other words, universal provision, incorporating the middle and higher income groups in state welfare services, is necessary to ensure high quality of provision. The 'sharp elbows of the middle class' – middle-class pressure to improve services – are necessary to maintain high levels of state spending. The belief in universalism is also bound up with the issue of avoiding shame or stigma, which is what supposedly characterised such targeted services as the Poor Law.

Critiques of Le Grand

Le Grand's pessimistic conclusions about the welfare state have been challenged by other writers who noted that he ignored the impact of cash benefits in his analysis (O'Higgins, 1985; Hills, 1997; Glennerster and Hills, 1998). An analysis of the distribution of social security spending shows a clear redistribution from rich to poor; social security is 'pro-poor' in its impact.

A further, important, point is that it is debatable to what extent the welfare state was supposed to achieve the kind of equality Le Grand was talking about. Le Grand arguably misinterpreted Tawney's conception of equality (Tawney, 1964). Tawney was less concerned with distributive justice (equality of distribution) than with social relationships or with socialist notions of common culture and equal worth. For Tawney, equality of distribution was simply a means to an end (Powell, 1995: 166–169). What really mattered for Tawney was equality of citizenship.

Discuss and Do

Do you think the welfare state, and government more generally, should be focused on promoting:

- equality of opportunity?
- equality of outcome?

Does it depend on what services we are considering? For example, think about the principles underpinning the provision of health care, education or benefits – should the aim of each of these be to promote equality of opportunity or equality of outcome?

Citizenship

A concept which ties together some of the concepts and ideas discussed above, and which is important for understanding the meaning and purpose of the welfare state, is the concept of 'citizenship'.

The status of 'citizen' is constituted by the possession of a set of rights, which include civil rights (often referred to as 'natural' or 'human' rights), political rights, and in the twenty-first century, 'social' rights, which include rights to various forms of state-provided welfare services and perhaps also the right to work. To be a citizen is to be a full member of a national community.

Citizenship is, however, like every other political term, a contested notion. There are right-wing as well as left-wing variants of the idea of citizenship. The right-wing version traditionally stresses the importance of duties or obligations as well as rights. Citizens have duties to the national community as well as rights in relation to it; these might include, for example, an obligation to work, to do military service, to pay taxes, to contribute voluntarily to the welfare of others, to be law-abiding and keep the peace. Although associated particularly with the Thatcher and Major periods, the idea that citizenship involves duties and responsibilities as well as rights has been a particular feature of the New Labour governments' ideology and policy since 1997, particularly in relation to criminal justice policy and employment policy, symbolised by anti-social behaviour orders (ASBOs) and 'Welfare to Work' policies.

Citizenship and its implications for social policy were explored by T.H. Marshall in 1949, in an influential series of lectures (Marshall, 1950, 1964). In them Marshall interpreted the remodelling of the social services by the post-war Labour government in the light of an expanded conception of citizenship as an expression of social as well as other kinds of rights. Marshall proposed that the concept of citizenship had evolved, and that by the mid-twentieth century it had come to include entitlements to welfare. Marshall also examined the nature of modern capitalism and its relation to democracy, and of the opposed conceptions of equality and inequality that arise from the conjunction of these two. Marshall's contribution to the understanding of modern citizenship continues to be the subject of lively debate (Bulmer and Rees, 1996).

The key point about citizenship is that it embodies a notion of equality. Marshall's real insight was the idea that post-war citizenship, as a combination of civil, political and social rights, was a way of reconciling capitalism, which is unequal, with democracy, which involves equality. Capitalism, as an economic system based on private property and free markets, generates inequalities in material resources and corresponding inequalities of class or status. The status hierarchy generated by capitalism can be counterbalanced by a status equality produced by democratic rights to political participation, and social rights in the form of public social provision. Modern welfare systems are supposed to be the antithesis of Poor Law approaches to welfare. The latter was stigmatising and imposed loss of status on recipients of relief. Recipients were excluded from citizenship.

Do the formal rights of citizenship correspond to substantial rights, or the experiences people actually have when using health or social services, claiming benefits or trying to find work? Citizenship poses difficult questions about membership; to talk of citizens is to talk, by implication, of non-citizens, people defined as 'aliens' or excluded.

The revival of interest in the concept of citizenship has been assisted by a number of social and policy changes during the last three decades. One such change was the increase in income inequality in the UK and other Anglophone countries, resulting from greater inequality in earnings from paid employment, the growth of unemployment, and a growing polarisation between two-earner and no-earner households. Policy changes, such as the reduction in top rates of income tax and the shift from direct to indirect taxation, also helped to propel this increase in inequality. There was a growth, in the 1980s, of social polarisation and of social exclusion.

The 'underclass'

These changes were accompanied by the contentious (re)discovery of the so-called 'underclass', a class with, allegedly, limited connection with mainstream values, the labour market and paid work, and conventional family life. The American writer Charles Murray's prolific writings on the subject were particularly influential. He associated the underclass with the rise in criminality in this period, and defined it not merely in terms of poverty or unemployment but as a group outside, and sometimes in opposition to, mainstream society (Murray, 1990). Murray's arguments, although largely rejected by US and British social scientists, stimulated a debate about the degree to which some sections of the population had come to be viewed as 'non-citizens'.

'New social movements'

Another important social development of the last three decades has been the advent of social movements which have questioned the reality of citizenship rights for some groups. In Marshall's day class divisions were regarded as the major determinant of social inequality and the main challenge to citizenship. Marshall himself did not believe that the welfare state as established by the 1940s had brought equal citizenship rights to all. Social class differences and inequalities were still barriers to equality in the welfare state and in society generally. Civil rights, for example, were formally, but not genuinely, equal, given unequal access to courts and litigation because of the costs of legal services.

'New social movements' based on gender, ethnicity, disability and sexuality have, however, posed new questions, not considered by Marshall, about the boundaries of citizenship in contemporary societies such as Britain. How far is the equal status promised by citizenship matched by real equality of rights? Formally, every adult British national resident in the UK is equal in the possession of the basic citizenship rights, but real equality of status, it is suggested, is as far off as ever. The most substantial of these critiques is that developed by feminists, who have pointed out how gender inequalities compromise the attainment of equal citizenship (Lister, 1998). Marshall himself implicitly accepted that citizenship was vested in male heads of households and ignored the position of women (Pedersen, 1993: 5–6). He neglected, perhaps understandably, race, ethnicity and culture, since the UK's ethnic minority population was smaller at the time of his lectures than it has since become. These are issues of great significance because they are now recognised as sources of social division, not only in relation to established ethnic minority communities, but in relation to the social rights of migrants, refugees and asylum-seekers.

Discuss and Do — Is health care a social right?

Anne-Marie Rogers, a sufferer from breast cancer, initially failed and then succeeded in 2006 in her attempt to use the courts to force her local Primary Care Trust to fund the prescription of the anti-cancer drug Herceptin (Tait, 2006a, 2006b). The Primary Care Trust's refusal to allow prescription of Herceptin in this case was a clear case of so-called 'postcode rationing' inasmuch as funding for the drug was available in more than a dozen other areas (Jack, 2006; Tait, 2006a). The Trust defended its decision on the grounds that the clinical effectiveness of the drug for all patients had not been proven; it was known to work in some cases but not others.

What does this case tell us about rights to health care? Citizenship implies that citizens have rights to welfare services – social security, health and education. Health care, like other services, is subject to rationing by health professionals and health authorities, who may choose to withhold treatment on the ground that the benefit to the patient is insufficient to justify the cost. Furthermore, professionals and health authorities may not apply uniform standards – standards vary from authority to authority, so eligibility and entitlement vary. This is 'postcode rationing'. In other words, there appears to be no uniform 'right to health care'. What you receive will depend on where you live. Marshall viewed the creation of the NHS in 1948 as exemplifying the creation of social rights. So was Marshall right or wrong about social rights, at least with regard to health?

Conclusion

This chapter has sought to do a number of things. In the first place, it has tried to show that argument about principles and values in relation to welfare is important. It has tried to show how evaluation works in discussion about policies and of the welfare state generally. It has identified a number of important principles in terms of which policies and services can be appraised. It has suggested that the vocabulary of evaluation is a rich and complex one, and that a number of principles are important in evaluating welfare arrangements. There is no single principle in terms of which we can judge and evaluate institutions and policies. It has also tried to show that the vocabulary of welfare evaluation is not separate from, but overlaps with, and is part of, the vocabulary for political analysis in general. It has suggested that the welfare state can be interpreted at least in part as being based on values, and that it is not simply a manifestation of a 'will to power' on the part of elites, or of class struggle on the part of dispossessed groups. Policy is open to revision in the light of principles and values, and the values themselves are open to revision and critique.

This chapter has:

- introduced you to some concepts, principles and values used in welfare evaluation;
- demonstrated that such concepts and principles are important;
- showed how concepts, principles and values have been employed in policy evaluation and in debates about social policy and the welfare state;

- demonstrated the contested nature of these concepts and principles and suggested that argument about them is indispensable.

Annotated further reading

There are a number of general texts on political and welfare theory which can be recommended. David Miller has provided an excellent, up-to-date, very brief and very clear introduction to theory in his *Political Philosophy: A very short introduction*; see especially Chapters 4–7 (Miller, 2003). Jonathan Wolff's *An Introduction to Political Philosophy* is also excellent, brief and clear; Chapters 4–6 are especially useful (Wolff, 1996). Adam Swift's *Political Philosophy: A beginners' guide for students and politicians* is very clear and accessible (Swift, 2001). David Raphael's introductory book, *Problems of Political Philosophy*, now in its third edition, is still worth reading and can be recommended as an easy introduction to aspects of theory, with useful chapters on justice, freedom and rights (Raphael, 1990). Raymond Plant's book *Modern Political Thought* is excellent, with very comprehensive and detailed chapters on most of the topics we have considered, and some we have not, including justice, rights, freedom, need and utilitarianism (Plant, 1991). More advanced, harder going but outstanding is Will Kymlicka's *Contemporary Political Philosophy: An introduction*, second edition (Kymlicka, 2002). On particular concepts, Stuart White's *Equality* can be strongly recommended (White, 2007), as can Harry Brighouse's *Justice* (Brighouse, 2004). Readers wanting to explore the concept of power should try the classic discussion by Steven Lukes: *Power: A radical view*, second edition (Lukes, 2005). A very recommendable text on welfare theory is Robert Drake's *The Principles of Social Policy* (Drake, 2001). Tony Fitzpatrick's *After the New Social Democracy* provides a stimulating and wide-ranging overview of some current approaches and issues in social policy (Fitzpatrick, 2003). The third edition of Chris Pierson's *Beyond the Welfare State?* provides an excellent critical survey of interpretations and explanations of the welfare state (Pierson, 2006). Another wide-ranging examination of some interpretative approaches and issues is Powell and Hewitt's *Welfare State and Welfare Change* (Powell and Hewitt, 2002). Feminist analyses of welfare and citizenship are provided by Ruth Lister in *Citizenship: Feminist perspectives*, and Gillian Pascall in *Social Policy: A new feminist analysis* (Pascall, 1997; Lister, 1998). Carole Pateman's essay 'The patriarchal welfare state' is a notable statement (Pateman, 1988).

Chapter 10

Ideology, the state and welfare in Britain

Objectives

- To provide an insight into the role of ideas and ideologies in shaping social policies.

- To give an idea of the diversity of ideas, from right and left of the political spectrum, which have influenced welfare in Britain.

- To introduce the idea of the post-war 'consensus' which underlay social policy, and the limitations of the concept of 'consensus'.

- To offer an introduction to some critical perspectives on welfare which have developed in recent years.

- To give an insight into contemporary developments in thinking about welfare.

- To provide an account of policy change which complements the discussions in Chapter 9 on welfare concepts, and in the chapters on welfare history (Chapters 2 and 3) and policy-making (Chapter 5).

Introduction

The purpose of this chapter is to complement Chapter 9 on welfare theory by examining, in a historical way, the development of ideas about the state, society and social policy in Britain. In addition to this, we will assess various critical perspectives on the welfare state. We will also examine the extent to which ideas and values are important in influencing changes and developments in policy.

The relevance of ideas and ideologies

Why should we study social and political ideas in trying to understand social policy? One reason is that they provide a way of understanding policy change and development, not only in the past, but at the present time. Policies can be regarded as embodying ideas about society, the economy, the state, citizens and relations between these. They embody views about justice, equality and individual responsibility.

An ideology is a body or collection of ideas about the world, about human nature, morality, society and politics, often or usually having some kind of relation to institutions such as political parties, political movements or state regimes. An ideology, or tradition of thought, for those holding to that ideology describes, explains and justifies. It provides a more or less coherent understanding or interpretation of some aspect of social reality for those who hold to it. Ideologies tend to be action-guiding, inasmuch as they influence people's behaviour. An understanding of the belief systems or 'assumptive worlds' of political actors can contribute to an explanation of actions and behaviour, and to some extent of outcomes: '... political activity could not begin to be understood without the existence of concepts, ideas and principles, however well hidden'; and the purpose of studying theory is '... to articulate those assumptions which lie behind practical activity' (Pearson and Williams, 1984: 1). Policy change, therefore, can be explained by reference to changes in background ideas about the state, society and the individual held by influential individuals, groups, movements and political parties. When ideas change, policies change. (For a full discussion of policy making, see Chapter 5.)

It is not quite so simple, however, for two reasons. Firstly, the importance of ideologies as tools for explaining social and political change should not be exaggerated. Ideas shape practical action, but action also influences ideas; thinkers and ideologues respond to the social environment and pressures which surround them (Marquand, 1996: 6). With social change comes ideological change; ideological change and social change are interdependent variables, rather than one being dependent and the other independent. Secondly, the relationship between actors' beliefs and policy change may be an ambiguous one.

To illustrate the advantages and limitations of a policy analysis approach based on ideologies, let us take as an example the present Labour government's 'Welfare to Work' strategy, which was designed to foster, among other things, the more fundamental goal of *social inclusion*. (The details of this policy will be found in Chapter 16 on employment policy.) The sociologist Ruth Levitas examined New Labour's 'social inclusion' strategy, and concluded that it was a mixture of three ideologies – what she called 'SID' ('social integrationist', emphasising paid work), 'MUD' (moralistic, behavioural, essentially 'New Right') and 'RED' (redistributive, egalitarian, essentially Old Left/Labour). She argues that New Labourist inclusivism is an 'uneasy amalgam' of 'SID', 'MUD' and 'RED' (Levitas, 2005: Ch. 1). In other words, the ideology underpinning 'Welfare to Work' is complex or even confused, being a mixture of 'left' and 'right'.

It is also, in a way, saying no more than that any policy can have multiple objectives and be informed by multiple, and even competing, ideological perspectives. Most policies have a number of differing justifying rationales and supporting arguments in their favour. Policy makers and legislators can agree on a policy without agreeing on the underlying rationales for that policy. One contemporary policy analyst has observed that '... The connection between a policy and good reasons for it is obscure, since ... many participants will act for diverse reasons' (Lindblom, 1979: 523; Lindblom, 1982: 135). In fact, ideological ambiguity may be an advantage in policy making, since consensus may be easier to achieve.

Take the case of school feeding, a policy introduced, or at least fostered, by a reforming Liberal government in 1906. The answer to the question 'Why was this policy introduced?' is in one way an obvious and straightforward one: because a

Liberal government with a large majority in the House of Commons and an absence of sufficient opposition from a sufficiently acquiescent House of Lords permitted its legislation by enabling a private member's bill to go forward (Hay, 1975: 43–44). There was more to it than that, however. This was a policy that was attractive from a variety of points of view – 'New' Liberal reformism, 'social imperialism', Fabian socialism, the 'national efficiency' movement, the Social Darwinist belief in the improvement of the 'British race' – all views that could be found within the Liberal Parliamentary Party and Liberal Cabinet, as well as outside them. A lot of people, of diverse ideological points of view, could find something of value in the policy and agree on it (Hay, 1975: 29–38).

The points of view listed above do not correspond exactly to party political labels – more than one could be found within a single party, and even within the same individual. Regarding individuals, the historian José Harris remarks of the Fabian social reformers Sidney and Beatrice Webb that '... their approach to social welfare ... reconcile[d] elitism with equality, imperialism with nationalism, abolition of differentials with maintenance of incentives, Stalinism with quintessential Christianity, sexual puritanism with sexual permissiveness' (Harris, 1984: 53): ideological ambiguity indeed.

Regarding Labour's 'Welfare to Work' strategy, it is possible to identify a number of rationales for this policy, for example to reduce public spending, to reduce 'dependency', to foster 'inclusion', and to promote equality by raising the incomes of the worst-off. The policy is, in other words, ideologically ambiguous, or even muddled, but not, therefore, necessarily suspect. To demonstrate that 'Welfare to Work' (to take this as exemplifying Labour's inclusivism) is a mixture of SID, MUD and RED is certainly valuable, but does not by itself contribute to an evaluation of its merits.

What all this suggests is, firstly, the need for detailed historical research into the origins of policies; identifying the ideological positions of the political actors involved is certainly important in this, but not sufficient by itself. Secondly, it suggests the need for careful analysis of the effects, impacts and outcomes of policies, in terms of some values which can be made explicit and debated openly.

Political and welfare ideologies

We can identify a number of broad traditions of political and social thought, or ideologies, in Britain since the nineteenth century, including, most importantly, liberalism and socialism (Pearson and Williams, 1984). These can be roughly associated with major British political parties having some sort of institutional continuity over lengthy periods of time.

The approach followed in the rest of this chapter is highly selective, and what seem to be the most significant ideological traditions have been chosen for consideration. We begin with some nineteenth-century political and welfare ideologies.

Liberalism

Classical liberalism emerged in the early nineteenth century and is typically associated with an identifying cluster of ideas – *laissez-faire*, natural rights, individualism, freedom, the minimal state. Classical liberalism is associated with the developing social science of political economy – the forerunner of modern economics. From this it derived its ideas about economic organisation: the superiority of free markets over state planning or regulation. The most important value for liberals is *freedom*, and one way of defining liberalism is as the ideology of freedom (for detailed discussion of the concept of freedom, see Chapter 9). Another fundamental liberal idea is that of *individualism*. The advantages of a free-market economic system stem from its individualism; the blindly self-interested behaviour of a myriad of individuals interacting as buyers and sellers in a variety of markets – for labour, capital and goods – results in beneficial 'unintended consequences' for all. Individual action is deemed to be superior to collective action (at least in the form of government action). Individualism is expressed morally through the typical liberal belief in individual '*natural*' or '*human*' rights. Freedom in the moral as opposed to economic sense is construed as the possession and enjoyment of a bundle of rights – freedom of speech, freedom of association, freedom of conscience and religious worship, freedom from arbitrary arrest and imprisonment, the right to a fair trial and so on (Gray, 1986; Bellamy, 1992; Vincent, 1992: Ch. 2; Freeden, 1996: Part II).

Classical liberals held that the role of the state should be minimised – reduced so as to intervene and regulate as little as possible and to concern itself with the smallest possible area of social life. The state is a coercive force. Coercion is an evil. On the other hand, the state is also essential. The state secures the general welfare by providing a general framework of laws, administered impartially and uncorruptly and by defending life and property. The state is not necessary to provide welfare, however. Beyond a basic minimum, general and individual welfare is best promoted by allowing individuals to associate and contract and exchange freely with one another through markets or other forms of voluntary action. Most social and welfare goods are more effectively provided by encouraging individual self-help and self-reliance, commercially via markets, and by various forms of voluntary action and association for charity and mutual aid purposes. The best state is one that does as little as possible directly for what we generally call welfare. The state might need to provide some kind of safety-net minimum for the really destitute and incapable, such as a Poor Law, but no more.

Individualism and collectivism: 'new' liberalism and social reform

From being an ideology supportive of capitalism, individualism and *laissez-faire*, liberalism in Britain developed in the latter part of the nineteenth century to produce a variant more conducive to an active role for the state, usually referred to as '*new*' *liberalism*. This development is associated also with changing conceptions of freedom and individualism. Individualism came to be viewed as individual self-development rather than simply as assertion of individual rights and negative liberty. Associated with these intellectual influences is a critique of *laissez-faire* in economics and of the sanctity and overriding importance of freedom of contract. These changes in the content of liberal ideology are linked with the politics and policies of the reforming Liberal governments of 1906–14, which are usually viewed as laying the foundations of the modern welfare state. Some of the thinkers particularly associated with these developments are the Oxford philosopher T.H. Green (1836–82), the political theorist and sociologist L.T. Hobhouse and the radical economist J.A. Hobson (Clarke *et al.*, 1987: 35–47; Bellamy, 1992: Ch. 1; Freeden, 1996: Ch. 5).

Twentieth-century 'new' liberals: Keynes and Beveridge

Two influential later representatives of this 'new' liberalism were John Maynard Keynes (1883–1946) and William Beveridge (1879–1963). Both could be described as 'new' liberal critics of *laissez-faire* capitalism. Neither of them was a socialist or an egalitarian. Both were concerned with the problem of unemployment, offering differing prescriptions for its solution. Both have been described as 'reluctant collectivists' by George and Wilding (George and Wilding, 1985: Ch. 3, 49). They were defenders of capitalism, believers in individualism and prepared to accept only a qualified notion of equality. They were, however, critics of unregulated capitalism.

Keynes remained a lifelong liberal in an era when the Liberal Party was undergoing disintegration and decline after the First World War. Keynes emphasised the importance (and possibility) of an 'active' state in relation to economic management; he developed his views on the basis of an analysis of the inter-war UK depression and slump, which he construed as arising from a deficiency of 'effective demand' and in relation to which orthodox liberal capitalist remedies seemed ineffective. There was a need for substantial state intervention and regulation in the context of a basically capitalist system of property relations and competitive markets (Moggridge, 1976; Skidelsky, 1996).

The critique of capitalism in terms of its supposed inefficiency, and the associated active state prescription, were acceptable within a wide range of ideological viewpoints and political opinion, including conservatism; the Edwardian obsession with 'national efficiency' only makes sense in this light.

Beveridge was a liberal social policy thinker, social reformer, government official, academic and university administrator, active throughout the first half of the twentieth century. He was, like Keynes, always associated with the Liberal Party. He was especially famous for the report *Social Insurance and Allied Services* of 1942 to which his name became indelibly attached, and which is often erroneously supposed to be the foundation document of the British welfare state. He also made studies of and wrote books about unemployment (1909), employment policy (1944) and the role and importance of voluntary action and the voluntary sector (1948) – a classic liberal theme. He was an advocate of family allowances, social insurance and labour exchanges. The Beveridge Report of 1942 was a triumph of public relations; in substance it was largely concerned with administrative rationalisation and the tidying-up of existing social security programmes, but Beveridge succeeded in giving the impression that it was about much more. The Report embodied the basic idea of the 'social minimum' and advocated flat-rate contributions and benefits rather than earnings-related ones, one reason for which was the encouragement of individual thrift and self-reliance; social security should provide no more than a floor upon which individuals could build (and would not be discouraged from building) their own welfare edifices (Lynes, 1984; Clarke *et al.*, 1987: 89–99; Harris, 1997).

Beveridge has been much criticised by feminists, who view the Beveridge Report as licensing the post-war confinement of women to the domestic sphere, treating them for social security purposes as dependent on men (see, further, Chapter 17 on pensions). Beveridge's report, it is argued, embodied assumptions about male and female roles – men as workers and earners, women as carers and homemakers – which have long since lost any relevance they may have had and were largely untenable even at the time. Beveridge's favoured social insurance model of social security provision had sexist implications, since it is an employment-based system of welfare entitlements, so an assumed context in which married women will not be working and earning necessarily makes them appendages of men. Furthermore, Beveridge took no account of family breakdown in his proposals and the position of separated and divorced women with children. The post-war social assistance scheme, National Assistance, now Income Support, similarly disadvantaged women by aggregating the income of a household, in the case of an unrelated man and woman living together, for calculating benefit entitlement, rather than treating benefit claimants as individuals. (Beveridge was in fact less concerned with social assistance in his proposals, treating it as a residual, fallback and relatively unimportant part of the income maintenance system.) Beveridge's assumptions no longer hold good, with the rise of female employment, family breakdown and single parenthood, and an individualist, rights-based culture.

These criticisms are partially justified. The social insurance system is an inflexible one which, although not formally exclusionary, must disadvantage those outside the labour market, who include, and are likely to continue to include, a substantial minority of women. (The system has been 'tweaked' to some extent to remove some of its sexist features and, for example, to enable married non-earning women to acquire some pension entitlement while outside the labour market; see Chapter 17.) A qualified defence of Beveridge might be that he certainly was aware of and concerned about the position of separated and divorced women with children and did give consideration to this issue at an early stage in his work on the report, but dropped them, considering them too controversial to be sold to policy makers (Harris, 1997). A second point is that the Report was necessarily of its time. It gave expression to a genuine desire on the part of many people for a return to 'normal' family life after the disruptions produced by war.

Socialism

Socialism, another ideology which emerged in the nineteenth century, is associated with the development of a kind of economic system and society based on capitalist industrialism. The conditions of this type of production – factory wage-labour – eventually generate the rise of social movements such as trades unions and eventually also political parties. Socialism is the ideology associated with these movements. Socialist ideology offers a critique of capitalism in moral or scientific terms or both (Vincent, 1992: Ch. 4; Freeden, 1996: Part IV). Marxist socialism claimed to be scientific and revolutionary. 'Social democracy', on the other hand, is the reformist tradition of socialism and is distinguished from revolutionary socialist traditions (Gamble, 1981: 175; Clarke *et al.*, 1987: 48–61). It arguably contributed more to social policy developments than the Marxist variety. Key social democratic ideas include those of '*public goods*' and '*collective consumption*' (public goods are discussed further in Chapter 8). Social democratic thought was sympathetic to the treatment of a wide range of goods as public goods to be provided collectively by public agencies, hence the idea of 'collective' as opposed to individual consumption.

The key socialist value, arguably, is that of *equality*, which was operationalised in terms of the concepts of social rights and the 'social minimum' (for detailed discussion of the concept of equality, see Chapter 9). Equality in either of these senses does not imply a mathematical equalising of condition (Gamble, 1981: 181).

Twentieth-century socialist thought in Britain

In talking of socialist ideology in twentieth-century Britain, we are to some extent referring to the ideology of the Labour Party, but there is a problematic connection between this and socialist ideology. There were and are various currents of thought or intellectual tendencies within and outside the Labour Party. We might refer to the ideology of the Labour Party as 'Labourism', although the Labour Party, like other political parties, is a coalition of various interests and points of view. This ideology is (or was) broadly representative of, or gives expression to, the interests of the working class, although it might not necessarily be socialist. In its earlier years the Labour Party was only doubtfully a socialist party (McKibbin, 1990: Ch. 1). Components of this ideology include, consistent with the close connection between the Labour Party and trades unions, a legally untrammelled system of industrial relations, independent trade-unionism and free collective bargaining.

Between 1918 and Tony Blair's and Gordon Brown's remodelling of the party's doctrine after 1994 to create 'New Labour', the party appeared more authentically socialist; its constitution, drafted by Sidney Webb and adopted in 1918, committed the party to extensive public ownership. The Labour Party was obviously, therefore, committed to changing the relationship between state and society and reconfiguring the role of the former in the interests of working people.

There are a number of significant figures in twentieth-century British socialist and social-democratic thought. Three will be considered here. The Webbs, Sidney (1859–1947) and Beatrice (1858–1943), a husband-and-wife couple, were writers and publicists of independent means – neither held any formal academic appointment – who contributed much to a distinctive British version of socialism, as well as to the development of sociology and social policy as academic subjects of study. They wrote copiously on the history of local government, the history of trade unionism, on social questions and, in later years, on the Soviet Union, served on committees of inquiry (Beatrice was a member of the Royal Commission on the Poor Laws 1905–1909, submitting an important minority report arguing for the break-up of the Poor Law). They formulated the influential concept of the 'social minimum' in their joint work of 1897, *Industrial Democracy*. Their careers and concerns make clear the close, if confused, connection between socialism and social policy in the influential British variant of socialism, as do those of R.H. Tawney. Beatrice has been praised as a writer and as possessing a novelist's talent for description and for depicting character and motive. As Charles Booth's assistant on his survey of poverty in London, she wrote, among other things, the deservedly celebrated chapter on the Jewish community of East London. Her first volume of autobiography, *My Apprenticeship* (1926), was commended by the critic F.R. Leavis as one of the great Victorian memoirs, along with John Ruskin's *Praeterita* and J.S. Mill's *Autobiography* (Harris, 1984; Clarke *et al.*, 1987: 48–61).

R.H. Tawney (1882–1962) was an academic economic and social historian. As well as writing works of history such as *Religion and the Rise of Capitalism* (1926), which deals with the same issues that had concerned the sociologist Max Weber in his essays on *The Protestant Ethic and the Spirit of Capitalism*, he wrote famous works of social criticism, including *The Acquisitive Society* (1921) and *Equality* (1931). The latter has continued to be reprinted and discussed. In some ways his social criticism and his history are hard to disentangle. The source of his social and political commitments was a profoundly held Christian belief. He had a very close association with the Labour Party and was in some respects the leading Labour ideologue of the first half of the twentieth century. His book *Equality* developed a view of the relationship between state social welfare provision and the achievement of equality which was to be very influential, as well as being an eloquent statement of the case for equality (Terrill, 1974; Winter, 1984).

Tawney also concerned himself with economic life and organisation, and *The Acquisitive Society*, much less read now than *Equality*, is a tract on the need to transform business into something like a social service guided by 'professional values' of, allegedly, disinterested service to others, rather than commercial ones like profit. Tawney took it for granted that 'professional values' – the supposed values of professional occupations like medicine, law and teaching – were noble and beneficent and that commercial, profit-making ones were otherwise, a point of view which seems a little quaint today in the light of sociological and other critiques of professional power (Wilding, 1982: Ch. 4). The book can be regarded as marking a stage in the twentieth-century extinction of the ideal of *laissez-faire* as a form of economic organisation, until its revival in the 1980s.

The 'end of ideology' and the post-war consensus

From the 1940s onwards there was the development of a mood or intellectual attitude in many Western, and particularly Anglo-Saxon, countries by the late 1950s referred to or characterised by the term '*end of ideology*'. This refers to, or is a shorthand way of referring to, the decline of ideologies, of strong ideological adherence on the part of substantial proportions of the populations of Western countries, to the rise of stable two-party or multi-party democratic politics in these countries and of a corresponding decline in political and social conflict. There was general society-wide agreement among all social groups about political and social fundamentals in a way that there had not been before 1945, at least in Europe. There was a decline in overt political and social class-based conflict, and this was associated with the construction of the post-war welfare state, agreement about political constitutions, social welfare and the economy.

In short there was what has been called a '*consensus*'. The consensus rested on a supposed political and social 'settlement' negotiated in the 1940s and henceforward accepted by both the main political parties. A term which has been used to refer to the dominant political economy in this period is that of the 'Keynesian social-demo-cratic state', which summarises the combination of economic, political and social elements in the consensus (Kavanagh, 1987: Chs 2 and 3; Marquand, 1988: Ch. 1; Marquand, 1996: 6–8). Major social problems, such as poverty and unemployment, appeared to have been solved. There was broad agreement between the Conservative and Labour parties about the parameters of state action and interven-tion in the economy and society, about the boundaries between private and public ownership, between the market and planning, and about the boundaries of state and individual responsibility. This view has recently been subject to a degree of challenge by some 'revisionist' historians, who argue that the consensus was a myth (Pimlott, 1988, 1994: 229–239; Webster, 1994; Lowe, 2005: 98).

Post-war social welfare thought

In the 30 years after 1945 there were a number of writers and theorists whose ideas were influential, at least in shaping debate, in the post-war period. Of these, some were clearly identified with the Labour Party, others less so. Three will be discussed here: T.H. Marshall, Richard Titmuss and Anthony Crosland.

T.H. Marshall was an academic, initially a social historian and then a sociologist. His party-political affiliations are unclear, but he was particularly important as a social theorist in developing an influential characterisation of the post-war British welfare state, or the system that emerged from the reform and reshaping of the 1940s, in terms of the concepts of 'citizenship' and social rights (Marshall, 1950, 1964). In his social theory he was concerned to identify the role of the 'social minimum', via the instrumentality of universal and comprehensive social services and spending programmes, in conferring a certain degree of egalitarian status on individuals and thereby counteracting the inegalitarian tendencies of the labour-market-determined position of individuals. Marshall's theory of citizenship is more fully considered in Chapter 9 (Bulmer and Rees, 1996).

R.M. Titmuss (1908–73) was a social policy academic, researcher and consultant and adviser to governments, more closely associated with the Labour Party than Marshall was. Although much of his work appears narrowly concerned with par-ticular social policy issues, he was a social theorist of some importance, articulating a view of the relationship of social services to the wider society. His theory of the welfare state, condemned by some commentators as lacking political and theoretical consistency, is unsystematic and involves a number of elements (Kincaid, 1984: 114). One element is a functionalist account of social policy as a means of bringing about *social integration* (Titmuss, 1968: 116). The welfare state is also, in Titmuss's view, an expression of the idea of gift-exchange or unilateral unconditional transfer, exemplified by the UK's blood transfusion service with its unpaid blood donors (Titmuss, 1970). A summary statement of these aspects of Titmuss's views is con-tained in his famous remark that 'All collectively provided services are deliberately designed to meet certain socially recognized "needs"; they are manifestations, first, of society's will to survive as an organic whole and, secondly, of the expressed wish of all the people to assist the survival of some people' (Titmuss, 1958: 39). Titmuss also, however, occasionally made use of a political conflict model of social policy change (Titmuss 1987: 122). Another element in Titmuss's thinking about welfare was the idea of *compensation*. Again and again he described collective welfare provision as 'compensation' to individuals for the 'diswelfares' caused by social and economic change (Titmuss, 1968: 63–64, 131; Titmuss, 1974: Ch. 5).

Titmuss may be regarded as a social democratic thinker in the mould of Tawney. His focus is narrower than Tawney's in that he had little, beyond occasional scattered remarks, to say about the economy and economic organisation; his focus is almost exclusively on social policy and the welfare state, a product, perhaps, of the disciplinary specialisation which began to overtake the subject after the war.

Anthony Crosland (1918–77) was an Oxford academic, socialist thinker, Labour MP and minister, dying in office as a senior member of the Callaghan Cabinet. His most influential book was *The Future of Socialism* (Crosland, 1964, 1982: Ch. 7). He is often referred to as a 'revisionist' in relation to core Labour Party doctrine. *The Future of Socialism* contains a number of themes: equality, especially as equality of opportunity; a defence of public spending; and an endorsement of Tawney's 'strategy of equality'. He sought to move Labour Party concerns away from an emphasis on public ownership, central planning and the economy towards a concern with how the fruits of economic growth might be distributed (Jenkins, 1989: 5–8; Plant, 1996). His general view about business and the private sector of the economy was that it was now, in the wake of the reforms of the 1940s, essentially benign.

The revival of ideology

From the late 1960s there appeared to be a revival of overt political and social, class-based, conflict in many Western countries, including Britain. A deterioration in industrial relations began in Britain in the late 1960s and continued and intensified into the 1970s. There was an apparent decline in stable majoritarian two-party politics after 1970 and a rise in the importance of third parties (nationalists and the Liberals). There was the rise of so-called '*new social movements*', associated with gender, ethnicity, sexuality and ecology amongst others. In the 1970s radical critiques of the post-war political economy – the 'Keynesian social-democratic consensus' – began to develop from both the orthodox left and right and from the various perspectives of the 'new social movements'. Substantial critiques of the post-war welfare state settlement emerged from both a resurgent Marxist left and a revived 'liberal' New Right.

These intellectual and ideological critiques accompanied what appeared to be a growing crisis in the systems themselves. A full-blown 'crisis' in the Western political economy had emerged by the mid-1970s (for detailed discussion of the 'crisis', see Chapter 4). A key year in this context is 1973, with the quadrupling in the price of oil by the cartel of oil producers following the Arab–Israeli war in that year triggering worldwide economic instability, which in countries like the UK produced a simultaneous combination of economic slump, involving falling levels of output, unprecedented and growing levels of unemployment and balance of payments crises, together with historically high levels of inflation. By the late 1970s the post-war consensus appeared to be dead, its ideological underpinning – Keynesian social democracy – was also dead or dying, and neo-liberal approaches, offering radical critiques of economic and social policy, were in the ascendant. These changes were marked at the party-political level in Britain by the election of the first Thatcher-led Conservative government in 1979 (Gamble, 1985, 1988; Kavanagh, 1987; Marquand, 1988, 1996; Pierson, 1996).

Critical perspectives: neo-liberalism and the 'New Right'

'Neo'-liberalism is an updated version of the classical liberalism of the nineteenth century. There is in a sense very little that is new about 'neo'-liberalism; it is essentially a restatement of old ideas in an up-to-date and more sophisticated form. Major contemporary neo-liberal thinkers include Friedrich Hayek (1899–1992), an Austro-British economist and political theorist who spent much of his later career at the University of Chicago after a period at the London School of Economics in the 1930s and 1940s. He was the author of, among many other works, *The Road to Serfdom* (1944), a book admired by Keynes, *The Constitution of Liberty* (1960) and the three-volume treatise *Law, Legislation and Liberty*, published in the 1970s (Hayek, 1944, 1960, 1982). Hayek was particularly sceptical in his later work about the concept of social justice, dismissing it as an illusory ideal.

Another significant figure is the University of Chicago economist Milton Friedman (1912–2007), who was especially associated with the revival of interest in monetary policy and with the doctrine of 'monetarism', which asserts that inflation is a purely monetary phenomenon which can be tamed by controlling the supply of money in the economy. His most politically influential book is probably *Capitalism and Freedom*, published in 1962 (Friedman, 1962). Most of this is devoted to exploring the supposedly negative effects of government in trying to regulate society, and how free markets and voluntary action could be used to solve a variety of social problems, including, for example, racial discrimination and professional dominance in health care (Friedman, 1962: Chs 7 and 9).

Another significant thinker was the American philosopher Robert Nozick (1939–2002), whose closely argued treatise *Anarchy, State and Utopia* seemed to some people to provide the philosophical underpinnings for a theory of the 'minimal' state (Nozick, 1974). These three thinkers differed in their basic assumptions, but all shared a scepticism about, or even a hostility to, the contemporary active, 'enabling' and interventionist state as had developed in the twentieth century, and particularly since the Second World War. With the possible exception of Nozick, they did not say that the state should have no role at all in providing welfare, only that any such role should be limited largely to the relief of destitution; the state should provide a safety net, but no more.

Friedman and Hayek in particular were hostile to the idea of monopolistic, state-provided welfare services. If the state must underwrite citizens' consumption of welfare services in kind, such as education or health care, then such assistance should be given in a form which maximised consumer choice and competition among providers, by providing people with either cash or vouchers. Finally, they were largely indifferent to equality, other than a liberal version of equality of opportunity. Socio-economic inequality resulting from the workings of the free market was not something that the state needed to do anything about, and in any case it could not appeal to a shared, consensual theory about what justice, in the sense of a fair distribution of resources, required. Such a theory did not exist.

For contemporary liberals, there is a contradiction between the logic of a capitalist economy and the logic of a welfare-promoting state (Skidelsky, 1997). For the neo-liberal, the state is a 'disabling' rather than an 'enabling' state. It has undermined the foundations on which capitalist prosperity depends. It has created a situation in which a multitude of competing special interests – trades unions, business lobbies, pressure groups – all attempting to capture influence with policy-makers, can flourish. It has usurped a wide range of welfare-maintaining and enhancing activities, in relation to income maintenance and health care, for example, which ought to be left to private markets or to individual initiative of various kinds. For some neo-liberal writers, the critique of the welfare state is linked with a critique of modern representative democracy (Brittan, 1976).

Critical perspectives: the Marxist left

Marxism may be regarded as the ideology of a class-based social movement, the labour movement, represented by trades unions and political parties. Marxism as an ideology had a substantial institutional base in mass political parties in some European countries, such as France and Italy, for much of the post-war period, although much less so in the Anglophone countries. With the questioning of Stalin's legacy in the communist countries that occurred after 1956, Marxist thought underwent a revival. Marxists have sought to understand the changes in capitalism that have taken place since the Second World War, and particularly the transformation of the state and its role. From being a 'committee for managing the common affairs of the whole bourgeoisie', which is how Marx and Engels conceived the role of the state in the mid-nineteenth century, the capitalist state appeared to have mutated into something more benign (Marx and Engels, 1968: 37).

Marxist attempts to theorise the welfare state began in the 1950s, although it is fair to say that social policy and the welfare state did not loom very large in Marxist thinking as a whole. Significant work was done, however, by a number of writers (Saville, 1957–58; Wedderburn, 1965; O'Connor, 1973; Gough, 1979; Offe, 1984). There is no unified Marxist theory of the welfare state and the authors cited differ in their interpretations (Klein, 1996c). In general, however, contemporary Marxists have dismissed the benevolence of the modern state as appearance; the reality is that it is a new way either of integrating a propertyless proletariat into a social system in which social divisions based on class remain substantial, or alternatively of providing the social underpinnings (such as health care, education, income support) for a labour force subject to unemployment or ill-health as a result of the effects of capitalist production (Gough, 1979: Ch. 3; Pierson, 2006). The welfare state is in fact a form of large-scale social control.

An alternative Marxist view is that the welfare state does represent a real achievement by the working class, at the expense of the capitalist class. It is the outcome of successful class struggle by that working class in support of its own interests. All Marxist views imply, however, that in some sense the 'real' interests of the working class are not being served by welfare-capitalist states and would be better served by some alternative arrangement of society (Gough, 1979: Ch. 4; Pierson, 2006).

The most sophisticated Marxist interpretation of the welfare state is that provided by O'Connor and the German sociologist Claus Offe (see Chapter 4 on the welfare state 'crisis' for further discussion of these writers). Their view is essentially that the welfare state is simultaneously necessary and damaging to capitalism; on the one hand, the welfare state is necessary to buy legitimacy and the acquiescence of the working class in the capitalist system; on the other, the expense of the welfare state undermines the system. High levels of taxation and generous welfare provision undermine the incentives – to work, save and invest – on which capitalism depends (O'Connor, 1973; Offe, 1984). The welfare state is therefore, in their view, a self-contradictory institution which cannot survive in the long run. Marxists and neo-liberals agree here in their views about the damaging effects of welfare.

The views described above can be associated with what is called the 'New Left', which in Britain was mainly an ideological movement among university academics and intellectuals, grouped around magazines like *New Left Review* and the annual *Socialist Register*. It would be wrong to say, however, that they were completely without political influence. Although most adherents of New Left views distanced themselves from the Labour Party, others chose to join the Labour Party and their influence permeated it, to some extent, in the 1970s and early 1980s, helping to explain the leftward shift in the party's policies at that time.

Critical perspectives: 'new social movements'

Feminism

Feminist ideology is now a substantial subject in its own right with a voluminous literature. It would be better to speak of the subject in the plural, rather than the singular, since various schools of thought, dimensions or tendencies within feminism have developed (Vincent 1992, Ch. 7; Freeden, 1996). Feminism(s) may be regarded as the ideology of a 'new social movement', one of a number that have appeared since the 1960s. Others include movements based on sexuality, disability, ethnicity and ecology or environmentalism. Feminism is associated with a movement for gender equality. Its central organising frame of reference is the interests and needs of women. As far as the welfare state and social policy are concerned, feminism's message is ambiguous and, as one might expect from the diversity of feminist viewpoints, there is no agreed view. Feminism arguably helped to build the welfare state in the twentieth century, as something in the interests of women and children. More recently, feminist theorising has become more critical.

Feminist thought of the first half of the twentieth century can be credited with a positive impact on social policy. In Britain, particularly noteworthy was the work of Eleanor Rathbone, who published what can be regarded as a major contribution to the economics of the family in 1924, *The Disinherited Family*. This was an argument for the introduction of what was called 'family endowment', or family allowances. This was important because it was a demand for a breaking of the link between paid work, wages and family welfare. The prevailing orthodoxy at the time was that the welfare of families and children was mainly a matter for the individual family. Some departures from the principle had been allowed in the first two decades of the twentieth century in the form of, for example, school feeding, school medical inspection and needs-based allowances for the families of men in the armed forces during the First World War. Insofar as family income figured in political demands at that time, it was in the form of trades union demands for a 'family wage', to be secured through free collective bargaining.

This was criticised by feminists like Rathbone as inadequate for two reasons. In the first place, wages took no account of family size and needs; what might be an adequate wage for a childless couple or small family might be inadequate for a large family. Secondly, the demand took no account of the division of household income among family members, simply assuming that the division of income was fair. This was often not the case. Rathbone's proposal was that the costs of child rearing should be accorded some recognition and partly socialised through the provision of a cash benefit paid to the mother. This represented an important departure from *laissez-faire* principles. The principle was eventually recognised, rather inadequately, in the family allowance legislation passed by the wartime coalition government in 1945, prefigured in remarks by Beveridge in his Report of 1942. This survives, alongside the various family-oriented tax credits introduced since 1997, as the universal Child Benefit (Pedersen, 1993).

What is called 'second wave' feminism developed as a movement in the late 1960s. Although not associated with a mass political movement or party, feminism is in practice an ideology of some variant of the political left, liberal, Marxist or 'radical'. Contemporary feminists have paid a great deal of attention to social welfare institutions because they impinge on the lives of women to such a great extent. Many of them have advanced a critical view of the welfare state. It is criticised as oppressive and patriarchal and as reinforcing a patriarchal organisation and domination of society. This occurs in a number of ways. Welfare policies and practices may be viewed as disadvantaging women; women are, for example, at greater risk of poverty in many welfare states than men. Welfare institutions may also be seen as agents of social (that is, patriarchal) control and as helping to reinforce gender stereotypes, both via service delivery policies and practices (ideas, for example, about women's roles as members of conventional nuclear families and as carers) and as large employers of female labour (Pateman, 1988; Williams, 1989: Ch. 3; Pierson, 1998: Ch. 3, 66–76).

Feminism has had a substantial influence on the political agenda, particularly in the years since 1997, but also in the 1970s with some notable anti-discrimination legislation such as the Equal Pay Act 1970.

Ethnicity and culture

The ethnicity perspective is one which takes ethnic or cultural identity as primary and as a foundation for social division. On this basis, Western welfare states may be viewed as racially, ethnically or culturally oppressive and exclusionary, and as stratified by ethnic or cultural group, with ethnic and cultural minorities occupying subordinate positions. Welfare institutions themselves may be viewed as playing roles in this, in terms of their own inegalitarian exclusionary service delivery policies and practices and their role as employers of low-wage migrant labour. This perspective might also, more broadly, draw attention to cleavage and division on an international scale, to histories of imperialism and colonial oppression, to such issues as developing-country poverty and underdevelopment, and population migration from less-developed to developed countries. The tendency is, again, to undermine the optimistic view of the Western welfare state as uniformly benevolent or uniformly and impartially concerned with the rights of all persons (Williams, 1989: Ch. 4; Pierson, 1998: Ch. 3, 76–88).

An ethnicity perspective had, arguably, limited influence on social policy until the 1990s, becoming more significant after 1997, when ethnicity became a mainstream issue for the Labour Party in the wake of the Macpherson Inquiry Report on the Steven Lawrence murder, published in 1999. Legislation followed in 2000 prohibiting public bodies from discriminating in their treatment of ethnic minority individuals. The Macpherson Report was also influential in its endorsement of the concept of 'institutional racism' as something which organisations, public and private, must avoid. These initiatives can be regarded as aspects of a liberal approach to equality as equality of opportunity and non-discrimination.

An interesting and significant aspect of a culture- and ethnicity-based approach to social policy is that of *multiculturalism*. Multiculturalism implies accommodating, respecting or recognising 'difference' in relation to minority communities. It can be viewed as an alternative or additional dimension of equality to the liberal emphasis on equality of rights and opportunities, one which stresses the importance of *'identity'*. Policy in the UK has been broadly multiculturalist, by comparison with that in other countries such as France.

On one level liberalism and a liberal conception of citizenship appear to be compatible with multiculturalism. Policy dilemmas arise in relation to identity politics, because in the first place liberalism seems to imply tolerance or acceptance of differences, given that the liberal state is supposed to be 'neutral' or non-prescriptive between competing conceptions of the good life, as instantiated, for example, in particular religious traditions and ways of life; all are supposed to be equally valid or worthy. On the other hand, liberalism is committed to basic values of equality and the equal worth of all individuals, and difficulties arise when particular cultural traditions appear to deny this, for example, in relation to such issues as forced marriage (Phillips 1999; Miller 2000; Barry 2001).

A further ethnicity- and culture-related issue is that of migration and what it implies for citizenship. On the whole, the UK has pursued a progressively more restrictive policy towards immigration from the 1960s until recently, and policy from 1971 until recently distinguished between immigrants on the basis of ethnic background, between 'Old' and 'New' Commonwealth migrants, for example. On the other hand, formal citizenship has been relatively easy to acquire (Hansen, 2000). Policy has relaxed since 1997 in some respects, as a booming British economy and strong demand for labour has drawn in workers from abroad, but has become more confused. The issue of expansion in the numbers of economic migrants from eastern Europe in the wake of EU enlargement, and elsewhere, has become mixed up with that of the growth in the number of refugees and asylum-seekers in the late 1990s and early 2000s. Social citizenship rights for the latter have become more restricted.

The Greens

The green or ecological perspective is in some ways a more radical critique than the others, although it has had less to say in detail about welfare institutions, since its tendency is to question basic features of a capitalist economic and social order and that order's conventional justification in terms of welfare maximisation (for detailed discussion of environmentalism, 'green' politics and social policy, see Chapter 21). The green perspective has drawn attention to the inadequacy of conventional definitions of welfare measured in terms of national income (GNP/GDP) and therefore of the complacent assumption that higher national income – economic growth – is equivalent to higher levels of 'real' welfare. The green perspective also, insofar as it involves assumptions about 'limits to growth', questions the supportability of a particular conception of capitalism and of a social and political order (the welfare state) based upon it (Pierson, 1998: Ch. 3, 89–92).

The green perspective has become more publicly salient in recent years, with the growth of concern about global warming and the long-term consequences of climate change and environmental degradation. These issues were highlighted by the Stern Report in 2006. Policy responses in the domestic sphere have been limited, and much energy has focused on trying to achieve international agreements relating to, for example, emission controls. These issues are discussed further in Chapter 21.

Critical perspectives: postmodernism

'Postmodernism' as an intellectual style or point of view has its origins in the realm of literary and cultural study. It has subsequently been extended to sociology, philosophy and history. Postmodernism is not a single unified viewpoint or analytical approach and there is no agreed view about who the significant or influential postmodernist 'thinkers' are supposed to be.

As a substantive point of view about modern society and culture (the 'postmodern condition'), perhaps the most significant and distinctive contribution is its identification of the ending of the organising intellectual frameworks, all-embracing 'world views', major secular ideologies such as liberalism and socialism, 'grand narratives' bequeathed by three centuries of the European Enlightenment as the main characteristic of modern culture (Lyon, 1994). There are no longer generally accepted explanatory or narrative frameworks which account for and describe the social reality that we know. The perspective draws attention to the diversity, fragmentation and incoherence of modern life, to the chaotic variety and irreducibility of competing viewpoints, theories and intellectual perspectives that exist in modern societies, to cultural differentiation, plurality and diversity. This is not necessarily something to be deplored, however; it can be something to celebrate.

For social policy the challenge of this perspective lies in the possibility that the ideas that underpin the modern welfare state are such a played-out 'grand narrative'. Postmodernist styles of thinking have influenced social policy analysis in a number of indirect ways, although the flurry of interest in the academic journals in the 1990s seems to have been short-lived (Taylor-Gooby, 1994; Penna and O'Brien, 1996; Carter, 1998). The continuing interest in 'social construction' and 'social constructionist' methodological and theoretical approaches in some recent writing and some academic sociology and social policy degree programmes is an example (Saraga, 1998).

The politics and ideology of Thatcherism

> The new Tory leader interrupted the seminar by reaching into her handbag and hauling out a copy of Hayek's *The Constitution of Liberty* ... she banged the book on the table and announced, 'This is what we believe.' (Jenkins, 1995: 1)

A Conservative Party led by Margaret Thatcher won, narrowly, the 1979 General Election, ushering in a period of 18 years of Conservative rule. Thatcher had succeeded to the Conservative Party leadership in 1975. The Conservatives had lost two elections in 1974, and under Thatcher the party began a process of policy rethinking. An important influence here was Sir Keith Joseph, in some respects Thatcher's mentor. Thatcher and Joseph founded a Conservative think-tank, the Centre for Policy Studies, in 1975. This became a vehicle for promoting new ideas, or at any rate recycling old ones.

This was a period when 'think-tanks' became important in generating ideas for policy making. The left-inclined Fabian Society, perhaps the oldest think-tank, had been founded in the 1880s. The Institute of Economic Affairs (IEA) had been founded in the 1950s to promote free-market ideas. The founding of new think-tanks became a minor industry in the next few years, with the founding of, amongst others, the right-wing Adam Smith Institute, the centre-right Social Market Foundation, the centre-left Institute for Public Policy Research, and the left-inclined DEMOS (Cockett, 1994).

What was 'Thatcherism'? In ideological terms it is convenient and conventional to label Mrs Thatcher's politics as 'anti-collectivist' (George and Wilding, 1985) or '*laissez-faire*' (Clarke *et al.*, 1987), in other words, as a manifestation in practical politics and policy making of neo-liberal, free-market liberal or 'New Right' ideology. This involved an attack on, or 'rolling back' of, the role and functions of government and expansion of the role of markets and the private sector. This implied limiting the state's responsibilities for welfare, cutting public spending and, where possible, privatising nationalised industries and other state-owned assets. Economic policy focused on the attempt to control inflation through monetary targeting – so-called 'monetarism'. Controlling inflation took priority over reducing unemployment. Other components of this view included a relative indifference to equality and the outcomes, in terms of inequality, generated by the free market.

However, 'New Right' ideology was or is more complex than that and also included non- or even anti-market elements (Gamble, 1988: 54–60). Together with the free-market liberal component, which might be labelled a 'libertarian' tendency, there is also a traditionalist conservative tendency, which stresses traditional values of family, nation, authority and hierarchy. This tendency was associated with the conservatism of periodicals like the *Salisbury Review* and writers like the philosopher Roger Scruton (Scruton, 1980). Individuals of a 'libertarian' persuasion might be inclined to believe in and support 'doing your own thing' and might accept or welcome permissiveness in personal behaviour such as drug-taking and the cultivation of alternative lifestyles. This is the individualism of the free market applied to personal life. The traditionalist tendency, on the other hand, would place stress on the importance of the traditional family, would oppose its break-up through easier divorce, and in general would be opposed to the adoption of alternative lifestyles associated, for example, with sexuality. This tendency is to that extent anti-individualist and more 'communitarian', opposed to permissiveness and tolerance in personal relations.

Both tendencies could agree, however, on the need to limit the extent of state involvement in society and both would be accepting of inequality as either 'natural' and inevitable (conservative traditionalist, with its belief in natural hierarchy) or the unintentional outcome of free-market processes which generate wealth that eventually 'trickles down' to benefit the less well-off (free-market liberal or libertarian).

'There is no such thing as society'

'There is no such thing as society', a remark made by Thatcher in a magazine interview (she went on to say that there are individuals and their families), has been taken to encapsulate a fundamental social philosophy underpinning her government's policies (Willetts, 1992: 47–48). Thatcher obviously did not mean what she literally said. The remark is essentially about the boundaries of individual and social or government responsibility, and Thatcher was saying that individuals and families should do more, government less, a point of view certainly at odds with post-war 'consensus' thinking.

Stop and Think

When Mrs Thatcher said 'There is no such thing as society', was she simply debunking and dismissing a popular 'social construction', a myth or figment of the left-wing imagination, which there is no good reason to 'believe in' (after all, when we look around us, there are 'only individuals', aren't there)?

The mainstream view is that Thatcher was a radical innovator who changed the character of British politics and social policy and ended the post-war consensus. On the other hand, there is a view which plays down the radicalism of Thatcher, emphasising either policy continuity or implementation failure (for example, the failure of the Thatcher government's 'monetarist' economic policy). Connections and comparisons may be made between the Callaghan-led Labour government of the 1970s and what followed; it can be argued that the unravelling of the consensus began before 1979, with Labour's public spending cuts after 1976, the adoption of a quasi-monetarist economic policy, acceptance of high unemployment levels, and Callaghan's rejection of Keynesian demand-management at his party conference speech in 1976, among other things. On the other hand, it can be said that what Labour in the 1970s did reluctantly, Thatcher-led governments did enthusiastically and with conviction.

During the Conservative governments' first two terms (1979–83, 1983–87) policy was dominated by economic issues, industrial relations and defence and foreign affairs. Social policy change certainly featured in the first two terms, but largely as a dependent variable of public expenditure policy. In Thatcher's third term, from 1987 onwards, public policy switched emphasis away from these to a concern with major welfare state spending programmes and their restructuring (for more on '*restructuring*', see Chapter 4) (Glennerster *et al.*, 1991; Le Grand and Bartlett, 1993). The Thatcher governments' views were characterised by, as well as a desire to control public spending, hostility to the public sector's alleged 'waste' and 'inefficiency', and a preference for market-type solutions (Seldon, 1994: 154–155). The term 'new public management' came to be applied to the broad reform agenda. Reform was applied to the NHS, education, housing and social care services. Policy was driven by a concern with efficiency and value for money (Le Grand and Bartlett, 1993).

The Central Policy Review Staff (CPRS), the government's own Cabinet-level think-tank, had conducted a review of long-term expenditure options which appeared in 1982. The report's proposals were radical, suggesting that, given likely assumptions about economic growth and the government's priorities of reducing taxation and public expenditure, much of the welfare state would have to be dismantled and privatised. The government was obliged to disown the report. A Treasury Green Paper on spending options for the next 10 years was subsequently published in 1984. This was more moderate in its conclusions and suggested stabilising public spending in real terms as a share of national income, or alternatively, that it should grow more slowly than the economy. The full neo-liberal programme had thus been ruled out. This might be regarded as exemplifying the triumph of politics over ideology.

From Thatcher to Blair: the politics of New Labour

'What counts is what works.' This slogan is supposed to encapsulate New Labour politics and policy under the party's leader from 1994 to 2007, Tony Blair. It implied a party and a government that is ideology-free: pragmatic and unconcerned with traditional Labour dogma. The ideology of New Labour is often dismissed as 'social democracy-lite', watered-down Thatcherism 'with a human face', or mere electoral opportunism. The party's ideology since the mid-1990s has been labelled 'Third Way' (Hale *et al.*, 2004; Lowe, 2005: 32–35). In fact, there has been little reference to the Third Way by Labour politicians in recent years, after an initial bout of enthusiasm following Labour's election victory in 1997. Before examining Third Way doctrine, we will look at the evolution of Labour thought since the 1980s.

Discuss and Do

What is the ideological content, or orientation, of the expression 'What counts is what works'? Does it, in your view, provide an accurate characterisation of 'New' Labour's policies since 1997?

New Labour and 'modernisation'

From the mid-1970s the Labour Party experienced a loss of ideological nerve; mainstream social democratic ideology was increasingly questioned and increasingly held to be irrelevant in the troubled times of that decade. The Wilson and Callaghan governments of the 1970s lurched from crisis to crisis, governed only by expediency rather than principles, so their critics claimed. The narrow election defeat of 1979 ushered in a period of left dominance in the party and the retreat of the right, ending in a second, disastrous, election defeat in 1983. The party began to move back to the ideological centre under the leadership of Neil Kinnock, from 1983 to 1992.

The pace of party 'modernisation' was stepped up after 1994 (Kavanagh, 1997: Ch. 10). One landmark in this process was the rewriting of Clause IV of the Labour Party constitution, forced through by the leadership. Clause IV was the clause, adopted in 1918, which committed the party to a socialist programme of nationalisation and public ownership. The revised clause dropped this commitment, replacing it with a more anodyne commitment to opportunity and equality. The change was marked by the party's change of name from 'Labour' to 'New Labour' at this time.

The Commission on Social Justice

John Smith, briefly Labour leader from 1992 to 1994, set up a semi-official inquiry into the party's values, principles and policies, the Commission on Social Justice, in the wake of the party's fourth election defeat in 1992; this reported in 1994. The Commission's report distinguished between three approaches to social and economic policy: those of what it called the *'levellers'*, *'deregulators'* and *'investors'*. The first, 'levellers', approach, is that of the 'Old Left', who ignored the production of wealth and concentrated on its distribution; the second, the 'deregulators', is that of the neo-liberal right, who ignored issues of equality and promoted free markets and deregulation; finally, there are the 'investors', who strike a balance between wealth production and values such as community and equality. The rethinking that resulted endorsed this 'investors' perspective: recognition and acknowledgement of the importance of the market, the importance of successful economic performance as a prerequisite for social justice and the need to reward effort and enterprise (Commission on Social Justice, 1994: 19). The Commission's report was critical of aspects of the 'Old Labour' welfare state.

The 'Third Way'

The *'Third Way'* is the term often used to refer to New Labour's ideology. It has been presented as a 'middle way' between Old Labour-style statism and Thatcherite individualism, in which there is a role for both state and market. At the same time, it claims to be committed to basic Labourist values or ideology, but with a change in the means of implementing them. Various other currents of thought have fed into the New Labour project and in some ways New Labour ideology in the mid-1990s was a mish-mash of disparate elements, as the party leadership thrashed around looking for the 'big idea' with which the party could connect with the electorate. On the one hand there was the Conservative, Thatcherite inheritance, which the Labour leadership did not wish entirely to repudiate. There were traditional Labour values such as equality. A variety of other concepts jostled for attention in books, articles and policy statements: 'community', 'social capital', 'stakeholding', 'social cohesion', 'responsibility'.

'*Community*' was a value which New Labour seized on. Even Conservatives had become unhappy, by the 1990s, with certain aspects of the Thatcherite legacy in social philosophy. A critique of Thatcherite individualism had been articulated by the ex-liberal, ex-Conservative thinker, John Gray, in a debate with the Conservative politician David Willetts; he remarked that the 'Maoism of the Right ... the paleo-liberal celebration of consumer choice and market freedom as the only undisputed values has become a recipe for anomie, social breakdown and ultimately economic failure' (Gray, 1994; Willetts, 1994).

The label '*communitarian*' became loosely applied to an intellectual group or movement in the 1990s. The idea of community was explored on the one hand by social scientists like Etzioni (Etzioni, 1994) and on the other hand, more abstractly, by a group of North American philosophers (Mulhall and Swift, 1996).

Communitarianism of either variety is a critique of liberalism and individualism. Sociologists like Etzioni were concerned about the apparent decline in communal life and in the family, a growth in immoral or illegal behaviour, rising crime rates, and family breakdown and dysfunction. They discovered a supposed 'parenting deficit' in society. For these they blamed the excessive growth of a 'rights' culture, and were critical of the individualism and selfishness of markets, competition, acquisition and consumption. On the other hand, theorists like Etzioni claimed to distinguish themselves from conservative 'moral majority' politics of the American variety, a claim that was received sceptically by many on the left.

As well as the idea of community, that of '*responsibility*' figures strongly in New Labour thinking. The state has the social responsibility of preventing social exclusion and the creation of an underclass, and the promotion of work, wealth and opportunity. In return, the state is entitled to ask and expect reciprocal responsibility from citizens. People should work if opportunities are available; parents have caring and educational responsibilities to their children, and people should be 'good neighbours' (Wright, 1997: 78). These ideas are encapsulated in Blair's comment in 1993 when shadow Home Secretary that a Labour government would be 'Tough on crime, tough on the causes of crime' (Blair, 1993).

Stop and Think

Should responsibilities go with rights to welfare, or should rights be 'unconditional'?

The most coherent attempt to pull together the concept of the 'Third Way' was probably that elaborated by the sociologist Anthony Giddens, allegedly Tony Blair's favourite 'guru'. Giddens was concerned with recreating a viable social democratic politics in an era in which the left was on the defensive, the communist model had collapsed after 1989 in eastern Europe, right-wing parties were in the ascendant in many countries, and economic life had become more globalised. Giddens offered an account of the broad sociological changes which underpinned these developments. The message was not dissimilar to that of the Commission on Social Justice.

Giddens' views about social policy involve, among other things, a reformulation of the goal of equality in terms of '*exclusion*' and '*inclusion*'. These two concepts relate to both the top and the bottom of society, to the poor and the rich. Inclusion as a value requires not only employment strategies but also universal social services (Giddens, 1998: 102–111). He accepts some aspects of the neo-liberal critique of the welfare state, which must be remodelled to some extent to be compatible with wealth creation and an economically more globalised world. This requires a greater focus on work-friendly strategies of 'social investment' (a term recalling the Commission on Social Justice's 'Investors' Britain') or investment in 'human capital' – education and training (Giddens, 1998: 111–128).

New Labour and equality: social 'inclusion' and 'exclusion'

New Labour has been concerned about *equality*, although not necessarily in the sense of trying to limit the overall degree of socio-economic or income inequality. The government has concentrated its efforts on improving the position of the poor relative to the average (Diamond and Giddens, 2005: 103). Labour has also pursued equality in the sense of equality of opportunity and equality of status or citizenship. There has been, since 1997, the vigorous pursuit of equality agendas in relation to gender, race, disability, sexuality and age.

New Labour policy language has made heavy use of the terms 'inclusion' and 'exclusion'. An advantage of these terms is that they have a clear relationship to other widely employed concepts and values in social science and social policy. 'Inclusion' has a broader and a narrower connotation, which are related, the former being close to such concepts as 'citizenship' and 'community' as aims and goals of the welfare state, and the latter implicit in the concern in poverty research and policy with poverty as relative deprivation.

A disadvantage of a focus on inclusion and exclusion might be that it disguises a retreat from traditional and more radical goals and values, and it has been condemned on these grounds by the left (Levitas, 2005). On the other hand, however, 'inclusion' might just be a less contentious way of referring to the same values and goals. An inclusivist social and political programme will arguably be egalitarian in some sense and to some degree (Dahrendorf 1998: 6; Diamond and Giddens, 2005: 110–111).

It is a mistake to assume that New Labour's inclusion strategy has been concerned only with work as a route to inclusion. The prevailing mood is intolerant of status inequality, at least, and this is reflected in New Labour's policies affecting, for example, race, disability, sexuality and age (Giddens, 2000: 91). 'Taken in this broader sense, this is a time of greater egalitarianism, not less' (Phillips, 1999: 131). The larger question, whether social cohesiveness and common citizenship can survive a state of affairs in which incomes become more unequal and the top few per cent of the income distribution – the rich – continue to pull away from the rest, remains unanswered. This is the question of 'social exclusion at the top' identified by Giddens (Giddens, 2000: 116–120).

From Blairism to Brownism?

Gordon Brown succeeded Tony Blair as Labour leader and Prime Minister in June 2007. It would be wrong to see substantial differences between the two. Brown was as much involved as Blair in New Labour's 'modernising' project and has as much responsibility for it. It is probably fair to say that Brown is more statist, less market- and choice-oriented, than Blair and seems to be more sympathetic to traditional models of public service delivery such as that of the pre-1979 NHS (Brown, 2003). Resemblances and differences between Brown and Blair in their attitudes to values like 'community' and 'responsibility' have been noted by some observers, Brown appearing to be somewhat more traditionally Labourist (Goes 2004: 115–116).

Stop and Think

What is the 'new' in 'New' Labour?

Conclusion

This chapter has tried to provide a short overview of the ideas that have in various ways underpinned, or challenged, welfare policy in the UK, from the free-market classical liberalism of the early and mid-nineteenth century to the varieties of social democratic thinking which have influenced British social policy since the mid-twentieth century. Much of the chapter has focused on the period since the 1970s and the shifts in thinking that have taken place since then. The first 30 years after the Second World War, the period of so-called 'consensus', has given way to a period of ideological fractiousness and contestation. The chapter has tried to indicate how policy has changed in response to changes in ideas, but also to suggest the limits of explanations presented in such terms.

In this chapter, you have been:

- provided with an insight into the role of ideas and ideologies in shaping social policies;
- introduced to the diversity of ideas, from right and left of the political spectrum, which have influenced welfare in Britain;
- introduced to the concept of the post-war 'consensus' which underlay social policy, and the limitation of the concept of 'consensus';
- given an insight into contemporary developments in thinking about welfare.

Annotated further reading

There are plenty of books on political and welfare ideologies. Clarke, Cochrane and Smart's *Ideologies of Welfare* (Clarke *et al.*, 1987), Vic George and Paul Wilding's *Welfare and Ideology* (1994) and Rodney Lowe's *The Welfare State in Britain since 1945* (2005) all present useful and accessible overviews of welfare ideologies.

Michael Freeden's *Ideologies and Political Theory: A conceptual approach* (1996) and Andrew Vincent's *Modern Political Ideologies* (1992) offer sophisticated discussions of political ideologies, although less focused on welfare issues. A good book on twentieth-century British political ideologies is Rodney Barker's *Political Ideas in Modern Britain* (1997).

An outstanding collection of articles on post-war ideas is that edited by David Marquand and Anthony Seldon, *The Ideas that Shaped Post-War Britain* (1996). Useful books on Thatcherism include Peter Jenkins' *Mrs Thatcher's Revolution* (1989), Dennis Kavanagh's *Thatcherism and British Politics: The end of consensus?* (1987) and the same author's *The Reordering of British Politics: Politics after Thatcher* (1997), Robert Skidelsky's *Thatcherism* (1988), an edited collection of articles, David Marquand's *The Unprincipled Society* (1988) and Andrew Gamble's *The Free Economy and the Strong State* (1988).

On New Labour and the Third Way, see the two books by Anthony Giddens (1998, 2000) on the subject, which are clear and accessible. Critical commentaries on Blair, the Third Way and New Labour ideology generally are provided by Stephen Driver and Luke Martell's *Blair's Britain* (2002), by a collection of articles, *The Third Way and Beyond*, edited by Sarah Hale and others (Hale *et al.*, 2004), and by Ruth Levitas in *The Inclusive Society? Social exclusion and New Labour* (Levitas, 2005). There is a useful chapter by Raymond Plant, 'Blair and ideology', in *The Blair Effect*, edited by Anthony Seldon (Plant, 2001). Very useful on social policy and the Third Way are Martin Powell's 'Introduction' to *New Labour, New Welfare State?*, a collection of articles he edited (Powell, 1999), and his article 'New Labour and social justice' in another of Powell's edited collections, *Evaluating New Labour's Welfare Reforms* (Powell, 2002).

Chapter 11

Doing social research

by Tony Colombo

Objectives

- To explain the purpose of social research.

- To discuss the relationship between theory and research.

- To understand how research helps us search for the 'truth'.

- To explore the extent to which doing social research is scientific.

- To explain the language of research or 'how to speak researchese'.

- To understand why sampling is important.

- To appreciate what the tools of the research trade are.

- To understand why ethical considerations are important.

- To explain how to start planning a social research project.

Introduction

A defining feature of any scholar is their ability to use their imagination as a tool in order to better understand the social world in which we live. Imagination is a cognitive faculty that we all possess but seldom employ to its fullest advantage. It involves taking an active interest in all aspects of society so that nothing is ignored or taken for granted. In other words, having an active imagination enables scholars to be curious about social phenomena to the extent that they are even prepared to become critical about their own thoughts and experiences (Mills, 1970). This willingness to think critically is achieved by asking questions, often difficult and challenging questions that are usually taken for granted by politicians and the public when reaching apparently obvious, common sense solutions about how to resolve particular social problems. Moreover, once scholars start asking these questions they then need to develop some way of coming up with answers. This involves knowing how to carry out or do social research.

The aim of this chapter is to provide students with a brief overview of the key issues involved in the process of doing social research. In particular, it provides enough practical information to help you start to understand something about the methodological approaches adopted in the research articles that you will come across in your particular field of study, and offers some ideas on how to begin thinking about planning your own research project. It is important to note that within the limited space available only a brief introduction to the subject can be presented here, and students are encouraged to build on their knowledge by referring to other more detailed research methods texts, a selection of which are provided at the end of this chapter.

Box 11.1	Bullying

Bullying is exaggerated, says childhood expert

Anushka Asthana, *The Observer*, Sunday 28 October 2007

The level of playground bullying is being exaggerated and children must learn to cope with name-calling and teasing to help them develop resilience, a childhood expert says.

... Tim Gill, a former government adviser who led a major review into children's play, argues that mollycoddling children by labelling 'unpleasant behaviour' as bullying is stopping them from building the skills they need to protect themselves. 'I have spoken to teachers and educational psychologists who say that parents and children are labelling as bullying what are actually minor fallings-out,' said Gill, the former director of the then Children's Play Council, who is currently advising the Conservative Party's childhood review.

'Children are not always nice to each other, but people are not always nice to each other. The world is not like that. One of the things in danger of being lost is children spending time with other children out of sight of adults; growing a sense of consequence for their actions without someone leaping in.'

... But his views on bullying are likely to cause most controversy. 'What may seem like minor name-calling to an adult could be devastating to the child,' said Liz Carnell, director of the charity Bullying UK. 'Bullying can start with one incident, and if you nip it in the bud straight away, it will not grow into a problem.'

[However] Gill has ... encountered a significant amount of support among both parents and head teachers. John Peck, the head of Peafield Lane Primary School in Mansfield, Nottinghamshire, said: 'To some extent the word bullying is over-used and sometimes people fail to differentiate between a normal fall-out between two human beings and something that is bullying.'

Reprinted with permission.

In discussing the many aspects of social research, the example of the social phenomenon of school bullying, widely debated (see Box 11.1), will be used throughout the chapter as a vehicle through which the multi-faceted nature of social research will be explored.

What is the purpose of social research?

Finding a subject

The actual process of doing social research may be defined as a logical and systematic approach that starts by selecting a social problem appropriate for study and then formulating a series of critical questions to be investigated (Bryman, 2004). At this early stage it is important to note that the subject you select for study is not drawn from a predefined list of topics stored in the darkest recesses of your university's vaults. Instead, you should be aware that potential areas of research interest are all around us; it is about using your imagination. Ask yourself what social issues are of current concern and what questions need to be addressed regarding these issues.

For example, you might recall the recent popular and political unease provoked by the media coverage of several incidents involving school bullying and violence. One such case was that of Natashia Jackman, a 15-year-old schoolgirl from Collingwood College in Surrey, who was stabbed several times in the eye, head and chest with a pair of scissors. Her attacker was a 14-year-old girl from the same school (BBC News, 11/11/2005). Now, it is likely that everyone has experienced bullying at some point in their lives, either directly as a victim or a perpetrator, or indirectly through knowing a third party who has had to deal with the problem. Moreover, for most of us such violence in our schools is a matter of concern and we try to make sense of our experiences. However, for some scholars the problem of school bullying is considered to be such a significant issue that they become motivated enough to carry out research into this social problem in order to gain a better understanding of the subject (Pitts and Smith, 1995).

In order to focus our discussion on *doing social research*, we will work with the subject of school bullying as an illustrative example throughout this chapter.

Stop and Think　　　Researching school bullying

- How would you set about researching school bullying?

- How easy do you think it is to get the facts on school bullying?

- Do you think the school you attended as a child would be happy for you to investigate the prevalence of bullying in the school?

Asking specific questions

Once you have decided on a suitable subject for study, the next task is to decide what it is you wish to know about the subject. In other words, it is important to determine the purpose of your study, which is defined by the types of question that you want answered. Most research can usually be categorised in accordance with one of four primary functions (Jupp, 2006): descriptive, exploratory, explanatory or evaluation research.

Descriptive research

This type of research is principally concerned with attempting to describe and define specific aspects of the phenomena being studied. For example, some of the main questions to be addressed in descriptive research concerning school bullying might include: How many children are bullied at school? How many children are the perpetrators of bullying? What are the most common forms of bullying? How many incidents are dealt with by the school, the police, or go unnoticed? What is the range of sanctions imposed by schools on those involved in bullying? How many parents are aware of the problem of school bullying?

Exploratory research

The primary aim of this type of research is to find out how people operate within a specific setting, especially the meanings and motives associated with particular actions. For example, in order for researchers to find out what is going on with regards to the phenomenon of school bullying, they may decide to observe closely how children interact with one another in the playground during break time; talk to children about their experiences as a victim or an offender; and observe or discuss with teachers their experiences of dealing with school bullying. The researcher should approach the subject to be investigated without any prior expectations about what they might find. Their task is to collect large amounts of information which will help build up a picture about what is actually happening.

Explanatory research

For many researchers, being able to explain in precise terms what causes a particular phenomenon to occur, or how to predict what the likely outcome will be within a given situation, is the ultimate goal of research. For example, in the case of school bullying, scholars engage in explanatory research when their studies try to address questions such as: Why do some children bully others? Does gender or class influence the likelihood of becoming a bully? Is there a relationship between TV violence and school bullying?

Evaluation research

This is a category of explanatory research which is set up in order to determine the effectiveness of particular social policy interventions. For example, in the case of school bullying such studies would be concerned with investigating the impact various anti-bullying programmes might have on actual rates of victimisation. This type of study is considered as having direct relevance to the real world and so is often referred to as *applied research*, a term sometimes used to distinguish this type of research from *pure research* – studies that do not seem to provide any immediate tangible benefit to society.

What is the relationship between theory and research?

Facts and theory

Scholars should do more than simply set the record straight by doing research in order to gather facts about a particular social phenomenon. Researchers must also analyse, interpret, systematically organise and in turn evaluate the various meanings associated with the factual information they have collected. In other words, facts and the meaning attributed to those facts are two different things.

To help scholars engage in the practice of evaluating facts, they must become familiar with the process of developing *theory*: a way of thinking about things which helps scholars join together isolated facts in order to develop statements which provide rational explanations of reality (Bryman, 2004). Thus, giving meaning to facts obtained through scientific research is the job of theory, and it is the use of theory in this systematic way that differentiates academic study from political, religious, journalistic or other approaches towards understanding social problems.

To elaborate on this point, an important contribution of social scientists to our understanding of social problems is the use of theory in order to make sense of the world around us. In its broadest sense theory addresses the 'why?' and 'how?' questions of a particular subject: Why do some children bully others? Why do some schools experience more problems of bullying than others? How can we prevent bullying within schools? Without such theoretical insights the social sciences would be intellectually bankrupt; an encyclopaedic mass of factual information, devoid of any attempt to summarise, explain or capture the essential nature of its subject matter.

Deduction and induction

Actually, scholars are not only concerned about giving meaning to facts through the development of theory, they are also interested in extracting insights from theory to use as the basis for future research. Thus, scholars tend to develop their understanding about social issues by moving back and forth between facts and theory using a scientific approach known as *logical reasoning*, which takes two forms: deduction and induction (Jupp, 2006).

Deduction or deductive thinking

Deduction or deductive thinking is a type of logical reasoning that involves taking the broad ideas within a general theory and applying those ideas to a more limited situation. For example, we might start with the general idea or hunch that 'boys are more likely than girls to become involved in bullying at school'. This is a wide claim covering the entire school population. We might then try to test this general idea, or deduce if this statement is correct, by setting up a research study to collect data on samples of male and female respondents within the school population who have been involved in bullying.

One of the main reasons for doing a literature review prior to a study is to help you become familiar with the bigger picture associated with your subject. From this mass of information you should then use deductive reasoning in order to decide on the precise nature of your research project, especially the specific questions that you wish to investigate.

Induction or inductive thinking

The second type of logical reasoning works in the opposite direction. Thus, induction is a type of logical reasoning that involves transforming a specific observation into general theory. This way of thinking is usually found at the end of a study, and is the point where the researcher uses their specific findings in order to develop more general conclusions. For example, if our earlier study did in fact show that boys are more likely than girls to become involved in bullying, then we have produced some very specific evidence to support a more general theory about the relationship between gender and bullying within schools.

Researchers typically work with both types of logical reasoning during the course of trying to make sense of social issues. In fact, the interplay between fact and theory may be regarded as a way of thinking that is in perpetual motion, which continuously refines our knowledge about social phenomena.

To conclude on this issue, you may be interested to know that a good way of remembering which way round these terms go is to think of the Arthur Conan Doyle stories involving the famous detective Sherlock Holmes. From close examination of something small, such as a walking stick or a handwritten note, he was always able to make grand statements about the owner of the item or how the crime occurred. In admiration, his friend and associate Watson would often say 'brilliant deduction Holmes'. Of course this remark is in error, as what in fact Watson should have been saying in response to the detective's efforts to reason logically from the specific to the general is 'brilliant induction Holmes!'

| Discuss and Do | Theorising school bullying – deductive and inductive approaches |

How would you set about using deductive and inductive reasoning in researching school bullying?

A deductive approach would start with a general idea such as: 'School bullying is predominantly conducted by boys on other boys'.

What other general ideas might one explore? (They could include theorising over the relationship between age or class and bullying.)

In an inductive approach you would build up a theoretical explanation from a specific observation. What might these observations include? (They could include specific examples of boys' involvement in bullying.)

How does research help us search for the 'truth'?

Matters of epistemology

The findings from every piece of research ever carried out on the subject of school bullying collectively provide us with our current state of knowledge or information about this particular social phenomenon. Moreover, the results from each study completed in the future will add to this knowledge-base, moving us closer to understanding the *truth* about what is really going on concerning the social problem of violence within schools. However, a very important question to ask about any research is: what kind of *truth* are we looking for? In other words, what should be regarded as acceptable *knowledge* within any given discipline? Such questions are important considerations which emerge from a branch of philosophy known as *epistemology*: an area of study essentially concerned with investigating the nature of knowledge and truth (Bryman, 2004).

Our first concern is to recognise that there are various kinds of *truth* and so what you believe to be true may not be supported by others. A good example is the different types of truth obtained through the use of either common sense or scientific evidence.

Common sense versus scientific evidence

On occasion it is claimed, most notably by politicians and some sections of the media, that the findings of social scientific research often amount to little more than good old common sense that has been embellished in a confusing and intimidating array of academic concepts, which seem to serve little purpose except to hide the obvious (Lee and Newby, 1983).

However, according to the influential American sociologist Peter Berger (1963: 14) an important starting point for any social science discipline should be to recognise that '... things are not what they seem'. Thus, the social scientist's key task when carrying out research should be to look beyond the familiar and question taken-for-granted common sense assumptions about social problems such as school bullying. To put this point another way, things are rarely as straightforward as they often appear to be and it is the role of social scientists to understand what is really going on. For example, in response to the media coverage concerning several incidents of school bullying, the children's commissioner, Al Aynley-Green, was quoted in *The Guardian* newspaper (Tuesday 15 November 2005) as blaming 'an increasingly violent society for the rising incidents of bullying in schools'. Most people would probably agree with this remark. However, the difficulty for researchers is that in the absence of appropriate scientific research evidence we just do not know whether this assertion – that we live in an increasingly violent society – is true.

The commissioner's statement is based on a number of common sense assumptions which academic theory and research has not confirmed to be true, namely that there is in fact more violent behaviour within contemporary society and that this apparent increase in violence has started to permeate into our schools. Moreover, consider the equally plausible common sense possibility that modern societies are no more violent than in the past, but simply less tolerant of violent conduct. Consequently, because people are no longer prepared to put up with acts of violence, they are more likely than in the past to report such incidents to the police, and in the case of school violence less likely to allow the matter to be dealt with behind closed doors. The point is that doing social research may help us come closer to the truth about what is actually happening, and represents a significant challenge to our common sense.

Ultimately, the facts and theories generated through doing research are not founded on either unsubstantiated assumptions or guesswork. Instead, scholars aim to use a range of scientific principles and methods in order to generate reliable and verifiable knowledge about their subject matter and its implications for society.

Discuss and Do	Common sense versus evidence-based explanations of school bullying

Can you think of a number of common sense versus epistemologically based explanations of school bullying? These may include a consideration of:

- whether boys are more violent than girls

- whether girls are more likely to be involved in bullying than they were 20–30 years ago

- whether society as a whole is more violent now than it was previously

- whether there are fewer 'no go' areas in towns and cities than there used to be.

Is doing social research scientific?

A tale of two sciences

Most academics would agree that the principles of science offer researchers a systematic way of producing knowledge; of collecting and analysing data so that theories can be tested (Sedlack and Stanley, 1992). However, not all scholars agree on precisely what doing scientific research should be about. The difficulty stems from the fact that there exist two distinct ways of thinking about *science* which have influenced the development of two very different research traditions within the social sciences. This distinction is between *positivists* who advocate the objective principles of the nature sciences and the use of quantitative methods, and *interpretivists* who support the use of subjective-based qualitative methods for studying social phenomena such as school bullying (Bryman, 2004).

The positivist tradition of doing social research

The epistemological position known as positivism states that social issues should be studied by employing the same principles and procedures that are used within the natural sciences such as physics, chemistry and astronomy. This approach to science starts from the assumption that there exists an objective reality to the social world which is *out there* waiting for us to come along and discover (Durkheim, 1964). In other words, positivists believe that there are definite answers to all our questions, and it is the job of scholars to carry out scientific research, in the positivist tradition, in order to uncover and make sense of these external truths. To elaborate further on this point, science does not make up these facts as a work of fiction; the task of research is simply to reveal their existence. Moreover, it does not matter whether scientists approve or disapprove of what they find, as human opinions or feelings about how things ought to be are irrelevant. Thus, we may not like the fact that leaves are green or that children are at risk from being bullied at school; for positivists these facts are simply naturally occurring features of our existence which amount to universal truths that need to be drawn together and made sense of by the academic community.

Positivist research is carried out through the use of either an experimental or a cross-sectional approach (see below) which is designed to collect quantitative (numerical) data about the empirical world around us. Thus, positivists are only interested in collecting *empirical data*: information about social phenomena that can be verified through our senses of touch, taste, smell, sight or sound. In these terms, abstract concepts such as intelligence exist because they can be empirically measured through the use of numerical IQ tests. However, the existence of phenomena such as God or the Devil would be challenged because their presence could not be empirically verified by the use of scientific data collection methods.

The ultimate goal of positivist science is to create law-like statements about social issues. These statements can only be confirmed if they exist universally: they are shown to be true across different social cultures and throughout different periods in time. With regards to our current state of knowledge, no universal laws have been established within the social sciences.

Finally, positivists assert that during the course of collecting empirical data researchers must be *objective*: they must remain value-free and have no biased thoughts or feelings about anyone or anything. When we think of science and the meaning of being objective, we generally have an image of people in white coats mixing chemicals in a laboratory, working endlessly in search of the *truth*. In reality, however, it is an attitude we all should adopt when we are about to do any kind of research, the aim being to ensure that our findings are not contaminated by our own biased or prejudicial view. We need to be able to deal strictly with the empirical facts before us. It is not scientific to carry out research with the sole intention of proving a point; that is the job of politicians and the media. They can be as biased as they like, and as vociferous as they need to be in order to put forward their point of view. As scientists we let the facts speak for us, they lead and we follow. It is not our job to manipulate (or fudge) the facts to suit our personal opinion.

The interpretivist (or humanist) tradition of doing social research

The interpretivist epistemology starts from the assumption that society operates very differently from the natural world. Consequently, it is argued that we cannot *do research* on people in the same way that biologists might study bacteria that swarm and multiply under a microscope. The fundamental distinction between social and physical phenomena is that unlike all other natural, physical and material things in the world, human beings enjoy a *conscious existence*: we try to make sense of our world and act in accordance with our interpretation of events. Interpretivists argue that it is this conscious awareness of life which makes the social sciences more difficult to study than the physical sciences.

Thus, while the philosophy and methods of scientific positivism may well be suitable for the study of natural science objects, humanity requires the production of a different kind of knowledge, one based on understanding the subjective meaning of human actions (Hammersley and Atkinson, 1995). To put this point another way, objects of the physical world such as plankton, plants and planets are not conscious of their surroundings, but simply react to external forces such as temperature, gravity and light. They react in this way because their behaviour is to all intents and purposes meaningless. However, because people are conscious of the world around them, it means something to them and they use these meanings in order to actively construct their own social reality.

Moreover, the meanings we attribute to things do not have an objective existence independent from people which are forced on us by society; instead we create our own unique, personal views through socially interacting with others. As a result of people's ability to attribute meaning to their actions, they can make choices. Predictably, bacteria swarm and multiply, plants grow and die, planets revolve and evolve, but because people are consciously aware of their environment they can do pretty much what they like. Consequently, the social world becomes a more difficult place to study because the only way to explain human behaviour is through gaining some understanding of people's subjective state of mind.

Interpretivists are interested in collecting empirical data, but in the form of qualitative (non-numerical) information that will help researchers gain insight into different cultures, people's subjective perceptions, and the ways in which humans socially interact with one another. For example, the act of school bullying must be understood from the point of view of the bully, especially the meanings and motives they attribute to their own actions: does a bully physically hurt his or her victim in order to obtain money, to exert revenge, to keep fit(!) or for some other reason?

The best way of collecting empirical data on people's subjective interpretation of the world is through scholars actively engaging in the research process. Thus, rather than see themselves as objective, impassive observers of events, interpretivists argue that researchers should engage in what the German sociologist Max Weber calls the act of *verstehen*: placing yourself in the position of (or empathising with) the person whose behaviour you are attempting to study. Subjectivity should not be viewed as a source of error within a study, but as virtue that enables the researcher to develop a more meaningful understanding and explanation of the social reality they are attempting to investigate (Weber, 1949).

Bridging the gap

In order to prepare a decent meal, you need quantitative instructions on the measurement of different ingredients that should be included and the skills to be able to judge the quality of the food you are preparing. Hence, just as we know that successful cooking requires both a recipe and a competent chef, so scholars are starting to realise that productive research requires both quantitative and qualitative methodologies. The point is that although the aim of this section has been to impress upon you the difference between the two epistemologies of science, we should not hammer a wedge too deeply between them.

Most social scientists tend to adopt a critical realist approach to doing research. This perspective still holds that there exists an objective truth about our existence, but recognises the complexities of the social world and the fact that the special difficulties of studying people only enable us to develop a partial understanding of this reality. Thus, most researchers recognise that universal laws tend not to hold and instead settle for *inter-subjective agreement*: a definition of reality which is accepted as existing when the observations from different researchers agree on what is happening in the natural and social world around them.

It is now also recognised and accepted by most researchers that there exists a great deal of merit in the investigation of people's subjective interpretations of their social actions. This is viewed as especially important in helping researchers to recognise that they themselves exist as part of the human world they are trying to investigate and so must reflect on how their personal world-view influences the interpretation of their research findings. As Max Weber observes, all knowledge is the product of a particular point of view. Ultimately, it is recognised that the philosophy and methods of the natural sciences are not sufficient to study the subject of human behaviour. More constructively, it is generally acknowledged that interpretive qualitative approaches should be used in conjunction with quantitative measures in order to gain a truer picture of socially complex phenomena (Bryman, 2004).

How to speak 'researchese' – the language of research?

Parlez-vous *researchese*? Learning to do social research is in some respects like being exposed to a foreign language. In fact, many students when confronted with *researchese* (the unfamiliar language of research) for the first time often experience a sense of disorientation and frustration at the seemingly incomprehensible way in which many studies are presented. However, it is important to be aware of the fact that the style of writing you are reacting to is not complex and beyond your ability to understand, it is simply unfamiliar to you at the present time. Hopefully, after reading the remaining sections in this chapter you will start to become more aware of some of the key terminology and *tricks of the trade* employed by researchers, which in time will help you to become more proficient at reading, writing and thinking in *researchese*.

Concepts and variables

The starting point for all scientific activity is the *concept*: a name or label given to phenomena which helps us to describe and understand what it represents in the real world. For example, *bullying* is a concept, as are related phenomena such as *bully*, *violence*, *oppression*, *terrorise* and *victim*. Social scientists also use concepts in order to describe people by observing psychological and socio-demographic characteristics such as *age*, *sex*, *race*, *intelligence*, *personality type*, *religion* and *social class*. Concepts are important because they help us to think about and discuss ideas concerning social phenomena. Interpretivist science works with concepts all the time, and the purpose of using qualitative methods is to help develop new and more sensitive concepts that will enhance the researchers' understanding and explanation of reality (Burgess, 1984).

However, positivist science is more interested in measuring concepts, a task which cannot be performed unless the concepts which are of interest to the scientist are empirically defined or operationalised. In other words, because concepts exist simply as abstract ideas which we are unable to experience with our senses (to touch, taste, see, smell or hear), they cannot be measured. We, therefore, need to be able to describe concepts in such a way that we will be able to answer questions about them such as: How much? How often? Does one concept increase at the same time as others? Thus, *operationalisation* involves converting concepts, which function as theoretical ideas, into quantifiable (numerical) and hence measurable elements known as variables.

Conversely, after concepts have been operationalised we are left with *variables*: concepts which are now definable in terms of specific categories or numerical values which change or vary from person to person. Perhaps a simple example will help clarify the process of operationalising (converting) concepts into variables.

Let us start by considering the concept of *school bully* and theoretically define it as *any pupil whose physical behaviour causes harm to another*. By doing so we have simply defined one concept, *school bully*, in terms of other concepts: *behaviour*, *harm* and *pupil*. However, as we pointed out earlier, you cannot measure such concepts because they are only words, or abstract ideas. Thus, if you were asked to go and pick out some *bullies* from a group of school children that you had never met, what would you look for? Can you see a *bully* in a crowd of strangers? No. Could you hear a *bully*? No. What does a *bully* smell, taste or feel like? We don't know because it is not possible for the concept *bully* to possess such attributes. It exists simply as a name, which just like other concepts such as *occupation*, *age*, *income*, *religion* or *social class* cannot be empirically identified (through our senses) from a group of people. To labour this point slightly: what does *occupation* or *religion* look like?

Therefore, in order to be able to pick out some bullies from a group of strangers, our definition of a *bully* as *any pupil whose physical behaviour causes harm to another* has to be translated or operationally defined into a form that can be picked up and measured by our senses. Let us do this by stating that a *bully is anyone under 16 years old at school who has ever been caught by a teacher inflicting physical pain on another person under 16 years old who attends the same school*. Thus, we now have a variable *bully* with two distinct *values*: (1) has been caught by a teacher, and, (2) has not been caught by a teacher. Armed with this new variable, we could ask our group of children the question: *Have you ever been caught by a teacher inflicting physical pain on another person under 16 years old who attends the same school*? We could then select those who answered *yes* as the bullies within our group.

It is important to point out at this stage that researchers must clearly state how they have operationised their variables, otherwise different definitions would produce different results. It is also worth emphasising here that such an approach will not identify those bullies who have not been caught; this is an obvious limitation which researchers will need to be conscious of when transforming concepts into variables.

Cause and effect relationships

The philosophical notion of causality is highly complex and represents the very essence of scientific research. Basically, science assumes that the world is made up of a series of *cause and effect* relationships and that the goal of scientific investigation is to discover how variables are related so that we can predict how change in one variable causes change in another. For example, if Mr Smith jumped out of an aeroplane at 1,000 feet and realised half way down that he had inadvertently forgotten his parachute, then we might reasonably conclude or predict, on the basis of what science already knows about gravity and solid objects, that the *effect* of falling such a distance will be to *cause* our absent-minded friend's demise. Thus, *causality* refers to the ways in which different variables are related to one another. Linking variables in terms of cause and effect relationships is important because it helps us to make *predictions*: to use what we do know about the world in order to predict or make forecasts about things that we currently don't know.

For example, let us scientifically test the possibility that school bullying is linked to TV violence. We might operationalise the variable *school bullying* as *the number of times (if any) each pupil in our study had been formally warned or punished for such conduct by their school*, and we might measure *TV violence* by *counting the total number of hours spent watching programmes that involve violent behaviour*. In terms of the scientific idea of cause and effect we would expect that change in one variable will cause change in another. The variable that is believed to be causing the change, which in our example study is exposure to TV violence, is called the *independent* (or *predictor*) *variable*. The variable that changes and the one we are attempting to predict, namely rates of school bullying, is referred to as the *dependent* (or *outcome*) *variable*.

We would conclude from the findings of our study that these variables are related if we can show that rates of *school bullying* are higher among those pupils who also have higher levels of exposure to *TV violence*. But can we generalise further and conclude from this that TV violence (our independent variable) is responsible for causing school bullying (the dependent variable)? No, not really. Why not? Well, to understand why, we need to know something about correlation.

A *correlation* is said to exist when a change in at least one variable is associated with a change in at least one other variable. From our fictitious study we could conclude that *TV violence* and *school bullying* are correlated because the two variables appear to be related in the sense that they change together. From this data we might reasonably predict that watching violent programmes is likely to cause children to become violent and so bully other children. Great! In order to solve the problem of school bullying, all we have to do is introduce a range of social policies and laws that prevent children from watching violent programmes.

However, social life is rarely so straightforward, and it is often the case that other factors are at work which cause change in both variables being studied. If you think about it, children who live in dysfunctional families may learn, from watching their parents, to resolve their problems through the use of force and, because family conflict is a way of life for them, be either directly or indirectly encouraged to watch more programmes containing violence. Thus, in contrast to our initial finding of a relationship between *TV violence* and *school bullying*, they may in fact turn out not to be connected with one other. Instead, a third variable, *poor parenting*, may actually be responsible for causing the increase we observed in both of the study variables. In other words, what we originally believed to be a relationship between our independent and dependent variables may actually turn out to be a *spurious correlation*: an apparent association between at least two variables which after further investigation is shown to be false because it was caused by another variable.

In order to determine the existence of spurious relationships, we might use a technique called *control*: holding constant (the same) relevant variables which are believed to be spurious in order to measure their effect. Thus, if we suspect (perhaps from previous research) that *poor parenting* may be generating a spurious (false) relationship between *TV violence* and *school bullying*, we could check for this by controlling (or holding constant) the variable *poor parenting*. This is achieved by setting up a separate study in which we only include in our research children from dysfunctional families and look again for a correlation between our original independent and dependent variables. If the findings from this second study still show that an increase in exposure to *TV violence* is linked to an increase in *school bullying*, then we can be more confident about the correlation observed in our original study. If, however, the relationship disappears or is much weaker when controlling for *poor parenting*, then we can be more certain that we have been dealing with a spurious relationship.

Reliability and validity

Researchers must check that the data they collect is accurate. In other words, they must make sure that the information obtained from *respondents* – the people participating in the study – has not been distorted by the method used in order to gather the required details.

For example, one way to find out how often children have bullied others within the last year is to ask them to recall (or self-report) the number of times they have committed this offence over the past 12 months. The problem with this approach, however, is that our memory often plays tricks on us, which may result in participants not accurately recalling all the instances of bullying that they were involved in. In order to check for this, researchers carry out reliability tests on the way in which the data was obtained. Thus, *reliability* refers to the replication of research and involves making sure that our method of collecting data will produce similar results if repeated on the same group of respondents. Usually researchers employ *the test–retest reliability procedure* which involves doing the initial study and then at a later stage, perhaps after an interval of a week or so, repeating the study with a sample of respondents who participated earlier. If the answers given to the same set of questions are similar to their first set of responses, we can be confident that our research is producing reliable results.

This, however, is not the same as saying that the quality of the data we have collected is any good. For example, a researcher might ask a respondent about their annual income. Now, if their income level was very low or very high, the temptation would be to lie to the researcher and over- or under-inflate the true figure. Moreover, during a retest the respondent may remember the income figure they gave the first time round and repeat their original false answer. What the research is left with is data which is accurate in terms of its reliability, but inaccurate in terms of its actual validity. In other words, it is not a valid representation of this person's annual income. Thus, researchers must test for *validity*, which refers to ensuring that the method used for collecting data is actually measuring what it claims to measure; that it is gathering the information that it is supposed to. Consider again our bullying self-report study. People may be embarrassed about or proud of the offences they have committed and so distort what they report to the researcher, or they may simply have forgotten about certain events. One way to check on the validity of our respondent's answers might be to check what they say against school records, or ask other people such as their friends and teachers to verify that particular incidents took place.

In sum, the findings obtained from social research are no better than the methods used for gathering the data to be collected. If the process turns out to be unreliable and/or invalid, then the study's findings will be inaccurate. Remember, just because your data is reliable this is no guarantee that it is valid, though if we can be sure that our data is valid then we can assume it to be reliable.

Why is sampling important?

Making sense of the terminology

A *population* (or *census*) is the total number of respondents who exist at the time of the study and who possess some characteristic which is of interest to the research. For example, if a researcher was interested in studying school bullying, then the population appropriate for study would include all those who fit the theoretical definition established for the purpose of the research, which may be *all pupils who have been caught causing harm to other pupils within all secondary schools in England and Wales*.

A *sample* would be some part or portion of the research population. It is made up of a smaller number of people who have been selected from the population for inclusion in the study. *Sampling* refers to the theoretical and practical processes used by researchers in order to select the study's respondents. There are two main types of sampling: a probability sampling design and a non-probability sampling design. Each design is organised around a specific set of procedures and methods which will be discussed shortly.

Why bother obtaining samples?

There are five main reasons why researchers prefer to deal with samples rather than the entire study population. Essentially, samples are used because the actual population to be investigated is often too large, making it impractical for everyone to be included in the research; there may not be adequate time to carry out research on every respondent within the population; the researcher may not have sufficient funds to be able to include everyone; a complete census of the study population may not be available or known to the researcher; and finally the study may be destructive or alter the object of interest in some way, such as testing each match to see if it lights.

Probability and non-probability sampling designs

Probability sampling design is a process of selecting a sample in which the chances of selecting any one respondent from the study population is known and is equal. For example, picking coloured discs out of a hat satisfies this condition, as we know that if there are ten different coloured discs then each disc has an equal one-in-ten chance of being selected This type of sampling design enables us to use statistical data obtained from the sample as the basis for making conclusions about the larger study population. Two of the most common sampling methods that follow this probability law are simple random samples and stratified samples (Bryman, 2004).

Non-probability sampling design is where the probability of selecting any one element from the population is *not* known. This type of sampling design restricts the range of statistical procedures that can be used, so no statistical inferences can be made from the sample to the wider population. However, these methods of sampling offer important economic advantages in terms of time, effort and cost, and so are very popular with researchers. Two of the most common non-probability sampling methods are judgemental or purposive samples, and snowball samples.

In *judgement/purposive samples* the researcher selects any element that is considered appropriate to their study. All that the researcher requires is knowledge about the population to be studied. For example, to do research on school bullying a researcher would probably simply attempt to gain access to several comprehensive schools in their locality in order to obtain their sample of respondents.

Snowball sampling occurs where a respondent who has been involved in the research is asked to help find other people who would be relevant to the study. Developing such a referral process is often the only way to do certain types of research, such as investigating the experiences of prostitutes or heroine users.

What are the tools of the research trade?

There is nothing mystical about the way in which scholars collect their research data. In fact, the methods they use are similar to those employed during the course of our everyday lives, such as asking questions, observing the behaviour of others, or counting how often a particular event occurs. The only difference is that when social scientists collect data, they follow a specifically defined research approach which is organised around a logical and systematic set of procedures that you will become familiar with. The five most common *research designs* (frameworks for the collection and analysis of data) are *experimental, cross-sectional, longitudinal, case study* and *secondary source*. No single approach should be considered as better or worse than the others; they simply represent different ways of helping scholars obtain meaningful answers to the questions they have set themselves.

Experimental designs

True or classical experimental designs are used for testing *hypotheses*: unproven statements about the cause and effect relationship between two or more variables under highly controlled conditions. Experiments are considered as explanatory research, as the aim is to find out not just what is going on, but why things happen in the way that they do. Such designs involve randomly assigning respondents (usually referred to as subjects) to either a *treatment* or a *control* group. For example, in a study on the relationship between TV violence and aggression, subjects in the *treatment* group may be asked to watch a violent programme while subjects in the *control* group watch something that contains no violence. Afterwards levels of aggression within both groups of subjects are measured. If subjects from the *treatment* group show more aggression than those in the *control* group, then we can be confident that the difference was due to TV violence (the study's independent variable).

Quasi-experimental designs are more commonly used in social research and involve setting up experimental conditions within normal social settings. These studies are quasi (or partial) in the sense that they do not fulfil all the strict requirements found in true laboratory-based experiments. For example, researchers may take advantage of the fact that a school is about to introduce CCTV surveillance and carry out a study concerning its impact on reducing incidents of bullying. Thus, a quasi-experimental design would be set up in which data is collected on incidents of bullying at two separate schools: one in which cameras are used and another where they are not. Of course, such studies would ensure that the two schools could be matched in terms of their rates of bullying prior to the quasi-experiment taking place.

Cross-sectional designs

This approach to doing research is also often referred to as a *survey design*. It involves the collection of primarily descriptive data on a large cross-sectional (or representative) sample of respondents who have been randomly drawn from the study population. The qualitative or quantitative information that is collected usually relates to a wide range of variables regarding the subject under investigation, and the purpose of analysing this data is to find patterns of association between variables. For example, a sample of pupils at a large comprehensive school may be asked a range of questions about their TV viewing habits, music influences, diet, relationship with parents, friendships, attitude towards teachers, views of violence, ethnicity, sex, financial allowance, etc., in order to better understand what factors might be associated with school bullying.

Cross-sectional survey designs employ variations on either the questionnaire or the interview technique for gathering data. A *questionnaire* is a measuring instrument that contains a series of written statements or questions which are answered by respondents. The responses that are given may be open-ended, which produces qualitative data such as a reply to the question: *What does the term 'school bully' mean to you?* Or the questions may require a fixed quantifiable response such as the following:

> *How many times have you been punched or kicked by another pupil at your school in the last 6 months?*

or

Sometimes you need to bully other pupils in order to get respect

Strongly Agree – Agree – Disagree – Strongly Disagree

(PLEASE CIRCLE THE ONE RESPONSE THAT MOST CLOSELY REPRESENTS YOUR VIEW)

An *interview* is a measuring instrument that contains a series of statements or questions which are answered by respondents within a face-to-face conversational situation. Interviews may be either *structured* or *unstructured*. The former usually involves the researcher asking a predefined series of questions in a particular order which require either quantitative or qualitative responses. Such data can also be obtained by carrying out an interview over the telephone or through various means of real-time communication such as e-mail, chat-rooms, or video conferencing. *Unstructured* or *in-depth interviews* are more informal and are guided only by a series of general themes that the interviewer wishes to explore with the respondent (or interviewee). Such an unstructured approach may be used in order to investigate sensitive subjects such as victims' experiences of bullying, or if detailed information on a particular subject is required, such as descriptive data from bullies on how they target their victims and the methods they use to avoid getting caught.

Longitudinal designs

This is an extension of the cross-sectional survey using questionnaires or interview data collection methods, but actually constitutes a distinct form of research design. In *longitudinal designs* a sample of respondents is surveyed and then the survey is repeated at several points in the future. The samples selected for inclusion in such studies usually represent a *cohort*: a group of people who have in common a particular characteristic such as all being born within the same year, or sharing a particular experience such as all being victims of school bullying.

Case study (or ethnographic) designs

This type of research design usually involves the detailed and intensive investigation of a single *case study*, which could be a single community, school, family, organisation, person or event. Most case study research is designed to collect either explanatory or descriptive information, and usually employs either interviews or *participant observation*: a data gathering technique in which researchers systematically observe people while at the same time becoming involved in the routine activities and general way of life of those being studied. For example, in order to study school bullying using the case study approach, a researcher might get a job (either overtly or covertly) as a teaching assistant. If the data to be collected on a case study involves the life history of a particular person, then a range of different methods may be employed, including unstructured interviews, diaries, biographies, photographs and letters.

Secondary source designs

This is an approach to research that is organised around the use *of secondary sources*: data already in existence which has been collected by others for reasons that may or may not be directly related to the process of doing research. For example, the content of newspapers or magazines is a secondary source of data which may be used in order to investigate popular attitudes towards events such as school bullying. Essentially, the researcher would employ various sampling techniques in order to obtain a sample of articles on a particular subject and then analyse their content for particular words, phrases or meanings. Another popular secondary source of data is the information collected by various government agencies such as the Home Office, the Department of Health, or the Department for Children, Schools and Families.

Stop and Think	Strengths and weaknesses of various research tools

For each of the various research tools, list their strengths and weaknesses in relation to researching school bullying.

Why are ethical considerations important?

Discussions concerning ethical considerations in social research generally revolve around four key issues: the lack of informed consent, the use of deception, harm to respondents and invasion of privacy. Let us briefly consider each issue in turn.

Informed consent

The principle of informed consent states that anyone who is asked to participate in social research should be given as much information as they need in order to help them decide whether or not they wish to get involved in the study. In particular, the researcher should do the following.

1. Inform potential participants that their involvement in the study is voluntary and that if they decide not to take part no adverse consequences will follow. This issue is especially important when dealing with powerless groups such as children who may feel that because the study is being carried out by adults, with the agreement of their teacher, they will be viewed negatively if they refuse to get involved. This raises the question as to whether children can ever be considered as truly voluntary participants in research.

2. Inform potential participants of the most important issues that might influence their decision about participating in the study. However, there are two key problems with this requirement, as follows: (a) In covert research which may involve observing people in their natural environment, such as the behaviour of children in a classroom, respondents are not given the option of taking part in the study; they are involved whether they like it or not. The difficulty here is that any

attempt to elicit their cooperation would contaminate the natural setting, as the children would then know they were being watched and so would behave very differently. (b) The second problem is that it is often difficult for researchers to provide all the information that the potential respondent might need. For example, it is often unclear even to the researcher whether the potential participant is likely to find the subject matter of the study upsetting, or precisely how long interviews will last. Moreover, sometimes it is necessary for researchers to withhold certain information, as such knowledge may impact on the kind of response that is given to important questions. Thus, if the potential respondents of a study on school bullying were told directly what the research was about, then it is likely that those who do bully others and the victims of bullying would refuse to get involved, or provide very guarded responses to particularly sensitive questions.

3. Inform potential participants that they have a right to withdraw from the study at any time. The potential downside to this ethical consideration for researchers is that a great deal of time, money and effort may be spent on securing a respondent's involvement only for them to withdraw from the study at a later stage. For captive audiences such as school children, the question should be raised as to whether they would find it difficult to withdraw from a study, given the lack of power they have to make such decisions during the course of normal classroom activities.

Deception

This is a related issue and essentially amounts to the researcher failing to obtain informed consent either by directly lying to potential respondents about the nature of the research, or by omitting to tell them about issues that the researcher knows would increase the potential participants' likelihood of refusing to cooperate. Such unethical conduct is typically associated with qualitative research where the researcher either directly or indirectly gives the impression that they are anything but a researcher. Instead, they may deceive the study group into believing that they are perhaps a teaching assistant or trainee teacher. Quantitative research can also involve methods of deceiving participants. For example, unknown to the respondents, lie scale items are sometimes included in attitudinal questionnaires in order to test whether they are providing honest answers. Thus, although the realities of doing research mean that respondents are often deceived to one degree or another, the researcher should make every effort to rule out acts of deception. Ultimately, such conduct should be considered as a form of abuse which is potentially harmful to respondents and, if not taken seriously, can severely undermine the professional integrity of future social research.

Harm

The lack of informed consent and degree of deception employed by researchers should never be so serious as to deliberately place respondents in harm's way. Thus, studies should not subject participants to any physical injury, psychological distress (such as through creating states of fear or anxiety) or social difficulties (such as through causing embarrassment, jeopardising friendships, social status, income, etc.). However, harm is an ethical principle more easily accepted in theory than in practice, as all research carries some degree of unforeseen risks. For example, if deception is used to encourage children to talk about bad behaviour in school, then it is possible that some respondents, especially those who, unknown to the researcher, are the victims of bullying, may well be psychologically harmed by the interview experience. Consequently, researchers should make every effort to ensure that they are aware of the potential dangers associated with their study and do all that they can to mitigate its potential impact. For example, research on school bullying may be done in cooperation with the school's counselling service.

Privacy

One of the main concerns potential participants have about becoming involved in research relates to the issue of privacy; will what a particular respondent says or does during the course of the study be made public? There are three steps researchers should take in order to allay potential respondents' fears with regards to this ethical issue.

1. It is important to emphasise to all respondents that they have the right to refuse to answer any questions that they feel may reveal potentially sensitive information about themselves. For example, often pupils may refuse to discuss their involvement in bullying or their experiences of being bullied. The researcher can manoeuvre around such problems by asking for general answers, or asking questions which encourage the respondent to answer in terms of a third person. For example, questions about bullying might be phrased in terms of the respondents' views of others who bully or who are victimised by bullies. Overall, however, if a respondent is reluctant to answer a particular question, the researcher should not place them under any undue pressure to respond.

2. If possible, it is important to give respondents assurances about *anonymity*: that the research is designed in order to make it impossible to identify individual respondents. This is usually achieved through assigning a code number or a pseudo-name to the information provided by respondents and/or by ensuring that the research data is collated in such a way that it would be impossible to determine the nature of any individual contribution.

3. If, however, anonymity cannot be achieved, then researchers have a duty to uphold their respondents' right to *confidentiality*, which involves the researcher agreeing to keep the identity of their respondents a secret. In such situations, the study participants and their responses are known only to the researcher and perhaps a small team of research associates. Keeping information in confidence also means ensuring that data is securely stored and only accessible to the research team. However, with the advent of networked databases, computer hacking and the theft of mass storage devices, the task of protecting research data often presents challenges that researchers seldom consider.

Stop and Think **Ethically researching school bullying**

What do you think are the various ethical considerations that a researcher would face in researching school bullying?

How to plan a social research project

In an attempt to draw together and make sense of many of the key issues discussed throughout this chapter, we will conclude by offering some advice on how you can start to organise a small research project. If you can give a positive response to each of the 10 questions below, then you should consider yourself well on the way to producing a sound piece of social research.

1. *Have you found a research problem?* This is a broad social issue that interests you and that causes social difficulties. *Have you found a topic worth studying within this research problem?* Use your imagination to draw out specific concerns which need to be more thoroughly understood. The list of possibilities is limitless.

2. *Have you decided on the research questions/issues to be addressed in the study?* These relate to your topic of study and help to focus the aims of your research. The questions/issues you focus on will depend on whether your project is descriptive, exploratory, explanatory or evaluative.

3. *Have you given some thought to your epistemological orientation?* In other words, are you approaching your research project from either a positivist or an interpretivist point of view? Will you be collecting qualitative or quantitative data, or a combination of the two?

4. *Have you started to review previous literature on your research problem and topic of study?* Your aim should be to learn about the different theories and methods that have already been employed in your area of interest. This literature will help you find questions to ask and decide on the design of your research. Look again at our earlier discussion on deduction and induction.

5. *Have you worked with your supervisor on considering how realistic the parameters of your research project are, given the time and resources available?* Most students start by wanting to solve all the world's problems in one go. This is a healthy sign, but you will need to get control of your research project before it takes control of you.

6. *Have you thoroughly considered the difficulties associated with obtaining access to research populations?* This usually involves completing ethical application forms and seeking permission from *gatekeepers*: the people who have the authority to grant researchers access to a specific research population such as schools, prisons or hospitals. *Have you decided on what sampling design to use?* As we discussed earlier, this will be either a probability sampling design using methods such as simple or stratified random sampling, or a non-probability sampling design using methods such as purposive or snowball sampling.

7. *Have you considered the key concepts and variables to be studied?* If you are working with variables, how will they be operationalised? Are you clear about which are the dependent and independent variables?

8. *Have you decided on the most appropriate research design for your study?* See our earlier discussion on experimental, cross-sectional, longitudinal, case study and secondary source designs. *Have you decided on which methods you are going to use in order to collect your data?* See our earlier references to questionnaires, interviews, participant observation, etc.

9. *Have you given serious consideration to testing the reliability and validity of the data obtained from your research?* This is an important task which tests the accuracy of your findings and is often overlooked in social science research.

10. *Have you given serious consideration to the ethical consequences of your research?* Especially in terms of informed consent, deceit, harm and privacy? How did you resolve any conflicts or justify any potentially unethical practices?

Conclusion

This chapter has aimed to explore the various key aspects to social research as applied to social policy and welfare, with explicit reference to the social phenomenon of school bullying. As such it has:

- explained the purpose of social research;
- discussed the relationship between theory and research;
- explained how research helps us search for the 'truth';
- explored the extent to which doing social research is scientific;
- explained the language of research;
- explained why sampling is important;
- introduced some of the various tools of the research trade;
- explored why ethical considerations are important;
- described how one would set about planning a social research project.

Annotated further reading

One of the most useful textbooks dealing with all aspects of social research is Alan Bryman's *Social Research Methods* (third edition, 2008). The key text for social policy students and practitioners is Becker and Bryman's *Understanding Research for Social Policy and Practice* (2004). It shows the importance and place of research, as well as offering guidance on carrying out good quality research in social policy. For information on specific research terms and issues, a particularly helpful reference is Victor Jupp's *The SAGE Dictionary of Social Research Methods* (2006). Steinar Kvale's *Interviews: An introduction to qualitative research interviews* (1996) discusses in an accessible way a wide range of qualitative issues and interviewing methods. An interesting introduction to feminist methodologies is presented by Liz Stanley and Sue Wise in *Breaking Out Again: Feminist consciousness and feminist research* (1993). For information on doing research via the web see Clive Hewson *et al.*, *Internet Research Methods: A practical guide for the social and behavioural sciences* (2003). Official government statistics can be accessed via http://www.statistics.gov.uk. Finally, the site http://www.data-archive.ac.uk is managed by Essex University and sources a significant amount of information on social research conducted in the UK.

Concluding comment to Part III

This part has introduced the reader to the nature and range of ideological, theoretical and methodological perspectives used to analyse welfare provision and direct its practice. These perspectives are employed to justify state intervention in welfare policy and moreover are used to prescribe the level and extent of that intervention. What each of the different positions outlined allows us to do is to evaluate, against different criteria, the relative success or failure of (particularly government) social policy.

We have presented an account of the more traditional set of explanations and theories. Secondly, we discussed more recent and radical theoretical departures and newer strands of welfare theory, including new social movement, feminist, post-modern, anti-racist and green perspectives. The ideological underpinnings of New Right and New Labour have also been explored, since an understanding of these perspectives is key to being able to understand, analyse and critique contemporary British social policy. Thirdly, we have examined how social polices can be examined and evaluated by applying the principles of research.

Although this is often difficult material to absorb, looking at social policy and welfare developments through such different theoretical lenses allows us to perceive social policy as a whole as well as partially and allows us to develop our critical analysis and explanation of social policy.

Part IV

Welfare themes

Introduction to Part IV

Part IV explores in more detail the key social policy areas in Britain. We will consider the big areas of social policy: health, social care, housing, education, work and pensions, but will consider also wider policy areas such as family, social divisions, criminal justice, the environment, and the impact of Europe and the international dimension. Some of these areas are often not considered to be part of social policy but are dealt with in texts more normally associated with economics, law or political science. However, we consider them to be central to the making and understanding of social policy.

Many of the chapters take as their starting point the Beveridge Report or the other policy initiatives that helped to establish the post-war welfare state, examining major policy developments since Beveridge and the legacy of the post-war settlement. Subsequent Acts of Parliament and their effects will be examined and placed within their contemporary political, socio-economic and policy-making contexts which face contemporary social policy makers, service providers and service users. Each chapter will conclude with an explanation and analysis of current developments and thinking and with a discussion of the key issues faced by that particular service sector or policy area.

Chapter 12

Health policy

Objectives

- To provide an overview of, and introduction to, health policy and the health system in the UK.

- To provide a basic account of some key concepts, themes and issues in health policy.

- To provide a brief account of the origins, development and structure of the UK system.

- To examine recent reforms to the UK health system.

- To analyse the health policy of the present ('New') Labour government.

- To provide an account of achievements and problems of the UK system.

Introduction: What is health policy?

In 2005, intense media scrutiny was directed at two issues: adult and childhood obesity, and the quality of children's school meals. It had been suggested that childhood obesity is a serious and growing problem for the nation's children, and not only in this country. The latter issue was highlighted in 2005 by the popular TV chef Jamie Oliver, in a series entitled Jamie's School Dinners, in which it was suggested that the quality of food was poor; that basic nutritional standards were absent or ignored; that poor nutritional quality was implicated in impaired learning and behavioural problems as well as overweight, itself a source of present or future health problems (Boone, 2005; Editorial, 2005). Both of the issues referred to were viewed as health issues, broadly conceived, in the public debate which developed (Toynbee and Walker, 2005: 303–304).

An assumption of participants in the debate was that 'something must be done' by the government. At one time these nutrition issues were not 'issues', or at any rate they were not public issues in the sense of being the object of sustained attention by the media and policy-makers. They *became* issues, that is, they became topics to which policy-makers were expected to respond.

This suggests a number of things about health policy:

- Firstly, it suggests that there is some connection between issues of health and the responsibilities, presumed or actual, of governments.

- Secondly it suggests that it is something dynamic and changing and is open to redefinition.

- Thirdly, it suggests the difficulty and complexity of issues and the appropriate response to them.
- Fourthly, it suggests a connection between diverse fields and policy areas. Although the connection of food and nutrition with health is obvious and accepted in a general way, this is not something normally considered to be part of health policy conventionally defined – it may be thought of as having more to do with agricultural policy, trade policy or EU relations.
- Fifthly, and finally, it suggests that health policy is more than a concern with health services, health care and the NHS.

What is health? Models of health

Let us begin by examining the concept of *health*. Health, like most concepts in the social sciences, is a disputed, contested, fuzzy concept. There is a variety of concepts of health (and its correlate, *illness*). We can distinguish between the so-called '*medical*' (or '*biomedical*') and '*social*' (or '*socio-medical*') models of health.

The *medical model* sees health as the absence of disease. Disease is interpreted as a physical malfunctioning of the organism as a result of invasion or attack by pathogens or by other disease-causing agents or processes, such as smoking, for example (Nettleton, 1995: 3–4). This model is associated with a 'scientific' view of medicine, health, illness and disease and has been the 'privileged', mainstream view of health and illness for much of the post-war period.

The '*social*' *model* of health embodies the view that health is more than the absence of disease. The range of factors affecting health is wider and includes, for example, material and social circumstances, such as income, working conditions, housing, education, environmental quality and the degree of social cohesion. (Relatively) poor material and social circumstances lead to (relatively) poor health outcomes. Chadwick's famous report of 1842 on public health, with its account of the poorer health of urban working-class populations in Britain's industrialising cities, by comparison with the middle classes, exemplifies the historical importance and influence of the social model (Fraser, 2003: 66–71).

Important restatements of the social approach are those of the World Health Organisation in the 1970s, which advanced an ambitious and demanding conception of health as a state of complete physical, mental and social well-being (Nettleton, 1995: 41), and the Black Report on health inequalities in Britain (Townsend and Davidson, 1982).

Health and illness in the United Kingdom

During the course of the twentieth century, there have been changes in disease patterns, from short-term, acute, infectious illness to long-term, chronic and degenerative conditions. The predominant causes of death in developed countries such as the UK are now cancers and cardio-vascular diseases, by comparison with the period before the Second World War, when the principal killers were infectious diseases, bacterial or viral in origin – for example TB, diphtheria, measles and polio (Webster, 1993; Jones, 1994; Porter, 1997).

Two important aspects of the contemporary health of the UK population are the continuation in the significant long-term *improvement* in the health of the population since records began in the mid-nineteenth century, and, at the same time, the persistence, and perhaps even worsening, of *health inequalities* of various kinds (Sassi, 2005: 70–73).

Figure 12.1 provides a convenient visual representation of one way of illustrating the improvement in UK health for men and women since 1901, as measured by life expectancy. (Life expectancy can be regarded as an indirect or proxy measure of health.) First of all, the graph shows a clear improvement in life expectancy since the beginning of the period, although the graph is rather more jagged and discontinuous during the first half of the twentieth century. It will also be seen that over the entire period, women's life expectancy has exceeded men's, and that the overall rate of improvement in population life expectancy and health was greatest during the first half of the twentieth century (the graph is steeper); the rate of improvement has levelled off since the middle of the last century.

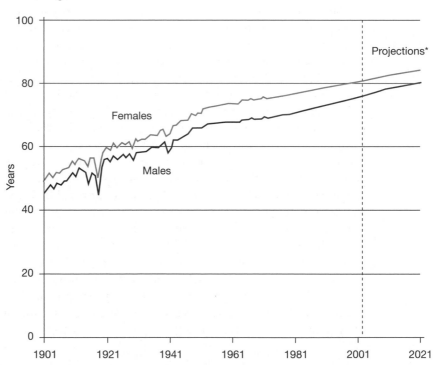

Expectation of life is the average number of years a new-born baby would survive if he or she experienced age-specific mortality rates for that time period throughout his or her life. * 2004-based projections for 2005 to 2021.

Figure 12.1 Expectation of life at birth: by sex
Source: Office for National Statistics (2006a) *Social Trends No. 36*, Figure 7.1, p. 100, London: ONS. Crown copyright material is reproduced with the permission of the Controller of HMSO and the Queen's Printer for Scotland under the terms of the Click-Use Licence. *Original source*: Government Actuary's Department.

Figure 12.2 shows the improvement in infant mortality since 1921. It reveals a fairly consistent improvement over the period, although there is a steady levelling-off in improvement since the middle of the twentieth century. This too is an indirect measure of general improvement in the health of the population. This graph in fact correlates quite well with Figure 12.1. This is because most, though not all, of the improvement in life expectancy has been driven by improvements in infant mortality. The improvement in UK life expectancy during the twentieth century is in fact due to a higher proportion of babies surviving their first year of life. This has been due partly to improvements in maternal and infant care – developments in ante-natal care, midwifery and health visiting services – but probably mainly to general improvements in living standards, reflecting improvements in wage levels, nutrition, housing and education.

Figure 12.3 illustrates the extent of social inequalities in health in the 1990s, giving life expectancies for men and women for each of 10 subdivisions of the population from the most to the least deprived. The graph reveals a clear pattern of persisting inequalities. Health inequalities have persisted, and indeed worsened, in a context of steadily improving population health as a whole (Sassi, 2005: 72–73, Figures 4.1 and 4.2). A pattern of widening health inequalities does not necessarily imply that the health of the

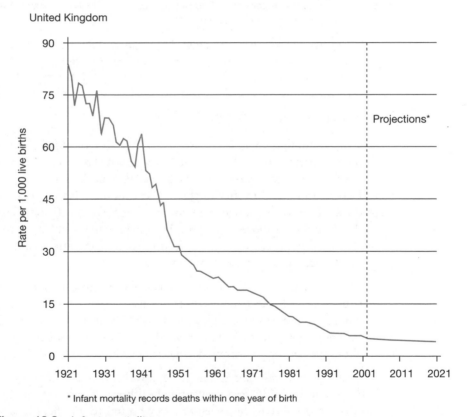

* Infant mortality records deaths within one year of birth

Figure 12.2   Infant mortality
Source: Office for National Statistics (2005a) *Social Trends No. 35,* Figure 7.5, p. 98, London: ONS. Crown copyright material is reproduced with the permission of the Controller of HMSO and the Queen's Printer for Scotland under the terms of the Click-Use Licence. *Original sources*: Office for National Statistics; General Register Office for Scotland; Northern Ireland Statistics and Research Agency; Government Actuary's Department.

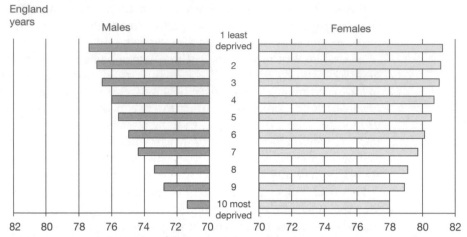

Figure 12.3   Life expectancy at birth: by deprivation group and sex, 1994–99
Source: Office for National Statistics (2006a) *Social Trends No. 36,* Figure 7.2, p. 100, London: ONS. Crown copyright material is reproduced with the permission of the Controller of HMSO and the Queen's Printer for Scotland under the terms of the Click-Use Licence. *Original sources*: Health Survey for England, Department of Health; Census 1991, Office for National Statistics; Small Area Health Statistics Unit, Imperial College.

most deprived groups has worsened. There is in fact little evidence for this. It may simply be that their health is improving, but at a slower rate than that of better-off groups.

Health policy and health care policy

It is important to distinguish between *health policy* and *health care policy*. The course of the twentieth century has, in the UK as elsewhere, seen a shift from health policy to health care policy, corresponding to a decline in the acceptance of the social model of health, and a rise in that of the medical model. Health policy is broader, having to do with the whole range of factors that impinge on the health of a population.

Health policy is more important, but health care policy is more salient for voters, public opinion and governments. Rudolf Klein drew attention to this paradox with his acute observation some years ago that

> The NHS has . . . a political constituency: those whose income comes from working in it and those who, as patients, derive some direct benefits from its services. Prevention has no such constituency. Those who will benefit cannot be identified; moreover, the benefit itself is uncertain. For prevention is about the reduction of statistical risk, not about the delivery of certain benefits to specific individuals (Klein, 1989: 173)

In other words, politicians might very well believe that public money would be better spent on public and preventive health measures, but the demands of winning elections require that they spend money on improving health services, for example by shortening waiting lists, increasing the numbers of doctors and nurses, and increasing the availability and uptake of new medical technology.

There is an uncertain relationship between health care and health. Improvements in the health of the British population (measured by reference to improvements in mortality and life expectancy) have taken place continuously since records began 150 years ago, but it is hard to correlate this with improvements in the amount, quality or availability of health care or health services. Figure 12.1, above, suggests that the rate of improvement in UK health was faster during the first half of the twentieth century, *before* the creation of the NHS and the universal availability of health care which it brought about, than subsequently. During the first half of the twentieth century, the UK added, on average, around 20 years to the life expectancies of both men and women, but only 10 years in the subsequent half-century. Mortality and life expectancy are, however, crude measures of health. If we define health broadly as something like 'quality of life', then health services may be more significant, but of course this is harder to measure.

Stop and Think

How should a population's health status be measured? Typically, mortality (death) rates and morbidity (illness) rates are used. What are the advantages and disadvantages of each of these measures?

Health policy-making

Governments do not create and shape health policy on their own. 'Health policy' can involve, in principle, a wide range of issues and participants. Organisations shaping and influencing health policy include, for example, health care professions, local government, trade unions, voluntary organisations, the World Health Organisation, the European Union, pharmaceutical companies, private health insurers, private health service providers, Parliament, and the higher education sector. Most health policy-making is the outcome of a complex process of bargaining and negotiation between the government and these various interest, pressure and lobby groups that comprise the health policy 'community' (for more on policy-making, see Chapters 5 and 6).

Power in health systems: professionals, patients and the state

The interpretation of power relations in the UK health care system has been controversial and disputed. Earlier commentators argued that there is an equal, or *'pluralist'*, distribution of power among the various interests in the system. More recently, it has been argued that groups and interests in the health policy community are not necessarily equal in their power to influence policy. On the whole, it is suggested, policy has been dominated by *producer* rather than *consumer* or user interests. *Producer power*, or *professional power*, is an important issue in many areas of social policy, especially, perhaps, in health policy (see Chapter 6 for more on professionals). 'In sociological terms, medicine, with law, was the paradigmatic profession, a publicly-mandated and state-backed monopolistic supplier of a valued service, exercising autonomy in the workplace and collegiate control over recruitment, training and the regulation of members' conduct' (Elston, 1991: 58). Since the 1970s there have been important critiques of mainstream medicine, 'radical', Marxist and feminist, part of a general critique of professions and professional power in social welfare services (Wilding, 1982).

The medical profession, it is argued, has been the dominant interest group in relation to health policy, because it has the power to determine health priorities. Its priorities are those of a focus on acute care and a 'medical model' approach to sickness and ill-health.

The existence of this medical power and its priorities is suggested by the existence of a variety of inequalities in provision and treatment, including, for example, the lower priority given to long-term illness and disability by comparison with acute and short-term conditions, the lower priority given to public and preventive health, and the relative neglect of health inequalities (Ham, 2004: 217–220).

The power of the medical profession does not imply complete ability to block all change and define agendas. The past 20 years in British health policy have seen a determined attempt on the part of politicians to subject the profession to some degree of control, to reshape agendas and priorities and to shift resources in new directions (Ham, 2004: Ch. 10).

'Consumerism'

A further development which has begun to challenge medical power is the rise of the *patient-as-consumer*. In recent years patients have become more demanding and active in challenging professional and policy decisions, for example over the availability of particular treatments (for more on this, see the section later in the chapter on 'rationing') (Ham, 2004: 247–251). Some of this activism is individual – examples include people using the Internet to inform themselves about medical conditions and treatments and using the information gained to challenge professional decisions – and some of it collective, via voluntary organisations of various kinds, including patients' associations and self-help groups for particular, especially long-term and chronic, medical conditions (Kelleher, 1994).

Origins and development of the UK health care system

The state has been involved in health at least since the nineteenth century in Britain, earlier in some other countries, and has grown steadily in importance, becoming a major player since the First World War. The Poor Law, reorganised in 1834, provided some basic medical assistance to recipients of poor relief ('paupers') and in the later nineteenth century developed a more specialised concern with health care, opening up to non-pauper poor and building specialised facilities for in-patient care. State involvement in public health took the form of a series of Public Health Acts, beginning with the famous Act of 1848. These were concerned with such matters as clean water and sewerage.

Hospital care was relatively unimportant before the later twentieth century. Health care was mostly unspecialised general practice, provided, apart from provision under the Poor Law, privately on a fee-for-service basis for those who could afford the doctor's fees, but also to working-class wage-earners who were members of 'friendly societies', which were mutual aid organisations and an important aspect of nineteenth-century 'self help' (De Swaan, 1988: Ch. 5).

Significant developments followed in the Edwardian period and during the First World War, influenced by concern about the poor health and physical condition of urban industrial populations (Thane, 1996: Ch. 3; Fraser, 2003: Ch. 6). There were innovations in infant, child and maternal health and in relation to the funding of health care, with the introduction of a social insurance-based scheme in 1911 –

National Health Insurance – which covered insured workers, but not their families, for primary care and provided a cash benefit where sickness resulted in interrupted earnings (Thane, 1996: Ch. 3; Fraser, 2003: Ch. 7). Some of these developments were influenced by foreign models, notably the German social insurance scheme introduced in the 1880s (Thane, 1996: Ch. 4).

The inter-war period was characterised by some expansion of NHI coverage and developments in local authority hospital care and of community-based medical and preventive services, but the system remained fragmented and uncoordinated, with substantial inequalities resulting from gaps in coverage and serious territorial inequalities in provision. There were serious problems of underfunding.

The outbreak of the War in 1939 helped to precipitate change. The Beveridge Report of 1942 famously proposed an assault on the 'five giants', one of which was 'disease'. 1944 saw the publication of a White Paper on health system reform by the Churchill-led coalition government. The task of reconstructing and remodelling the health system, however, fell to a Labour government elected in July 1945.

Creating the National Health Service

There is argument and debate among historians about the origins of Labour's reforms of the health system, and whether the creation of the NHS was the product of a 'consensus' in health policy between the political parties or major social interests. Some have argued that the reform was essentially professional, bureaucratic and technical in origin and inspiration, and the subject of broad agreement; others have argued for a more conflictual and partisan process in which consensus was initially absent, only becoming established later (Webster, 1998; Klein, 2006: Ch. 1). Legislation was passed in 1946, and the NHS came into being in 1948. Between these two dates there was intense conflict between the medical profession and the Government over the terms and conditions on offer, and almost until the last moment there was doubt about whether the doctors would join the new scheme.

There were reforms in *coverage*, *eligibility*, *governance* and *funding*. Coverage became *universal*, with no exclusions on grounds of income or wealth. Direct payments for health care – fees and charges – were abolished. Hospitals – local authority and most voluntary – were nationalised, in the sense of being taken into national public ownership. Local authorities thereby lost many of their major health responsibilities, but retained important responsibilities for community medical services and public health. The GP service, created under NHI in 1911, was left largely unchanged. Hospital specialists became salaried employees, with a generous system of merit awards to reward the most able and with the right to treat private patients in their now publicly owned hospitals. Funding was simplified, now coming from central government, made up of general tax revenues and National Insurance contributions. Levels of and increases in health care funding therefore became entirely subject to central government discretion.

After its creation the new system settled down for a period of 30 years or so of consolidation and piecemeal development driven by improvements in medical technology and largely under the control of a hegemonic medical profession (Klein, 1990, 1996d).

The 1970s saw the beginnings of attempts to deal with long-standing problems of poor-quality services experienced by certain low-priority groups. These, the so-called 'Cinderella' services, which included services for the mentally ill, mentally handicapped and elderly, were the object of neglect in the NHS, which had developed in ways that focused on acute and short-term illness.

Conservative health policies, 1979–97

The three decades that have elapsed since the election of the Conservative government in 1979 have been a period of radical upheaval in and questioning of many taken-for-granted aspects of the structure and organisation of the health care system. Why is this? In order to understand recent policy developments, we must examine some general issues facing all contemporary health systems.

There are a number of critical problems and pressures facing most health care systems at the present time, including those in the UK. Three important pressures are those of *demography*, *medical technology* and *public expectations* (Blank and Burau, 2004).

The first refers to the ageing of populations in many countries, and changes in population structure. Population ageing is associated with increases in health services expenditure, because older people tend to be heavy users of health services. As populations age, therefore, an upward impulse is given to health care spending.

A *second* factor that health systems have to deal with is that of innovation and growth in medical technology. The adoption of new technologies, which includes diagnostic equipment and procedures, and new drugs as well as surgical interventions, also imparts an upward momentum to health expenditures.

Thirdly, there are rising public expectations about health care and its presumed benefits. Populations in many developed countries have in recent years been demanding more in the way of quality, availability and amount of health care. Such elevated expectations are fuelled by the media and their coverage of health issues, and by rises in income and in educational levels (Blank and Burau, 2004).

Reform of the health system since the 1970s, both Conservative and Labour, has been to a considerable extent an attempt to confront the issues of the relentless upward pressure to spend more, and enhanced expectations about what the system should provide.

The Conservatives early on ruled out substantial privatisation of health care funding and claimed to defend, in its essentials, the basis of the system as it had existed since 1948. The 1980s was nevertheless a decade in which the private sector, in both funding and in the provision of services, was encouraged to expand. Private health insurance, private hospital care, private residential and long-term nursing care, and the contracting-out of a variety of ancillary, non-core hospital services, all developed in this period.

Management and markets

'Value for money' in public services was an important issue for the Conservatives in the 1980s, in a context of tight control of public spending. Achieving it required change in managing these services (for more on management and governance changes in this period, see Chapter 6). Management reform of the NHS began in the 1980s in the wake of a report by Sir Roy Griffiths, a businessman and friend of the Prime Minister, in 1983 (Department of Health and Social Security, 1983). More significant still were developments after the 1987 General Election. A White Paper, *Working for Patients* (Department of Health, 1989a), and subsequent legislation in 1990 envisaged the creation of a 'purchaser–provider split' in NHS organisation and the creation of a competitive market in the production and allocation of health services (a 'quasi-market' or 'internal market' as it came to be called). The aim was to decentralise the system, to move services closer to the patient, to make the system more responsive to the patient, and also to enhance efficiency in the sense of reducing variations between areas in the quality and availability of hospital treatment. The reforms were implemented in 1991 (Klein, 2006: Ch. 6).

Evaluating the Conservative reforms

The verdict of evaluative research on the Conservative reforms is mixed (Robinson and Le Grand, 1994; Le Grand *et al.*, 1998). Some improvements were noted, but criticism centred on the alleged creation of a 'two-tier' service, in part following from one of the most dynamic elements of the reforms, GP fundholding and commissioning. The conclusion of one critically sympathetic observer, reflecting other findings, is, however, that 'the change in behaviour and culture was nevertheless tangible ... the separation of purchaser and provider responsibilities altered the organizational politics of the NHS leading to changes in the balance of power both within the medical profession and between doctors and managers' (Ham, 2004: 46–47).

The public health agenda

The public health agenda, relatively neglected by the Conservatives, developed in a piecemeal way in the 1980s in response to particular emergencies, such as the advent of the HIV/AIDS crisis. The early 1990s saw the beginnings of a general strategy for population health, with the publication of a White Paper in 1992 (Department of Health, 1992). This proposed targeting a limited number of health conditions, with numerical targets for improvements in a given time-period. Another important aspect of this was the idea of collaborative working amongst agencies, organisations and groups, national, local, statutory, and private – voluntary and commercial – to achieve these goals.

Recent developments: 'New' Labour health policy

The 'New' Labour Party headed by Tony Blair won the General Election of 1997 and two subsequent elections in 2001 and 2005. In some respects it has carried forward the revolution begun under the Thatcher and Major governments. At the same time, there have been departures from Conservative policy. New Labour health policy is, however, hard to interpret. There have been changes in direction since 1997, and disagreements within the government over the direction of change. Change has continued to come fast and furiously despite an implied 1997 election manifesto promise of a quieter life for the NHS.

Devolution

Importantly, in this context, there have been major constitutional changes in the UK since 1998 (see Chapter 7). There are now devolved governments, with varying degrees of autonomy and responsibility, in Scotland, Wales and Northern Ireland, and four UK health systems, each with its own policies. It is no longer possible, if it ever was, to talk about UK health and NHS policy. English and Scottish policies for the NHS, for example, now seem to be quite different (Ham, 2004: Ch. 5). In what follows we shall focus on English developments, occasionally noting policy variations in the other three countries (Peckham, 2007).

Health policy in England: NHS funding

One of the government's key aims has been to improve and modernise health services by increasing the volume and improving the quality of NHS care (Klein, 2005: 52). This 'supply side' strategy has required more generous funding. The early years of New Labour from 1997 to 1999 were, however, years of relatively low growth in funding as a result of New Labour's election pledge to adhere to Conservative public spending targets.

There was a significant change in January 2000, with the Prime Minister's announcement, on television, that spending levels would be substantially increased. The annual rate of increase would be doubled with the aim of matching the European average by 2008 and of increasing funding by one-third in real terms in five years. Here perhaps is an example of the impact of crises on policy-making. The immediate background to the announcement early in 2000 was an influenza epidemic in the winter of 1999–2000, which increased pressure on NHS hospitals, resulting in bed shortages and trolley-waits for patients in hospitals.

An expert inquiry was established under the chairmanship of the banker and statistician Derek Wanless to report on NHS funding and to make recommendations. Wanless's first two reports in 2001 and 2002 essentially ratified and provided an analytical foundation for the funding decision that had already been taken (H.M. Treasury, 2002; Chen, 2003) and that would be formalised in the Treasury's 2002 Spending Review.

Extra resources for the increase were found by increasing National Insurance contributions. The rise in contributions was explicitly linked to the need to provide extra funding for the NHS. In this context it should be noted that the funding of other NHS systems in the UK, notably the Scottish and Northern Irish, has always been more generous than that of the English system.

Much of this funding increase was spent on employing more staff and raising staff salaries. Health care is a labour-intensive activity, and around two-thirds of health care budgets is spent on staff salaries. More staff needed to be recruited, educated and trained. There have been increased intakes in medical school numbers and an increase in the number of new medical schools (Toynbee and Walker, 2005: 16).

Questions remain about how effective these funding and resource increases have been in terms of securing improvements in volume and quality of patient care. The Conservative opposition questioned the government's strategy, claiming that 40% more was spent on the NHS between 1998 and 2003, but that this resulted in only a 5% increase in in-patient activity (Toynbee and Walker, 2005: 38).

Figure 12.4, adapted from the 2007 Wanless Report, provides an overview of health spending in the UK and in EU countries since 1960, as percentages of GDP, with spending projections to 2030. The lines that matter are the two dense lines for EU and UK spending. The graph reveals that spending on health has increased over the period in both the UK and the EU as a whole – it has more than doubled as a percentage of GDP. It will be seen that since the early 1960s UK spending has been below the EU average, but that since 2000 there has been a convergence of the two lines, resulting in UK spending matching the EU average at around 9% of GDP by 2007. Although EU and UK spending steadily diverged over most of the period, the fluctuations and discontinuities in spending revealed by the two lines are fairly closely correlated, suggesting that the factors that govern trends in health spending operated both for the UK and for the EU as a whole.

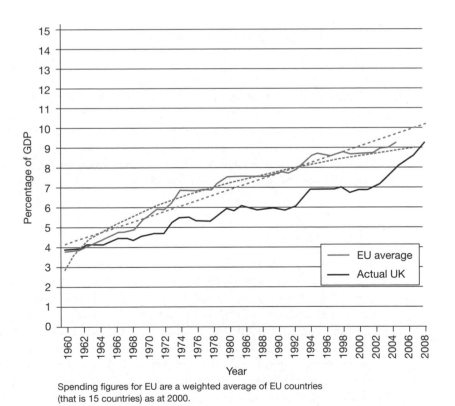

Spending figures for EU are a weighted average of EU countries
(that is 15 countries) as at 2000.

Figure 12.4   Historic and projected UK and EU spending on health care, 1960–2007
Source: Adapted from D. Wanless (2007) *Our Future Health Secured? A Review of NHS Funding and Performance*, Figure 14, p. 86, London: King's Fund.

Governance and management

Labour initially rejected the Conservatives' internal market experiment, with its allegedly poor consequences for equity, coordination and planning (Department of Health, 1997). There was also an efficiency objection to the internal market, which drew attention to the administrative costs of commissioning and contracting. The stated intention in 1997 was a return, not to the supposed 'command and control' system that prevailed until the 1980s, but to cooperation, coordination and joint working.

The Conservatives' concept of a 'primary care-led NHS' was, nevertheless, one that New Labour found congenial (Department of Health, 1997). All GP practices would henceforth become members of collective commissioning entities called Primary Care Groups (PCGs), later to become Trusts (PCTs), with devolved budgets which would be used to commission care from secondary (mainly hospital) providers. This was an implicit acknowledgement that the GP fundholding scheme had brought some benefits for those patients whose GPs were members of the scheme. PCTs would control 75% of the NHS budget by 2004.

Other innovations presented in the 1997 White Paper included NHS Direct, a 24-hour telephone and online consultation service, and the introduction of local walk-in centres, staffed by nurses, providing basic advice and care. These were 'modernisation' measures aimed at increasing public access to health services.

National Service Frameworks

Another important innovation, connected with the 1997 White Paper's commitment to make the NHS once again truly 'national', was the introduction of so-called National Service Frameworks (NSFs). These lay down, for a range of conditions, minimum appropriate standards of care and treatment. As well as specifying standards of care and treatment, the underlying idea is to eliminate variations in treatment between areas and localities, a vexed issue, and to ensure that quality of treatment does not depend on where a patient lives. One effect of this is to encroach on and limit the area of clinical freedom.

New agencies

Other policy initiatives involved the creation of special-purpose agencies (or 'quangos'). These arms-length agencies are designed to devolve decision-making away from central government. Examples include the National Institute for Health and Clinical Excellence (NICE) and the Health Care Commission, formerly the Commission for Health Improvement (CHI). NICE is concerned with evaluating medical technology (which includes all types of therapeutic interventions, drugs, procedures, surgical and other) in terms of effectiveness and efficiency, permitting their use by the NHS or alternatively rejecting and prohibiting it. The existence of NICE also implies, like NSFs, some limitation of clinical freedom. Doctors are no longer free to prescribe for their patients according to their own independent professional judgement as to what is appropriate. The HCC is an inspectoral body which has the task of monitoring standards of provision in NHS hospitals.

Targets

A major development in the management of the NHS is the use of *targets* of all kinds. These represent an attempt to strengthen control from the centre – that is (in England) the Department of Health. Such 'top-down' control is particularly associated with the former Chancellor Gordon Brown and the enhanced power of the Treasury over all aspects of domestic policy. The biennial Spending Reviews incorporate Public Spending Agreements which draw up and list targets for service improvements. These are usually numerical, with a target date by which an improvement is to be secured.

An example of a Department of Health target is that of reducing waiting times to 18 weeks from initial GP consultation to in-patient hospital operation put forward in 2004, this to be achieved for all conditions and specialisms by 2008 (Timmins, 2005b).

Waiting lists are typically associated with elective, non-urgent, surgical procedures. Waiting lists and waiting times have been a key area for service improvements in the NHS since 1997, and the government has striven, even more than its predecessors, to bring about reductions. Money has been directed at these, possibly to the detriment of care and treatment in other areas. The policy has had some success.

The Department of Health has recently given the impression of moving away from the 'command and control', top-down managerial approach associated with the regime of targets and public service agreements towards a looser, more arms-length regulation, relying on monitoring and inspection by agencies such as the Healthcare Commission to maintain and improve standards (Klein, 2005: 52).

The NHS Plan 2000

The enhanced NHS spending programme announced in 2000 was accompanied by the NHS Plan 2000, which put forward a 10-year programme of development for the NHS. The Plan enunciated the basic aim of creating a health service 'designed around the patient'. The NHS by implication had failed to create a health service focused on individual patient needs.

The emphasis was on investment and reform. Reforms included increased staffing, reduction in waiting times, more training, and 'joined up' working with social care. Specific commitments included cleaner hospitals, better hospital food, improved pay and working conditions, new consultant and GP contracts, more information and greater choice for patients, and commitment to cut waiting times.

There was a renewed emphasis on decentralisation, with the proposal in 2002, enunciated in the document *Delivering the NHS Plan*, for so-called 'foundation' hospitals (Department of Health, 2002). 'Foundation' hospitals are supposed to enjoy a degree of independence and freedom from central control. This was a controversial issue within the health policy community and the government's supporters in Parliament. Foundation hospitals resemble the NHS hospital trusts promoted by the Conservatives in 1990, and have been construed as 'back-door' privatisation, just as the Conservative trusts were.

'Choice' in health care: a 'patient-led' NHS?

Choice is a significant element in the 2000 reform package. Choice of provider, whether primary care doctor, specialist or hospital, is something which people in many European and other countries take for granted, but has never figured prominently among the goals of the NHS. Patients are now to be allowed to choose their hospital provider from a list of four or five, and it is intended that from 2008 choice will be unlimited.

'Choice' is a controversial policy, rejected by traditionalist defenders of the NHS, who argue that it is incompatible with the basic goal of the NHS to provide equality of access to health care for all on the basis of need. Not everybody can choose, it is suggested, and 'choice' is a policy that can only lead to a 'two-tier' service.

Discuss and Do

How important is 'choice' in health care? Does it matter to you personally whether you can choose your hospital, GP or consultant, the dates and times of appointments, consultations and treatment? Do you think, for example, that you should have the right to second or third opinions if you disagree with your doctor's diagnosis and prescription?

'Payment by results'

In 2004 a new system was introduced for paying providers – mainly hospitals – by results. This important innovation involved the construction of a reimbursement schedule of tariffs or fees for every medical procedure based on average costs for each procedure. Providers with below average costs can keep the surplus; those with above average costs will suffer a shortfall which will supposedly induce them to improve efficiency, but might have implications for long-run financial viability of some providers (Klein, 2005: 59–60). By this means, money is supposed to 'follow the patient'.

The private sector and public–private partnerships

A further, highly controversial issue is that of public–private partnerships. These take a variety of forms.

One area of public–private collaboration is that of the Private Finance Initiative (PFI), which involves the use of private capital investment in the building and equipping of NHS infrastructure, such as hospitals (for more discussion of PFI, see Chapter 8). The PFI programme was launched by the Conservatives in 1992 but bore fruit under Labour. By 2005 a large number of PFI deals had been signed with private sector consortia; 52 PFI schemes had opened, while another 80 or more, with a capital value of £18 billion, were in the pipeline (Timmins, 2005a).

By 2005 the value of the PFI programme was being questioned by Department of Health policy-makers who realised that many PFI hospital schemes were too large and inflexible for a rapidly changing health care market, in which traditional hospital services will increasingly be delivered outside hospitals and lengthy hospital stays become less prevalent. Day surgery, for example, will become more important, reducing the need for in-patient care (Timmins, 2005a).

New Labour initially shunned collaboration with private sector health care providers in 1997. The policy was reversed in 2000 when the Department of Health agreed a 'concordat' with the private sector, involving an agreement for the NHS to use independent sector facilities, hospital and other, to treat NHS patients. The policy has developed further since then with the introduction of independent sector treatment centres (ISTCs), some supplied and staffed by commercial groups from overseas, to provide specialist treatment for routine elective conditions, such as hip replacements and cataract operations, where there are substantial NHS waiting lists (Allsop and Baggott, 2004: 37).

In this section we turn to examine two important issues in some detail – the issue of *public health* and that of *rationing* of health care, and how these have fared under New Labour.

The public and preventive health agenda

The public and preventive health agenda received early attention from the new government, with White Papers in 1998 and the Acheson inquiry into health inequalities in the same year. A Minister for Public Health was appointed. The creation of so-called 'Health Action Zones' in 1998 exemplified both New Labour's 'social exclusion' agenda and its aspiration towards 'joined-up' government. The government stepped more gingerly around a number of other issues, for example smoking and alcohol, although a White Paper on the former appeared in 1998 and legislation in 2002 which prohibited tobacco advertising in certain contexts. Campaigns on diet (the 'Five-a-day' fruit and vegetable campaign, for example) seem to reflect an individualist–behavioural model of health rather than the structural–material one that might have been expected.

The creation of Health Action Zones (HAZs), area-based strategies for health interventions in areas of high deprivation, exhibited one government response to the health inequality issue, as well as its interest in 'joined-up' strategies for social interventions generally, since HAZs required multi-agency partnerships and working. Twenty-six HAZs were eventually introduced, by 1999. The main participants were health authorities and local authorities. An enormous variety of local initiatives was initiated, including, for example, attempts to promote the health of excluded groups such as travellers, street drinkers and prostitutes. The schemes were closed down earlier than expected, in 2003. Evaluation suggests that the schemes were unsuccessful in one of their basic aims of reducing health inequalities, but that, on the other hand, such schemes may, if given the opportunity, have some value. There is scope for interventions that target 'place', as well as people, as a locus of deprivation (Bauld *et al.*, 2005; Sassi, 2005: 82–83; Klein, 2006: 226).

The term 'social exclusion' has been used by the present government in preference to poverty or inequality in various areas of public policy. A focus on social exclusion would seem to have implications for health policy different from those of a focus on inequality. It would imply a policy of targeting resources and interventions on the 'excluded', the deprived, the marginalised, and would not necessarily have larger implications for the overall distribution of resources throughout society. Of course, poor health is itself a cause of social exclusion, so the relationship is a two-way one (Sassi, 2005: 69–70).

If, on the other hand, it is inequality across the range that matters, the issue is not simply the health status of the bottom 10% or 20%, say, of the income distribution. A focus on health inequality in general would imply a more radical approach to public policy, involving an attempt to shift the pattern of resource distribution within society, a more sharply redistributive tax regime and redistribution towards those below the median via increases in a range of social benefits (Wilkinson, 1996).

In fact, Labour governments since 1997 have simultaneously pursued both kinds of strategy. The HAZ strategy seemed to imply a more limited, 'exclusionist' focus, since it implied targeting geographically identifiable areas, populations or communities characterised by multiple deprivations, and allocating resources accordingly. On the other hand, more radical strategies have also been pursued; the tax and benefit systems have, for example, become more redistributive towards some of the less well-off, principally families, since 1997 with the introduction and advance of so-called 'stealth taxes' and increases in social security benefits for the retired and families with children. Not all groups of the poor and excluded have, however, benefited from this strategy (Glennerster, 2001; Hills, 2004; Hills and Stewart, 2005; Toynbee and Walker, 2005).

Priorities, rationing and health care

An issue that has emerged in the last decade is that of the non-availability of certain treatments. There has, for example, been controversy over the decision by the drug regulation and authorisation agency NICE, the National Institute for Health and Clinical Excellence, to restrict the use of drugs for treating Alzheimer's Syndrome. NICE had originally decided in 2001 that such cholinesterase inhibitors as Aricept should be available to Alzheimer's sufferers and be paid for by the NHS. In 2005, after further research, NICE reversed its decision and stated that the drugs should no longer be paid for by the NHS, as they were only marginally beneficial and were not cost-effective. There was strong opposition to this decision from the pharmaceutical industry, from patients' groups representing Alzheimer's sufferers and from the Royal College of Psychiatrists (Timmins, 2005c). In 2006 NICE again changed its position and declared that the drugs could be available to those with a moderate form of the condition (Jack and Timmins, 2006).

Discuss and Do

Should such organisations as NICE be able to restrict the availability of such drugs as those used for treating Alzheimer's sufferers on the grounds of 'cost-effectiveness'? (Remember the economist's principle of *'opportunity cost'*: money spent on one thing cannot be used for something else. Overall, resources are scarce and we must choose. NICE was saying that in terms of improving the health of the whole population, Alzheimer's drugs are worth less than treatments for other conditions.)

A recent, much publicised example of this kind of issue was the case of Anne-Marie Rogers, a sufferer from breast cancer, who initially failed and then succeeded in her attempt to use the courts to force her local Primary Care Trust to fund the prescription of the anti-cancer drug Herceptin (see Chapter 9) (Tait, 2006a, 2006b). Yet another example of this kind of issue is that of the decision some years ago by the then Secretary of State, Frank Dobson, to restrict the availability of the erectile dysfunction drug Viagra. These are all examples of what is called *rationing* (Klein *et al.*, 1996; Ham and Pickard, 1998).

The word 'rationing' in this context means allocating or distributing health care, in a context where ability to pay for treatment no longer operates, and where demand by professionals to drive up spending on health care is limited by fixed or 'global' budgets. 'Rationing' has unfavourable connotations, derived from some people's Second World War experience or image of ration books and shortages. It seems to imply the sharing-out of a meagre, restricted resource by bureaucratic authority. In fact rationing is inevitable and has always existed in health care systems governed according to principles of need and equality, rather than ability to pay. The most visible manifestations of rationing are waiting lists for out-patient and in-patient non-urgent care and the time delays involved in consulting GPs; this is 'rationing by delay'.

Many of these cases exemplify what is called *'postcode' rationing*, a state of affairs in which the availability or quality of treatment varies from area to area. The availability of some procedures or interventions (IVF, abortion, tattoo removal) has been restricted in particular areas, or been subject to varying criteria of eligibility. The PCT's initial refusal to allow prescription of Herceptin in the case of Anne-Marie Rogers was a clear case of 'postcode rationing' inasmuch as funding for the drug was available in more than a dozen other areas (Jack, 2006; Tait, 2006a).

All this seemed to have the worrying consequence for the public that fundamental principles of the NHS – universality, comprehensiveness, need and absence of direct payment for treatment – appeared to be being called into question. It has seemed to many that cost and affordability have become criteria for treatment rather than need.

Discuss and Do

What is wrong with 'postcode rationing'? Shouldn't local areas or communities have the responsibility of deciding on the treatments that will be available locally, in the light of local needs and priorities? (Remember that postcode rationing exists in any case within the UK as a whole, since the Scottish, Welsh and Northern Irish Health Services are substantially devolved. Remember also that although the question refers to 'local areas and communities', there is in fact no local electoral accountability in the NHS. Memberships of PCT and Foundation Hospital Boards are appointed, not elected.)

Financial crisis once more

In 2005–06 the headlines appeared to be dominated by a number of issues of what looked like policy failure. The main one was the growth of financial deficits among hospitals and PCTs (Timmins, 2005d). It was forecast that the deficit could be as high as £600–£700 million by the end of the 2005–06 financial year (Adams, 2006). By the summer of 2006, job losses, and even redundancies among hospital staffs, were occurring. This was embarrassing for the government because it occurred after years of much higher than average funding increases, and because opponents of the reforms have been able to suggest that some of the reforms themselves, for example 'payment by results', produced overspends and lack of financial control.

Other observers denied this and suggested that the deficits resulted from generous pay deals stemming from new contracts, the lack of good-quality financial management in NHS organisations, and the existence of too many hospitals in many areas, such as the Home Counties, in a context where patterns of care were changing and moving away from expensive out-patient and in-patient care (Timmins, 2006a, 2006b).

The service reconfiguration issue was a politically sensitive one for health ministers, because of the 'Kidderminster effect'. In 2001 an incumbent Labour MP and junior minister had lost his Wyre Forest seat to an NHS consultant who had led a successful local campaign to save Kidderminster Hospital's emergency department from closure (he won again in the 2005 election). Ministers feared that hospital closure plans elsewhere would face similar opposition (Timmins, 2006a).

Critiques of recent policy

By 2006 the NHS in England appeared to be evolving steadily in a market-like direction. (Developments in other parts of the UK, especially in Scotland, appeared to be in the opposite direction.) It was being suggested that the NHS might disappear as a health care provider, simply becoming a commissioning agency for care provided by independent providers. At the same time, there was ambiguity about the extent and direction of change and disagreement about how far and in what way the emerging NHS market was to be regulated (Timmins, 2006c, 2006d).

For many critics of the government's NHS modernisation strategy on the left, market-type reforms were to blame for financial deficits and other failures and shortcomings. A sharply polarised debate has developed about the government's NHS strategy in England. The left oppose any kind of private-sector involvement, whether in terms of finance or provision, in health care and what it sees as a compromising of basic NHS values, essentially the ideal of a planned, publicly owned economy of health care (Leys, 2001: Ch. 6; Pollock, 2005). Health Service trades unions are also naturally hostile to recent developments.

On the other hand, the government has also come under fire from those sympathetic to the new direction in policy for not going far enough. A King's Fund Report in 2006 described the reforms as 'half-baked' and insufficiently market-like. This report was the product of a group of senior NHS managers with a few individuals from the voluntary and private sectors and might be taken as representing a mainstream NHS provider position (Hall, 2006b; Timmins, 2006c). There are also groups further to the right such as the Reform and Adam Smith Institute think-tanks which broadly support what is happening and call for a more vigorous pursuit of the current line (Goldsmith and Gladstone, 2005).

The future

The Treasury's long-awaited 'Comprehensive' Spending Review was published in October 2007. The NHS was treated relatively well, and better than had been expected (H.M. Treasury, 2007: Annex D2). For the UK as a whole, budgets were planned to increase by £22 billion over the following three years, to £126 billion. For the NHS in England the planned rise is from a total of £90 billion in 2007–08 to £110 billion by 2010–11, a 4% per year rise in real terms; these are expectation-beating figures, but contrast with the experience of the last seven years, when expenditure has grown by an average of 7% per year (Timmins, 2007a).

After Gordon Brown's replacement of Tony Blair as Prime Minister at the end of June 2007, the competition and choice agenda appeared to lose focus and become indistinct. Mixed messages were sent out about the role of the private sector in provision and commissioning. New contracts for diagnostics and independent treatment centres remained under seemingly permanent review in the Department of Health (Timmins, 2007b).

Reviews of the NHS, one official, one unofficial, were published in the autumn of 2007, one by Lord Darzi, the first report of a two-stage review (Department of Health, 2007: 6). Derek Wanless contributed yet another review of the NHS, published in September 2007, this time sponsored by the King's Fund, an independent health policy think-tank and management education body (Wanless, 2007). This unofficial review was essentially an attempt to measure progress in the NHS and population health against targets proposed in Wanless's 2002 report (H.M. Treasury, 2002). It described modest progress, but at the same time provided fairly severe criticism of the quality of policy-making and implementation by the Department (Wanless, 2007: Ch. 3).

The review warned that the consensus about the NHS could break down if improvements in performance and in individual health failed to match improvements in funding – an extra £43 billion – that have taken place over the last five years. Individuals needed to take more responsibility for their own health and the NHS needed to extract better performance from its investment in new staff contracts and higher staff salaries. Without this, the costs of NHS care would rise more steeply in future (Wanless, 2007: xix).

Stop and Think

'New' Labour claimed to be 'new'. In what respects is this true in relation, at any rate, to the NHS and health policy?

UK health policy and the NHS: an assessment

The UK health system was remodelled and the NHS created in 1948 with a variety of objectives in mind. An important one was to secure a degree of equality in access to health care, and implicitly, to reduce inequalities in health. There was also a strong 'preventive' component in the rationale for the creation of the NHS. Early diagnosis and treatment, important for successful (and lower-cost) outcomes, would not be inhibited by a patient's inability to pay (Titmuss, 1958: 140–114). Other objectives included giving health care providers, such as hospitals, a degree of financial security, and providing health professionals with a working environment in which they could exercise their professional skills free from financial considerations. This is not the place for a full assessment of the health system's performance in all of these respects, and we will concentrate on inequalities in health care.

In relation to equality, the NHS has been subject to considerable evaluation during the past quarter of a century. Most evaluative studies agree that the NHS has reduced the financial insecurity associated with ill-health. Its system of funding, via (mostly) general taxation, is 'fair' by comparison with many other systems, such as those that rely on employment-related social insurance or private insurance, because the risk pool is large, the funding base wide, and tax contributions are roughly proportional to income.

In relation to the larger issue of inequalities in health, the NHS cannot be expected to make much difference. The health inequalities issue – a component of the broad public or preventive health agenda – is a large one which requires coordinated government action across a wide policy field, including, importantly, social security and taxation, as well as education and employment policies. Public policy has moved in a more egalitarian direction since 1997 in various respects, although reductions in overall socio-economic inequality as measured, for example, by Gini coefficients, have so far been modest (Hills and Stewart, 2005).

The narrower issue of access to and utilisation of health services – allocating health care according to medical need – seems a more promising ground for evaluation. It had long been argued from various points on the political spectrum, left and right, that the middle classes had actually been the main beneficiaries of the creation of the NHS; Richard Titmuss, for example, had suggested this in the 1960s (Titmuss, 1968: 196). Studies published in the 1990s, however, based on GP consultation rates and self-reported sickness among adults consulting a doctor – admittedly imperfect measures – suggested, firstly, that there has been a consistent 'pro-poor' bias in use of NHS facilities at least from the 1970s to the 1990s, and, secondly, that the NHS became more 'pro-poor' between the 1970s and 1990s (Hills, 1997: 57–58, Figure 40).

A criticism of these studies is that they involve aggregation, which may conceal the experience of particular social groups and also variations in use of particular services. In any case, consultation and use of facilities do not provide evidence about people's experience of health services or of the more nebulous dimensions of service 'quality'.

For example, with the rise of the women's movement since the 1970s, there has been the development of a strong critique of health care provision for women (Doyal, 1994). Women were, of course, one of the groups that benefited from the creation of the NHS because the previous NHI system was focused on the breadwinner. The NHS improved women's access to health care, but on terms dictated by a male-dominated medical profession, and in recent decades discontent with the quality of some of what was available has grown (Doyal, 1994: 140).

The poor quality of much long-term care and treatment for chronically sick and disabled groups provided by the NHS has been something of a scandal, recognised as an issue since the 1960s and partially addressed since then by, for example, the development of social 'care in the community' and the closure of long-stay hospitals. More recently, ethnic and cultural dimensions have been added to the debate about equality (Smaje, 1995).

More recent analysis, focusing on 'micro'-level access to and utilisation of particular services by different socio-economic groups, as well as 'macro' studies of utilisation using aggregate data, provides a complex picture of health care inequality (Le Grand and Vizard, 1998: 107; Dixon *et al.*, 2003: 18). Earlier macro-level studies mostly suggest that the system is equitable, while micro-level studies of particular services, such as cardiac care, cancer care, elective surgery, preventive, chronic disease and maternity services, uniformly suggest the opposite. In the light of these findings, it can be assumed that, for example, minority ethnic groups will experience poorer service from the NHS than the white population, simply because of their greater concentration in lower socio-economic groups, higher levels of manual employment and higher levels of unemployment.

Explanations for these inequalities include local accessibility of health services – mediated by variables such as distance, travel and transport, and employment and personal commitments, such as caring responsibilities, and 'voice'. Local availability of services is unlikely to be generally important, contrary to the famous suggestion many years ago by Julian Tudor Hart that there is an 'inverse care law' in health care provision (Tudor Hart, 1971). Transport and travel issues were more significant, with car ownership, for example, influencing use of facilities. Employment status was also significant, with manual workers less able to take time off work to see doctors, compared with non-manual workers (Dixon *et al.*, 2003: 22–25). 'Voice' is the idea that the middle classes are able to work the system to get more out of it; they are more articulate, better able to express need, and culturally have more in common with middle-class professionals providing the services (Dixon *et al.*, 2003: 26).

Critiques of the health system's performance in relation to various dimensions of equity have fed, in a confused way, into contemporary 'consumerist' agendas on the one hand, and rights- or citizenship-based agendas on the other, about health care and indeed about other public services (on citizenship, see Chapter 9). They can be found underpinning some of the impetus towards reform of public services which policy-makers have undertaken in recent years. It is interesting that some observers have suggested that the health needs of ethnic minorities and women, as well as lower socio-economic groups in general, might in some respects be better served in more market- and choice-oriented health systems – an implication being that the English NHS's current 'choice' agenda may actually be a way of improving the system's equity (Doyal, 1994: 141; Dixon *et al.*, 2003: 5, 30; Phillips and Reid, 2004). The contrasting, opposed, 'citizenship' agenda for health has also received recent intellectual support (Commission on the NHS, 2000) and some policy attention, although arguably more in the other UK countries than in England.

Conclusion

In this chapter we have tried to provide you with an outline of the UK health system, focusing on the English system, and an overview of developments in health policy, mainly since the Second World War. We have examined the distinctive features of the UK public health care system, the NHS, and explored the changing relationship between the State, the medical professions and the public. We have identified different models of health, social and medical, and considered their relationship to dominant post-war styles of health policy. We have examined changing agendas in health policy and health care policy and considered some of the explanations for these changes. We have seen how all governments, regardless of political party, have faced certain intractable and perennial problems: appropriate levels of NHS funding; a sometimes fraught relationship with the health care professions; problems of the system's accountability, both to government and to the public; and the long-running conflict between the achievement of equity or equality in terms of health care accessibility, treatment and outcomes on the one hand, and local autonomy on the other. We have explored some particular issues, including recent developments in the public health agenda, and the rise to prominence of the 'rationing' issue. Finally, we have identified a wider health policy agenda, embracing such issues as the persistence of inequalities in health between social groups, which lie beyond the remit of the Department of Health. In this sense, health policy poses enormous challenges for any government, of 'joined-up' governance and policy coherence across a wide field of government and extra-government activity.

In this chapter, you have:

- acquired a basic understanding of some key concepts, themes and issues in health policy;
- learnt about the origins, development and structure of the UK health system;
- examined recent reforms to the UK and especially the English health system;
- examined and analysed the health policy of the present ('New') Labour Government;
- acquired some knowledge and understanding of some problems and achievements of the UK health system.

Annotated further reading

A sophisticated and extremely well-written book on health policy and the NHS is Rudolf Klein's now classic *The Politics of the NHS* (1989; fifth edition entitled *The New Politics of the NHS*, 2006). This is indispensable reading (Klein, 2006). Chris Ham's *Health Policy in Britain* (5th edition, 2004) is a highly recommendable text, which presents a valuable policy-making perspective on health policy and the NHS and discusses a variety of current issues sensibly and very lucidly. It also provides some coverage of the devolved health systems of the UK in Scotland, Wales and Northern Ireland (Ham, 2004). Another good text is Rob Baggott's *Health and Health Care in Britain* (3rd edition, 2004). Updates on UK health policy are provided in regular articles in the annual series of *Social Policy Reviews*. On health policy in the devolved countries of the UK, see also the recent book by Scott Greer, *Territorial Politics and Health Policy* (Greer, 2005), and the article by Stephen Peckham in *Social Policy Review 19* (Peckham, 2007).

For a major contemporary restatement of the social model of health, see the outstanding recent text by Michael Marmot, *Status Syndrome* (Marmot, 2004). This book is aimed at a non-specialist audience and is accessibly written. See also most textbooks on the sociology of health and illness, such as Steve Taylor and David Field's *Sociology of Health and Health* Care (Taylor and Field, 2007) and Sarah Nettleton's *The Sociology of Health and Illness* (Nettleton, 1995), all of which discuss the social determinants of health and illness and examine the issue of health inequalities. The Acheson Report is essentially an update of the famous Black Report on health inequalities (Department of Health, 1998c). This and Margaret Whitehead's follow-up *The Health Divide* have been reprinted many times (Townsend and Davidson, 1982; Whitehead, 1987).

For official and unofficial reviews of the state of the NHS, see the series of reports by Sir Derek Wanless (H.M. Treasury, 2002; Wanless, 2004, 2007). See also the interim report of the Darzi review (Department of Health, 2007). Darzi's final review should appear in early 2008. All this material is downloadable from appropriate websites.

Evaluation of the performance, achievements and shortcomings of the NHS is controversial and subject to disagreement. Martin Powell's *Evaluating the National Health Service* is an attempt at a comprehensive evaluation of the NHS (Powell, 1997).

Chapter 13

Social care

Objectives

- To outline the developments of social care provision for children and adults from its charitable foundations through to contemporary state-regulated provision.

- To outline the development of social care policy during the 'post-war consensus period'.

- To explain how child and adult social care policy was reconstructed under the Conservative administrations of Margaret Thatcher and John Major.

- To explain how social care policy has developed since the election of New Labour in 1997, not least with the re-emergence of separate children's and adults' social care services.

Introduction

The aim of this chapter is to explain the nature of social care policy and how it has developed over the twentieth century and into the first part of the twenty-first century.

Typically, social policy texts have contained a chapter on the personal social services as, indeed, did previous editions of this text. However, one of the significant social policy developments, in England and Wales at least, of this century has been the dismantling of local authority social services departments (and local authority education departments) and the creation of separate 'Children's Services' and 'Adult Services' departments. This has been partly in an attempt to ensure the provision of 'joined-up' services for both children and adults. Any analysis of social services needs to take account of this context. Therefore, the chapter provides:

- an historical background to social care provision;
- an account of the post-war settlement in relation to social care for children, young people and adults;
- an account of the changes to child social care implemented by the governments of the New Right and New Labour over the last 30 years;
- an account of the corresponding changes to adult social care implemented by the governments of the New Right and New Labour over the same time period.

The arrangements for social care in Scotland, Wales and Northern Ireland are increasingly different from those in England as the impact of devolved government increases (see Chapter 7).

Defining social care

Before exploring policy developments and changes in relation to social care, it is worth considering a definition of social care. For the purposes of this chapter social care relates to 'caring support' (as distinct from health care – though this is a very precarious distinction) received by various service user or client groups – children, older people, children and adults with physical and/or learning disabilities, children and adults with mental health problems. This care may be provided in a variety of ways or settings: in residential homes, in day centres or (increasingly) in people's own homes. Such care may be provided by local authorities (though this is decreasingly the case) or by the independent sector (private and voluntary sector agencies). As we will explore in this chapter, the last 15 to 20 years has witnessed an emphasis on encouraging provision by the independent sector and a related reduction in local authority-provided social care. As has been discussed in other chapters (for example, Chapter 6) local authorities have been encouraged to be enablers or purchasers of services rather than direct service providers. This holds for certain aspects of social care probably as much as if not more than it does for other areas of social policy. In addition, there is a policy imperative for service users to be able to decide on what care and assistance they want to be provided and how and by whom that care would be provided.

The Poor Laws

Depending on how far one chooses to go back, of course, most commentators would regard social care provision as having its origins in the charitable voluntarism of the 1601 Elizabethan Poor Law (see Chapter 2). Over 200 years later, with the Poor Law Amendment Act of 1834, the emphasis on the 'deserving' and 'undeserving' poor remained – with the deserving individuals being able to receive charitable assistance from Victorian philanthropy and charity as opposed to the 'undeserving' individuals, judged to be responsible for their own plight and not, therefore, deemed to warrant others' charitable support. The residue of this distinction between the 'deserving' and 'undeserving' poor arguably remains with us to this day when we consider what society's response should be to those who require support and assistance, whether in relation to social care or to housing, health care or income support.

The first Poor Law in Elizabethan times stemmed from the recognition that there was a need for a national set of arrangements to deal with the problems of the poor within a context of increasing movement in populations, more people living in towns, developments in agricultural processes, and the enlargement of towns and cities, and the associated growth of populations living in them. Under such circumstances the charitable and voluntary, often church-based, arrangements that had existed up until then needed to be augmented. The response, the first Poor Law, gave the parishes the responsibility for 'their own' poor and, if necessary, this meant the returning (resettlement) of poor people to their parishes of origin where they would be provided with relief. Such poor relief was to be funded by a local tax on properties – a property rate. While these arrangements worked, of a fashion, for the best part of 250 years, by the beginning of the nineteenth century it was recognised that they needed amending. By this time, the process of industrialisation was impacting significantly on cities, towns and villages. People were increasingly moving into urban areas. The processes of industrialisation and urbanisation were creating their own problems, for example poor public health and impoverishment. The 1834 Poor Law Amendment Act was, therefore, an attempt to respond to this changing context. Amongst other things, it established the 'workhouses' (though many already existed) where those unable to support themselves would be sent for 'indoor relief'. Underpinning these arrangements was the notion of 'eligibility' – mentioned above – that is, those 'sent to' the workhouse were judged to be more badly off and destitute than anyone in receipt of outdoor relief – that is, the least eligible.

Stop and Think

How useful is it to distinguish between those people who deserve state care support and those who do not? What is problematic about such a distinction?

Twentieth-century reform

In terms of the care of children and adults, the developments in the mid- to late nineteenth century included the public health initiatives of local authorities, the regulating of children's and women's working hours, and the entitlement of children to schooling. By the beginning of the twentieth century, the Liberal government had established school medical services and schools meals services within state education. The Liberal government of 1906–14 was also, as discussed elsewhere, responsible at the time for other significant social policy legislation, not least the non-contributory and means-tested Old Age Pensions Act and the contributory but non-means-tested 1911 National Insurance Act for those working who became unemployed or sick (but not their families). All of these had an impact on the care and welfare of children and adults. In 1929, with the 1929 Local Government Act, local authorities inherited responsibility for the old workhouses. While many of these would pass to the health service as part of the creation of the NHS in 1948, post-war local government continued to have a public health role as well as increased responsibilities for the care and welfare of children, young people and adults (Means and Smith, 1998).

Moving to the post-Second World War social care arrangements, one observes that, though not often regarded as part of the headline swathe of post-war welfare reform, relevant legislation was passed. The 1948 Children Act promoted the further development of the existing arrangements for child care in that it gave local authorities specific responsibilities for establishing Children's Departments within local authorities within which professional social workers would take the lead in protecting vulnerable children from abuse, neglect or delinquency. In addition, local authorities also established departments for the welfare of adults, including disabled and elderly people. As mentioned above, the 1929 Local Government Act had given local authorities the responsibility for housing and caring for such individuals when the workhouses were passed to them. However, two pieces of post-war legislation set out a significant demarcation between health care and social care: the NHS Act 1946 and the National Assistance Act 1948. The NHS Act 1946 (as Chapter 12 explores fully) enabled the provision of health care to everyone, free at the point of delivery, irrespective of their ability to pay, on a universal and uniform national basis. On the other hand, the National Assistance Act 1948 constructed social care (of older people who needed sheltered or residential care) as local provision, subject to means testing and local variance (see Means and Smith, 1998). Therefore, from the start of the post-war welfare state, a wedge was inserted between means-tested social care and free health care.

In the late 1960s and early 1970s, with the 1970 Local Government Act for England and Wales and the 1968 Social Work (Scotland) Act in Scotland, the separate Children's Departments and Personal Social Services Departments were merged. In addition, and more specifically, the 1970 Chronically Sick and Disabled Persons Act placed a responsibility on local authorities to assist disabled people. At the same time, local authorities expanded their support for older people in terms of the provision of residential care homes, day care and home care. However, the statutory duties of much of this 'long-term social care' provision were uncertain and led to legal difficulties in the 1980s and 1990s when local authorities started to 'withdraw' or 'ration' their provision (see Means et al., 2002). However, it is to children's social care that the chapter now turns.

Children's services

As we have already mentioned, the care of children, by social workers and others, and through social departments and elsewhere, can be seen to have its roots in the Christian philanthropy dating back to the mid-nineteenth-century Victorian period, if not before. Others may argue that attention was motivated less by a concern with the moral well-being of children and more by a concern with the need for an orderly working class (not least its children). This tension between support and control remains as part of the background to welfare provision generally. Therefore, whether as a result of philanthropic concern for the moral well-being of children, or from the recognition that state-coordinated action was required, by the start of the twentieth century the state was taking a direct interest in the well-being of children judged to be neglected, abused or unruly. However, it was not really until after the Second World War and the late 1940s that a coordinated approach appeared when local authorities were charged with establishing children's departments (along with corresponding departments for the physically and mentally sick and disabled as well as for the elderly). Much of this care for children (and also for older people and those with physical disabilities, learning disabilities or mental health problems) was of an institutional nature. During the 1960s, these services were reviewed by the Seebohm Committee (Seebohm, 1968) and resulted in the 1970 Local Authority

Social Services Act which paved the way for the establishment of generic, multipurpose social services departments responsible for providing personal social services. This structure remained in place until the 2000s and the separation once again of children and adult services (see below).

Developments in children's social care under the New Right

The rights of children and the Children Act 1989

Arguably the key legislation under the New Right governments of Margaret Thatcher and John Major was the Children Act 1989, and the equivalent legislation in Scotland in 1995. Indeed, one could go so far as to argue that this is the key piece of post-war policy affecting children's services, as it sought to bring together previous pieces of policy and legislation on the protection of children. The Children Act 1989 sought to offer greater protection to children. For parents, the emphasis was on their responsibilities as opposed to their rights. As such, the main principles of the Act were:

- to protect the rights of children;
- to make children's welfare a priority;
- to seek children's views according to their age and understanding;
- to recognise that wherever possible children should be brought up within their families;
- that the local authorities could provide services for children and families in need;
- to promote partnership between children, parents and local authorities;
- to improve the way courts dealt with children and families with their having rights of appeal against court decisions;
- to ensure that children and families would have access to effective independent representations and complaints procedures.

Where it was felt that a child had suffered, or was likely to suffer, significant harm by their family or was beyond parental control, the Act gave local authorities the power, via the courts, to place a Care Order on the child. The consequence of this was that the child was placed in the care of the local authority, with parental responsibility being shared between the parents and the local authority. The Act also set out arrangements whereby children could be 'looked after' by the local authority with the agreement of their parents. Such accommodation would include residential or foster care. The Act did, therefore, stipulate that parents continued to have parental responsibility for their child, even when they were no longer living with them. This included being kept informed of their child's situation and being able to participate in decisions made about their child's future.

The legislation therefore endeavoured to enshrine the rights of children, with the main aim being to protect the child as a priority. However, this was to be balanced against the aim of trying to ensure wherever possible that children should remain within their family. This obviously throws up the inherent tension when caring for children or other vulnerable individuals of, on the one hand, wanting to protect the individual (for example from abuse, mistreatment or neglect) and, on the other, not wanting to remove the individual from their 'natural' family setting. Where children are judged (by a variety of agencies, including the courts and criminal justice system, or health and education professionals) as being at risk of abuse, neglect or harm in other ways, then local authorities do have powers to protect the child. Ultimately, this can mean the removal of the child from their family and being taken into 'the legal care of the local authority'.

Discuss and Do

When should the state step in? There is an inherent tension in child protection between, on the one hand, the state and its agents (social workers, police, doctors, nurses, teachers) standing back and not interfering with the lives of individual families and, on the other hand, stepping in because it is believed that a child is in danger of neglect or abuse.

- What are the sorts of criticisms that are made, for example in the media, when the state 'gets it wrong'?

- Is this an inevitable and insurmountable problem or are there things that could be done to improve the situation?

Social workers are usually the professionals who oversee this process, though the decision to take a child into the 'legal care' of the local authority is one made by the courts. Where a child is 'taken into care', the aim is still to ensure that the child remains wherever possible with their family (in a supervised manner) or with a foster family. Fostering has increasingly been used as a more appropriate arrangement then other forms of institutional care. As can be seen from Table 13.1, the vast majority, that is nearly two-thirds, of 'looked-after children' are cared for in foster homes. Foster parents are paid for their services by a local authority and social workers supervise the foster care. It may be that children who are fostered then go on to be legally adopted on a permanent basis by the foster or another family.

Table 13.1 Children looked after by local authorities, year ending 31 March 2001

	Total children looked after per thousand resident population			Manner of accommodation (percentages)			
	Children admitted	Ceased to be looked after	Looked after	Foster homes	Children's homes and hostels	Other	Number of children looked after (= 100%)
England	2.2	2.2	5.2	65.1	11.5	23.4	58,900
Wales	2.4	2.2	5.5	73.8	6.4	19.7	3,644
Scotland	4.2	4.2	9.7	28.3	14.5	57.2	10,900
Northern Ireland	2.4	2.3	5.2	63.3	11.3	25.4	2,400

Source: Office for National Statistics (2005b) *Children Looked After by Local Authorities, Year Ending 31 March 2001*, London: ONS. Crown copyright material is reproduced with the permission of the Controller of HMSO and the Queen's Printer for Scotland under the terms of the Click-Use Licence.

Why do you think most looked-after children are cared for in foster families?

Since the 1969 Children and Young Persons Act, local authorities have also had responsibility for caring for children who are judged by the courts to be beyond parental control. Such 'young offenders' are under the supervision of the local authority via a 'care order'. This process is an attempt to avoid the criminalisation of young people and tries, instead, to provide adequate supervision that, it is deemed, the child's family is unable to provide. Such children have been cared for in 'remand homes', 'community homes' or 'secure' institutions. These are increasingly provided by 'out of authority' providers – from the voluntary and private sectors – to a number of local authorities.

Child care

A key part of children's services has been and remains that of preventative services and interventions. Social workers, along with other professionals, will provide advice and support to families in terms of day care, counselling, parental advice, financial/benefit advice, and referral to other services and agencies, e.g. housing, health care and education. Day care and children's nurseries, for example, have grown out of a residual state provision often traditionally provided by social services departments for families regarded as in significant need. Universal statutory children's day care (nursery provision) was not promoted by the New Right, unlike New Labour which has made significant advances in this area (see later in this chapter for a discussion of this development). The New Right preferred to encourage individual families to be responsible for their own arrangements and to encourage (though not financially other than with its introduction of nursery vouchers) a plethora of non-statutory child care provision – private nurseries, registered (and unregistered) child minders, pre-school nursery schools, voluntary play groups and so forth. This section of the chapter will now move to consider New Labour's approach to the care of children.

New Labour and children's social care

Child protection, 'Every Child Matters' and the Children Act 2004

New Labour has looked to reorganise children's services as its response to the perceived failure in providing effective child protection and as part of its 'modernisation' (Department of Health, 1998a), 'social inclusion' (Department for Work and Pensions, 2001) and 'respect' agendas (Home Office, 2003) as they impact on child care more generally. There are two aspects to New Labour's approach to child social care that will be the focus of this section: child protection and child care more generally. In relation to child protection, probably the key piece of policy was the 2004 Children Act which was a response to the 2003 *Every Child Matters* Green Paper (Department for Education and Skills, 2003), itself a response to the Lord Laming Report (2003) into the investigation of the enquiry into the death of Victoria Climbié while she was under the care and protection of her local social services department (Box 13.1). The death of Victoria Climbié was arguably only the latest (though tragic) high-profile case of the state 'failing' to protect children it knew were liable to harm or abuse, a list that includes and goes back to Maria Colwell in the 1970s and Jasmine Beckford in the 1980s.

Box 13.1	Victoria Climbié

Timeline for the Climbié case

David Batty, *The Guardian*, Monday 24 September 2001

Nearly three years after Victoria Climbié's parents sent her to Britain from Africa in the hope of a better life a public inquiry begins into her murder. The investigation will determine why the horrific abuse she suffered was never tackled despite repeated contact with social services, the NHS and the police.

November 1998 Seven-year-old Victoria Climbié left her parents' house in the shanty suburb of Abobo in the Ivory Coast. She was 'happy and excited' about her new life with her aunt Marie Thérèse Kouao in Britain. Her parents hoped she would get a good education. Instead she was kept prisoner in the tiny studio flat in Tottenham, north London, shared by her aunt and her boyfriend Carl Manning who brutally tortured her.

July 15 1999 A cut and bruised Victoria was seen by consultant paediatrician and child protection doctor, Ruby Schwartz, at Central Middlesex hospital. But she was released back into her aunt's care as the doctor was persuaded that her injuries were self-inflicted – a result of scratching because of itchiness from scabies. Haringey Council social worker Lisa Arthurworrey and child protection officer PC Karen Jones later cancelled their August 4 home visit when they heard Victoria had scabies.

August 6 1999 After two weeks in North Middlesex hospital, Victoria returned to her aunt's flat. In a meeting at Haringey's social services department on the previous day, Kouao had told Ms Arthurworrey and PC Jones that she poured hot water over her niece's head because it was itchy and that the girl injured herself with a fork and spoon.

November 1 1999 Victoria made an unfounded sexual allegation against Manning, withdrawn the next day. Ms Arthurworrey believed Kouao put the child up to it in order to get housing. PC Jones was assigned to find out why the false allegation was made. Although her letter to Kouao was ignored, no further action was taken.

February 25 2000 After months of torture, Victoria died of hypothermia at her aunt's flat. She had 128 injuries all over her body. The Home Office pathologist who later examined her corpse described the case as 'the worst case of child abuse' he had ever seen.

November 20 2000 The trial of Marie Thérèse Kouao and her boyfriend Carl Manning for Victoria's murder opened at the Old Bailey, London. The court heard how the girl was beaten and tied up for 24 hours or more. The child protection team's investigation of Victoria's case, which allowed her to be returned to Kouao and Manning, was criticised as 'blindingly incompetent'. The National Society for the Prevention of Cruelty to Children called for a complete overhaul of child protection procedures.

January 12 2001 Marie Thérèse Kouao and her boyfriend Carl Manning were jailed for life for Victoria's murder. Judge Richard Hawkins said: 'What Anna endured was truly unimaginable.' [Victoria was called Anna by Kouao and Manning.] The health secretary, Alan Milburn, ordered a statutory inquiry into her death headed by former chief inspector of social services, Lord Laming. The government also placed Haringey social services department under special measures requiring close supervision by the social services inspectorate.

April 22 2001 The government announced that the inquiry into Victoria's death will be public. John Hutton, then the health minister responsible for children's services, said it would be the first 'tripartite' investigation using powers under the Children's Act, the NHS Act and Police Act. In effect there would be three simultaneous inquiries, producing a single report in spring 2002 to the health secretary and the home secretary.

May 7 2001 Lord Laming appealed for witnesses to give evidence at the inquiry. Speaking to the Guardian, he disclosed that ministers believed her death may have been the result of 'a gross failure of the system' rather than the failings of individual staff.

Reprinted with permission.

The *Laming Report* had argued that children were not adequately protected and cared for due to a number of factors, including:

- fragmented services;
- lack of integration between 'crisis intervention' and general care provision;
- confusion of professional boundaries and responsibilities.

The *Every Child Matters* (ECM) Green Paper duly set out a series of recommendations that the government believed would reduce the likelihood of failures to protect vulnerable children from abuse and neglect in the future. It recommended doing this by reshaping children's services into holistic, joined-up provision that would focus on:

- the child's well-being as a whole;
- outcomes of service intervention;
- the maximisation of children's life-chances.

The ECM Green Paper stated that in the future children's and young people's services (social care, education, leisure, youth services, health services) should focus on children's well-being in relation to five key objectives:

- Health
- Safety
- Contribution to society
- Enjoyment and achievement
- Economic well-being.

The ECM Green Paper recommended the establishment of integrated children's services departments. The 2004 Children Act duly gave local authorities the responsibility for establishing children's and young people's departments. In addition, local authorities were obliged to establish local safeguarding children's boards. Local authorities have, therefore, integrated their education departments (the Local Education Authority) with the children and families part of their social services departments into single children's and young people's departments. (At the same time they have created separate adult services departments – see below.) These children's and young people's departments are being led by a Children's Director. The Children's Director is also responsible for establishing a local children's trust (a strategic partnership) in order to ensure effective co-operation and partnership, working between the local agencies responsible for the well-being of children in their locality such as the health service, police, schools, youth offending teams and voluntary sector organisations. Within this, partnership working, budget pooling, horizontal and vertical integration are all to be encouraged to ensure seamless, joined-up services for children.

Discuss and Do

Do you think the establishment of Children's Services Departments by amalgamating those parts of the old social services departments that were responsible for children with local authority education departments will:

- help to avoid or make less likely a repeat of cases such as that of Victoria Climbié?

- promote joined-up children's services provision?

Can you see any disadvantages of such a reorganisation?

Time will tell as to whether or not these structural changes will be effective. Criticisms have been made, such as that child protection will be only a very small (and potentially marginalised) part of these large children's departments. Second, some have suggested that structural and organisational changes would not be sufficient in themselves to lead to improvements in child protection.

Promoting child care provision

In tandem with its policy changes in relation to child protection and children's well-being more generally, New Labour has sought to expand child care provision in a variety of ways. It established the 'Sure Start' programme early in its first term of government, which has led to the establishment of multi-disciplinary (health, social care, education and so forth) children's centres in socio-economically deprived areas of the country. These are an attempt to provide young (pre-school) children with a better economic, social and emotional start in life. By 2008 New Labour hoped to have had in place some 2,500 Sure Start centres across the country. In addition, under the 2006 Childcare Act, local authorities have been charged with providing all parents (particularly working parents) with information on child care and nursery provision and with ensuring that sufficient provision is in place (though not as a key provider themselves). Such provision will be liable to inspection by Ofsted (the agency responsible for inspecting primary, secondary and tertiary education provision – see Chapter 15). Meanwhile, parents of pre-school age children have been provided with nursery vouchers and tax credits to assist them in paying for child care. Historically, the UK has had minimal pre-school provision and parents have faced paying some of the highest child care fees when compared with other European (EU and OECD) countries. However, the UK continues to under-fund child care in comparison to other countries – 0.8% of GDP by 2008 (Toynbee, 2006). Child care provision remains a sector made up of poorly paid staff, and those families arguably most in need, non-working families, are not eligible for the state subsidies because these are directed at those in work. In addition, whilst local authorities are responsible for overseeing and promoting provision, they are discouraged by central government from actually providing child care themselves, even though this is an area of social welfare where, arguably, the public has most confidence in actual state provision (Toynbee, 2006).

New Labour had also proposed changes in how social care would be provided to 'look after children'. In its *Care Matters* Green Paper (Department for Education and Skills, 2006a), the government also recognised weaknesses and failings of service provision for 'looked-after children', not least when one looked at their disproportionately low educational achievement rates and disproportionately high criminal justice encounters. Looked-after children would therefore be provided with services that would be focused on preventing children entering care, providing appropriate care for those who are in receipt of formal care, and support in moving on and out of formal care. As part of this, local authorities would have responsibility for providing a dedicated social worker who would act as a guardian and commissioner of care and support for the child or young person, to ensure that looked-after children receive the same educational opportunities as other children and young people, including at higher education level.

From the above, it is possible to argue that New Labour's emphasis has been on ensuring that services for children and young people have been focused on:

- the safety and protection of children;
- the general well-being of all children;
- adequate provision of child care, particularly for working parents;
- emphasising that provision is provided through partnership working;
- encouraging private and voluntary sector provider agencies;
- encouraging the pooling of budgets;
- emphasising that local authorities have a duty to coordinate children's services and act as strategic leaders and enablers of these partnerships but not necessarily as providers of such services.

Adult social care

This section explores the developments in adult social care. What was described in the 1980s and 1990s as 'community care' is dealt with here as adult social care, though one needs to note that they are not entirely synonymous with each other, for example 'community care' was and is care that children and adults may have received. However, for the purposes of this section of the chapter, adult social care and 'community care' will be treated as one and the same thing. As mentioned above, the post-war welfare state constructed health care, via the NHS Act 1946, as free at the point of delivery. However, social care, via the National Assistance Act 1948, was to be the responsibility of local authorities and, as such, subject to means testing and local variance. As Means observed: 'Such tensions over the health and social care divide have never been resolved, but the overall trend has been towards [local authorities] taking responsibility for more and more dependent elderly people' (Means, 1995: 205), not least as a means for containing public expenditure on social care.

Adult social care policy was further developed post-war as part of the 1968 Seebohm report and the establishment of local authority personal social services departments. The 1970 Chronically Sick and Disabled Persons Act placed a responsibility on local authorities to assist disabled people. Local authorities expanded their support for older people in terms of the provision of residential care homes, day care and home care. However, the statutory duty of much of this 'long-term social care' provision was uncertain. At the same time, adult social care has been subject to a number of policy imperatives, particularly since the mid-1980s. These have included a desire to:

- deinstitutionalise social care provision and provide it in more community-like settings;
- promote service users' independence and responsibility;
- promote service user 'choice', not least via quasi-markets;
- reconstruct long-term care as social care rather than health care;
- contain the overall level of expenditure on community social care.

Adult social and community care under the New Right

Expansion of state-funded private residential care

Adult social care policy in Britain underwent significant changes in the period 1979–97. This section examines the changes which occurred to adult social care policy over this period under the New Right governments of Margaret Thatcher and John Major. Arguably the key policy development under the New Right was the NHS and Community Care Act 1990 (Lewis and Glennerster, 1996). There had been a number of drivers for changes to adult social care policy since the mid-1980s, including those listed above. Indeed, by the mid-1980s the Conservative government was arguably facing a crisis in social care policy and provision, in particular with regard to the costs of private residential care. A change in social security policy in the early 1980s had resulted in people being financially advantaged if they went into residential care (rather than being cared for in the 'community') since they could claim social security supplementary benefit assistance towards their residential care costs. Essentially, a large part of the budget of the (as then) Department of Health and Social Security (DHSS) was going towards paying for individuals to be cared for in private residential homes. What made the situation 'perverse' was that if individuals chose instead to be cared for in the community, they faced the possibility of receiving no assistance whatsoever and the likelihood of being charged for any state support which they received. (Adult social 'community care' such as domiciliary care, day care, meals-on-wheels, cleaning and laundry assistance were provided by local authority social services departments (SSDs), for which they were permitted to charge and means-test individuals in receipt of their assistance.) The budgetary problem had escalated over the period 1979–85 such that DHSS funding for private residential care had increased exponentially during this period. In 1979 the DHSS spent £10 million in assisting 12,000 people with their residential care costs. By the mid-1980s it was estimated that it would be costing around £2,000 million in 1991 (assisting over 230,000 people) and nearly £2,500 million by mid-1993 (with 270,000 claimants) (Wistow *et al.*, 1994; Lewis and Glennerster, 1996). Therefore by the mid-1980s the government recognised that it needed to review its social care policy and duty and asked the Audit Commission to undertake the review.

Review of community care

The Audit Commission's report of the effectiveness of community care policy was damning. It identified policy failure as far as community care was concerned, placing the responsibility for this with central government. It reported that community care policy was failing because of '"policy contradictions" and "perverse incentives" for which central government bore substantial responsibility' (Wistow *et al.*, 1994: 4). Its Report concluded that:

> If nothing changes the outlook is bleak ... [with] a continued waste of resources and, worse still, care and support that is either lacking entirely or inappropriate to the needs of some of the most disadvantaged members of society and their relatives who seek to care for them .... (Audit Commission, 1986: paras. 4–48)

The government responded by setting up a strategic review which resulted in The Griffiths Report (Griffiths, 1988). As the name suggests, the review was chaired by Sir Roy Griffiths, who had a few years earlier reported to the government on the state of the organisation and management of the NHS (see Chapter 12). Griffiths' scope was restricted, particularly in terms of any analysis of the adequacy of community care funding, though this did not stop him from suggesting that funding was a problem. Griffiths concluded that the state of community care policy and provision was at such a low level that 'in few areas can the gap between political rhetoric and policy on the one hand, or between policy and reality in the field have been so great' (Griffiths, 1988: iv). His Report concluded that community care policy was in need of significant reform, recommending the following actions: the creation of an internal or quasi-market in the provision of social care services, with social service departments being given the lead role locally for planning and coordinating social care; local authorities would act as enablers in organising and purchasing services but not necessarily in providing them; local authorities should have transferred to them earmarked resources to fund these new responsibilities; and a new Minister with specific responsibility for community care should be appointed at national level (Griffiths, 1988). These proposals were designed to achieve a number of policy objectives. First, it was hoped that the 'perverse incentives' currently within the system and the consequent escalating costs of private residential care would be curtailed. Second, a mixed economy of social care provision would be encouraged, whereby SSDs would take the lead role in coordinating social care provision, although they would not be the main providers, making them enablers rather than providers of care. The Griffiths Report therefore set out the framework for the Thatcher government's community care policy, in which 'choice' and 'markets' were to be central tenets. These were to be enshrined within the subsequent legislation, initially set out in the government's White Paper: *Caring for People: Community care in the next decade and beyond* (Department of Health, 1989b).

What the government found particularly useful within Griffiths' proposals was the suggestion to shift the responsibility for long-term care from the health service to SSDs, along with suggestions of how to stem the flow of resources out of the Department of Social Security that had been paying for residential care up until then. However, less pleasing to the government was the recommendation that SSDs should be responsible for the strategic planning of community care provision. SSDs would act as the gatekeeper and budget holder and be held accountable for provision. However, the government's concerns at giving SSDs this responsibility were assuaged, because SSDs were only allowed to take on an enabling rather than a providing role and the vast majority of 'community care' funding would continue to be spent in the independent sector. Local authority SSDs would not be allowed to expand their provision significantly. Rather, the private sector would continue to be encouraged to provide social/community care and SSDs would be instructed that they had to spend a significant proportion (at least 85%) of their funds in the private sector.

Community Care White Paper 1989 – 'Caring for People'

The government therefore duly approved the main proposals within the Griffiths report, after some delay, with the publication of the White Paper (Department of Health, 1989b). Reflecting the Griffiths report, the White Paper emphasised the government's policy intention that community care was not just to be provided *in* the community but also *by* the community:

> ... most care is provided by the family, friends and neighbours. The majority of carers take on responsibilities willingly, but the government recognises that many need help to be able to manage what can be a heavy burden. Their lives could be made much easier if the right support is there at the right time, and a key responsibility of the statutory service providers should be to do all they can to assist and support carers. (Department of Health, 1989b: 9)

The key objectives of the White Paper set out the government's intentions in terms of its social community care policy: to promote the development of domiciliary, day and respite services to enable people to live in their own homes wherever feasible and sensible; to ensure that service providers made practical support for carers a high priority; to make proper assessment of need and good care management the cornerstone of high-quality care; to promote the development of a flourishing independent (that is, private and voluntary) sector; and to secure better value for taxpayers' money by introducing a new funding structure for social care. These proposals were duly incorporated into the NHS and Community Care Act 1990 (referred to below as the NHS&CCA 1990).

The NHS and Community Care Act 1990

As the title suggests, the NHS and Community Care Act 1990 dealt not just with the enactment of the government's community care policy but also with its reorganisation of the health service. However, while the health service aspects of the legislation were implemented quite speedily, the implementation of the changes in community care policy was delayed until April 1993. This was partly due to the difficulties of implementing the health aspects of the new legislation and partly because of difficulties in implementing another major piece of legislation directly impacting on local government, namely the Community Charge or 'Poll Tax'. However, once implemented, the NHS&CCA 1990 passed even more of the responsibility for long-term care to local authority SSDs in that care that had previously been defined as health care was now redefined as social care, therefore becoming means-testable and subject to rationing.

> Throughout the 1980s and 1990s, boundaries between health and social services were being redrawn. As social services became responsible for assessing access to care under the new community care policies laid down in the 1990 NHS and Community Care Act, the health service was pulling out of responsibility for long-term (continuing) care. The issue for the consumer was that this meant care was no longer free at the point of use. Moreover this change was being accomplished by stealth. (Dalley, 1999: 535)

Service users were faced with a situation where the policy rhetoric said they were to have choice and independence but in reality they only received support if judged to be in need and without sufficient independent means.

Discuss and Do	Health and social care – whose responsibility?

Since the 1940s there has arguably been a differentiation between health care and social care, with health care being provided free at the point of delivery and universal whereas social care was to be means-tested and targeted. The NHS and Community Care Act 1990 consolidated this distinction and emphasised that care *in* the community was to be provided *by* the community.

- In what respects does it make sense for government to claim that there is a difference between health care and social care?

- Is this really simply a device to pass the costs of long-term care to individuals or their families?

- Should families be expected to fulfil the responsibilities of caring for family members with long-term care needs?

- Can you see any difficulties or tensions arising when individual family members do take on caring responsibilities for other members of their family?

Following the implementation of the NHS&CCA 1990, the Conservative governments did make some further policy adjustments during the remainder of their time in power in the 1990s, not least in relation to carers' rights and support and the further promotion of service users' empowerment. Although the government did provide some additional policy guidance on supporting and including carers after the implementation of the 1990 Act, it became apparent that it had neglected the needs of carers to such an extent that further legislation was required. This was addressed with the Carers (Recognition and Services) Act 1995, which concerned itself mainly with the needs of informal carers who provided 'regular' or 'substantial' care, though it was left up to local authorities to define both these terms. The NHS&CCA 1990 also had the empowerment of users and carers as part of its intentions, for example via the development of social care markets. Even so, users and carers had not necessarily been put in control. The disability movement in particular had pressed for greater independence over how their care packages were set up and managed. Such pressure to amend the NHS&CCA 1990 eventually resulted in the passing of the Community Care (Direct Payments) Act 1996. This allowed local authority SSDs (though it did not make it a statutory duty) to transfer the responsibility for care packages to users themselves, who could then set up their own care arrangements by making 'direct payments' to third parties to provide them with care. However, the entitlement was initially restricted to people under 60 years of age, though more recently it was extended to people of 60 years and older.

Evaluating the Conservatives' adult social care reforms

In terms of evaluating the Conservatives' reforms to adult social or community care, one can reach a number of conclusions. As mentioned near the beginning of this section, the New Right's social care policy was focused on a desire to:

- promote deinstitutionalisation, where care *in* the community was constructed to mean care *by* the community;
- contain expenditure and tackle the 'perverse incentives' of DHSS-funded residential care, where long-term care would be redefined as social care rather than health care;
- promote service user involvement, empowerment, independence and responsibility;
- promote service user 'choice' via a mixed economy of provision;
- develop social care quasi-markets in which local authorities' SSDs would act as 'purchasers' of care from independent sector providers.

As to an evaluation of the level of success of these various policy intentions during the period of the New Right, research (for example, Rummery and Glendinning, 1999, 2000) indicates that users had not been provided with choices. Rather, their horizons are restricted by a policy whose impact has been to control expenditure, by assessment processes that slotted users into existing services rather than developing services around their needs, and by provision that was restricted in terms of which of their needs were met, when and by whom. Research also indicated that SSDs had not been developed as 'enablers' of social care particularly. Neither social care markets nor a mixed economy of provision have been developed significantly. This in turn meant that there were only limited opportunities for service users to shape and direct community care provision (Daly, 2001).

Adult social care under New Labour

To a large extent, the policy intentions set out in the NHS&CCA 1990 by Margaret Thatcher's Conservative government have remained in place under the Labour government. New Labour has certainly continued to espouse a belief in community-based care, service user involvement, and a mixed economy of provision delivered via social care markets. Indeed, according to Rummery (2007: 67), the legacy of the NHS&CCA 1990 '... remains a powerful driver in social services: policies designed and implemented by the New Labour government since 1997 have never strayed too far [from the original aims] to control public expenditure, facilitate joint working between health and social care and empower service users'. What is different is that New Labour has arguably placed an increased emphasis on accountability through performance measurement and management (part of its modernisation agenda), as well as a change in emphasis concerning participation and involvement which extended to other stakeholders, not just service users. This section of the chapter now looks at this in some detail.

New Labour's 'Third Way' – modernising social services

Personal social services (including adult social care) were arguably not at the top of New Labour's social policy agenda when it returned to power in 1997 (Johnson, 2001), though this lack of attention changed by its second term (Means *et al.*, 2002). However, New Labour did see the need for *Modernising Social Services* (Department of Health, 1998a) along with other parts of the public sector, declaring, for example, that as far as mental health users were concerned, 'Care in the community has failed' (Department of Health, 1998b: 4) and, more generally, that 'Social services are often failing to provide the support' which people deserved and expected (Department of Health, 1998a: 5). The government's analysis was that social services, including adult social care, were failing in a number of ways, including the following:

- lack of protection – users had been exposed to abuse and neglect;
- lack of coordination between the various agencies responsible for provision;
- inflexibility and a tendency for the persistence of supplier dominance;
- lack of clarity concerning what social services should provide and the quality of that provision;
- inconsistency in service quality;
- inconsistency in terms of costs and 'best value'.

New Labour's priorities, therefore, were for social services that promoted service users' independence, were consistently of good quality and value, were convenient, and were user-centred (Department of Health, 1998a).

However, New Labour's adult and social care policy can be seen to some extent as a continuation of the Conservatives' approach. New Labour wished to promote the following:

- independence;
- user involvement;

- support for carers;
- social (not health) care that is open to means testing and rationing;
- control of costs through the pursuit of 'best value';
- a mixed economy of provision;
- care provided via (quasi-)markets;
- accountability through standards and inspection (Department of Health, 1998a).

In promoting a mixed economy of provision rather than a return to publicly provided social care, it argued that this was part of its 'non-ideological' *Third Way* (Blair, 1998; see Inman, 1999; Langan, 2000). New Labour found no difficulty in supporting the promotion of the market or quasi-markets if this meant good quality social care provision (Johnson, 2001).

Long-term care remains social care

New Labour has chosen to continue with the construction of long-term care as essentially social care and therefore open to rationing and means testing, in England at least (see Chapter 7 for consideration of the situation in Scotland, Wales and Northern Ireland). As such, it rejected the recommendation of the Royal Commission on the Funding of Long-term Care (Sutherland, 1999) to have long-term care (whether 'social' or 'health' care) paid for out of general taxation; nor did it choose to implement the recommendation that living and housing costs should be eligible for co-payment but subject to means testing. Instead the government responded to the Royal Commission by agreeing to nursing care only being paid for out of taxation (Department of Health, 2000). Personal care (bathing, feeding, dressing) would remain defined as social care and therefore not available as of right. The situation is different in Scotland where, via the enactment of the Scottish Parliament's Community Care and Health (Scotland) Bill, older people are entitled to free personal care (see Inman, 2002) (see Chapter 7). Therefore, New Labour can be seen to have continued with the New Right's agenda to control (adult) social care costs.

However, certain policy differences are increasingly apparent. First, New Labour extended the support offered to carers. As part of the Carers and Disabled Children's Act 2000, carers' needs were now assessed in their own right, and local authority SSDs had to provide prescribed services for them such as home helps, assistance with travel and mobile phones (Department of Health, 2001). In addition, as part of the extension of Direct Payments, carers were able to purchase services to meet their own needs. Second, regarding service user involvement, while supporting the New Right's belief in involving users, New Labour also emphasised the involvement of other citizens too: 'the Best Value regime will place a requirement on local authorities to find out what local citizens' service needs are, and what they think of how the council is doing' (Department of Health, 1998a: 34). Langan (2000) for one has suggested that the major difference between New Labour and the New Right as far as personal social services is concerned is New Labour's greater emphasis on the requirement for social services to be accountable to taxpayers and citizens (and therefore not just users).

> The innovations of New Labour have concentrated on ... accountability. The modernizing White Paper proposes initiatives in a number of areas to render social services more answerable to the mythical taxpayer/citizen who ultimately foots the bill, to the clients and carers who rely on social care – and to the rest of us who may well, at different times, or indeed at the same time, occupy any of these categories. (Langan, 2000: 160)

Similarly, Braye has observed that New Labour: '[seeks] to engage a wider constituency of people in dialogue about traditionally marginalised services, in effect to enhance the participation of people as citizens rather than as service users' (Braye, 2000: 12).

However, it is more in its second and third terms that New Labour's particular approach to adult social care has appeared, not least in relation to, firstly, the continued pursuit of service user choice and, secondly, the further encouragement of social care markets and a diversity of supply.

Adult Social Care Green Paper 2005 – 'Independence, Well-being and Choice'

The promotion of service user choice can be seen in the 2005 Adult Social Care Green Paper *Independence, Well-being and Choice* (Department of Health, 2005) and the pronouncements around adult social care articulated in the subsequent White Paper, *Our Health, Our Care, Our Say: A new direction for community services* (Department of Health, 2006). In the Green Paper, the then Secretary of State, John Reid, set out the New Labour government's ambitions for adults in receipt of social care:

> We want to give individuals and their families and friends greater control over the way in which social care supports their needs. We want to support ... individuals to live as independently as possible for as long as possible. (Green Paper – John Reid, Foreword, Department of Health, 2005: 6)

The White Paper (Department of Health, 2006) further espoused the rhetoric of both choice and voice in social care provision:

> This White Paper confirms the vision in the Green Paper of high-quality support meeting people's aspirations for independence and greater control over their lives, making services flexible and responsive to individual needs. We will [put] people more in control .... We will move towards fitting services round people not people round services .... We will give people a stronger voice so that they are the major drivers of service improvement. (Department of Health, 2006, Executive summary, Sections 5–12)

The intention was that social care markets were to be further developed to provide greater choice and that direct payments (an initiative of the mid-1990s and the previous Conservative government) would be extended to other social care service users:

> In talking to people who use services and to carers, it is clear that direct payments give people that choice and control, and we think that this is a mechanism that

should be extended and encouraged where possible. (Department of Health, 2005)

Consequently, in the White Paper, it was proposed to extend direct payments but also to introduce another mechanism, 'Individual Budgets' or 'Personal Budgets', to empower service users:

> ... we will increase the take-up of direct payments by ... extend[ing] their availability to currently excluded groups and will pilot the introduction of individual budgets, bringing together several income-streams from social care, community equipment, Access to Work, Independent Living Funds, Disability Facilities Grants and Supporting People. (Department of Health, 2006: 7)

Discuss and Do

Does providing adult social care service users with 'choice and independence', for example through the promotion of direct payments or individual budgets whereby service users are given their own budgets to plan and pay for care in the way they want it, seem a sensible policy development to you?

- Why might adult service users be attracted by such a policy aim?

- What difficulties can you envisage with this policy?

- Do you think all service users would want to take it up?

Evaluating New Labour's adult social care reforms

New Labour has continued to espouse the discourse of choice, voice, social care markets and a mixed economy of provision that ensures 'services fit round people not people round services'. In bringing this chapter to a close, a brief evaluation will be provided of the extent to which we are able to judge whether these policy aims have been achieved. Whilst it is the case that a mixed economy of service provision now exists in various social care areas, e.g. in residential and home care, this does not automatically or necessarily mean that service users are provided with greater choice or autonomy. Rather, it can be argued that the promotion of social care market is part of the government's 'managerialist' approach explored in Chapter 6.

The mixed economy of social care providers and social care markets has been developed (see Netten, 2005; Rummery, 2007). For example, Netten (2005: 91–93) suggests that there has been a 'substantial shift to independent rather than in-house provision of services and a shift to people being increasingly cared for in their own homes .... The shift between in-house and independent provision that took place in the late 1980s and early 1990s in residential care [under the Conservative governments] has been mirrored in home care in the subsequent decade'. However, the number of people receiving social care purchased by local authorities is *decreasing*, as it is increasingly only those most need who receive support. However, these individuals are receiving more hours of care (see Figures 13.1 to 13.3, in which 'CSSRs' stands for Councils with Social Services Responsibilities).

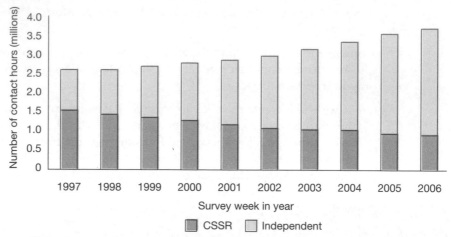

Figure 13.1   Estimated number of contact hours of home care by sector, 1997–2006
Source: The Information Centre (2007) *Community Care Statistics 2006: Home Help/Care Services for Adults, England*, Figure 1, London: The Information Centre (Adult Social Services Statistics). Crown copyright material is reproduced with the permission of the Controllor of HMSO and the Queen's Printer for Scotland under the PSI Licence. *Original source*: Department of Health, *HH1 Return*, Table 1, London: Department of Health.

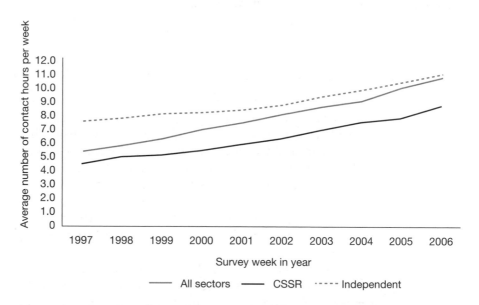

Figures for 2000 onwards for All Sectors exclude double counting.
Households receiving care purchased with a direct payment are excluded.

Figure 13.2   Average number of hours per week of home care provided by each sector, 1997–2006
Source: The Information Centre (2007) *Community Care Statistics 2006: Home Help/Care Services for Adults, England*, Figure 2, London: The Information Centre (Adult Social Services Statistics). Crown copyright material is reproduced with the permission of the Controllor of HMSO and the Queen's Printer for Scotland under the PSI Licence. *Original source*: Department of Health, *HH1 Return*, Tables 1, 2A, 2B and 3A (for 2000 onwards), London: Department of Health.

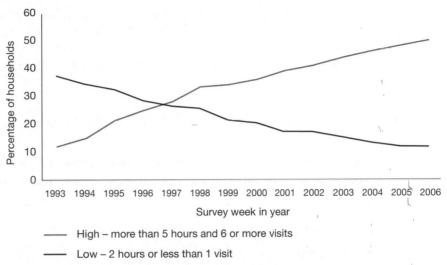

Figure 13.3 Intensity of home help/home care: percentage of households, 1993–2006
Source: The Information Centre (2007) *Community Care Statistics 2006: Home Help/Care Services for Adults, England*, Figure 4, London: The Information Centre (Adult Social Services Statistics). Crown copyright material is reproduced with the permission of the Controllor of HMSO and the Queen's Printer for Scotland under the PSI Licence. *Original source*: Department of Health, London: Department of Health.

> The combination of maintaining people at home, who would previously have been in residential care, and increased targeting of services has led to considerable intensification of services. [Figures 13.2 and 13.3] demonstrate the increase in intensity of home care provision. In recent years, the number of commissioned home care hours has been rising rapidly, but the number of households receiving home care and the number of care places has been falling. As a result, the average number of publicly funded home care contact hours per household more than doubled from 3.5 hours per week in 1993 to 8.2 hours in 2003. Consequently, those with lower levels of need are increasingly purchasing support services independently .... (Netten, 2005: 93–94)

Therefore, a trend that was arguably started under the New Right social care reforms has continued, that is, those adults in receipt of social care are more needy and are receiving more hours of social care. However, the overall numbers in receipt of adult social care have decreased. Therefore, a somewhat paradoxical situation has arguably emerged with regard to adult social care provision in England at least. If one is judged to be in need of social care support, one may be provided with both a greater voice and greater choice over provision. However, this is at the expense of the numbers deemed not entitled to receive adult social care (Daly, 2001). And so, when returning to the aims of social care reforms over the last 30 years, that is:

- to deinstitutionalise social care provision;
- to promote service users' independence and responsibility;
- to promote service user 'choice', not least via quasi-markets;
- to reconstruct long-term care as social care rather than health care;
- to contain the overall level of expenditure on community social care;

it is possible to suggest that while care was deinstitutionalised outside the old care institutions, these have arguably been replaced by other forms of institutional arrangements, and that service user choice remains a far-off goal while cost containment remains a key focus of social care policy implementation (see Rummery, 2007).

Conclusion

This chapter has explored how children and adult social care services have developed, particularly over the last 20 to 30 years under the governments of the New Right and New Labour. For both sets of provisions, there are examples of continuities and discontinuities during this period. As far as children's and young people's services are concerned, government has emphasised:

- the general well-being of all children;
- the safety and protection of children;
- the need to overcome the state's failings in this arena.

However, in addition, New Labour has:

- promoted local authorities as coordinators of children's services and as strategic leaders and enablers of these partnerships, but not necessarily as providers of such services;
- emphasised that children's social care is provided through partnership working;
- promoted the need for adequate provision of child care, particularly for working parents;
- encouraged private and voluntary sector provider agencies.

For adult social care, one can see the following continuities over the last 30 years:

- an emphasis on a discourse of service user choice and voice;
- the promotion of a mixed economy of provision and promotion of the independent sector as provider;
- the defining of long-term care as social care, not health care, and therefore not universally available or free at the point of use;
- a policy imperative that only the neediest are permitted to receive state-supported social care.

However, in addition, New Labour has:

- extended the scope of Direct Payments and supplemented this with the introduction of Individual Budgets or Personal Budgets;
- promoted to an even greater extent the discourse of user and other voices in shaping service provision;
- been even more managerialist and preoccupied with performance in relation to social care provision.

Annotated further reading

Adult social and community care

Robin Means and Randall Smith have written extensively on the historical development of social care policy and provision. One of their texts provides a very useful account of the development of social care from the start of the Second World War through to the early 1970s with the establishment of social services departments (Means and Smith, 1998, *From Poor Law to Community Care*), whilst another (Means, Morbey and Smith, 2002, *From Community Care to Market Care?*) explores the restructuring of community care from the 1970s to the early 1990s. Jane Lewis and Howard Glennerster provide a very readable account of the aims of Conservative community care policy (the 'new community care') in the 1980s and 1990s (Lewis and Glennerster, 1996, *Implementing the New Community Care*). Peter Sharkey provides a useful guide to current community care policy and practice (Sharkey, 2006, *Essentials of Community Care*). Jon Glasby and Rosemary Littlechild provide a useful analysis of the challenges of trying to work across the health and social care divide (Glasby and Littlechild, 2004, *The Health and Social Care Divide*) as well as writing on the effectiveness of direct payments in promoting independence for social care service users (Glasby and Littlechild, 2002, *Social Work and Direct Payments*). Kirstein Rummery provides a recent analysis of New Labour's adult social care policy (Rummery, 2007, 'Modernising services, empowering users? Adult Social Care in 2006', in Clarke, Maltby and Kennett, 2007, *Social Policy Review 19*).

Children's social care and welfare

Harry Hendrick provides a useful introduction to the various concepts, issues, policies and practices affecting child welfare, with a particular emphasis on the changing nature of the relationship between child welfare and social policy (Hendrick (ed.), 2005, *Child Welfare and Social Policy*). Barry Goldson and colleagues provide a useful contemporary analysis of the society and the state's relationship to children from a Marxist perspective (Goldson, Lavalette and McKechnie (eds), 2002, *Children, Welfare and the State*). In terms of specific work on social inclusion, the text by Roger Matthews and colleagues is a useful recent assessment of the impact of anti-social behaviour orders (Matthews, Easton, Briggs and Pease, 2007, *Assessing the Use and Impact of Anti-Social Behaviour Orders*). Finally, Harriet Churchill presents a helpful analysis of New Labour's social policy in relation to the development of children's services (Churchill, 2007, 'Children's services in 2006', in Clarke, Maltby and Kennett, *Social Policy Review 19*).

Chapter 14

Housing policy

Objectives

- To outline the development of state involvement in the provision of housing.

- To examine the development of different housing sectors — private rental, public rental and owner occupation.

- To consider the Conservative New Right's housing policy of 1979–97, including:

  - the residualisation of council housing

  - the development and operation of the private housing market – and the aspiration to promote a 'property owning democracy'.

- To consider New Labour's housing policy, including:

  - the refashioning of the public rented (social housing) sector

  - the continued promotion of the private housing market

  - the support for homeless and other vulnerable individuals and groups.

Introduction

Housing is a crucial aspect of people's welfare. Having inadequate housing or being homeless is a terrible predicament in which to find oneself, as can be seen from the newspaper article (Booth, 2007) in Box 14.1 about Ed Mitchell, who had previously been a successful television journalist for ITN until debts and alcohol problems had such an impact on him and his family.

This chapter therefore examines the development of housing policy since the creation of the British welfare state. As such, housing has increasingly come to be seen as the 'wobbly pillar' (Harloe, 1995; Malpass, 2003) of welfare state provision, in that while state health and education provision have been constructed as universal (that is, provision for all), housing policy has been focused on (a) public provision for the most needy, and (b) the promotion of the private market for the majority (for example, through mortgage income tax relief, the promotion of the 'right to buy' for council tenants and the promotion of the notion of a 'property owning democracy'). This chapter therefore provides an overview of British housing policy, initially via an account of the historical background and then by exploring more recent trends of home ownership and rented provision.

Box 14.1	**Ed Mitchell**

ITN man once interviewed the influential, now he sleeps rough

Journalist homeless for 10 months after losing job and going through divorce

Robert Booth, *The Guardian*, Saturday 15 December 2007

He was the ITN broadcaster who interviewed Margaret Thatcher, John Major and Tony Blair. But not for Ed Mitchell the knighthoods, celebrity and bestselling books that have come to other leading broadcasters. Mitchell said yesterday he had been homeless for the last 10 months, sleeping on a bench next to a nightclub on the windblown seafront at Hove, Sussex.

'It's a bit bleak,' the 54-year-old said as he surveyed his view across the Channel. 'But at night the constellation of Orion rises clearly over there above the Babylon Lounge.'

It was one poetic thought in an otherwise desperate story of increasing credit card debt and alcoholism that has taken Mitchell from his status as a broadcaster earning £100,000 a year with a wife and two children, to divorce, bankruptcy and homelessness.

He admitted yesterday that his decline has left Frederick, 22, and Alexandra, 24, ashamed of him, and his 83-year-old mother unable to understand how her son's 'fall from grace should be so sharp and steep'.

He told how he sleeps fitfully in fear of attack, shaves in public toilets and tries to survive on just £52 a week in jobseeker's allowance . . .. Now, he wants to get back to work and find housing. 'I know so much about the pain of being homeless, I want to give back through volunteer organisations my time and expertise.'

Reprinted with permission.

Stop and Think

Why is housing so crucial to an individual or a family's welfare? What do you think are the consequences of being homeless or inadequately housed?

Historical background

Historically the question of housing policy was one of the last areas of social provision to attract the attention of a nascent and developing welfare state. It was not until the years of the First World War that the question of housing for the working classes received serious attention on the British political agenda, when the protests of workers against the profiteering of their landlords, in sensitive industrial areas such as munitions and shipbuilding in and around Glasgow, forced the Lloyd-George government to act. Initially the political response was to subsidise rents in order to buy industrial peace, and it was not until the years following the war that the state's interest in the construction and management of public housing projects began in earnest. Even then the response was short-lived as public expenditure restrictions in the early years of the 1920s restricted the ability of local municipal authorities (councils) to finance house building.

As Malpass and Murie (1999) indicate, before 1914 there was barely a recognisable housing policy. However, the years of the First World War (1914–18), during which housing production fell, meant that by 1918 there existed a severe housing shortage that the private building sector was unable to address. During the inter-war years housing policy developed on two fronts: the control of rents in the private rented sector and the subsidy of local authority building, partly prompted by the various programmes of slum clearance, particularly after 1930. Emphasis, however, remained with the private building sector which alone constructed 100,000 dwellings every year from 1925 to over 250,000 annually between 1934 and 1938, with local authorities averaging only 25,000 completions annually during the same period (Malpass and Murie, 1999). Thus housing policy as a part of the formative welfare state remained hardly recognisable, but there was nonetheless a shift in the pattern of tenure as private ownership began to take over from private rentals as the preferred option – herein, arguably, lies the roots of Britain's 'property owning democracy'.

Public housing was therefore, at this time, very much a minority undertaking with many local authorities reluctant to enter the property development market. But those that did, especially those controlled by Labour councillors, sought to show that workers' housing needed no longer to be slums, and in so doing mirrored works undertaken by the cooperative and trades union movements. They sought instead to install the range and type of facilities that they considered were the best that could be bought, and the space available in many early public housing projects was generous. They were keen to show that a future Labour government could construct and successfully manage quality homes for their working-class constituents at affordable rents. However, the building costs of those early projects were high as authorities sought to maintain high quality and at the same time were forced to pay high labour costs to attract skilled building workers away from the private sector (Malpass and Murie, 1999).

This general picture remained largely unaltered during the inter-war years as the majority of newly built houses were, as we have seen, in the privately owned sector. Government interest in housing instead focused on the question of inner-city congestion and slum clearance. It was only really as a result of the Second World War (1939–45), and the effects of civilian bombing together with the desire to fulfil the promises of the 'khaki election' to build homes for heroes, that housing policy was placed more centrally on the policy stage. The programmes of slum clearance continued, although priorities began to change as building standards were gradually lowered in an attempt to accelerate the building programme. Urban planning, as a result, became chaotic as towns began to spread as new suburbs sprang up and the back-to-back terraces of the town centres disappeared. Local authorities were, as Malpass and Murie (1999) indicate, fulfilling a residual role at this time, as they sought to rehouse those people displaced by slum clearance, while for those who had the resources and opportunity a privately owned suburban semi-detached became a realisable dream.

The early years of the 1940s were witness to a radical shift in housing priorities for the policy makers of the post-war years. Some 3.5 million dwellings were either wholly destroyed or substantially damaged by air raids by 1945 and the slum clearance programmes, which had temporarily halted, could renew apace. The housing crisis facing this generation's set of returning war heroes was thus far more severe than that seen in 1918–19 and the incoming government was required to act quickly and moreover to build quickly. Both the major political parties (Labour and Conservative) promised rapid completion rates in house building to replace those properties damaged or destroyed and to allow slum clearance to resume, and visionary urban architects were able to find ready employment within local authorities and to give life to their creations in places like Portsmouth and Coventry. However, there was a difference in emphasis, with Labour favouring public building projects and municipal management of new estates and with the Conservatives retaining their traditional loyalty to the private building industry and adopting the new slogan that promised the creation of a 'property-owning democracy'. We are thus, from these rather different ideological stances, able to identify clear periods in the development of post-war housing policy and priorities:

- The period from 1945 to 1953 saw a rapid growth in municipal housing developments.
- The mid-1950s to mid-1960s was a period of growth in private sector developments.
- The mid-1960s onwards saw an emphasis on improvement to existing housing stock.
- The 1980s into the 1990s was a time when public housing was no longer seen to be effective.
- The late 1990s into the 2000s has been a time where public or social housing has become a residual sector, the political consensus is one of home ownership as the aspiration for most households, and the vast majority of households are housed privately.

The first period, that is the first eight years of the post-war welfare state (1945 to 1953), were characterised by rapid growth in municipal housing projects, in part attributable to the creation of new towns. The emphasis was very much one of rapid construction to meet short-term need in the face of shortages of both materials and labour. The second period, from the mid-1950s for a decade, saw the rapid pace of building continuing but the responsibility for that building was laid squarely at the feet of the private building industry. In the third period, that is through the 1960s, perspectives appeared to change yet again and it was belatedly realised that the war against slum clearance could never be won as social standards in housing continued to grow, thus always leaving a proportion of housing in the category of 'unfit'. Emphasis once again shifted as the principle of 'renewability' was adopted and government monies made available for, initially, the renovation of poor quality housing stock and latterly of inner-city environments, as governments defined both General Improvement Areas and later Housing Action Areas. By this time Britain had established a firmly polarised housing sector dominated by powerful lobbies for both municipally controlled rented stock and private ownership. The private rented sector underwent a decline, squeezed out by successive governments' preferences for alternately public and private housing.

Housing, then, at least as an identifiable area of government policy, is almost exclusively confined to the post-1945 era and may be characterised by an air of euphoria, at least on the part of the housing bureaucracy, as they reached successive construction targets. However, dramatic failure, particularly in municipal projects, was always just around the corner, and in the 1980s the ground was laid bare for a revolution in property ownership and the large-scale disposal of council-owned property. The dominant policy rhetoric by the early to mid-1980s was that local authority-run municipal housing had by now come to embody inefficient, ineffective and unpopular provision – that is, not very dissimilar to the privately rented stock it had been designed to replace. Local authority housing departments were perceived to be as inflexible as any private landlord in their regulation of tenants. Local authorities were charged, not always unfairly, with replacing the inner-city slums with newer suburban or high-rise slums. These council houses and estates were increasingly regarded as poorly built, poorly maintained, inefficiently managed and/or used as dumping grounds for the local authorities' most troublesome tenants. On the other hand, after 1975 local authorities may justifiably point to increased central control over their finances which restricted their ability to act, for instance in controlling how capital from council house sales may be utilised. Even so, by the 1980s local authority council housing was increasingly seen by politicians and other policy makers to be no longer part of the solution to housing those in need but instead as a significant part of the problem.

The 1980s were to witness radical changes to British housing policy. The 1979 election returned a 'New Right' Conservative government, under Margaret Thatcher's leadership, which amongst other things promised to give council tenants the opportunity of joining the property-owning democracy by giving them the 'right to buy' their council house or flat. Indeed, the sale of council houses was one of the central planks of the Conservatives' election victory in 1979. The 1980s, as we have seen in other chapters in this book, was a decade in which the large-scale provision of state-funded welfare was increasingly questioned and challenged. In the field of housing we witnessed possibly the most successful attempt to alter radically the pattern of welfare provision. Public dissatisfaction with council housing was well publicised and local authorities were often regarded as landlords of the most poorly built and inadequately maintained stock. Local authorities were also accused of being over-bureaucratic and unresponsive to the needs of their tenants, not least by adopting practices which ghettoised ethnic-minority households and lone-parent headed households within the most inadequate, the least well maintained and the most unsuitable housing. It was in the 1980s too that the problems stored up by the previous rapid construction programmes in the early post-war years came to a head as many local authorities began to find it untenable any longer to maintain and renovate deteriorating stock. Indeed, many local authorities began to resort instead to the demolition not just of individual properties but also of whole estates, which were often little more than 30 years old and (ironically) had been built to house families moved out as part of slum clearance programmes.

Housing policy under the New Right – residualised state involvement and the promotion of the market

It is often tempting to begin a review of contemporary housing policy trends with the 1979 election and the manifesto promises of the first Thatcher administration. But we can detect the beginnings of policy change within the final years of the previous Labour government. Labour's traditional and ideological support for state-owned and subsidised rented accommodation was fundamentally questioned when it was unable to maintain commitments to expanding public expenditures in the middle of the decade and 'in its 1977 Green Paper, its endorsement of the balance between tenures was weighted towards home ownership' (Doling, 1993). Such consensorial support of home ownership had not been openly acknowledged by Labour until this point, although from the mid-1950s Labour had implicitly conceded the electoral popularity of home ownership.

However, the 1979 election victory for Margaret Thatcher heralded something of a revolution. The next 18 years would be a period in which home ownership was promoted as the preferred form of tenure, alongside the 'dismantling of the public rented sector' and the 'deregulation of private renting', by which process housing would be regarded less and less as a public or merit good (see the 'Discuss and Do' activity) and the provision of a decent home was no longer considered part of government's basic responsibility and came instead to be regarded increasingly as a private good with the government's role one of market regulation (Linneman and Megbolugbe, 1994; Malpass, 1996). The period of New Right Conservative rule began almost triumphantly as the 1980 Housing Act introduced the right of council tenants to purchase their homes at substantial discounts. This was made easier for these would-be home owners by the subsequent deregulation of financial markets which made the obtaining of a mortgage far easier. Local authorities would then be left to provide what was frequently referred to as 'residual housing, for the poorest of tenants, and specialist housing for particular needy groups, such as the elderly (although this too was to change with the impact of the 1990 NHS and Community Care Act and the implementation of 'community care policy' – see Chapter 13).

The right to buy was substantially buoyed by the economic boom of the mid-1980s and the general availability of low-cost credit. However, the picture changed rapidly and dramatically at the end of the 1980s as the economic boom turned to recession and the economy, controlled largely by interest rates, seriously undermined the efficacy of the burgeoning housing market. Mortgage default, negative equity and even repossession were experienced by millions of home-owners in the 1990s. In the private rented sector, the government sought to revitalise the market by deregulating and creating incentives for private landlords, whilst at the same time attempting to force the transfer of local authority housing stock into the hands of alternative landlords in the form of 'tenants' choice' and encouraging other social housing providers, particularly housing associations (see below). Perhaps most fundamentally, the 1980s heralded a shift in housing finance away from the subsidy of supply – house building – towards one built more around the subsidising of demand – via means-tested housing benefit in the rental sector and mortgage interest relief for owner occupiers.

Discuss and Do

From your understanding of the historical background to British housing policy, why might the consumption of housing be regarded as either a private or a merit/public good?

Reasons for constructing housing as a private good include:

- sovereignty of individual consumers – personal responsibility and autonomy
- belief in the supremacy of the market – responsive to demand, efficient and cost effective.

However, housing in particular can be regarded as a merit or public good for a number of reasons, including:

- housing markets cannot respond 'elastically' to demand simply by increasing supply – the production of new properties takes a long time, in part due to the limited availability of land that can be used for house building
- increases in demand therefore result in increases in house values – for both buyers and renters
- lack of an adequate supply of housing has consequences for wider society as well as the individual consumer – e.g. where key workers (teachers, health workers, fire fighters, police officers) cannot afford to live in areas of the country where their skills are scarce, and where the implications of poor housing or no housing are felt not just by the individual tenant or homeless person but by the wider society too.

Public housing under the Conservatives

The privatisation of public rented housing has been viewed by some as an attack on the welfare state at its weakest link, or on its wobbliest pillar (Harloe, 1995; Malpass, 2003). However, it was portrayed politically as the dismantling of a relatively unpopular service. It was here, therefore, where the market had already proved itself a popular success as people 'invested in bricks and mortar', that the New Right experiment may be said to have begun. 'Council housing was the perfect symbol for the failings of the public sector; unpopular, socially stigmatising, incompetently managed and oblivious to consumer preferences' (Cole and Furbey, 1994: 183–18). The consensus that previously accepted that there was a significant role for the local authority (or more generally the state) sector to play in the provision of low-cost rented accommodation had dissolved. Home ownership was accepted by both sides of the political divide as desired by the electorate and therefore politically supportable. The Conservative Party was able to exploit this by offering the prospect of the right to buy council houses.

So it was in 1980 that the Housing Act of that year introduced the right for council tenants, of at least three years' tenure, to have the option to own their own council home, by purchasing it at a substantial discount and so to benefit from rising prices in the housing market, which appeared set to continue *ad infinitum* (Malpass, 1996). The revolution in home ownership was supported by an equally dynamic revolution in the British financial sector which itself was to undergo the 'throes of deregulation' (Doling, 1993). The government felt that the privatisation of housing provision would serve a number of related purposes.

Stop and Think

Can you think of some of the reasons why the Conservative government might have wanted to 'dismantle' local authority controlled council housing?

Various reasons could have included:

- the belief in wanting individuals to have control and choice over their housing situation
- the belief in the supremacy of the market
- the belief that state-run council housing was and is inefficient and does not provide tenants with choice
- an antipathy to Labour-controlled local authorities with their ideology of state control.

First, and politically, it would break the political monopoly enjoyed by Labour councillors on Britain's inner-city housing estates – the logic of the time was that a council tenant was more likely to be a Labour voter whereas a home-owner was more likely to be a Conservative sympathiser. Secondly, the desperate condition of some of those same housing estates would be remedied by an injection of funds from new home-owners and the removal of the local authorities' bureaucratic stranglehold, which in turn would raise standards on those estates. Thirdly, many economic questions could be addressed as public expenditure would be more easily controlled by the Treasury and may even fall as revenues from council house sales began to accumulate. Finally, the overall economic picture could only continue to improve as a booming housing market stimulated other, related, sectors of the economy at large.

This scenario persisted throughout much of the 1980s, since between 1983 and 1989 both the economy and in turn the housing market enjoyed an unprecedented boom, during which time over 1 million council houses were transferred from state to private ownership, with tenants being encouraged by both continually rising rents and increasingly more generous discounts on sale price during this period. Government opted to use the mechanism of council house sales, first to individual tenants who were to be encouraged by a discounted price compared to the market value of the property and determined by the length of their tenancy (the maximum would be a 70% discount) and by the right to obtain a mortgage. Secondly, and later in the decade, sales to other landlords were encouraged either at the instigation of the local authority itself or at the initiative of the tenants.

Figure 14.1 and Table 14.1 illustrate the scale of the privatisation of public sector housing and indicate that between 1984 and 1997 the ownership of over 1.5 million public sector dwellings was transferred. (One should also note that since 1997 this trend of council house sales continued under New Labour's first two terms.) The transfers were almost all to owner occupation, and to sitting tenants. Despite the 'right to buy' scheme, however, local authorities continued to provide the majority of rental sector housing in the 1990s, with council house sales appearing to reach something of

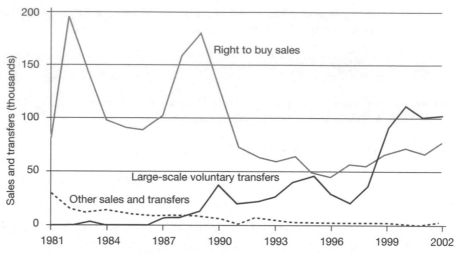

Figure 14.1 Sales and transfers of local authority dwellings, Great Britain, 1981–2002
Source: Adapted from Office for National Statistics (2004) *Social Trends No. 34*, Figure 10.2, p. 162, London: ONS. Crown copyright material is reproduced with the permission of the Controller of HMSO and the Queen's Printer for Scotland under the terms of the Click-Use Licence.

Table 14.1 Sales and transfers of local authority dwellings, Great Britain, 1981-2002 (thousands)

	Right to buy sales	Large-scale voluntary transfers	Other sales and transfers
1981	79.4	0.4	30.3
1982	196.8	0.9	16.2
1983	138.6	3.3	12.5
1984	100.6	0.9	14.5
1985	92.6	0.6	10.7
1986	89.3	0.2	9.7
1987	103.3	6.6	10.1
1988	160.6	8.6	9.6
1989	181.4	13.7	9.2
1990	126.2	38.4	6.7
1991	73.6	21.5	3.8
1992	64.3	21.9	6.9
1993	60.4	27.5	6.0
1994	65.2	41.0	4.6
1995	49.6	47.7	3.2
1996	45.0	29.9	3.0
1997	58.1	21.1	3.4
1998	56.0	36.9	2.7
1999	66.8	88.7	3.3
2000	71.3	111.4	2.4
2001	66.5	100.8	1.6
2002	78.3	102.5	1.4

Source: Office for National Statistics (2004) *Social Trends No. 34*, data from Chapter 10, London: ONS. Crown copyright material is reproduced with the permission of the Controller of HMSO and the Queen's Printer for Scotland under the terms of the Click-Use Licence.

an impasse (Whitehead, 1993; Linneman and Megbolugbe, 1994) in the 1990s. To overcome this stalling, first the Conservatives and latterly the Labour government have endeavoured to use 'stock transfer' (see discussion of this later in the chapter) as a means of accelerating and perpetuating the residualisation of council housing.

The development of this policy of council house sales in the 1980s showed a number of things. First, the numbers of sales remained relatively small and the new owner-occupiers were largely drawn from the financially more secure tenants, in particular those in secure employment. That group of tenants were encouraged to purchase their council houses by rapidly increasing rent levels and restrictions to housing benefit regulations. Secondly, the transfer of housing stock was of a particular type, and most typically of suburban houses with gardens rather than flats or homes located within the inner city (Doling, 1993; Malpass, 1996). Therefore, the stock that remained in the control of local authorities was often the least popular, least well maintained, and rented by tenants who were in less-secure employment or long-term unemployment. The policy of council house sales increasingly created a residualised public rented housing sector. This was exacerbated when from the mid-1990s the impetus, first by the Conservatives and then by New Labour, was to encourage local authorities to transfer their entire housing stock (stock transfer) to independent landlords. The matter of stock transfer is dealt with later in the chapter.

Government policy, under the Conservatives in the latter part of the 1980s and early 1990s, had thus changed course with the establishment, in many fields of welfare provision including housing, of the 'enabling' local authority. What this has meant for local government is a change of role away from direct provision of services towards one in which the authority oversees and regulates services provided by a range of different organisations, private, voluntary and charity (see, for example, Chapters 13 on social care and 15 on education). In terms of housing, the role of councils developed into a role involving the maintenance of standards and regulation of rents in the private rented sector, the administration of the housing benefits system, the enforcement of environmental health standards and the temporary accommodation of the statutory homeless.

Therefore, the story of council housing in the 1980s and early 1990s explains only part of the picture of public rental housing in Britain. A significant and growing, though still proportionately small, number of dwellings are available to rent within housing association control (sometimes described as Registered Social Landlords or RSLs), which are non-profit organisations and remain, largely at least, publicly funded. Indeed, of council house transfers over the period 1984–94, some 155,000 council houses in England were transferred to the control of housing associations, and therefore remained within the public rental sector. Over the decade of the 1980s and into the 1990s the Conservative government sought to expand significantly the role of housing associations within the housing sector, not least the number of housing association (RSL) properties (see Figure 14.2 and Table 14.2). This included encouragement and legislative recognition of those schemes which, usually at the initiative of local councils, effected the transfer of housing to association control. But, as part of this change of role, associations saw their revenue support from public funds fall as they were encouraged to seek private sources of finance to supplement public funds. As a result, and to encourage private investment, housing association rents rose to a market level in order to offer better rates of return to private investors.

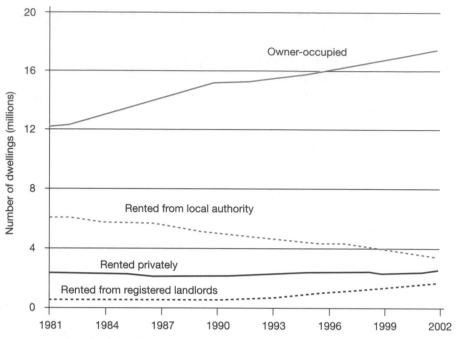

Figure 14.2 Stock of dwellings by tenure, Great Britain, 1981–2002
Source: Adapted from Office for National Statistics (2004) *Social Trends No. 34*, Figure 10.5, London: ONS. Crown copyright material is reproduced with the permission of the Controller of HMSO and the Queen's Printer for Scotland under the terms of the Click-Use Licence.

Home ownership

The availability of cheap credit and loans secured against homes ensured that the house market expanded and house prices rose rapidly. During the Conservatives' period of office, the housing market itself reached a peak during 1988/89 as the credit boom coincided with new government restrictions to mortgage interest tax relief and house sales reached a frenzy before the August deadline. The furore of the 1980s housing boom was, however, to end swiftly and dramatically. The end of the 1980s brought with it economic recession and as inflation began to rise the government's solution was to raise interest rates in order to slow down the economy. This recession brought with it numerous problems for the newly created 'mass' housing market. First, unemployment rose rapidly in the months and years of the late 1980s–early 1990s recession and in precisely those areas which had experienced the greatest housing market activity, such that increasing numbers of people who had recently become owner-occupiers could not afford to remain so (Malpass, 1996). Secondly, the recession introduced negative equity to the housing market on a massive scale and left many millions of home-owners unable to sell their homes as house prices fell, and saddled with mortgage debt which had now outstripped the market value of their homes (Malpass, 1996). As the recession continued, mortgage lenders increasingly resorted to litigation and began to repossess homes, a trend which reached an all-time high of over 75,000 repossessions in 1991. Even so, the decade of the 1980s had established, ideologically and politically, home ownership as the most desirable form of housing tenure (Doling, 1993), which,

Table 14.2 Stock of dwellings by tenure, Great Britain, 1981–2002 (millions)

	Owner-occupied	Rented privately	Rented from registered social landlords	Rented from local authority
1981	12.2	2.3	0.5	6.1
1982	12.3	2.3	0.5	6.1
1983	12.7	2.3	0.5	5.9
1984	13.0	2.3	0.5	5.8
1985	13.3	2.3	0.5	5.7
1986	13.7	2.2	0.6	5.7
1987	14.0	2.1	0.6	5.6
1988	14.4	2.1	0.6	5.4
1989	14.8	2.1	0.6	5.2
1990	15.1	2.1	0.6	5.1
1991	15.2	2.2	0.7	5.0
1992	15.3	2.3	0.7	4.9
1993	15.5	2.3	0.8	4.8
1994	15.6	2.4	0.9	4.6
1995	15.8	2.4	1.0	4.5
1996	16.0	2.5	1.1	4.4
1997	16.3	2.5	1.1	4.3
1998	16.5	2.5	1.2	4.1
1999	16.7	2.4	1.3	4.0
2000	17.0	2.4	1.5	3.8
2001	17.2	2.4	1.6	3.6
2002	17.4	2.5	1.7	3.4

Source: Office of the Deputy Prime Minister/National Statistics (2005b) *Housing Statistics*, Table 1.66, pp. 13–14, London: ODPM. Crown copyright material is reproduced with the permission of the Controller of HMSO and the Queen's Printer for Scotland under the terms of the Click-Use Licence.

as we have already witnessed, was encouraged by government policies which enforced the sale of public-owned and rented properties and forced rapid rent increases across the public rental sector. Allied to these policies, deregulation in British financial markets made mortgages, and loans secured against property, increasingly attractive.

By the time New Labour was to be elected into government in 1997, it had recognised and fully accepted the consensus of home ownership as the dominant form of tenure. When elected back into power in May 1997, Labour simply promised to manage the housing market better than the Conservatives by ameliorating the worst of the economic fluctuations affecting the housing market and reducing the boom-bust housing cycle. As we will see shortly in this chapter, Labour's period of office coincided with a further boom in the home ownership housing market.

The private rental sector

The private rental sector, over the course of the twentieth century, was arguably in a state of terminal decline. Governments over the years, particularly in the years after 1945, have promoted either public rented council housing or the private ownership (the property-owning democracy – which in the 1980s became firmly rooted in the popular imagination). Governments have variously sought to revitalise the private rented sector, whether to fill gaps in housing policy which were not met by other sectors or to promote private entrepreneurship and landlordship, or have sought to regulate what they perceived to be a firmly established relationship of exploitation, especially where the sector provided low-income tenancies. Responses to the private rented sector of British housing often depend upon political or ideological presuppositions; that is, whether one views the landlord as the exploiter of frequently poor tenants, or as a hard-working entrepreneur attempting to provide a much-needed service in an over-regulated housing market.

The Conservative government in the 1980s recognised that there would still be a demand for rented accommodation by people perhaps more mobile in their employment. Government therefore sought to develop strategies which would revive the private rental sector by making the development of rental accommodation a more attractive investment. This would involve, in line with the government's market ideology, attempts to deregulate control of the sector, allowing rents to rise in line with 'market' levels rather than the notion of a 'fair rent' which had been introduced in the 1972 Housing Finance Act. Secondly, this process would involve changes in the security of tenure offered to tenants, by allowing greater access of landlords to their property by the introduction of the assured shorthold tenancy. Additionally new landlords would be encouraged to enter the sector.

Despite this, there was little impact in terms of increasing the available rented stock, as Figure 14.2 and Table 14.2 illustrate, and the number of rental units available in the private sector changed little over the 10 years between 1984 and 1993 (and, indeed, since then). As a percentage of total available stock, the private rented sector continued to decline and, while housing association lets increased, this had not been enough to replace those units lost in the process of council house sales and the overall quantity of rented accommodation also declined.

Homelessness

Much of the 1980s and 1990s was characterised by what has been termed an affordability crisis in British housing (Bramley, 1994). Policies aimed at widening the base of home ownership, such as council house sales and financial deregulation, had been largely successful, but arguably at a price. The stock of affordable rented accommodation continued to decline, and the low-rent sector developed into low-quality housing for the poorest of tenants. Councils were left with stock which proved the most difficult to maintain successfully in a climate of continued financial restrictions. Housing associations were unable to fill the gap left in the provision of social housing. Similarly, as we have seen above, private landlords did not significantly expand provision as the government had hoped in the early part of the 1990s. Against this background we must now turn to what was one of the hallmarks of the housing scene in the 1980s and early 1990s (and has continued to be a persistent challenge for housing policy) – the rise in homelessness, and most visibly youth homelessness.

The rise in the homeless can be identified in a number of related areas. The economic downturn of the 1980s, as we have noted, severely curtailed the revolution in home ownership of the early years of that decade. Unemployment led to a rapid rise in mortgage arrears and ultimately repossessions. Dwindling stocks of low-rent accommodation, paralleled by rising rents in that sector, took rented accommodation beyond the reach of many poorer families. Most importantly, perhaps, changes in benefit regulations for young people virtually ended the possibility of young people obtaining rented accommodation until they reached their mid-twenties. The situation was exacerbated because single people were no longer regarded as a priority by local authorities when accepting claims for help.

These individuals also represented a demographic change in Britain as we entered a period in which more young people were entering the housing market and the desire for living singly continued to increase as people chose to marry later in life. Unemployment together with lack of access to cheap, low-quality accommodation and benefit reductions continued therefore to contribute to increasing numbers of homeless individuals in the Thatcher and Major periods of office (Bramley, 1994) and persisted under New Labour (as the newspaper story at the beginning of this chapter on the television broadcaster, Ed Mitchell, demonstrates). It is probably fair to say that by the end of the Conservative government's term of office in 1997, housing had become a key social policy issue not least in terms of affordable home ownership, an adequate supply of good quality social housing, and the persistent incidence of homelessness.

New Labour's housing policy

By the time, therefore, that Labour was elected back into government in May 1997, it was faced with a number of housing policy challenges, not least:

- what to do about a private housing market which had resulted in negative equity and significant levels of repossessions for some individuals and families;
- how to respond to the lack of supply of private housing and an associated increasing unaffordability for significant sections of the population unable to enter the housing market;
- a residual local authority housing sector that had divested itself of its better properties via the right-to-buy and stock transfer schemes;
- a private rented sector that remained a significant but proportionally small part of the housing scene;
- the persistent problem of homelessness.

Labour's housing policy has developed fitfully during its time in office as a response to these problems, with relatively little policy development in its first term (1997–2001) but from 2000 onwards becoming more active. As with other parts of New Labour's social policy, its housing policy has been based on an acceptance of the market, an advocacy of choice and an evocation of duty.

It is perhaps unsurprising that despite the policy challenges it faced on election in 1997 and thereafter, New Labour's housing policy has been fairly continuous with the preceding approach of the New Right governments of Margaret Thatcher and John Major, in as much as it has been possible to discern a thought-through housing policy under New Labour (Lund, 2006; Stephens and Quilgars, 2006). There was little mention of housing in its election manifesto in 1997 or in initial policy documents on returning to government (Mullins and Murie, 2006; Murie, 2007). However, since 2000 Labour has focused on housing to a greater extent. This could be seen initially by the publication of its first Housing Green Paper *Quality and Choice – A Decent Home for All* (Department of the Environment, Transport and the Regions, 2000) since its election in 1997, which concerned itself with the quality of housing and the promotion of choice. Subsequent policy initiatives have included the Treasury-commissioned Barker Report (Barker, 2004) on the supply of housing, and the more recent government-commissioned Hills review of the role of social housing (Hills, 2007) as well as the 2007 Housing Green Paper *Homes for the Future: More Affordable, More Sustainable* (Department for Communities and Local Government, 2007). In addition, Gordon Brown's statements on taking office as Prime Minister (Summers, 2007) – see Box 14.2 – suggest a more active housing policy being pursued latterly by the Labour government. As such, Labour's housing policy has developed in terms of:

- the promotion of non-local authority social housing and the continued residualisation of council housing during its first two terms of office;
- its promotion of home ownership and an associated drive to increase the supply of housing, including affordable housing;
- the support of the private rented sector;
- policy initiatives to support provision for homeless and other vulnerable individuals and groups.

Box 14.2 | **Gordon Brown's homes pledge**

Brown outlines legislative programme

Deborah Summers, *The Guardian,* Wednesday 11 July 2007

Gordon Brown today pledged to build 3 million new houses by 2020 ... . Unveiling a blueprint for his first year in power, the Prime Minister put housing at the top of the political agenda as he announced plans for three new bills to tackle the shortage of affordable homes. Announcing new laws to overhaul the planning system and to encourage local authorities to provide more affordable housing, Mr Brown demanded a 25% increase in the number of new homes being built over the next 13 years, bring the total to 3 million by 2020.

Reprinted with permission.

For writers such as Lund (2006) and Malpass and Cairncross (2006), Labour's approach prefaces a new phase. Historically, British housing policy had been concerned with public health, then adequate housing supply, followed by state control over production and consumption, and then the Conservatives' belief in the market solutions in the 1980s and 1990s. Labour's approach has been described by Lund (2006: 222) as 'characterized by a recognition that an ample housing supply is vital ... and hence a state requirement to ensure that supply is more responsive to demand; consensus on the virtues of home ownership; the selective use of state resources to supply the infrastructure for sustainable housing both in low-demand and high-demand areas; promoting social inclusion', whether that be in relation to homelessness or anti-social behaviour. This section of the chapter will now explore

Labour's evolving and emerging housing policy in relation to public housing, home ownership, the private rental sector, homelessness and other vulnerable households.

Public housing under New Labour

Labour's approach to public or social housing has been to focus initially on the quality of public housing stock, on providing tenant choice, and on housing associations as the preferred vehicle for new-build and the on-going management of social housing stock. Its 2000 Housing Green Paper (Department of the Environment, Transport and the Regions, 2000) concentrated on the poor quality of social housing, particularly council housing stock. Here it acknowledged the underinvestment in social housing and, as a consequence, its unpopularity. New Labour therefore chose to concentrate on improving the quality of the stock and providing greater opportunities for choice for social housing tenants. Regarding housing stock quality, it set a target that by 2010 all social housing would have to meet a 'decent homes' standard, a stiff target when one considers that in 2001 43% of council housing could not meet the decent homes standard. In the 2007 Housing Green Paper *Homes for the Future* the government adjusted the target to 95% of homes meeting the decent homes standard by 2010 (Department for Communities and Local Government, 2007). In 2000, it had estimated that there was a catalogue of outstanding repairs and underinvestment to the value of some £10 billion. Many local authorities judged that the government was reluctant simply to provide the funding to facilitate improvements, and so local government looked for other sources of funding. As such, local authorities had three main options open to them. First, they could transfer their housing stock ('stock transfer') to a registered social landlord (RSL) such as a housing association which could then borrow money commercially. Second, under the Private Finance Initiative, a local authority could enter into an agreement with a private company whereby that company provides capital funding in return for a contract to manage the housing stock for a considerable period, typically 25 years. Third, local authorities could set up Arms Length Management Organisations (ALMOs) that would manage their housing stock and, in so doing, be permitted to borrow additional funds. Of these three options, only stock transfer (a policy initially introduced by the Conservative government, as we have seen earlier in this chapter) manifested itself to any significant extent and it is this option that the Labour government has continued to pursue enthusiastically (Daly *et al.*, 2005). In its 2000 Housing Green Paper, the government argued for significant levels of stock transfer, aiming for 'the transfer of up to 200,000 homes each year from local authorities to registered landlords' (Department of the Environment, Transport and the Regions, 2000: 11). This was to be the main means by which local authorities could lever in housing investment, that is private (and, therefore, 'off balance sheet') funding.

Some local authorities, trades unions and tenants' groups (not least the Defend Council Housing pressure group) continued to press (unsuccessfully) for a 'fourth option' – whereby local authorities would be allowed to borrow funds directly themselves and be provided with Treasury assistance in paying off outstanding debts. However, the government continued to resist these demands even when they were expressed repeatedly by members of the Labour Party at the annual Labour

Party Conference. In part this was because of the government's desire to restructure the governance of public housing. As such, New Labour can be seen to be as antipathetic as the previous Conservative governments to local authorities as significant suppliers of social housing. Stock transfer has, therefore, been used not only as a mechanism to lever in private finance but also as a means by which local authorities are increasingly being regarded no longer as direct providers but instead as strategic enablers of the provision of housing in their areas.

Stock transfer has therefore continued steadily since transfers began in earnest in the mid-1980s under the Conservatives. However, by the mid-2000s, more than half of council housing stock remained with local authorities (Malpass and Cairncross, 2006), though the number of transfers grew significantly after the election of New Labour in 1997 and particularly since 2000. As one can see from Figure 14.1 and Table 14.1, stock transfer ('large scale voluntary transfer') rose significantly in the years 2000–02, averaging out at over 100,000 properties per year – though this was considerably fewer properties than the 200,000 per year aimed for by the government. Where stock transfer has occurred, it has frequently been transferred to, and therefore created, an expansion in housing association provision.

Housing associations have also continued to be the preferred source of new-build and management arrangement for public housing under Labour (Murie, 2007). Housing associations have seen their provision increase – from 1,147,000 units in 1997 (4.6% of all housing stock in the UK) to 2,001,000 (7.7% of housing stock) in 2004 (Office of the Deputy Prime Minister, 2005b). As we have seen above, this is partly through stock transfer but it is also due to housing associations being encouraged by government to build new stock. Housing associations have seen significant numbers of new-build completions each year during Labour's rule since 1997, with 28,554 new-build completions in its first year of office (1997/98) and 22,682 more recently (2004/05). And yet, neither of these years compare favourably with the numbers of new-build completions under the previous Conservative government which, for example, saw 30,951 completions in its last year of government (1996/97) (Office of the Deputy Prime Minister, 2005b). Nor are such completion rates adequate by the Labour government's own target, which states that there needs to be an increase of new-builds of 17,000 per year, a virtual doubling of current rates (Malpass, 2005). New Labour recognised in its 2007 Housing Green Paper *Homes for the Future* (Department for Communities and Local Government, 2007) the need to increase the amount of social housing new-builds. Indeed, it set itself and the social housing sector significant targets for social housing new-builds – with a target of at least 45,000 new social homes a year by 2010–11, a more than doubling of new stock when compared with 2004–05.

Labour's social housing policy has also striven to promote 'choice' for public housing tenants. It has sought to do this via three main policy reforms: 'choice-based lettings', 'market-based rents', and reforms to housing benefit. Choice-based lettings (CBLs) is a scheme that the Labour government expected all local authority housing providers to have adopted by 2010. Traditionally social housing has been allocated broadly according to need, with applicants typically being awarded points depending on their circumstances. For example, homeless applicants have been treated as some of the neediest applicants. Other criteria have included the awarding of points for the length of time an applicant had been on the waiting list, for how many children they had, whether they were living in an overcrowded situation, and so forth. Once an applicant had enough points they would be offered a suitable property when one became available. Labour housing policy has endeavoured to move to a situation where applicants are consumers who will be offered a choice of properties. Therefore, under CBLs housing vacancies are to be advertised such that would-be tenants could apply for a property that they would like. However, critics of this quasi-market, consumerist approach argue that it would not necessarily result in a demand for properties in less popular areas, whereas in popular areas and for popular types of property demand will remain greater than supply. Therefore, what would happen is that instead of properties being allocated according to need, they would be allocated to those applicants wiling to wait the longest (Stephens and Quilgars, 2006).

Stop and Think

- How do you think social housing should be allocated?

- If you were to design a points system to assist in allocating social housing, what would your categories be for allocating points and which categories or criteria would have the most points set against them?

Market-based rents is the second facet of Labour's choice agenda in social housing policy. As part of its 2000 Green Paper (Department of the Environment, Transport and the Regions, 2000), the Labour government proposed to restructure social housing rents. Unlike the previous Conservative government, Labour did not propose that social housing rents be set at the same levels as the market would charge. However, the government believed that rents should reflect more closely the size, quality and location of homes, taking account of local property values so that tenants would pay a comparable rent for a comparable property. However, property values would not be the only consideration such that rent calculations could take account of other factors, such as regional earnings and running costs. Paraphrasing the government's own words, it was proposed that social housing rents should be both 'affordable and fair'.

The third aspect of the Labour government's housing policy choice agenda has been their proposals to reform housing benefit with the intention that it reflects the rent that a household would typically have to pay in a particular region, in much the same way that market rents (explored above) would take account of context. In this way, it was intended that recipients of housing benefit could make choices about their housing costs, for example whether they wished to add to their housing benefit in order to access more expensive housing or, instead, to rent something cheaper and to retain the difference in cost to spend on other priorities. This initiative fits in with the Labour government's advocacy of welfare choice (White and Wintour, 2005) since the government believes that tenants would be able to choose the quantity and quality of their housing (Stephens and Quilgars, 2006). However, there are certainly two potential weaknesses with the policy. First, it assumes that social housing consumers have surplus income which they can use to supplement their housing benefit if they want to consume more housing, arguably an unlikely scenario particularly for citizens in receipt of benefits. Second, the policy assumes that there is a sufficient supply of social (and/or privately rented) housing at a variety of prices and of various stock types from which housing consumers can choose. Neither of these – surplus income or adequate supply – would seem to be in place. This second matter, that of housing supply, also relates to the next area of the Labour government's housing policy, home ownership, to which we now turn.

Home ownership under New Labour

New Labour, on entering office, continued with the previous Conservative government's commitment to promoting home ownership as the main type of housing tenure. It confirmed this commitment in both its 2000 Housing Green Paper (Department of the Environment, Transport and the Regions, 2000) and again in its 2007 Green Paper (Department for Communities and Local Government, 2007 where it declared its intent to increase home ownership to some 75% of households). According to *Social Trends* (Office for National Statistics, 2005a), by the end of New Labour's second term, that is 'in 2003/04, 70% of dwellings (18 million) in Great Britain were owner-occupied. This was an increase of 45% from 12 million in 1981' (see Figure 14.3). But as the bar chart in Figure 14.3 also shows, 'Tenure ... varies regionally. In 2003/04 owner-occupation was highest in the South East, East

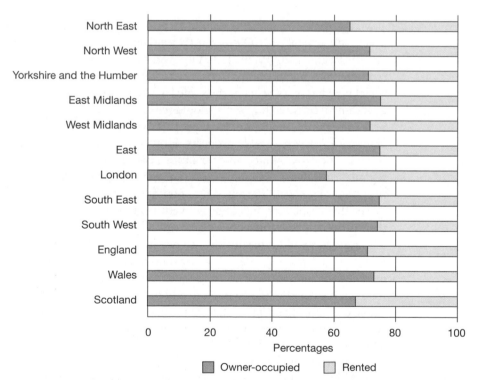

Figure 14.3   Housing stock in 2003 by region and tenure: 70% of dwellings in Great Britain are owner-occupied

Source: Adapted from National Statistics website, http://www.statistics.gov.uk/cci/nugget.asp?id=1105 (last accessed 6 February 2008). Crown copyright material is reproduced with the permission of the Controller of HMSO and the Queen's Printer for Scotland under the terms of the Click-Use Licence.

Stop and Think

What do you think are some of the reasons for the regional differences in levels of home ownership across Great Britain (i.e. England, Scotland and Wales)?

Midlands and East (75%) and lowest in London (58%) and Scotland (67%) ....'
(*Social Trends*, Office for National Statistics, 2005a).

In its first term of office, the Labour government concerned itself mostly with ensuring that home owners did not suffer from the high interest rates which had jeopardised mortgage repayments for many home-owners during the latter part of the previous Conservative years of government. Early into its first term, New Labour hived off responsibility for determining interest rates to the Bank of England Monetary Policy Committee (MPC). Meanwhile, the Treasury saw its role as being to ensure low inflation and economic growth and stability to ensure that low interest rates would not be threatened. However, the low interest rates perversely assisted a boom in house prices, whereby the average house price increased from £70,000 in 1997 to £195,000 in 2007 (Collinson, 2007). Within these increases were significant regional differences, such that the increases in the south-east particularly in London (see Box 14.3), were more marked than in the Midlands and the North.

Box 14.3   Crisis warning over house prices

Rocketing house prices in London are creating a social housing crisis, the Housing Federation has warned. Its report showed first-time buyers need to earn more than £100,000 a year to buy an average priced home – of £318,000 – in 25% of London's boroughs.

But it said an estimated 330,000 families were registered on waiting lists for social housing in the city. According to the Federation this has grown by 57% in five years with the highest levels in Newham, east London. The report, *Home Truths London: The real cost of housing 2007–2012*, showed there were almost 30,000 households on the waiting list for Newham last year.

Top five boroughs
Newham – 29,574
Haringey – 24,939
Lewisham – 17,535
Barnet – 16,470
Brent – 16,398

In the same period the waiting list in Barking and Dagenham, east London, showed the biggest increase, rising 250% to 7,689 households.

Only in three boroughs – Enfield, Merton and Westminster – did the numbers waiting for an affordable home decrease, figures revealed.

Olivia Powis, of the London Housing Federation, said: 'Despite fears of a drop in the market, house prices remain beyond the reach of many Londoners and the capital faces nothing short of a social crisis .... We must tackle the housing crisis head on to halt this growing social divide.'

Source: BBC News (27.11.2007).

Stop and Think

- Why do you think London and the south-east has experienced higher house prices increases than other parts of the UK?

- Do you think this is inevitable?

- What, if anything, should government do to tackle the problems of lack of affordability in the private sector and lack of supply in the social housing sector?

In addition, house price increases have also meant both a reduction in the numbers of first-time buyers and an increase in the average age of first-time buyers, indicating increased difficulty for young people in particular to enter the housing market (Murie, 2007). The government hoped that the increase in demand for home owner-ship would lead to a corresponding increase in supply by the house-building industry, but this has not materialised sufficiently to stabilise house prices or cope with demand and need. It was in part the dislocation between demand and supply and associated house price inflation that led the Treasury to establish the Barker Review into housing supply. The Barker Review (Barker, 2004) concluded that the lack of supply of new homes was a major cause of high house prices, that the demand for housing was outstripping supply and, as a consequence, that this was driving UK house prices ever higher. The lack of supply was due, in part, to fewer homes being built in Britain in 2003/04 than at any time since the 1920s (see Figure 14.4).

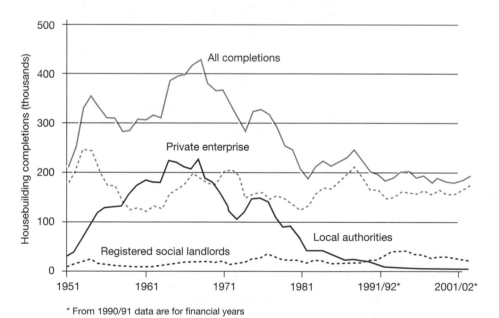

* From 1990/91 data are for financial years

Figure 14.4 UK housebuilding completions by sector, 1951–2003/04
Source: Adapted from Office for National Statistics (2005a) *Social Trends No. 35*, Figure 10.3, London: ONS. Crown copyright material is reproduced with the permission of the Controller of HMSO and the Queen's Printer for Scotland under the terms of the Click-Use Licence. *Original sources*: Office of the Deputy Prime Minister; National Assembly for Wales; Scottish Executive; Department of the Environment, Northern Ireland.

The other main reason for the mismatch between supply and demand in housing provision is the impact of the demographic changes in the number and types of households. For example, in 1991 there were just over 19 million households in England (of which 11.7 million were married couples or co-habitees, 1 million were lone parent and 5.1 million were one person households) whereas in 2006 it was estimated that there were likely to be nearly 22 million households (of which 11.8 million were married couples or co-habitees, 1.3 million were lone parent and 8.5 million were one-person households). The overall number of households in England is estimated to increase by a further 1 million by 2016 (Office of the Deputy Prime Minister, 2005a). As a consequence, the Barker Review recommended that Britain needed to build up to 140,000 extra new homes a year in order for housing supply to match demand. The government's response to the Barker Report was to commit itself to an even more exacting target of 200,000 new properties per year over a 10-year period, that is 2 million new homes by 2016 and 3 million by 2020, mostly provided by the private sector (Office of the Deputy Prime Minister, 2003, 2005a; Department for Communities and Local Government, 2007).

As well as attempting to attend to the supply of homes, the government also attempted to address the problems of home-ownership affordability. It established and extended its HomeBuy scheme which is designed to allow key workers in the public sector, along with social housing tenants and others, to gain access to owner-occupation via part-ownership schemes where participants are able to buy up to 75% of a property's value, with the government taking up the remaining commitment. However, whether this helps tackle problems of affordability is debatable, as an (unintended) consequence is that it may simply facilitate even greater house price inflation.

The private rental sector

The private rental sector has continued to remain static as a proportion of housing tenure, remaining fairly constant at 10–11% of overall housing provision while Labour has been in government (Office of the Deputy Prime Minister, 2005a; Lund, 2006; Murie, 2007). However, the Labour government has tried to promote the private rental sector. It saw the private rental sector as being a key provider for those individuals not wanting, or not able, to enter owner-occupation. The private rental sector is seen by the government as accessible and flexible housing provision, particularly attractive to younger people (Department for Communities and Local Government, 2007). As such, the government has distanced itself from the Labour Party's previous antipathy to this part of the housing sector. In so doing, the government attempted to assure private landlords that it did not intend to make any changes to the structure of assured tenancies or assured shorthold tenancies (terminated after six months) and it would not reintroduce rent controls. This Labour government therefore saw the private rental sector as an integral part of housing provision.

What one has seen during Labour's period of office is an increase in the numbers of 'buy-to-let' providers. According to Lund (2006), in the period from 1998 to 2004 there was an 18-fold increase in the number of mortgage loans on buy-to-let properties, with approximately half a million outstanding loans in 2004. This was partly as a result of low interest rates as well as due to the availability of 100% mortgages, which made it easier for more people to buy up properties in order to rent out. (This does, consequently, act as a further pressure on supply and helps fuel house price inflation.) Indeed, an aspect peculiar to British housing provision is its reliance on small-scale landlords (Stephens and Quilgars, 2006). Rather than large-scale business conglomerates being the financiers and managers of private rental stock, much is owned and managed by individual landlords who own a few properties, the median average of properties owned by a landlord being four in number (Lund, 2006). This makes the sector liable to volatility and means that the individual tenant may normally be likely to enter into only short-term tenancies.

Many of the issues traditionally associated with the private rented sector persist, whether that is in terms of rent levels, the demographic spread of tenants, length of tenancies, or the quality of rental property (Office of the Deputy Prime Minister, 2005a; Lund, 2006). Firstly, rents are significantly higher than in the social housing sector – the average rent in 2004/05 in the private rented sector being £523 per month as against an average social housing rent of £293 per month and an average council tenant rent of £255 per month (Office of the Deputy Prime Minister, 2005b). Secondly, unlike in the social housing sector, a significant majority of tenants continue to be employed and are often young professionals. Thirdly, private tenants tend to rent a property for a relatively short period of time, that is less than a year. Finally, the quality of the private rented sector continues to be below that of the other housing sectors when measured against the Labour government's 'decent homes standard' – with 17% of private rented stock falling below the standard as compared to 8% of owner-occupied stock, 9% of local authority stock and 5% of housing association properties. Accordingly, the private rental sector is not without its issues and arguably remains a marginal, though significant, part of housing provision.

Homeless and other vulnerable individuals and households

In exploring Labour's housing policy in relation to homelessness, the first thing to note is that any examination of statistics on homelessness is problematic not least because of the difficulties of definition. The definition of homelessness has been liable to change with the passing of new legislation. For example, in the 1977 Housing (Homeless Persons) Act a homeless person was someone who did not have a legal right to occupy a dwelling. The Act then went further by distinguishing between those who were and were not intentionally homeless as well as those in priority need. The 1986 Housing and Planning Act widened the definition of homelessness to include those people who are living in unfit accommodation, while the 1996 Housing Act altered things so that local authorities were only obliged to provide temporary accommodation to homeless people. More recently the 2002 Homeless Act expanded the category of priority need to include those leaving care, prison or the armed forces or those who were vulnerable because of domestic violence or the threat of domestic violence. Therefore, attempts to analyse the levels of homelessness are difficult since the definition of homelessness is subject to change.

Even so, two main measures are now typically used to compare changes in the levels of homelessness: first, the number of households judged as unintentionally homeless per year who are in priority need, and second, the numbers of households in temporary accommodation. Using the first set of statistics, the number of households judged to be unintentionally homeless who are in priority need, we have seen the numbers of homeless increase during Labour's rule, and almost return to the numbers experienced in the early 1990s. Therefore, not long after Labour returned to power (that is, 1997/98) the numbers unintentionally homeless in priority need amounted to some 102,400 households. By 2004/05 this had increased to 120,860 (Office of the Deputy Prime Minister, 2005b). The second measure of homelessness, the numbers of households in temporary accommodation, has also seen significant increases year on year since 1997; indeed, there has been a doubling in the numbers during Labour's first two terms of office – from 41,000 in 1997 to 97,000 households in 2004 and, of these, the numbers being accommodated in 'bed and breakfast' accommodation have increased from 4,000 (1997) to 7,000 (2004) (Office of the Deputy Prime Minister, 2005b). However, balanced against these increases in homeless numbers is that the Labour government's more liberal definition of homelessness helps to explain, in part at least, the increase in the numbers of homeless during their time in office; for example, it should be noted that in 2002 the definition of 'unintentionally homeless and in priority need' was extended to include additional priority needs such as young homeless people and people who are homeless who had been 'in care'.

As a response, the Labour government has undertaken a number of initiatives during its time in office to address the problems of homelessness. The 2002 Homelessness Act was an attempt to coordinate provision for homeless people, not least those leaving care, prison, the armed forces or vulnerable because of domestic violence or the threat of domestic violence. Local authorities have been required since 2002 to have in place a homelessness strategy to tackle the problems of homelessness, including proactive preventative measures. It set out to tackle the problem of people sleeping rough and the overuse of bed and breakfast as temporary accommodation. The government's 'Sustainable Communities' plan (Office of the Deputy Prime Minister, 2003) and 'Homes for All' (Office of the Deputy Prime Minister, 2005a) included proposals to reduce homelessness, not least by halving the number of households in insecure temporary accommodation by 2010. As such, the government has provided additional funding to increase the supply of new social housing and to expand preventative services (National Audit Office, 2005). The National Audit Office judged that the Labour government had made good progress in addressing the problems of homelessness. (National Audit Office, 2005)

Since coming to power, New Labour has also focused its housing policy on 'rough sleepers', that is individuals who find themselves sleeping outdoors. In 1998 it was estimated that there were 1,850 rough sleepers in England (National Audit Office, 2005). The government's Social Exclusion Unit (1998) stated that many rough sleepers have had troubled personal backgrounds, such as difficulties with leaving care, the armed forces or prison, or personal difficulties that caused them to leave home. Indeed, the example provided at the start of this chapter of Ed Mitchell's situation illustrates the detrimental impact of such personal difficulties on an individual's housing situation. The government's approach has included providing three sorts of accommodation for rough sleepers: initial hostels and shelters, specialist hostels and shelters to meet particular needs, and more permanent accommodation once an individual is able to manage this. By 2004, in part because of these initiatives, the numbers of rough sleepers in England had reduced to just over 500. Even so, there has been less success in tackling the issue of rough sleepers in London, where half of England's rough sleepers are located. In London, the number of rough sleepers has been reduced by 50% but not by the government's own target of 66%.

One further area of housing policy that it is important to mention is in relation to provision for other 'vulnerable people'. One such policy is the 'Supporting People' initiative which aims to provide support to vulnerable people (older people, people escaping from domestic violence, people with learning difficulties or mental health problems) to continue to live independently in their own homes. According to the government, Supporting People has enabled over 1.2 million people to continue to live independently.

A final area of policy pursued by Labour since returning to power is its approach to dealing with the perceived problem of anti-social behaviour, arguably an area related as much to criminal justice policy as to housing policy. Even so, anti-social behaviour is believed to have a detrimental effect on the reputation of a locality and the desire of people to live there. Labour's housing and wider policy has sought to emphasise the renewal of local environments, for example through its 'New Deal for Communities' neighbourhood renewal initiative and the 'Respect' agenda (Home Office, 2006) rather than solely the repair of housing stock or the demolition of whole estates. The government therefore linked its neighbourhood renewal strategy to that of tackling anti-social behaviour. Managing anti-social behaviour has presented local authorities, the police and the criminal justice system generally with challenges for some considerable time. Even though local authorities have long had powers to evict 'troublesome' tenants, this was often difficult to operationalise as it required statements from witnesses and getting a court conviction. However, in 1998 the Labour government passed the Crime and Disorder Act which included the power for local authorities and the police to place an Anti-Social Behaviour Order (ASBO) on any individual, aged 10 years or more, who was judged in a civil court to be a violent threat. The law was strengthened in 2003 with the Anti-Social Behaviour Act which gave the police and local authorities the powers to disperse individuals from particular neighbourhoods or move them back into a particular area. It also gave RSLs the power to prohibit anti-social behaviour by its tenants, through placing restrictions on the tenancy and removing from the tenant the 'Right to Buy'. However, views on the merits and effectiveness of ASBOs are mixed. On the one hand, some writers suggest that they have improved the quality of life of communities blighted by anti-social behaviour, whilst on the other, ASBOs have also been seen to be part of an anti-civil liberties enforcement agenda (Stephens and Quilgars, 2006) which is actually counter-productive as it is as likely to provide young people on whom an ASBO is placed with local notoriety rather than make them curb their behaviour.

Conclusion

What, then, are we able to conclude from this review of changing housing policy over the last 60 years and, particularly, over the last 30 years? According to Malpass and Cairncross (2006), there has been a rise and then more recently a decline in the prominence of housing policy. We will return to this alleged decline in housing policy shortly. As this chapter has explored, what we have arguably witnessed in Britain over the last 60 years is:

- a fairly constant and persistent increase in the numbers of households year on year, for example an extra one million households in Great Britain from 1997 to 2002;
- a significant increase in the supply of housing, though not sufficient to meet demand (with current government estimates of a need for an extra 200,000 properties per year until 2010);
- an increase in the quality of housing for most people whereby 90% of households could be judged as living in adequate housing as opposed to 80% of households living in either overcrowded, substandard or unfit accommodation in 1951;
- a shift in the patterns of tenure, from a small minority of people living in owner-occupied households (10% in the 1910s) to the vast majority of the population being so housed nowadays (70% in 2005) and its general acceptance by the majority of people as the preferred type of tenure;
- a consensus across all the major political parties in the support of owner-occupation as the main form of tenure;
- an associated shift from local authority rented housing as being the dominant form within the rented sector to one where council housing has decreased from 30% to around 10% of tenures over the last 25 years;
- a corresponding (though not proportionate) increase in social housing being provided by Registered Social Landlords (e.g. housing associations) from just over 2% to 7% of all tenures (over the last 25 years);
- the decline of the private rented sector to a fairly constant 10% of stock over the last 20–30 years.

Therefore, the picture of housing in Britain is somewhat mixed, in which there have been winners and losers. As such, there remains a need for government to have a clear housing policy. Borrowing from Malpass and Cairncross (2006), it is possible to draw the following conclusions:

- Affordability remains a barrier to decent housing for significant sections of the population, particularly in south-east England.
- While some parts of the country experience excessive demand, such as the south-east, other areas and regions – for example, parts of the Midlands and North and South Wales – suffer from insufficient demand.
- Lack of supply remains a key problem, with the government predicting the need for 200,000 new homes per year over the next 10 years, that is an extra 2 million homes by 2016 and an extra 3 million by 2020.
- Social housing remains residualised, as a result of successive governments' lack of adequate investment and support.

- As a consequence, many communities where social housing is dominant or prevalent continue to experience social disadvantage and exclusion.

Therefore, even though the housing problems now experienced by the majority of British citizens are not as acute as they were at the end of the Second World War, it is highly likely that housing policy will need to continue to be an aspect of British social policy and government activity. Governments will continue to be required to attend to the matter of housing as issues of affordability, lack of supply, homelessness and poor quality of provision all continue to persist. Therefore, while housing policy has been described as the wobbly pillar of the British welfare state, it remains an important part of British social policy, a fact recognised rhetorically at least by the current Labour government which has described its more recent policy initiatives as a 'step change in housing policy' (Office of the Deputy Prime Minister, 2005a).

Annotated reading

Perhaps the most useful and enduring overview of British housing policy is the volume by Malpass and Murie (1999), *Housing Policy and Practice*, now in its fifth edition. Also useful is the text by Malpass and Means (1993), *Implementing Housing Policy*. For an account of the decline of (municipal) public sector housing see Cole and Furbey's *The Eclipse of Council Housing* (1994). Books that provide general overviews include those by Brian Lund (2006), *Understanding Housing Policy*, and by Mullins and Murie (2006), *Housing Policy in the UK*. An interesting discussion of the place of housing policy and state involvement in housing provision is provided by Malpass (2003) in his article 'The wobbly pillar? Housing and the British postwar welfare state' in the *Journal of Social Policy*. Indeed, to obtain up-to-date accounts of housing policy developments, it is useful to refer to the general social policy journals such as *Critical Social Policy*, the *Journal of Social Policy and Society*, the *Journal of Public Policy*, The *Journal of Public Administration* and the journal *Social Policy and Administration*. In addition, the more specific academic housing journals such as *Housing Studies* and the *European Journal of Housing Studies* are useful sources, as are other journals such as *Local Economy and Urban Studies*. The 'trade' journal *Inside Housing* provides useful contemporary commentary and analysis of developments in housing policy and practice.

Chapter 15

Education

Objectives

- To outline the developments of state education provision during the first part of the twentieth century.

- To outline the development of education policy during the 'post-war consensus period'.

- To explore how education policy changed under the Conservative administrations of Margaret Thatcher and John Major.

- To examine contemporary education policy since the election of New Labour in 1997 and how this compares with the policies of the New Right.

Introduction

'... *if you think education is expensive, try ignorance. ...*'

Tony Benn

The aim of this chapter, therefore, is to explain the nature of education policy and how it has developed over the twentieth and into the first part of the twenty-first century.

The news report in Box 15.1 highlights how important and emotive issues about education can be in the UK. Parents, particularly, can become very concerned about the education of their children and some will do all that they can to get their children into what they regard as a good state school.

This chapter examines what we understand to be the socio-political developments of education provision in the UK over the last 100 years. In doing this, the chapter explores:

- education policy and provision in the nineteenth century and the first half of the twentieth century;

- the nature of the post-war settlement in terms of education policy;

- the development of education policy and provision under the Conservative governments of Margaret Thatcher and John Major;

- more contemporary education policy under New Labour and how this compares with the policies of the New Right.

Box 15.1	The school place lottery

'War over school boundaries divides Brighton

Council brings in lottery for sought-after places; Parents in old catchment area threaten court action'

Sandra Laville and Rebecca Smithers, *The Guardian*, Thursday 1 March 2007

The middle classes of Brighton are locked in a bitter war involving death threats, espionage and allegations of gerrymandering over whose children have the right to go to the best schools in the city. Two factions of parents have been split by controversial plans to award school places based on a lottery system, confirmed by the town's Labour council. On one side are the parents of 'muesli mountain', families who live in period houses and name their community website the 'caring corner'. On the other are the well heeled of the 'golden halo', couples who have paid up to half a million pounds for homes in the catchment of the two leading secondaries. And on the sidelines, critics say, are the most deprived children of the city, who have been left voiceless and marginalised.

A two-year discussion, involving parents, teachers and city councillors, about the admissions policy of the eight state secondaries in Brighton and Hove culminated on Tuesday night in a narrowly won vote, on the casting hand of the Labour chairman of the children, families and schools committee, to change the system. No longer will parents who live nearest the two most sought after schools – Dorothy Stringer High and Varndean – be guaranteed a place in the high achieving schools. Instead the catchment areas of all eight schools have been redrawn to reflect a better social mix. If schools are oversubscribed there will be a lottery for places.

Reprinted with permission.

Stop and Think

- Was it important to you and your family what school you attended or to which you sent your children? Why was it important?

- Were you able to choose which school to attend? If you were unable to obtain the school you wanted, why was this?

- Presuming you did exercise some choice, what were the reasons for your choosing the school that you did?

Education was seen to be one of the five key tenets of the post-Second World War welfare state settlement in that it was seen to be crucial in tackling one of Beveridge's 'Five Evils' – that of 'ignorance' (see Chapter 3). This chapter explores how free elementary schooling up to the age of 14 had been provided in the UK from the latter part of the nineteenth century. The chapter then maps out how education policy and provision have developed over the last 100 years by looking at education policy and provision before the Second World War, how this changed as part of post-war welfare state settlement, how it developed further with the break-up of this consensus in the 1980s and 1990s, and, contemporaneously, how it is seen by the current government as being key to providing equal opportunities and social justice for all citizens and, at the same time, ensuring the UK is able to compete in the global marketplace by having a suitably knowledgeable and skilled workforce.

Education provision in the nineteenth century

In the nineteenth century education policy developed incrementally, that is in a bit-by-bit manner (see Hill, 2003). During that century Christian elementary schools ('voluntary schools') began to be established. In the 1830s the government started to provide funding assistance, which then led the government to establish a Schools Inspectorate in 1839 in order to monitor the effectiveness of state-funded schooling (see Table 15.1). By the second half of the nineteenth century, society had become concerned with the lack of education of the poorer parts of the population. The concern was largely articulated in two respects. First, with the expansion of indus-trialisation, there was a greater appreciation of the need for an educated workforce. Second, with the widening of the franchise (those eligible to vote in elections), there was a concern that these new voters would not be sufficiently well informed to exercise their vote properly.

Table 15.1 Key education policy dates

1830s	Start of state funding for elementary schooling
1839	Establishment of Schools Inspectorate
1880	Education Act – compulsory education 5–10 years
1890s	Establishment of free elementary schooling
1902	Education Act – local councils take over responsibility for education from local school boards and permitted expenditure on secondary and tertiary education
1900s	Free school meals and schools medical service
1918	Free state education up to 14 years of age
1944	Education Act – universal free state education and proposed tripartite secondary education system (grammar, technical and secondary modern)
1950s	Introduction of comprehensive schools
1963	Robbins Committee – expansion of higher education provision
1973	Raising of school leaving age to 16 years
1976	Legislation (under the Labour government) to abolish grammar schools; repealed in 1980 (under the Conservatives)
1980	Education Act – expansion of parental choice in secondary schools, e.g. state funding to attend private schools; repeal of legislation to abolish grammar schools
1988	Education Reform Act – introduction of national curriculum and testing at ages 7, 11, 14 and 16 years; establishment of local management of schools and the option for independence through the establishment of grant maintained schools
1988 and 1992	Further and Higher Education Reform Act and Further and Higher Education Act – polytechnics and further education colleges given independence from LEAs
1990	Education (Student Loans) Act – higher education students allowed to take out loans to support their maintenance
1997	Excellence in Schools – NLS and NNS launched
2001	White Paper: 'Schools Achieving Success'
2003	Higher Education White Paper 'The Future of Higher Education' – higher education participation rate target of 50%, funded by top-up fees
2006	Education and Inspections Act – proposed expansion of city academies and the option for schools to apply for trust status
2007	Education and Skills Bill proposes to raise school leaving age to 18 years

Education provision pre-war

The period from the last quarter of the nineteenth century to the end of the First World War in 1918 was a period in which state education provision for most people meant free 'elementary' schooling up until 14 years of age (see Hill, 2003). Those that went on to school for the most part had to pay school fees unless they were very fortunate to be awarded a scholarship. The picture of provision was a confusing one, with a mixture of state-provided and 'voluntary assisted' (usually 'church') schools. Therefore the majority of the population during this period received an elementary education based around the 'three Rs' of reading, writing and arithmetic. The teaching was provided along what many of us would now consider to be very traditional lines in which pupils were instructed to 'rote learn'. The teaching methods of today, where school children learn via 'child-centred' (pedagogical) and focused classes, often in 'ability sets', are very different from the approaches of the latter parts of the nineteenth century and first half of the twentieth century.

Attempts were made after the First World War (1914–18) to extend state schooling up to the age of 16, but cuts in public expenditure in the early 1920s and then the recession and depression of the 1930s blocked this from happening. Therefore, whilst a small proportion of working-class children might have been fortunate enough to win a scholarship to enable them to progress onto post-elementary education with their middle-class peers, it was not until after the Second World War that secondary education for all (let alone the possibility of a university education) became a reality.

The post-war education settlement and period of consensus

During the Second World War, the coalition government did set about planning the reform of education provision (see Timmins, 1995). The (Conservative) Minister of Education, R. A. (RAB) Butler, was responsible for overseeing the development of policy that would result in the 1944 Education Act which set out the structures for education in the post-war period. Central government would oversee primary and secondary education in that the Treasury would provide a significant proportion of the funding and the Ministry of Education would provide the policy lead. Local councils, via the local education authorities (LEAs), would manage provision locally in that they would be responsible for strategic oversight of educational provision in their areas. In addition, the LEAs would be responsible for actually managing the schools at primary (5–11 years of age), secondary (11–16 or 18 years) and tertiary (16 years upwards) levels. At the time of the 1944 Act, LEAs had no responsibility for higher education (universities and polytechnics) but would have for a limited period with the establishment of the polytechnics in the 1960s. The 1960s also saw an expansion of university higher education provision as a result of the proposals within the Robbins Committee report. The significant changes in the 1970s were the legislating for the raising of the school leaving age to 16 years and, under the Labour government at the time, the abolition of selective grammar schools. However, the period between the 1944 Education Act and the election of the 1979 Conservative government has generally been regarded as a period of political consensus and education policy consolidation (see Chapter 3). However, as with other social policy changes, the election of Margaret Thatcher's Conservative government arguably witnessed the coming to the end of that period of policy and political consensus (see Chapter 4).

During the period of 'post-war consensus', the main point of difference between the Conservative and Labour governments from 1945 to 1979 was arguably over selective grammar schools (see Sullivan, 1996). Labour increasingly saw the existence of grammar schools as being inequitable and divisive and, therefore, promoted comprehensive schools for all state-funded secondary school pupils. Initially the move away from selection to comprehensive schooling was on a voluntary basis for each LEA and local authority. However, in the 1976 Act, under the Labour government of the 1970s, funding of grammar schools was restricted, thus forcing many of them to close, convert to comprehensive schools or move into the private sector. The private sector (that is, 'public schools') had not been affected in any significant way by any government during the post-war period, though it had seen the numbers of children it educated as a proportion of all children fall from over 10% in 1947 to around 6% by the beginning of the 1980s (Glennerster and Low, 1991).

An area of consensus was the desire to expand higher education (university) provision during the post-war period. By the 1960s the proportion of school leavers entering higher education in the 1940s had remained relatively small at 6%, with the vast majority (80%) coming from middle and upper class families (Scott, 2002). The Conservative government of the early 1960s established the Robbins Committee (Robbins, 1963) to review higher education provision and, when it reported in 1963, it recommended the doubling of higher education participation. Partly as a response to this, the then Wilson Labour government of the mid- to late 1960s established the vocationally and technically focused polytechnics, controlled by local authorities. Harold Wilson's ambition was for a country that led in the fields of technology and innovation, driven by a highly educated workforce (see Pimlott, 1993). Related to this, Wilson also encouraged the establishment of the Open University (OU) in the 1960s. Indeed, it has been said that he regarded the establishment of the Open University as one of his greatest achievements. The Open University provided distance-learning higher education for adult learners who had not had the opportunity to gain a university education in their earlier years. OU students typically studied for their awards independently at home, supported by tutors and the necessary learning materials, including via television and radio broadcasts.

While the 1944-1979 period of education policy was arguably a consensual one in the main, not least in terms of a belief in free state schooling through to secondary level and a belief in expanding higher education opportunities (and notwithstanding the party political divergence over secondary selection), by the end of the 1970s the political consensus had focused around a belief that UK state education was not producing a sufficiently skilled workforce that was able to compete with its economic competitors. The Labour Prime Minister at the time, Jim Callaghan, encapsulated these concerns over illiterate and innumerate school leavers in his 1978 Ruskin speech. In this speech, Callaghan suggested that the education system was not equipping school leavers with the education and training needed in order to take up the jobs needed in the modern age (see Riley, 1998). In some respects,

Callaghan's articulation of concerns over standards foreshadowed the discourse of the incoming Conservative government of Margaret Thatcher in 1979.

Education during the period of the New Right

When Margaret Thatcher returned the Conservative Party government in 1979, their concern for education focused around standards, choice and the empowerment of parents. Thatcher and her government, informed by the arguments put forward by New Right thinkers in the Black Papers (Cox and Boyson, 1975; see Chitty, 1989), thought that education policy and provision had been taken over by teachers and local authorities, with both groups pursuing their own 'progressive' agendas at the expense of sound, basic, essential education which every child needed and the country as a whole required if it was to have an appropriately educated workforce able to meet the challenges of competitive markets in the late twentieth century. The New Right government believed that control over education policy and provision, therefore, needed to be wrestled out of the hands of the teaching profession and its powerful trades unions (for example, the National Union of Teachers and the National Association of Schoolmasters and Union of Women Teachers) and left-leaning local authorities preoccupied with equality and political correctness. The Conservatives wanted a return to the days of the 'three Rs' (reading, writing and arithmetic) and the grammar school and to create a climate where parents and schools were empowered and local authorities' influence reigned back (Glennerster and Low, 1991).

Similarly to other aspects of its social policy agenda (Levin, 1997), significant policy change did not occur immediately. Indeed, the first two terms of Thatcher's Conservative government were most noteworthy for the level of expenditure cuts in education (Glennerster and Low, 1991). Indeed, it was not until the 1988 Education Reform Act (ERA) that we saw significant developments, most of which still remain (for example, the National Curriculum, testing, league tables, local management of schools, inspection). However, quite early on, Thatcher's government did legislate to allow for an element of 'parental choice' with the 1980 Education Act, in that parents of 'bright children' could opt to apply for their children to be educated in the private sector under the 'Assisted Places Scheme'. In addition, local authorities lost the power to determine the catchment areas of their schools, which had up until then allowed LEAs to determine which children would attend which schools. This was to be replaced by a 'quasi-market' system (see Chapter 6) whereby a parent could apply for their child to attend a school of their choice irrespective of whether or not it was their local school.

Stop and Think

- Do you think the state, that is public money, should be used to pay for 'bright' children from poorer backgrounds to attend private schools?

- Do you think children should attend their local school or the one that they and their parents choose for them?

In reality, selection was now determined by how near or far a child lived from a school. However, what it did mean was that 'good' schools became over-subscribed and 'poorer' schools had to try to improve to ensure that they did not wither away due to falling rolls (numbers of pupils enrolled at the school). In reality, those parents able to do so would move house to be near to a popular school, while those unable to move would have to make do with what was locally available. This continues to be an issue (see later discussion over school selection). Another policy change was in relation to the governance of schools. Prior to the Conservatives returning to power nationally in 1979, school governing bodies typically comprised a majority of LEA appointed governors (that is, local political appointees). The exception to this was the church schools whose governing bodies were made up for the most part of church appointees. The Conservatives altered the balance by increasing the number of parent and staff governors such that no one constituent part had a majority on the school governing body.

The 1988 Education Reform Act and the reform of schools

As mentioned above, the key piece of legislation during the 1980s affecting schools was the 1988 Education Reform Act (ERA), under the leadership of the then Secretary of State for Education, Kenneth Baker (Fergusson, 1994). The ERA was significant in six main respects:

- the promotion of Grant Maintained Status (GMS) schools;
- the establishment of Local Management of Schools (LMS) for all other schools;
- the establishment of a National Curriculum from the age of five until 16 years of age;
- the requirement for children to sit national tests – Standard Attainment Tests/Targets (SATs) – at Key Stages 1, 2, 3 and 4 (see below);
- the publication of a school's performance in these tests and national examinations (GCSEs and 'A' Levels) in 'league tables';
- regular inspection of schools by Ofsted (the Office for Standards in Education).

Grant Maintained Status (GMS) schools were to be established if and when a majority of the parents in such a school voted to 'opt out' of the local authority's control. The advantages to the school of doing this included the fact that it would then receive its budget directly from the Department for Education and Science rather than via the LEA (which had been able to exercise some discretion over levels of funding across and between its schools). In addition, a GMS school would be locally governed by its governing body and managed more directly by its head-teacher and senior staff. GMS schools would also have powers to borrow money for school developments and powers over pupil entry and selection. Those schools that chose not to 'opt out' were to be given greater budgetary control via LMS (local management of schools). This meant that rather than the LEA deciding on the levels of funding per school, all schools would receive a formula-based budget, that is initially 85% of the LEA's budget for schools would be devolved to its schools on a per capita (the number of pupils per school) calculation. This meant that each primary school in an area would be allocated the same level of funding as the other primary schools, and each secondary school would be allocated the same funding as other secondary schools, as indeed would be the case for the LEA's special schools. LEAs would retain control over capital funding (monies for buildings and other large projects) and LEA-wide services (for example curriculum advisors, school music and library services, educational psychologists, education grants, careers services).

Overall, the government argued that GMS schools and (to a lesser extent) LMS schools enabled the provision of education that parents, pupils and teachers wanted, as compared with the perceived interference by local authorities. The government hoped that GMS and/or LMS would facilitate the creation of a 'quasi-market' in primary and secondary education. Schools would have greater control over how to run their affairs. Successful schools would be rewarded by increased numbers of parents wanting to send their children to such schools, while less successful schools would need to work harder in order to attract sufficient pupil numbers to remain viable. In reality, it can be argued that GMS particularly would lead to a greater centralisation of power over education policy and provision, not least when one takes account of the implications of the National Curriculum, SATs and the regular inspection of schools by Ofsted (Glennerster and Low, 1991).

The National Curriculum

The ERA was also presented as an attempt to empower parents. This was to be done by a return to basic educational values – the 'three Rs' – and the establishment of a National Curriculum to which each child would be entitled, irrespective of where they lived and which local authority or LEA might oversee their school. (This did not apply to 'public', that is private, schools.) The National Curriculum was a prescribed set of subjects and content, initially determined by the DES with the responsibility later given over to the National Curriculum Council. Within the National Curriculum the then Secretary of State for Education, their ministers, civil servants and educational advisors could determine what subjects would be taught along with the precise content of each subject. There was to be an emphasis on mathematics, English, science, languages, history and geography, as well as a requirement for daily worship of a 'Christian nature'. In addition, it was proposed that pupils would be tested at four Key Stages:

- Key Stage 1 – for children aged 7 years at the end of their second year of primary school.
- Key Stage 2 – for children aged 11 years at the end of their sixth year of primary school.
- Key Stage 3 – for children aged 14 years at the end of their third year of secondary school.
- Key Stage 4 – for children aged 16 years at the end of their fifth year of secondary school. (The proposals for testing at Key Stage 4 were withdrawn as pupils would normally be taking GCSEs at this point in their schooling.)

The results of schools' SATs at Key Stage 2 were to be published in 'league tables' along with schools' GCSE and 'A' level results. It was argued that this information would help to inform parents of how successful individual schools were. Parents could make comparisons between the local schools in their area. This information, along with the publication of school inspection reports undertaken by Ofsted, would seemingly allow parents to make more informed decisions about the choice of schools they faced. However, the very opposite of this could be argued as resultant from these policy developments, and a distortion of what the aims of publicly provided schooling should be. Instead of empowered parents and empowering education, schools arguably became preoccupied with how their pupils were performing in national tests (SATs, GCSEs and 'A' levels), at the expense of broader educational aims. Interrelated with this, parents became even more concerned about which school to send their children to and whether it was a 'good' school. This, in turn, arguably put pressure on schools to consider whom they should 'select' or encourage to enrol – with some schools moving ostensibly to a selection process if they could, in order to ensure their league table position was not detrimentally affected by future intakes.

Further and higher education reforms under the Conservatives

Further education (FE) was the responsibility of LEAs when the Conservatives returned to power in 1979. FE colleges were responsible for providing 'post-16' technical and vocational education and training for young people wishing to pursue vocational careers. In addition, FE colleges did provide some academic subject provision at GCSE and A level. In certain parts of the country there were also in existence Sixth Form colleges or Tertiary colleges which generally provided GCSE and A level subjects. All of this provision tended to be under the control of local authority LEAs and this did not change throughout the 1980s. However, in the early 1990s the Conservatives did legislate to remove FE colleges from LEA control with the 1990 Further and Higher Education Reform Act. Prior to that, the New Right had made some policy changes to post-16 education and training. In the early 1980s (which was a period of significant increase in the actual numbers of unemployed, not least youth unemployed) the Youth Opportunities Scheme, later renamed the Youth Training Scheme, was established to provide training for 16–17-year-olds who would otherwise have been unemployed. Indeed, the entitlement to unemployment benefit was removed for young people. The YTS was soon extended to two years, that is 16–18 years. In the mid-1980s, with the 1986 White Paper 'Working together: education and training', National Vocational Qualifications (NVQs) were introduced, with the aim of ensuring that each sector had the skilled workers they required and the country had a skilled workforce more generally. In the late 1980s, Training and Enterprise Councils (TECs) were established to take over from LEAs the responsibility for planning and funding post-16 vocational training – yet another example of LEAs losing education and training responsibilities. The 1992 Further Education and Higher Education Act went even further by making FE colleges independent of LEA control. At the time, many FE senior staff and governors saw this as a liberating change. However, the Act presaged a period of staff cutbacks and poor industrial relations. In addition, staff in adult education provision saw their role being increasingly focused on 'vocational' outputs as opposed to 'education for education's sake'.

Higher ('university') education reform under the New Right was resultant from the 1988 Education Reform Act in that this resulted in the polytechnics gaining independence from the LEAs. However, the 1987 White Paper: 'Higher education: meeting the challenge' did present an increased emphasis on the purpose of higher education being to meet the needs of the economy:

> Meeting the needs of the economy is not the sole purpose of higher education nor can higher education alone achieve what is needed. But this aim, with its implications for the scale and quality of higher education, must be vigorously pursued …. The Government and its central funding agencies will do all they can to encourage and reward approaches to higher education institutions which bring them closer together to the world of business. (Department of Education and Science, 1987)

However, the significant changes occurred with the 1992 Further Education and Higher Education Act (FE&HE Act), whereby the polytechnics were allowed to take on the status and title of 'University' and the CNAA was abolished – with the ex-polytechnics thus being able to award their own academic awards (that is, degrees). A funding body for each of the four countries of the UK was established which allocated funds to higher education universities and colleges. In so doing, these new funding bodies attempted to equalise the funding between the historically better funded old universities and the historically poorer funded ex-polytechnics. Perhaps most significant of all, the FE&HE Act set a target of 30% participation rate for higher education. However, running counter to this policy imperative to increase the numbers of 18-year-olds and mature students participating in higher education, higher education experienced significant expenditure cuts, after previously overseeing a period of growth in student numbers (Sullivan, 1996). (One could regard the two developments as being related: an increase in higher education student numbers necessitated a reduction in the unit of resource if the overall budget for higher education was not to be increased significantly.) The increase in student numbers was to be achieved in part by moving from student maintenance grants to a system of student loans. In 1990 the Education (Student Loans) Act had given the power for students to receive loans rather than grants. In effect the maintenance grant was frozen and from then on any increases in students' entitlement to maintenance would be made up by an interest-free loan. Therefore by the end of the Thatcher–Major governments, one had seen an increase in higher education student numbers and an increase in the participation rate but a relative reduction in the 'unit of resource' (the amount that a university received per student) and an increase in the proportion of funds that students were expected to fund themselves either immediately or in the form of loans.

Evaluating the New Right's reforms of education – a managerialist approach

Overall, as we can see from what has been explored in this section, when one looks back at the Thatcher–Major period of government and its influence on education policy and provision, whether that be in relation to primary and secondary education (with the introduction of the GMS and LMS, the National Curriculum, SATs, inspections, league tables) or in relation to further and higher education where there was an increased emphasis on vocational and technical education, the New Right's agenda for education had been a managerialist one (Fergusson, 1994) (see Chapter 6 for a longer discussion of managerialism). As such, its agenda was one that was wrapped in a discourse focused implicitly or explicitly on:

- the needs of the economy;
- the empowerment of parents through choice;
- the introduction of market and quasi-market arrangements;
- the downplaying of the power and influence of teaching professionals (teachers and lecturers across the primary, secondary, tertiary and higher education sectors) and their trades unions;
- the removal of local authorities from many aspects of education, and the reduction of their role where they continued to have one;
- the associated centralisation of much of education policy and provision;
- the increased 'privatising' of education (that is, emphasising education increasingly as a private concern rather than a public good).

New Labour's approach, 'education, education, education', the number one priority

As most students of contemporary UK social policy are more than aware, when Labour was re-elected into government in 1997, it was in no small part on a platform of promising to renew educational policy and provision. In 1997, the Labour Party Manifesto for that General Election stated that:

> Over the five years of a Labour government ... we will increase the share of national income spent on education .... [As such] we will make education our number one priority. (Labour Party, 1997)

In essence, Labour's first term concentrated on education 'standards not structures' (The Labour Party, 1997). However, it was to be in its second (2001–05) and third (from 2005) terms that it concentrated to a greater extent on systems and structures (types of schools, and so forth).

Back in 1997 Labour promised to cut class sizes to 30 or under for all five-, six- and seven-year-old children; to provide nursery places for all four-year-olds; to tackle low standards in schools; to provide children with access to computer technology; to promote lifelong learning for adults through a new University for Industry; and to increase spending on education overall as the cost of funding benefits to the unemployed fell in line with the fall in the numbers unemployed. This section now goes on to explore Labour's policy developments as they have affected the pre-school, primary, secondary and higher education sectors.

Pre-school provision

New Labour has espoused the importance of pre-school provision for two broad policy imperatives: firstly, as a means of providing children with a satisfactory start in life, and secondly as a mechanism for supporting parents – not least those returning to work. As Dyson *et al.* (2006: 53–54) have observed, New Labour's pre-school provision encompasses:

> ... two ... strands of policy – the creation of a more extensive, coherent and accessible pattern of childcare to release parents for paid work, and the regulation of improvement of children's early learning experience as a means of equipping them with the necessary tools for tackling the school curriculum proper.

As such, New Labour has funded (via nursery vouchers and tax credits) nursery provision for three- and four-year-old children and established the 'Sure Start' programme in socially deprived areas to support pre-school children and their families, established an early years curriculum – the 'curriculum for toddlers' (Dyson *et al.*, 2006), and extended Ofsted's responsibilities to include the inspection of pre-school provision including in the private and voluntary sectors. According to Moss (2000: 70):

> ... policy has become firmly established in areas in which it had [previously] only a toehold, and which were constituted for many years as predominantly private areas, the responsibility of the individual parents or employers. Government has accepted a substantial measure of responsibility ... to actively promote supply and subsidise the costs [of childcare].

Labour's policy intentions have been to combat child poverty and, relatedly, to promote the engagement of women in employment.

While it has been recognised that Labour has at least provided a substantial increase in pre-school provision, it has arguably not radically altered the nature of that provision – rather it has been 'more of the same' (Moss, 2000). For example, unlike in other European countries, pre-school provision is still only part-time and thought of as being up to the age of four rather than full-time and from the first few months of life up until the start of school at six years of age. Alongside this, significant reform of the early years workforce has yet to materialise through, for example, the emergence of a specialist early years professional – the 'pedagogue', who would have the same status and level of training as teachers. Further, the funding of pre-school provision remains a mixed-bag of tax credits alongside publicly and privately funded provision. This in turn continues to result in a mixed economy of provision: child-minders, private nurseries, public sector nurseries, and state school provision in the form of nursery classes and reception classes within primary schools.

Primary education under New Labour

In primary education, New Labour had promised on its return to government to increase the funding for new teachers and other staff, and therefore decrease the average class size, so that no child would be taught in a class with more than 30 pupils. By 2007 it had made significant progress against this target in that, by 2007, 88% of primary school children were being taught in a class of no more than 30 pupils, compared with 72% of children in 1997. This was due in no small part to the fact that during this 10-year period the number of teachers had been increased by 9%. In relation to the primary school curriculum, New Labour introduced a National Literacy Strategy (NLS) and a National Numeracy Strategy (NNS) which very much directed *what* would be taught and *how* it would be taught for both literacy and numeracy in primary schools. By 2007 Labour was claiming that it had achieved the following in relation to primary literacy and numeracy:

- Literacy – 80% of children achieved the standards for their age at Key Stage 2 in 2007 as compared with 75% in 2000 and 54% in 1996.
- Numeracy – 77% of children achieved Level 4 and above in Key Stage 2 in 2007 as compared with 72% in 2000 and 54% in 1996.
- Progress in primary school English and Mathematics was fastest in the most disadvantaged areas of the country. (Crace, 2007; Department for Education and Skills, 2001a, 2001b; McNally and Vaitilingam, 2007)

Indeed, it can be demonstrated that there have been improvements in the achievements of children at the primary level following the introduction of the NLS and NNS. The improvements were most marked in the early years of the introduction of these strategies, whereas more recently there has been a levelling off in the improvement rate (see Figure 15.1).

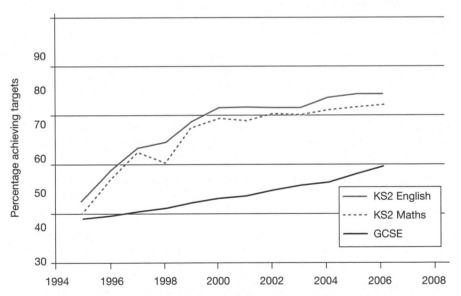

Note: The indicators for Key Stage 2 English and Maths show the percentage of students achieving Level 4 or above. The indicator for GCSE shows the percentage of students achieving five or more A*–C grades.

Figure 15.1 Percentage achieving target at age 11 (Key Stage 2) and age 16 (GCSE)
Source: S. McNally and R. Vaitilingam (2007) *Policy Analysis: Has Labour Delivered on the Policy Priorities of 'Education, Education, Education'? The Evidence on School Standards, Parental Choice and Staying On*, Figure 1, London: Centre for Economic Performance, LSE. Reprinted with permission.

As with any target, the improvements may, in part at least, be due to those being measured altering their behaviour in order to meet the target, in this case through children being increasingly 'coached' by their teachers to perform well in the tests. Indeed, disquiet has been expressed at the appropriateness and robustness of the SATs tests (Tymms, 2004; Statistics Commission, 2005; Curtis, 2007a, 2007b). It has been suggested that the increased improvement from 1995 to 2000 'was a reflection of schools getting better at teaching pupils to take tests' (Curtis, 2007a).

Box 15.2	Testing primary school children

Test results for third of primary students wrong, says study

Polly Curtis, *The Guardian*, 2 November 2007

As many as one in three primary school children is given the wrong marks in national tests, according to a report on standards in primary schools. Sats for seven- and 11-year-olds, which are used to assess their progress and feed into national school league tables, are unreliable, put pupils under psychological pressure and have had little impact, the report says. The researchers accuse the government of ignoring academic evidence, backed by the then Statistics Commission, that the dramatic rises in results in the run-up to 2000 were 'exaggerated'.

The report commissioned for Cambridge University's review of primary education comes after the prime minister pledged to put testing at the heart of the next phase of the government's plan to eradicate failure. Ministers believe that without nationally comparable tests teachers are not able to target pupils who are falling behind. The reports document research showing that up to one in three pupils is given the wrong mark at the end of the tests. Short papers with questions that have a narrow range of possible answers mean that pupils' skills are not rigorously tested, leaving a wide margin of error.

'It is estimated that for the end of key stage tests in England this means that as many as one third of pupils may be given the wrong "level",' the report says. 'Only an increase in length of test beyond anything that is practicable would materially change this situation. Thus there are limits to how accurate the results of tests can be.'

The report concludes that levels of literacy have remained almost static since the 1950s, while there has been a steady improvement in maths. Over the same period, enjoyment of reading has declined among pupils preparing to move to secondary school.

'Massive efforts to bring about change have had a relatively small impact,' the report says. 'These policies have cost many hundreds of millions of pounds but they have generally not had a sound research base and have not been systematically evaluated.'

It claims that the use of Sats to measure progress year to year is fundamentally flawed. The rapid rise from 1995 to 2000, often cited as evidence that the tests work, was a reflection of schools getting better at teaching pupils to take tests.

Reprinted with permission.

Secondary education under New Labour

In secondary education, New Labour has chosen not to take on the battles over grammar schools and selection, placing this tricky political issue in the 'long grass' by saying that it would be up to parents locally to vote on whether they wanted to retain existing grammar schools.

Discuss and Do

- Why do you think it might be useful to test children's numeracy and literacy abilities?

- What might be some of the problems associated with testing school children's literacy and numeracy levels?

- What do you make of the claim in the report in Box 15.2 that the levels of literacy have remained fairly static over the last 50–60 years?

> In [secondary] education, we reject both the idea of a return to the 11-plus and the monolithic comprehensive schools that take no account of children's differing abilities. Instead we favour all-in schooling which identifies the distinct abilities of individual pupils and organises them in classes to maximise their progress in individual subjects. In this way we modernise the comprehensive principle, learning from the experience of its 30 years of application. (Labour Party, 1997)

Politically, this may well have been a sensible move as can be seen from the controversy that the Conservative Party caused itself when it proposed to withdraw its support for an expansion of grammar schools – see Box 15.3.

New Labour later went on to say that it did not want to support 'bog standard' comprehensives (see Department for Education and Skills, 2001a, 2001b) but, rather, would revitalise secondary provision by allowing comprehensive schools to 'specialise', thus creating:

> ... a diverse system where schools differ markedly from each other in the particular contribution they choose to make but are equally excellent in giving their students a broad curriculum. (Department for Education and Skills, 2001b: 38)

As such, it has been argued that it has reintroduced or reinforced selection by stealth. It has arguably done this in its promotion of 'diversity' in the types of secondary schools that would be promoted. Secondary comprehensive schools would be able to apply to become 'specialist schools', for example in the arts, languages, sciences or sports. (By 2006, 80% of secondary schools in England were specialist schools.) Labour argued that rather than returning to selection, what it was doing was supporting 'aptitude' – aptitude in relation to the arts, languages, sciences or sports. Specialist schools were therefore to be allowed to select up to 10% of their pupils based on aptitude.

Academies

Labour's other major policy development in relation to secondary education has been in its promotion of 'academies', particularly as a result of the Education and Inspections Act 2006 (Ball, 2007). These can be seen as a development of the Conservatives' City Technology Colleges. Academies are independent from the LEA controlled schools. Usually, they have been established in parts of the country where the schools are 'underperforming' or 'failing'. They tend to be newly built or substantially refurbished schools. The level of expenditure tends to be significantly more than the norm in the state sector, with some of the money (about 10%)

Box 15.3	The Tories and grammar schools

Cameron faces Tory revolt after retreat on grammar schools

James Meikle, education correspondent, *The Guardian*, Thursday May 17, 2007

Tory MPs turned on their leadership last night after David Cameron ditched a party article of faith, the superiority of grammar schools. About a dozen backbenchers used a meeting … to attack remarks by the shadow education secretary, David Willetts, that 'academic selection entrenches advantage, it does not spread it'.

Mr Cameron had also asserted that 'a pointless debate about creating a few grammar schools is not going to get us anywhere', and pledged instead to concentrate on raising standards and improving discipline in all England's 24,000 state schools. The Tory leader said history had shown that establishing new grammar schools was extremely difficult and often unpopular. 'Parents fundamentally don't want their children divided into sheep and goats at the age of 11,' Mr Cameron told the BBC.

One backbencher said the stormy meeting lasted an hour, but that some colleagues had calmed down after it was made clear that the party was not, as they had feared, planning to scrap existing grammar schools.

Mr Willetts, addressing a CBI conference, outlined how Conservatives would adopt Tony Blair's academies – state schools outside local authority control – and run them better than Gordon Brown. The Tories would make it easier to set up academies, which Mr Willetts labelled a 'diluted' version of the Conservatives' earlier city technology college programme. This would include removing the requirement for outside sponsors to contribute £2m . …

'For those children from modest backgrounds who do get to grammar schools, the benefits are enormous,' Mr Willetts said. 'We will not get rid of the grammar schools that remain. But the chances of a child from a poor background getting to a grammar school are shockingly low. Just 2% of children at grammar schools are on free school meals, compared with 12% of the school population in their areas.'

Roger Gale, the grammar school-educated MP for North Thanet, said: 'The concept that only middle-class parents are able to "play the system" to get their children into grammar schools is bizarre.'

Reprinted with permission.

coming from private investment. In return, the private investors have a majority say in how the school is run. Since academies are outside of the control of the LEA, being 'publicly funded independent schools', they can select their own headteacher and staff, have their own pay and conditions arrangements for their staff, appoint the majority of the school's governing body, and have greater latitude over the requirements of the National Curriculum. The private funders of city academies are varied – some being faith based (Church of England, Catholic, evangelical), others being business-based with successful 'responsible capitalists' wanting to do their bit for local communities and society more generally. Many, though not all, of these private business interests have been Labour Party supporters. In addition, there has been controversy over the involvement of certain sponsors, for example those of a

Stop and Think

- Do you think that selective (grammar) schools provide opportunities for less advantaged children?

- Conversely, do you think selective schools are divisive and do not provide equal opportunities?

- Why do you think that parents living in those parts of the country that no longer have grammar schools, e.g. Solihull in the West Midlands, have not demanded a return to selective education at the secondary stage, and yet in other parts of the country where grammar schools still exist, e.g. Birmingham, which is a neighbouring local authority to Solihull in the West Midlands, there remains significant support among parents for the retention of the selective schools that remain in that area?

religious disposition (Ball, 2007). Whether or not private finances are involved, the majority of the funding still comes out of the public purse, though this in turn is often via the 'private finance initiative'. However, it has only been in Labour's second and third terms of government that one has seen the academies take off significantly – fewer than 50 had been established by the end of 2006. The Education and Inspections Act 2006 looked to increase the numbers of academies in that Labour policy is to have 200 academies in place by 2010. The then Secretary of State for Education, Ruth Kelly, praised the achievements of academies at the time:

> Attainment at academies, which have replaced failing schools, is rising at a much faster rate than in other schools. [Academies] and their pupils have benefited from greater autonomy, greater freedom, a strong individual ethos, and the involvement of community partners from business, charities and higher education institutions. (Ruth Kelly, Department for Education and Skills, 2002b)

In the meantime, academies remain controversial, not least in relation to whether or not their performance is any better than that of the schools they have tended to replace. Many commentators have argued that, when one takes account of the extra investment they receive, and the impact they have in relation to attracting 'bright pupils' who might otherwise have gone to other local schools, academies do not, relatively speaking, outperform other secondary schools (see Hatcher, 2005, 2006; Lee, 2005; Mansell *et al.*, 2005; Parkin, 2005; Paton, 2005; Stewart, 2005b).

Stop and Think

- Why might a government want to encourage the involvement of private sector and other interests in the establishment and running of academies?

- What problems might you envisage in the encouragement of such interests in the provision of primary or secondary education?

- What are some of the difficulties you would encounter when trying to measure the effectiveness of academies as compared with other schools in a particular locality?

New Labour's policy shift from 2005 onwards – bringing the market back in?

From 2005 onwards, one can arguably see a shift in Labour's education policy at secondary and primary levels. During this period one witnessed attempts to move from a 'national system of education, locally delivered' in which national policy was interpreted and implemented via LEAs, to a system where schools would be increasingly independent, perhaps as not-for-profit trust schools. This can be seen in the Education and Inspections Act 2006, legislation that was the result of both significant compromise and rebellion amongst the Parliamentary Labour Party in that despite large compromises over its content, 46 Labour MPs still voted against the legislation – seemingly, the biggest government rebellion since 1924. The Act set out arrangements for the increased marketisation of education, in terms of the types of schools that could exist within the state system, the continued espousal of parental choice, and the further diminishing of the powers of LEAs. In certain respects one can see this policy development as being a continuation and evolvement of the approach of the previous Conservative government in its promotion of quasi-market arrangements. Therefore, under New Labour not only have we seen schools continue to manage their own budgets (Local Management of Schools) which are allocated predominantly on a per capita (numbers of pupils) basis, and schools continue to 'compete' with each other for pupils, but in addition to this under the 2006 Act schools can set themselves up as individual trust schools. As such, trust schools can be seen as the next step on from the establishment of specialist schools and city academies. A trust school would be able to own its own assets, contract for itself on capital projects, and enter into partnerships with other schools. Similarly to city academies, a trust school can also establish a majority on the school's governing body and move to be independent from the exegesis of the LEA. In certain respects, the development of trust schools can be regarded as the re-emergence of the Conservatives' GMS schools. It is perhaps not surprising then that the proposal proved controversial to a significant number of the Labour government's own MPs. Indeed, the compromises which the government had to cede to its own MPs included not allowing trust schools to have control over their own admissions, and agreeing that LEAs would continue to have strategic responsibilities for schooling in their area in relation to the building of new schools and in intervening where schools were deemed to be 'failing'. Even so, there remained major concerns for many opponents of the proposals, not least being the worry that popular trust schools would 'cream off' affluent or more able children while less popular schools would become 'sink schools' for those unable to win the selection battle, and as a consequence any attempts at social mixing could be lost.

Part of the reason for New Labour wanting to introduce further market-type arrangements into school provision was because it believed that the improvements in school education that it sought had not been sufficiently achieved. In particular, the performance of both primary and secondary schools in the poorest local authorities had not improved to the extent that the government would have liked. Even so, over its three terms of office there had been certain improvements in secondary school performance such that the Labour government has claimed that:

- more young people were now achieving five or more higher grades at GCSE – 60% in 2007, compared to 49.2% in 2001 and 46.3% in 1998;

- the percentage of working-class children achieving five higher grades at GCSE had risen faster than the national average: (Department for Education and Skills, 2001b; Department for Children, Schools and Families, 2007).

However, it is generally recognised that some of this improvement is due to 'lower attaining students' being switched to courses and examinations where it is easier to obtain (GCSE equivalent) passes (Dyson *et al.*, 2006; Mansell, 2004). Even so, these claimed improvements in secondary school performance have led the Labour government to loosen certain aspects of the National Curriculum at secondary level, but more so for schools that were deemed to be succeeding. Conversely, for less successful (often poorer) schools the curriculum would be more prescribed than for other schools, not least in terms of a concentration on the basics at the expense of some of the extra-curricular activities.

Higher education policy under New Labour

New Labour has regarded higher education as one of the key drivers in the development of the UK as a 'knowledge based economy', that is an economy which is increasingly concerned with high-value products and services, since one of the impacts of globalisation is that it is increasingly difficult for developed countries like the UK to compete in the traditional industries with developing countries due to the significant differences in labour costs. In its 1997 manifesto, Labour proposed to expand higher education opportunities:

> In today's world, there is no such thing as too clever. The more you know, the further you will go . . . . Why is it only now, we have lifted the cap on student numbers and 100,000 more will go to university in the next 2 years, 700,000 more to further education. So today I set a target of 50 per cent of young adults going into higher education in the next century. (Blair, 1999)

Even though New Labour has expanded higher education provision, it created a good deal of controversy by arguing that this expansion could not be funded out of general taxation and, therefore, students would have to pay for their own maintenance out of loans which they would be required to pay back once they were in work earning a particular level of salary – £15,000 per annum.

> The improvement and expansion of higher education cannot be funded out of general taxation. Our proposals for funding have been made to the Dearing Committee, in line with successful policies abroad . . . . The costs of student maintenance should be repaid by graduates on an income-related basis from the career success to which higher education has contributed. (Labour Party, 1997)

Labour duly asked Lord Dearing to look into the matter of higher education financing once again (he had done so for the Conservatives in 1996–97) and make recommendations on how HE could be funded. As a response to this (though it was not a recommendation of the report) the Labour government introduced tuition fees of £1,000 for all new undergraduates for the 1998/99 academic year.

In the 2001 General Election manifesto 'Ambitions for Britain', Labour proposed to expand higher education to 50% participation rate by 2010. No mention was made in the manifesto of any plan to introduce top-up fees (in addition to the

£1,100 fee students were by now paying) as the means by which this expansion would be funded:

> Our ten-year goal is 50 per cent of young adults entering higher education. By 2010, we want a majority of Britain's young people entering higher education. We will not introduce 'top-up' fees and have legislated to prevent them. (Labour Party, 2001)

However, not long into their second term, it became obvious that the government had changed its mind on variable top-up tuition fees, as it duly stated in its 2003 Higher Education White Paper 'The Future of Higher Education'. By then, it had decided that it would allow universities to charge variable top-up fees with a ceiling of £3,000 per full-time student per year. This was duly legislated for and implemented in 2006/07. There is the possibility that the cap of £3,000 may be lifted in 2010 when universities may be allowed to charge whatever fee they want, that is what the 'market' will bear. Alongside the power to charge significant top-up fees, universities were now expected to provide scholarships (against fees) and maintenance bursaries to assist students from poorer backgrounds in participating in HE. The government argued that these measures allowed for the reintroduction of maintenance support and fee assistance for poorer families which had previously disappeared. These measures were in part a response to concerns that the introduction of tuition fees in 1998 may have discouraged mature students, as well as students from working-class and ethnic minority backgrounds, from entering higher education (Goddard, 1999; Tomlinson, 2004).

Gordon Brown's agenda for education

Whilst it has been argued that New Labour's education policy, similarly to other areas of social policy, has been very much influenced by Gordon Brown during his time as Chancellor, Gordon Brown's premiership has been one where education is a key priority for him and his government:

> Our national mission is to be world class in education … We will bring together business, universities, colleges and the voluntary sector. Every secondary school – trusts, specialists or academies – linked to a business, every school linked to a college or university. I want for our young people the biggest expansion in educational opportunity our country has ever seen … We will launch a national campaign for thousands more to stay on after 16, to sign up to an apprenticeship, to study at university and college. (Gordon Brown, in Branigan, 2007)

As parts of its strategy for education and children's welfare more generally, the Brown government has set itself the following targets for 2020:

- two-year-olds from disadvantaged families to be provided with free nursery spaces;
- nursery provision for three- and four-year-old children will expand from 12.5 hours per week of free provision to 15 hours a week by 2011 and ultimately to 20 hours;
- a reduction in the 'overcrowded' curriculum in primary schools in order to make space for more literacy and numeracy;

- the possibility of flexible starting dates for summer-born babies to help them catch up;
- new measures to increase the progress in reading in primary schools, including the use of synthetic phonics;
- an overhauling of the SATs regime;
- the inclusion of foreign language teaching for all primary pupils;
- in secondary schools an expectation that 90% of pupils will achieve five A* to C GCSEs (60% of pupils achieved this in 2007);
- the raising of the school leaving age to 18 years;
- the provision of extra support for disabled children;
- the promotion of greater involvement of parents in their children's education and school life more generally;
- an increase in state education spending to levels that match per pupil spending in the private sector – the Institute of Fiscal Studies (IFS) has questioned the feasibility of this (Goodman and Sibeta, 2006);
- an increase in the number of extended schools with onsite provision of other services and professionals, including social work, police, sports and library facilities. (See Department for Children, Schools and Families, 2007)

Class, gender and 'race' inequalities

After 10 years of New Labour in government, inequalities in educational provision and opportunities persist (Tomlinson, 2001, 2005; Ball, 2003). Inequalities within the state sector continue with, as we have seen, competition to obtain a place in a 'good' primary or secondary school sometimes being very intense. At secondary level in particular there is competition: over grammar school places in areas that continue to have such schools, over places at faith schools or specialist and foundation schools as well as Academies where these exist. Furthermore, despite the rhetoric of 'choice', only 85% of families get their choice of school, meaning that 70,000 families did not in 2004 (Baker, 2005). In addition, despite Gordon Brown's pledge to increase the funding to state schools to the level enjoyed by privately educated pupils (circa £8,000 per year), state schools continue to receive significantly less (circa £3,000 per pupil in 2007 (Goodman and Sibeta, 2006). At the same time the 7% of children who are educated privately make up 26% of A level examination entrants (Tomlinson, 2004), a stark comparison with the 79% of the young people who had been in care and had no GCSEs or other educational qualifications when they left school (Barnardo's, 2006). In terms of gender, the trend for girls to perform better in the education system persists at primary and secondary levels and is starting to emerge in higher education, where more females than males are now entering higher education. And, despite Labour's rhetoric of inclusion, children from ethnic minorities (particularly African-Caribbean, Pakistani and Bangladeshi children) continue to underachieve relative to white children (Gillborn and Mirza, 2000). In higher education, there remain key class and racial differences (Archer *et al.*, 2003; Tomlinson, 2003), for example in degree choice (Reay *et al.*, 2001).

Conclusion

Overall, New Labour's education policy has demonstrated some fairly clear continuities with the previous Conservative government's education policy, such as the persistence with testing, league tables, the National Curriculum, and the marketisation of education provision via city academies and trust schools (Tomlinson, 2004). It has also overseen a significant expansion in higher education. Much of this has necessitated significant increases in expenditure. In summary, New Labour has:

- persisted with testing in England (though incorporated an element of 'value added' into their interpretation);
- continued with the national curriculum and augmented this with an emphasis on literacy and numeracy at primary level;
- continued to espouse parental choice;
- persisted with the quasi-market arrangements such as LMS;
- promoted city academies in the place of City Technology Colleges;
- espoused children's aptitude rather than ability and promoted specialist schools as a means of meeting these aptitudes;
- started to promote trust schools along similar lines to GMS schools;
- increased educational expenditure by more than 0.5% of GDP from 4.9% to 5.6% of GDP and, in so doing, has brought it near to the European (OECD) average levels of expenditure;
- overseen an increase in the number of teachers by 9% in the 10 years since 1997;
- seen class sizes fall;
- expanded higher education with a participation rate target of 50%;
- introduced tuition fees as a means of contributing to adequately funding higher education;
- extended student loans and, latterly, means-tested maintenance grants as the means by which students would support themselves.

In conclusion, many would see this as quite a list of actions, if not achievements, though whether it equates to 'education, education, education' will remain open to debate. And yet, Labour's education policy has a number of inherent contradictions within it (Tomlinson, 2004). Such contradictions arguably include:

- increases in the quantity of education provision but perhaps to the detriment of quality;
- increases in public expenditure on education but with increasing involvement of private funding and provision;
- promotion of diversity at the expense of increasing inequality;
- promotion of merit (for example through selection) at the expense of inclusion.

As Hulme and Hulme (2005: 33) have suggested:

> The tensions and contradictions [are] evident [in] a platform of education reform that is couched in the language of social inclusion, yet extends the market in education and regulates this through ever more intrusive instruments of 'governmentality' [that is, government regulation and control].

Perhaps what is immutable is the significance of education policy for individual children and young people, their families, and society more widely. As such, education remains, in part, a public good, irrespective of the degree to which it is constructed around a discourse of 'choice' and succumbs increasingly to market-type mechanisms and pressures. Both individual and societal interests are very much determined by the effectiveness of education policy.

Annotated further reading

Tomlinson (2005) provides an overview of education policy from the creation of the post-war welfare state through to policies of the New Right and then on to the policies of New Labour. Hill (2003) provides a useful overview of the development of education policy and provision in the nineteenth and twentieth centuries.

Sullivan (1996) offers an accessible but sufficiently detailed account of the development of educational provision and policy post-war through to the policies of the Conservative governments of Margaret Thatcher and John Major. For a deeper consideration of the educational policies of the New Right Conservative government, Chitty (1989) is a useful place to start. Fergusson (1994) provides an accessible account of how the New Right's education policy can be considered in relation to the 'managerialist' analysis.

As well as Tomlinson (2005), Chitty (2004) provides a useful analysis of education policy under New Labour, covering all parts of the education provision: pre-school, primary and secondary schooling, and higher education provision. Hatcher (2005, 2006) has more specifically analysed the development of Academies under New Labour. For analyses of inequalities in education, the works of Ball (2003) and Tomlinson (2005) are very useful.

Chapter 16

Work and employment policy

Objectives

- To examine the nature and purposes of employment policy, and the role of employment policy in relation to the pursuit of social welfare.

- To examine the relation between employment policy and other areas of social and public policy.

- To provide a brief examination of trends in the British labour market since the 1970s.

- To examine the development of in-work benefits and the partial integration of the tax and benefits system that has taken place since 1997 with the introduction of tax credits for the working poor.

Introduction

'Hain begins "crusade" for full employment' ... 'CBI backs 3.2% rise in minimum wage' ... 'Brown "wasted £9bn" on tax credits' ... 'Claims for pay equality swell tribunal cases' ... 'Child poverty sees shock increase' ... 'Work is the route claimants must take, says Murphy' ... 'Call to revamp "woeful" New Deal' ... 'Gay bias persists in banks says claimant'...

These are some headlines published in a national newspaper during 2007. The stories – about full employment, the minimum wage, tax credits, equal pay, child poverty, the importance of work, the 'New Deal', and alleged discrimination against gays in workplaces – are all to do with, in varying ways, employment and employment policy, but they touch on wider issues. They suggest, firstly, that issues of employment and employment policy have some relationship to social welfare, broadly conceived, and, secondly, that there is a relationship between employment and other areas of public policy, for example economic policy, equality policy, poverty policy and income maintenance policy. They suggest, therefore, that the world of work is not something entirely distinguishable from or separate from the world of social welfare and social policy. It is the purpose of this chapter to explore this relationship in some detail and thereby to throw light on contemporary UK social policy.

Why work? The connection between work and welfare

A systematic contemporary statement of the case for seeing economic and social policy as closely linked and mutually interdependent was made by the Labour Party's Commission on Social Justice, a semi-official inquiry, in its 1994 Report: '. . . economic and social policy are inextricably linked . . . An economic high road of growth and productivity must also be a social high road of opportunity and security' (Commission on Social Justice, 1994: 97). The integration of employment policy and social policy, always, however, implicit in the post-war Beveridgean welfare 'consensus', was made explicit after 1997 and the election of the 'New' Labour government, which, following the Commission, emphasised work as a source of welfare and as the most appropriate route out of poverty.

This view was reiterated, more starkly, by the then welfare reform minister, Jim Murphy, in a speech in March 2007, when he declared that 'Work is the only way out of poverty . . . the benefit system will never pay of itself [enough to lift people out of poverty] and I don't think it should', a comment which caused consternation in the academic social policy community and poverty lobby (Timmins, 2007d). His remarks about benefits were interpreted by critics as a departure from what had been understood to be traditional Labour Party policy. Whether this is the case or not, Murphy's, and the Labour government's, views about the importance of work are not peculiar to British welfare policy-makers; they are generally accepted in the European Union and more generally amongst members of the OECD group of countries, where the commitment has in recent years shifted decisively in the direction of what are called labour market 'activation' policies – roughly speaking, getting unemployed people off welfare and into work (Finn, 2003: 114; Bailey, 2006: 163).

The argument is not simply about income poverty, material deprivation and the value of work in overcoming these. A large body of evidence suggests that there is a connection between involvement in work and general well-being. 'Worklessness is associated with poorer physical and mental health and well-being. Work can be therapeutic and can reverse the adverse health effects of unemployment . . . Overall, the beneficial effects of work outweigh the risks of work, and are greater than the harmful effects of long term unemployment or prolonged sickness absence. Work is generally good for health and well-being.' (Waddell and Burton, 2006: 32). In this sense, therefore, a policy to enable or encourage people to engage in work is a welfare policy.

We will begin by examining a number of concepts and theories of employment and unemployment, then turn to look at the history of policies for employment and unemployment, drawing attention to their connections with broader welfare objectives. The focus will be on the period since the 1970s. We will examine recent trends and changes in the labour market, and glance briefly at the role of the European Union in relation to UK policy, before examining the policies of the present Labour government in some detail.

Some concepts and definitions

We can distinguish (at least) two dimensions of employment policy. '*Primary*' employment policy is concerned with employment and unemployment, with reducing the latter and creating the conditions which underpin high levels of employment, assisting job search and placement, paying cash benefits to the unemployed and, via links with the education and training sector, ensuring that there is an appropriately skilled workforce.

'*Secondary*' employment policy involves various kinds of labour market *regulation*. Workplace health and safety, limitations on hours of work, the pursuit of equal treatment and equal opportunities within employment, in relation to, for example, gender, race and disability, legislation for equal pay and minimum wages are all examples of the state's attempt to regulate the labour market in the pursuit of social objectives.

The quality of working life is an aspect of 'secondary' policy, which concerns the 'quality' of jobs – whether they are satisfying and fulfilling, or boring, repetitive, and so on – participation and opportunities for employees' 'voice' to be heard in crucial decisions, employees' degree of autonomy and control over work processes and hours of work, opportunities for training and development, and employees' sense of security and self-worth (Brinkley *et al.*, 2007: 4, 59).

Two concepts used in official statistics and official and academic discussion of employment policy are '*economically active*' and '*economically inactive*'. The 'economically active' are a combination of the employed and the unemployed – all people who are in some sense 'in' the labour market. The 'economically inactive' are those who, for various reasons, are outside the labour market, and include, for example, all those engaged in full-time education, people who are permanently retired and those who are engaged in unremunerated caring responsibilities for family members.

Concepts like employment and unemployment are open to interpretation, like most concepts in social life and the social sciences (Whiteside, 1991: 11–13, 126–130). A broad definition, now used in the UK, is that of the International Labour Organisation (ILO), a branch of the United Nations, which counts as unemployed 'those aged 16 and over who are without a job, are available to start work in the next two weeks, who have been seeking a job in the last four weeks or are out of work and waiting to start a job already obtained in the next two weeks' (Office for National Statistics, 2006a: 51). This is, however, as a definition, just as artificial as any other. A small child or an old person past retirement age, willing to work and looking for it, but unable to find it, will not be classified as 'unemployed' for official purposes (Glynn, 1991: 14). Another example is the argument over the employment status of women, and the circumstances in which they may be defined officially as 'unemployed' – that is, looking for, and available for, work. Policy-makers for much of the twentieth century were remarkably unwilling to afford women, especially married women, the status of being 'unemployed' (Whiteside, 1991: 11–12). Counting the numbers of unemployed people has also been something open to political manipulation; governments have sought to reduce the apparent numbers of unemployed by adopting narrower definitions.

Stop and Think

Why do you think policy-makers might have had difficulty with the idea of allowing married women to be classified as 'unemployed'?

It is important to distinguish between *long-term* and *short-term* unemployment. There is a difference between being unemployed for a week and being unemployed for a year or more. In any reasonably dynamic economy, there will be, at any given moment, a proportion of economically active people who are between jobs and therefore 'unemployed'. People are continually moving from one job to another and in and out of unemployment. This is not a problem. Long-term unemployment, on the other hand, is.

Theories of employment and unemployment

Contemporary policies for employment and unemployment should be related to changing theories about the causes of, and factors influencing, employment and unemployment. We can, following Bryson, distinguish between *'economic'*, *'behavioural'* and *'institutional'* theories about the causes of unemployment (Bryson, 2003: 79–81).

Economic theories are of two types – *'demand'* theories and *'supply'* theories.

- *'Demand' theories* emphasise changes in the demand for labour as influencing levels of employment and unemployment. The Keynesian approach described below is of the first type. Unemployment is due to a lack of demand for labour brought about by lack of 'effective' demand in the economy. This is the kind of unemployment that occurs in an economic recession. (Another term for this kind of unemployment is 'cyclical' unemployment.) Demand theories have fallen out of fashion since the 1970s. Since then, 'supply' theories have become popular.

- *'Supply' theories* draw attention to the characteristics and quality of the workforce, in terms of skill levels, and emphasise policy instruments such as subsidies, training, 'make work' schemes, or ways of improving the number of job offers individuals receive. Other supply-side factors include economic restructuring, involving the decline of manufacturing and the rise of the service economy, globalisation and the accompanying intensified international competition in the traded sector of the economy (Bryson, 2003: 79–80). (Such unemployment is also known as 'structural' unemployment.)

- *'Behavioural' theories* of unemployment emphasise either individual shortcomings – people's unwillingness to look for work or keep it – or, on the other hand, the demoralising effects of long-term unemployment on the unemployed and their motivation to seek work.

- *'Institutional' theories*, finally, stress the impact of institutions such as the welfare state itself, and place emphasis on unconditional entitlement to benefits, rather than making benefits conditional on appropriate job search behaviour – 'rights' without 'responsibilities' (Bryson, 2003: 80–81).

Of course, these theories of unemployment are not mutually exclusive, and policy may be underpinned by more than one view about causal factors and influences. In fact contemporary policy towards unemployment in the UK is probably a mixture of all three.

The economic policy of 'inflation targeting' for example, pursued informally from 1993 to 1997 and formally thereafter, has as one of its objectives the creation of a stable economic environment in which demand for labour is buoyant. Policies of removing barriers to freedom of trade, investment and (in a more limited way) movement of labour, associated with the UK's EU membership and involvement in the World Trade Organisation, are also in part designed to create conditions in which business and enterprise can flourish and employers are willing to hire.

Trade union reform, carried out by the Conservatives in the 1980s and largely accepted and retained by subsequent Labour governments, has been designed to create a more 'flexible' labour market and remove barriers to employers' rights to hire and fire. Changes in the administration of job search and placement services and the administration of benefits for the unemployed, associated for example with Labour's 'New Deals' and the creation of 'Jobcentre Plus', have been designed to ensure that benefit recipients engage with the labour market and that unemployed individuals accept some responsibility for seeking and retaining work, or at least seek to acquire work-relevant skills by engaging in training.

Background: employment policy from the beginnings to Thatcher

There is probably no earlier period of British history when governments have not sought to regulate the labour market in some way, whether through the Poor Law, apprenticeship laws or laws governing wages. Even the mid-Victorian liberal heyday was in reality characterised by a degree of state intervention. Factory legislation, for example, dates from 1800, and there were subsequently many other legislative interventions relating to employment in factories, mines and workshops, limiting hours of work, regulating the employment of juveniles and women, and other aspects of working conditions.

Governments hardly recognised, however, any responsibility for influencing the *level* of unemployment until shortly before the First World War. Free-market liberal ideas were dominant in economics and among policy-makers, who believed that the economy was a self-regulating mechanism which tended towards 'equilibrium', a state in which all 'factors of production', including human ones, would be employed at an appropriate price (wages in the case of labour). Unemployment could only be a temporary phenomenon (see Chapter 10). The Poor Law, which had existed since 1601, was, after its reform in 1834, an adjunct to this approach to the labour market. It was reconfigured as, essentially, a work-focused system of social security, designed to encourage engagement with the labour market and to ensure that support for out of work individuals did not discourage them from seeking work by being too generous (Harris, 1972: 1–2).

Discuss and Do

In terms of the three theories of unemployment described in an earlier section – 'economic', 'behavioural' and 'institutional' – what theory or theories do you think underlie the view of unemployment described in the previous paragraph?

Policy began to change in the early years of the twentieth century (see Chapter 10). Legislation passed by a Liberal government in 1909 created 'labour exchanges' – the forerunners of today's Jobcentres – providing basic job search and placement services, designed to aid the unemployed to find work, and employers to find workers. Another innovation in this period was the introduction of minimum wages in some low-paid sectors of the economy. A further innovation was the introduction of unemployment benefit, a social insurance-based cash benefit, outside the ambit of the Poor Law, in 1911 for certain limited classes of insured persons.

The optimistic free-market view of labour markets as always tending naturally towards full-employment equilibrium was dealt a final, fatal blow by the inter-war experience of high and persistent unemployment. A major redefinition of employment policy took place in the 1940s, under the influence of the ideas of economists like John Maynard Keynes, and of the impact of mass unemployment in the 1930s. Unemployment was seen as resulting less from labour market inefficiencies and imperfections than from the workings of the economy, and in particular, from a deficiency of aggregate 'effective demand'.

The Beveridge Report of 1942 took as one of its basic assumptions the creation and maintenance of high and stable levels of employment (Harris, 1997; Lowe, 2005: 118–119). The wartime Churchill-led coalition government's 1944 White Paper on employment policy demonstrated Keynesian influence and marked a change in élite opinion about the nature, causes and remedies for unemployment. Its view of the issue was to become a consensual one in post-war British politics (on the post-war 'consensus', see Chapters 3 and 10). Governments on both sides of the political divide sought to ensure steady growth, increasing prosperity and full employment along with low inflation. Unemployment rates remained low, at around 2–3%, from the 1940s to the 1960s.

Views differed about what constituted 'full' employment. The 1944 White Paper's notion of full employment was a rate of 8.5%. Beveridge and the Attlee government thought it was an unemployment rate of 3%, according to the traditional British measure of 'those out of work and claiming benefit' (Lowe, 2005: 382).

Discuss and Do

In terms of the three theories of unemployment described in an earlier section – 'economic', 'behavioural' and 'institutional' – what theory or theories do you think underlie the view of unemployment held by UK policy-makers in the post-war period?

The economic environment became much less favourable in the 1970s for the British economy, which from the 1960s onwards seemed to become less competitive and to fall behind those of other, especially European, countries in terms of productivity and innovation. Britain became known as 'the sick man of Europe' (Gamble, 1985). Both unemployment and inflation rose, and government management of the economy became much more difficult. The Conservative government of 1970–74 under Edward Heath was the last to try to operate an old-style 'demand management' policy, pursuing expansionary policies at a time when both inflation and unemployment were rising. This went disastrously wrong, and both inflation and unemployment rose sharply.

The succeeding Labour governments under Harold Wilson (1974–76) and James Callaghan (1976–79) fought simultaneously to control inflation, check the rise in unemployment and promote economic growth. These efforts were modestly successful; unemployment was stabilised at a little above 1 million and inflation was steadily reduced. These policies nevertheless represented a partial departure from those which constituted what has come to be called the post-war 'consensus' (Kavanagh, 1987: Ch. 5).

The 'social contract' drawn up between the Labour government and the unions broke down at the end of 1978 with breaches in the incomes policy as unions sought to protect their members' living standards, eroded by tax increases as well as price rises. There were strikes in both the private and public sectors during the winter of 1978–79, the (in)famous 'winter of discontent'. This was to cost Labour the election that took place the following May. At the same time, the climate of policy opinion was changing, and new ideas about economic management, employment and unemployment began to be entertained across the political spectrum, including, most importantly, in the Conservative Party (Gamble, 1988: Ch. 3).

The Thatcher governments, the unemployment crisis and employment policy in the 1980s

> ... mass, long-term unemployment is the worst breakdown a society can experience, the most damning evidence of political failure. (Glynn, 1991: 1, citing Hugo Young, 1987)

The Conservative Party under Margaret Thatcher's leadership won the General Election in May 1979, narrowly defeating Labour. The election of a new government brought about new approaches to the management of the economy, to employment and industrial relations (Kavanagh, 1987: 204–207; Gamble, 1988: Ch. 3). 'Monetarism', so-called, an approach to economic policy adopted by the first Thatcher government, is a short-hand term for an approach which emphasised the control of inflation as the prime economic objective.

The early years of the Thatcher government were a time of severe economic recession. The number of unemployed in Britain rose from 1.25 million in 1979 and doubled within 18 months; by 1985 it had reached 3 million. Previous Conservative governments would not have tolerated levels of unemployment of this magnitude, but the Thatcher government adopted a robust attitude, Margaret Thatcher stating famously that 'there is no alternative'. (For trends in employment and unemployment rates in this period, see Figures 16.1 and 16.2, below.)

The government's own policies worsened the effect of the recession. A highly deflationary monetary and fiscal policy brought down inflation, but at a high cost in business failures and redundancies, especially in manufacturing industry, which was, in international terms, uncompetitive. The experiment failed, not only because of the extremely high financial and social costs imposed by high unemployment, but because inflation was only temporarily and incompletely conquered, and took off again in the late 1980s (Kavanagh, 1987: Ch. 8; Gamble, 1988: Ch. 4; Smith, 1993).

It is difficult, from the perspective of today, to overestimate the salience of unemployment in the politics of the 1980s. For the numerous critics of the Thatcher governments, the extent and persistence of unemployment constituted those governments' major policy failure, as well as marking the definitive end to the post-war full employment 'consensus'. Critics lamented that the Thatcher governments had changed the agenda of politics so that unemployment no longer mattered for electoral success and failure. It is true that Conservative governments did not formally commit themselves to achieving some particular target rate of unemployment. (Note that if the 'full employment' rate is taken to be that envisaged in the 1944 White Paper – 8.5% – then there were only a relatively few years in the 1980s and 1990s when this target was not met.) Contrary to received wisdom, however, the Thatcher (and Major) governments did not succeed in changing the agenda of politics in such a way that unemployment no longer mattered. Their success in three general elections after 1979 does not prove that the full employment consensus of the post-war years had been replaced by a fatalistic acceptance of high levels of unemployment as the necessary price to be paid for long-term economic stability. Conservative thinking in this period involved a reformulation of the means, rather than the ends, of employment policy. They clearly believed that their legitimacy in the eyes of the electorate depended on being seen to do something about unemployment. To that extent a 'full employment' consensus remained in place. The 'something' was to take a variety of forms from the mid-1980s onwards. By 1983, for example, the Conservatives were already spending £2 billion per year on special employment and training measures for 850,000 people.

Discuss and Do

What do you feel about the status of unemployment as a voting issue? For you, is it high up the agenda or not in terms of which party to support in an election? Why do you think the Conservatives might have won three general elections between 1983 and 1992, despite high levels of unemployment?

One task the new government set itself was the deregulation of the labour market to make it more 'flexible', so that employment, and unemployment, could reach their 'natural' market levels. The Conservative Chancellor of the Exchequer from 1983 to 1989, Nigel Lawson, sketched out an employment agenda for government in his Mais lecture of 1984. In his view, unemployment was a microeconomic, not a macroeconomic, problem. Macroeconomic policy was concerned with creating economic stability and controlling inflation; it had nothing *directly* to do with employment and unemployment. Unemployment must be tackled through microeconomic policy interventions to improve the workings of the labour market and the quality of the workforce, so that employers would be more willing to invest and hire. This was the obverse of what had come to be understood as the 'Keynesian' position (Smith, 1987: 118–119; Keegan, 1989: 136–137).

Governments engaged in some presentational manipulation by changing the basis for counting the unemployed, for instance by removing the unemployed who were near to retirement (1981) and school leavers (1983); in all, 31 changes were made to the method of calculating unemployment by the Conservatives. The effect of these was to artificially reduce the number of officially unemployed and to disguise the rate of dependency on unemployment benefits. These changes, although condemned, were not reversed by New Labour after 1997 (Lowe, 2005: 498).

Youth unemployment was the focus of concern in the early 1980s, as it had been in the 1970s under the Wilson and Callaghan Labour governments. The Thatcher government introduced a range of measures intended to tackle it, building on the previous Labour government's Youth Opportunities Programme (YOP). A variety of schemes were introduced, including the Youth Training Scheme (YTS), the Community Programme (CP) for the long-term unemployed, and the Enterprise Allowance Scheme, which paid people Unemployment Benefit while setting up in business on their own.

Unemployed youngsters aged between 18 and 24 were offered a job training scheme which gave an allowance of £10 above benefit levels if the unemployed person participated in recognised training. Another direct subsidy scheme, the Jobstart allowance, offered the unemployed person an allowance, for six months only, for 18-year-olds who accepted work below a given wages ceiling. Such schemes sought to fill a perceived gap between the skills and training provided by compulsory education and those required by employers. There were also policies aimed at encouraging employers to take on unemployed workers, for example the New Workers' Scheme, which paid employers an allowance for each unemployed worker they took on at a rate under a given wage ceiling. This amounted to a direct wage subsidy.

Stop and Think

Why do you think policy-makers from the 1970s to the present have been so concerned about the unemployment of younger people ?

The older and long-term unemployed, those 'shaken out' and made redundant, mostly from manufacturing industry in the severe recession of 1980–83, received less attention at first. Between 1982 and 1986, for example, the government suspended the requirement that the unemployed should look for work as a condition of receiving unemployment benefits. Policy changed in 1986 with the introduction of the Restart programme for the long-term unemployed, which involved compulsory job search interviews for anyone out of work for over six months (Finn, 2003: 112). In 1989 the unemployed were required to actively seek work and the grounds for refusing job offers were restricted. An Employment Service (ES) was created at the same time, integrating jobcentres and unemployment benefit offices. The role of the ES was to develop in the direction of strengthening work incentives and monitoring job search behaviour. The ES also became involved in promoting the take-up of in-work benefits, such as the Family Credit, introduced in 1988, as a way of making low-paid work an attractive option. By 1996 some 600,000 families were in receipt of this benefit (Finn, 2003: 113). At the other end of the age scale, government favoured the promotion of early retirement above the retraining of the older unemployed.

The Conservatives also modified social security policies in various ways to encourage the long-term unemployed to seek work. The duration of contribution-based Unemployment Benefit was reduced from 12 to six months in 1996. At the same time, Unemployment Benefit was renamed Jobseekers' Allowance (JSA), and intended only for those 'actively seeking work'. The stricter job search regime accompanying the introduction of JSA helped to reduce the number of claimants by between 100,000 and 200,000 (Finn, 2003: 113)

Discuss and Do

In terms of the three theories of unemployment described in an earlier section – 'economic', 'behavioural' and 'institutional' – what theory or theories do you think underlie the Conservative governments' policies on unemployment described in the previous paragraph?

The latter half of the 1980s was a period of economic recovery and the resumption of growth, accompanied by falling unemployment (see Figures 16.1 and 16.2 below). Monetary policy had been relaxed; 'monetarism' in the strict, Milton Friedman, sense – control of the money supply – had been abandoned by about 1985 as being unworkable (Smith, 1987; Keegan, 1989: Ch. 9; Johnson, 1991). In fact policy became too relaxed and inflation began to take off once more. From 1990 to 1992 the economy lapsed into recession again, with a rising number of business failures, falling house prices, redundancies and rising unemployment, a period which coincided with Britain's brief membership of the Exchange Rate Mechanism of the European Monetary Union, a sort of forerunner of the Euro (Smith, 1993; Stephens, 1997). The UK's forced exit from the ERM in September 1992 – this was effectively a devaluation of the pound – gave an immediate boost to the economy through lower interest rates and export prices, bringing about sustained growth and falling unemployment, which has continued until the present.

Evaluating Conservative policies

Conservative policies for employment and unemployment are probably to be accounted a failure, at least until the last few years of the Major government. Macroeconomic policy was unstable for much of the period, leading to economic fluctuations and severe fluctuations in unemployment, as the Conservatives searched for an appropriate set of rules for the conduct of policy. The social (and fiscal) costs of this were high. The Conservative period is nevertheless one of considerable policy activism and innovation. We can trace the emergence of an active labour market policy in this period, and much of the Conservative legacy was to be an inheritance developed by successive Labour governments after 1997.

In the next section, we turn to consider, briefly, some basic changes and trends in the UK labour market from the 1970s to the 2000s, before commenting on the policies pursued by Labour governments since 1997.

Trends in employment and unemployment: the experience

Since the 1970s there have been significant changes in the British labour market. One long-term trend has been the long-term rise in the economically active population. Another has been the continuing shift away from employment in manufacturing industry and towards employment in services, coinciding with a shift away from manual and towards white-collar employment (Brinkley *et al.*, 2007: 12). Other trends include the relative decline in full-time male employment and the rise in women's employment.

From the 1980s to the mid-1990s it seemed as if the world of work was undergoing drastic changes, inspiring an outpouring of apocalyptic management literature which predicted and preached 'the end of work', forecasting the rise of temporary, part-time, fixed contract employment and an end to full-time, permanent jobs. Large companies were 'downsizing' their workforces, a process which affected white-collar and management work as well as manual work, as companies 'delayered' management hierarchies. There appeared to be growing insecurity among workers, fearful of losing their jobs (Brinkley *et al.*, 2007: 5–7). These trends were real. There was a growth in self-employment, temporary and part-time work, and in numbers of people with second jobs, but not in full-time jobs, where there was a reduction. Permanent employment also grew much more slowly than part-time employment (Brinkley *et al.*, 2007: 8).

These trends have been reversed since the mid-1990s. Total employment growth has been much greater, and most of it has been in 'traditional', full-time, permanent jobs. Numbers in temporary employment fell, and self-employment grew more slowly than the general trend. The 'proper' job therefore experienced something of a recovery in this decade, contrary to the forecasts of the doom-mongers (Brinkley *et al.*, 2007: 9–11). The labour market trends of the earlier decade were a specific, and temporary, response to the much harsher economic climate of that period.

Figure 16.1 shows long-term trends in economic activity and unemployment rates from 1971 to 2005. The difference between the 'economically active' and the 'in employment' lines is, of course, the unemployment rate, the dashed line at the bottom of the graph. As one might expect, the lines for the employed and the unemployed populations are almost mirror images. It is noticeable that both the 'economically active' and the 'economically inactive' populations have grown over the period 1971–2005. The economically active population is now around 30 million. The trend in employment broadly reflects that in the economically active population. The main factors influencing the rise in the economically active population include an increasing UK population arising from natural increase and immigration, and increases in the numbers of women entering the labour market. The growth in the economically inactive population reflects rises in the numbers of retired persons – people living longer and retiring earlier – and expansion in the numbers of people continuing in full-time education. It will be noticed that the graphs of all these trends are not smooth, but exhibit fluctuations and discontinuities. Thus there are dips in the numbers of employed and economically active persons in the first half of the 1980s and 1990s, periods of high unemployment, as shown by the lowest, dashed, line. Unemployment, in terms of the numbers, is approximately the same at the end of the period as it was in the later 1970s.

Figure 16.2 on page 346, with its exaggerated vertical axis by comparison with Figure 16.1, gives a rather clearer picture of trends in unemployment over the same period, broken down by sex. (The dashed line for 'all' is simply a spikier version of the 'unemployed' line in Figure 16.1.) Overall unemployment tripled between 1971 and the early 1980s, when it rose to over 3 million, and halved between 1993 and 2005 to its present level of about 1.5 million. The sharp increases in both male and

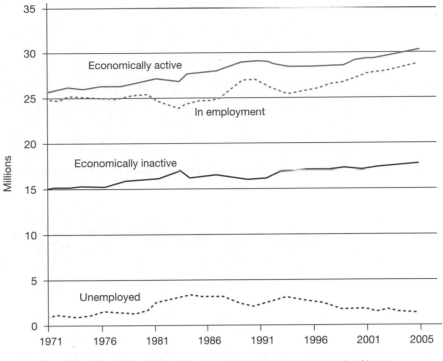

At spring each year. People aged 16 or over. Data are seasonally adjusted and have been adjusted in line with population estimates published in Autumn 2005.

Figure 16.1 Trends in economic activity levels, United Kingdom, 1971–2005 (millions)
Source: Office for National Statistics (2006b) *Labour Force Survey*, Figure 4.1, p. 50, London: ONS. Crown copyright material is reproduced with the permission of the Controller of HMSO and the Queen's Printer for Scotland under the terms of the Click-Use Licence.

female unemployment in the early 1980s and early 1990s are clearly shown. It will also be seen, however, that the graph for female unemployment is somewhat smoother than that for men. This is particularly the case for the early 1990s, where the increase in male unemployment is particularly marked. The unemployment experience for men was slightly worse, and that for women rather better, in the early 1990s than they had been in the early 1980s. These differences reflect the concentration of men in manufacturing industry, much more seriously affected by the economic downturns in these periods than were the service industries in which women are more likely to be found.

Table 16.1 overleaf provides some useful comparative data on unemployment among some EU member countries in 2004. It will be seen that the UK's unemployment performance is among the more successful, especially by comparison with the larger continental countries such as Germany, France and Italy. The UK performs well in relation to both male and female unemployment, and considerably better than the larger European economies. Rather surprisingly, perhaps, the UK's performance even appears more successful than Sweden's, the 'model' welfare state country which pioneered active labour market policies in the 1950s, and which had very low unemployment rates until the 1990s. More recent data would show some improvement in the figures for some of these countries. Germany's employment performance improved between 2005 and 2007, accompanying a revival in the German economy.

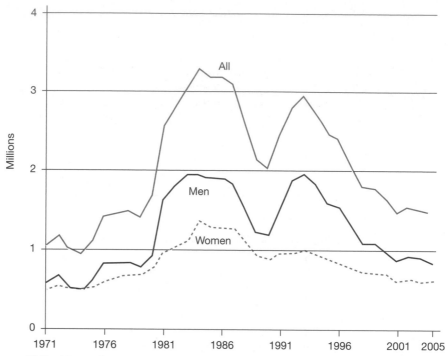

Figure 16.2   Unemployment trends by sex, United Kingdom, 1971–2005 (millions)
Source: Office for National Statistics (2006b) *Labour Force Survey*, Figure 4.19, p. 60, London:
ONS. Crown copyright material is reproduced with the permission of the Controller of HMSO and
the Queen's Printer for Scotland under the terms of the Click-Use Licence.

What looks like a relatively good UK employment performance should not lead
to a complacent assumption that all is well. There is arguably a good deal of hidden
unemployment in the UK among groups not formally labelled as unemployed, such
as people on incapacity benefits, lone parents and older people, as well as among
groups experiencing particular disadvantage, such as ethnic minorities.

Figure 16.3 provides a breakdown of unemployment by ethnic group and sex in
the UK. The bar chart exhibits clear patterns of employment disadvantage among

Table 16.1 Unemployment percentage rates by sex, EU comparison, 2004

	Men	**Women**	**All**
Netherlands	4.3	4.8	4.6
United Kingdom	5.0	4.2	4.7
Austria	4.4	5.3	4.8
Sweden	6.5	6.1	6.3
Belgium	7.1	8.9	7.9
Italy	6.4	10.5	8.0
Germany	8.7	10.5	9.5
France	8.7	10.5	9.6
Spain	8.1	15.0	11.0
EU-25 average	8.1	10.2	9.0

Source: Office for National Statistics (2006b) *Labour Force Survey*, Table 4.20, p. 61, London: ONS. Crown copyright material is
reproduced with the permission of the Controller of HMSO and the Queen's Printer for Scotland under the terms of the Click-Use Licence.

Discuss and Do

Figure 16.2 seems to show that unemployed men consistently outnumber unemployed women in the UK. Table 16.1 also shows that the unemployment rate for men is higher than that for women in the UK (unlike all other countries except Sweden in the table). What do you think might explain these differences between men's and women's unemployment?

ethnic groups. All ethnic groups have higher levels of unemployment than the 'White British' group. It also shows that the experience of different ethnic groups varies, and that there are interesting differences among ethnic groups in relation to both male and female unemployment. The male unemployment rate is highest for black Caribbeans at around 15%. The female rate is highest for women of Pakistani origin, at around 20% (that for Bangladeshi women is not shown, but is assumed to be comparable with that for Pakistani women). Those of Indian origin had the lowest unemployment rates among non-white groups. These differences between groups and between them and the majority white population reflect varying legacies, of concentration in declining industrial sectors and regions, and continuing experience of discrimination, direct and indirect. Many non-white ethnic groups, heavily concentrated in traditional manufacturing employment in particular regions and urban areas, have suffered disproportionately from the effects of industrial and employment 'restructuring' and resulting unemployment in the UK since the 1970s, and have subsequently

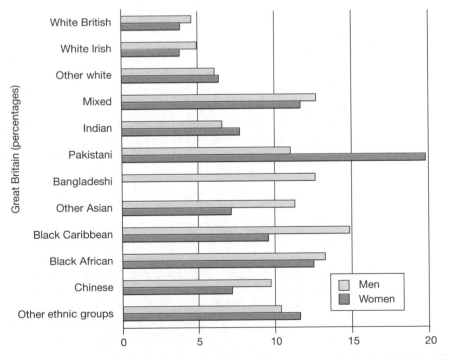

Figure 16.3 Unemployment percentage rates by ethnic group and sex, Great Britain, 2004
Source: Office for National Statistics (2006b) *Labour Force Survey*, Figure 4.21, p. 61, London: ONS. Crown copyright material is reproduced with the permission of the Controller of HMSO and the Queen's Printer for Scotland under the terms of the Click-Use Licence.

failed to share to the same extent as white groups in the economic recovery that has taken place. Relatively high levels of ethnic minority unemployment have also coexisted, paradoxically, with strong demand for labour in the economy since the mid-1990s and historically high levels of immigration responding to that demand.

One of the most fundamental changes in the post-war UK labour market has been the growth of women's employment. Since the 1960s there has been a growing demand for equality of access to the labour market and equality of treatment within the workplace. The treatment of women workers and the interplay of work and family responsibilities for men and women have become serious issues. Policy began to address questions of equality of reward, equal treatment in the workplace and pension provision in a system that had been based upon the outdated notion of full male employment. Early forays into equal opportunities were the Equal Pay Act (1970) and Sex Discrimination Act (1976), both passed by a Labour government. In addition, the increasingly complex relationship between work and family where both parents (assuming a two parent family) are in work began to pose new questions (see Chapter 18).

The European Union dimension

The role of the European Union (EU) has become important in shaping national employment policies via the social provisions of the European treaties (see Chapter 22). Conservative attempts to deregulate and 'flexibilise' the labour market in the 1980s and 1990s were thwarted to some extent by the European Union. In fact the period of the Thatcher and Major governments seemed to see an almost continuous struggle between Westminster and Brussels over social questions, insofar as they related to employment issues (MacInnes, 1987: 54, 104; Taylor, 1994: 259–263). The Conservatives refused to sign up to the Social Chapter of the Maastricht Treaty in 1991, which was about transforming the European Community into the European Union. (The Treaty was a consequence of the introduction of the Single Market, which the Conservatives had signed up to in 1986, before apparently realising what the implications for the social dimension of European integration might amount to. This decision was reversed by the newly elected Labour government in 1997.) The Conservative hope was that this would enable the UK to escape the regulatory burden of the European Social Charter, drafted in 1989. This proved illlusory.

In 1995 a House of Lords ruling on terms and conditions for part-time workers declared that existing UK policy was inconsistent with a 1991 EU regulation. The European Court of Justice ruled on the terms and conditions for workers subject to competitive tendering and contracting-out. European directives aimed at the control of social dumping, or the attempt to create a 'level European playing field' by preventing countries gaining a competitive advantage by reducing their own employment protection measures, were regarded by Conservative governments and employers as an attempt to impose a new quasi-socialist consensus. In fact the impression given is that the social philosophy, a mixture of social Catholicism and social democracy, underpinning the European Union was completely at odds with that of the 'Anglo-Saxon' model of free-market capitalism which Margaret Thatcher and her followers were seeking to develop in the UK.

From 'old' to 'new' Labour: employment policy since 1997

New Labour's approach to employment policy, work and welfare had its origins in the 'modernisation' of the party's ideology (see Chapter 10). The Labour Party modernisers were sympathetic to the Thatcher–Major 'flexible' employment approach (Whiteside, 1998: 104). At the same time, the focus on work also formed part of their new 'social inclusion' agenda. The modernisers were able to draw on ideas and proposals on the relationship between work and welfare put forward by its semi-formal inquiry, the Commission on Social Justice, whose approach emphasised that welfare and labour market interventions are forms of 'investment' which promote economic success, as well as being desirable on social justice grounds (Commission on Social Justice, 1994: 96–98). These are themes reiterated by such 'Third Way' commentators as Anthony Giddens (see Chapter 10) (Giddens, 1998: Ch. 4).

This work-focused welfare philosophy was criticised by some observers on the left for whom such approaches were uncomfortably reminiscent of American 'workfare'-style approaches to the poor and unemployed, in which the emphasis seems to be on re-moralising or re-socialising the unemployed. Such American commentators as Charles Murray and Lawrence Mead, especially the latter, who take the view that unemployment is a behavioural or cultural rather than a structural issue, were, it is claimed, influences on 'New' Labour thinking (Mead, 1997). It is also argued by some critics that a policy emphasis on paid work devalues other activities such as caring. New Labour's work-focused social inclusion agenda has been criticised by some writers, who have claimed to detect just such a moralising strain in its social philosophy (Levitas, 2005). The view that New Labour's policy has been 'anti-liberal' has been advanced by commentators such as Desmond King, who have argued that elements of compulsion in the Welfare to Work strategy violate a Marshallian 'social rights' perspective on benefits underpinning the welfare state since the 1940s (King, 1999).

There has certainly been an American influence on New Labour welfare and employment policy. There was a brisk trade in transatlantic policy learning, nearly all one-way, during the early and mid-1990s, and the Clinton 'New Democrats' provided models for export which New Labour modernisers were eager to acquire (King and Wickham-Jones, 1999). There has also, however, been a European (EU) influence on policy, which, in relation to work and employment, is close to the social 'investment' approach of the Commission on Social Justice (Annesley, 2003).

Stop and Think

Has New Labour been right to emphasise the importance of work as a principal component of its welfare strategy? Are there any dangers in such an emphasis?

The Welfare to Work strategy and the 'New Deals'

The Labour Party, in opposition for 18 years, won the General Election of 1997, as expected, with a large majority. Its welfare philosophy was summed up by the new Secretary of State, Harriet Harman, who was quoted as saying that 'We believe work is the best form of welfare for people of working age and that includes lone parents' (*Financial Times*, 3 July). The policy, labelled 'Welfare to Work', was designed to 'make work pay'. Gordon Brown, the new Chancellor of the Exchequer, and one of the party's principal modernisers, was quoted as saying that the government's objective was not just to 'alleviate the problem of youth and long-term unemployment for a few months' but to develop a 'welfare state built around the work ethic' (Deacon, 1997: xiii; *The Observer*, 11 May 1997).

The Labour Party had promised in its 1997 election manifesto to get 250,000 young people off benefit into work. The 'New Deal' was announced by the Chancellor in his first budget speech in 1997: £3.15 billion (later revised downwards to £2.2 billion) was made available, from a £5.2 billion 'windfall' (one-off) tax on the excess profits of the privatised utilities, to be spent over a five-year period on employment schemes. A number of different schemes were proposed, the main one being for 18–24-year-olds unemployed for six months or more. A further £350 million was provided for long-term unemployed people in other age groups out of work for two years or more. There was a separate but related New Deal for lone parents, for which £200 million was made available. Pilot schemes began in January 1998 in selected localities and the full scheme was rolled out nationally in April of that year. The programme began in a favourable economic climate, with falling unemployment.

There were a number of elements of the New Deal schemes. The 'Gateway' would prepare people for the labour market. It provided intensive job search with a personal adviser, and involved a combination of wage subsidies, training allowances, help with child care and access to material support from the Employment Service. Tailored advice would be available from Personal Advisers, followed by a move into an unsubsidised job or one of four options: six months in a subsidised job, with subsidy of £60 per week to the employer; six months with a voluntary sector organisation; six months with an environmental task force; or education and training. There would be no 'fifth option' of staying at home. Those refusing to cooperate faced loss of benefit.

In line with New Labour ideology as had been reshaped by the party's modernisers, the programme appeared to involve a 'Third Way'-ist linking of 'citizenship' responsibilities with rights (see Chapter 10).

The minimum wage

New Labour accepted the case for a uniform national minimum wage (NMW) and its 1997 election manifesto promised to introduce it for all occupations and industries (Labour Party, 1997: 17). The new government established an arms-length body, the Low Pay Commission, to make recommendations. The rationale for this was to, in some sense, 'take the issue out of politics'. Decision-making about rate-setting and enforcement of the minimum wage would, however, remain the government's responsibility. The LPC proposed the introduction of a minimum wage of £3.60 from April 1999. A lower rate should be available for young workers between the ages of 18 and 20. Young people between 16 and 17, the Commission recommended, should engage in education, training or apprenticeship, and therefore should be excluded from the provisions of the NMW. This policy was reversed in 2004 and the NMW introduced for this group at a low rate of £3 per hour.

The minimum wage was a constituent part of the government's work-focused, anti-poverty, social inclusion strategy, an aspect of its attempt to 'make work pay', in the same way that the new in-work benefits were to make work pay.

Employers argued that the minimum wage would have adverse effects on employment, and that it would in fact increase unemployment, by 'pricing workers out of jobs' (Lal, 1995). Trade unions favoured the minimum wage. They were, however, disappointed by the Low Pay Commission's recommended £3.60, having proposed a rate of at least £4 per hour. (Trade union support for minimum wages is not just an expression of altruistic social concern for workers unfortunate enough not to belong to a union. For unions engaging in collective bargaining, minimum wages provide a floor from which wage negotiations can begin, since a basic aspect of collective bargaining is the maintenance of pay differentials. The higher the floor, therefore, the higher the base from which wage bargaining can begin.)

Since 1999 minimum wage rates have risen substantially from what was perceived to be a low base, and have in fact grown faster than average earnings for much of this period. The adult rate was increased to £5.52 per hour in October 2007. This represented an increase of over 50% in the adult rate since 1999 (Taylor, 2007).

In fact the 2007 increase in the adult rate (from £5.35) represented a much lower than average increase in the minimum wage, of only 3.2%, the lowest rate of increase since 2002, and less than the average rise in annual earnings, running (in March 2007) at 3.7%. The Commission were clearly concerned about the impact of rate rises on employment opportunities in making their recommendation, given the then state of the labour market.

Discuss and Do

How should the level of the minimum wage be decided? What factors should the Low Pay Commission, and the government, take into account in deciding by how much the minimum wage should be increased every year?

Tax credits

One of the most distinctive of New Labour's policy innovations has been the introduction of tax credits for the working poor. Tax credits are part of the Welfare to Work strategy, and like other elements of it are designed to 'make work pay'. This topic is one in which social security policy and employment policy come together, since tax credits are a form of work-related social security. Another feature of these benefits is that they are paid through the tax system, by H.M. Revenue and Customs, not by a dedicated social security agency, as has been the case with all previous national cash benefits. Tax credits also reveal American influence, in the shape of the US's Earned Income Tax Credit (EITC). The principal focus of the Tax Credit regime has been on families with children, and the principal target has been child poverty. It is essentially a form of targeted assistance, and in this differs from the main form, hitherto, of cash assistance to families with children, Child Benefit, which has existed since 1945. This universal benefit is paid to all families with children, regardless of income level.

The first tax credits to be introduced were the Working Families Tax Credit and the Childcare Tax Credit. These two credits were introduced in October 1999, replacing the Conservatives' Family Credit, and paid to the main earner. Payment of the Working Families Tax Credit to the main earner represented a significant change from the payment of earlier in-work benefits, which had been paid to the carer, generally the mother. The justification for the new approach, which involved a shift of financial support from women to men, was, according to Gordon Brown, that it helped to reinforce the link between work and benefits. Further tax credits were introduced for children in 2001 and for babies in 2002. These two proved short-lived. A change came in April 2003 with their replacement by the Child Tax Credit, paid to the main carer rather than the main earner, and Working Tax Credit. The latter incorporates the adult element of the Working Families Tax Credit and the Childcare Tax Credit, and is also available for low-paid adults over the age of 25 without dependent children. From 2004 the Child Tax Credit also became available for non-working families, replacing the child elements of Income Support and Jobseekers' Allowance (JSA). The Treasury's change of policy in 2003 to credit the main carer rather than the main earner for children's cash support involved a recognition that cash given to the carer rather than the earner was more likely to be spent on the children. At the same time, of course, it also involved a reduction in earners' take-home pay.

Work–life balance and 'family-friendly' policies

An important aspect of employment policy is its relationship with policies for equality of opportunity. In this connection the family has been a particular focus of attention for New Labour. New Labour has been able to present itself as a 'pro-family' party, although in rather a different sense from that in which the Conservatives claimed to be the 'party of the family'. Labour's 'family-friendly' policies are probably better understood as woman-friendly policies, and as an aspect of its attempt to enhance its electoral appeal to women. The ideal of 'work–life' balance might be thought of as an attempt to rebalance work and home life and to mitigate the culture of excessive working hours characteristic of Anglo-Saxon capitalism, but it is as much to do with the expansion of work opportunities for women and an encouragement of men's greater participation in family life and sharing of domestic responsibilities.

These policies are, however, as much about recognising a changed reality as about influencing it. There have been dramatic changes in women's employment experience in the post-war period and Labour's policies can, as can the Conservatives' to some extent, be regarded as an acknowledgement of this. A range of policies has been pursued in connection with this agenda, including the expansion of state-subsidised nursery provision. These aspects of employment policy are explored more fully in Chapter 18.

Evaluating New Labour's employment policy

At the end of 2000, the government announced that the target of helping 250,000 young unemployed people to find work had been reached. A year later, it was claimed that 500,000 people had found jobs through the New Deal programme and that around 80% of jobs were sustained for over 13 weeks and that there was a high level of job satisfaction among those who had found work through the programme. Between 1997 and 2002 the number of 18–24-year-olds out of work and claiming

JSA for over 26 weeks fell by over 55% from 87,700 to 39,800; numbers out of work for over a year fell from 90,700 to 5,100, a 95% reduction (Finn, 2003: 123).

Such figures give a picture of unalloyed benefit from these programmes. Evaluation of the net positive effect of such policies is, however, more difficult, because of such background influences as the changing state of the economy and the demand for labour. A number of different organisations have concluded that the net effect is, however, positive. The National Audit Office, for example, reported in 2002 that the New Deal for Young People (NDYP) was 'cost-effective', had reduced youth unemployment and increased youth employment (National Audit Office, 2002). More recent evaluations of the NDYP estimate that the scheme has had a positive effect on unemployment. By 2004, according to one reported study, it had raised employment by 17,000 a year, and the social cost per job was outweighed by the social benefit (McKnight, 2005: 32–33).

Critics of the programmes have argued, on the other hand, that there has been a relatively high failure rate in terms of job placement and retention. Significant minorities of young NDYP participants return to unemployment or fail to retain it for 13 weeks. There are particular problems for ethnic minority unemployed young people and people living in economically depressed urban and regional areas where labour markets are weak, resulting in people being recycled and 'churned' through programmes (Finn, 2003: 124–125). More recent government policies have sought to address these criticisms.

The national minimum wage has, on balance, been judged a success, but it nevertheless remains controversial. Women have been among the principal beneficiaries of the NMW, unsurprisingly, given the concentration of women in low-paid sectors of the economy and in part-time work. Trade unions continue to argue that the NMW rate is still too low, while employer and business representatives suggest that larger increases would be unaffordable for firms in competitive sectors of the economy such as retail and hospitality (Taylor, 2006, 2007: 4). The Work Foundation, a left-of-centre think tank, published a glowing evaluation of the scheme in 2007 (Coats, 2007). Economists still argue, however, about the merits of such schemes, and those of a liberal market persuasion remain unconvinced (Buiter, 2006).

The tax credit regime, which had appeared to be working well during its first few years, came in for fierce and very public criticism in 2005, and some of the disadvantages of attempting to amalgamate taxes and benefits were revealed. There were substantial overpayments of tax credit to some recipients, which they were then required to repay, causing hardship.

The conclusions of recent evaluative comment on New Labour's labour market policies are that the government has succeeded, to a degree, in 're-regulating' the labour market and mitigating the worst effects of the flexible labour market regime sought by previous governments, but that there is still a long way to go in terms of achieving fairness, the creation and maintenance of workplace rights, and the general quality of working life (Brinkley *et al.*, 2007).

In terms of more fundamental issues – the impact of any of these programmes on poverty and social exclusion – the evidence is less clear. One recent poverty and social exclusion study of the effects of work and employment – not specifically concerned with evaluating New Labour's Welfare to Work programmes – suggests that work has a positive impact on poverty, but that its impact on social exclusion is less obvious. One reason why 'work pays' in the UK is that out-of-work cash support for the unemployed is so low (Bailey, 2006: 179–181). This study claims that poverty continues to be a serious problem in the UK, affecting around one-quarter of the population, and would therefore, by implication, be sceptical about the general direction of recent policy. If, on the other hand, social exclusion is identified with worklessness, then evaluation is more straightforward – policies have been successful to the extent that more people are in work. Another recent study is slightly more optimistic, claiming that poverty has been reduced among working families, although not for childless unemployed or workless families (McKnight, 2005: 43–45).

Although the government's employment strategies appear to have been successful, it is hard to disentangle the effects of these policies from the effects of the generally benign economic climate of the last 15 years. A substantial amount of the decline in unemployment that has taken place would have occurred anyway, regardless of the particular employment policies pursued, because the demand for labour has been buoyant, as the immigration influx since the mid-1990s shows. In this sense the context for employment policy has been quite different from that of the 1980s and early 1990s.

Recent developments

Employment policy continued to develop during the government's second term from 2001 to 2005. Tax credits were remodelled as described above and there was an intensification of New Deal programmes to reach 'harder to help' groups. The Employment Service (ES) and the Benefits Agency (BA) were replaced by a 'Jobcentre Plus' executive agency. This agency integrated job search support and benefit payments, in line with the views of academic advisers like Richard Layard who had criticised the separation of these two functions (Finn, 2003: 111–112, 122).

Since the 2005 General Election there has been a flurry of consultation documents ('Green Papers') and consultation exercises and special inquiries from the Department, as well as related inquiries such as the Leitch Review of Skills, sponsored by the Treasury and the Department for Education and Skills (Department for Work and Pensions, 2006c, 2007; H.M. Treasury, 2006b; Freud, 2007; Timmins, 2007f). The focus has shifted towards groups not customarily regarded as unemployed, such as disabled people on incapacity benefits.

In February 2005 the Department for Work and Pensions announced in its Five Year Strategy a long-term ambition of achieving an employment target of 80%. At that time the employment rate was about 75% (Department for Work and Pensions, 2005: 22). A target employment rate has therefore, apparently, replaced a target unemployment rate (Brinkley et al., 2007: 16). A Green Paper entitled A New Deal for Welfare: Empowering People to Work was published in January the following year (Department for Work and Pensions, 2006c; Hall and Taylor, 2006). This was essentially a strategy for developing the approach of the earlier New Deals and extending it to other groups of the economically inactive, in particular those on incapacity benefits, lone parents and older people. It reiterated previous declarations regarding the importance of work and the need to move from a 'passive' to an 'active' welfare and labour market approach, and the need to balance rights and responsibilities (Department for Work and Pensions, 2006c: 2, para. 2, 4–6). The document reiterated the ambitious 80% employment target, which will require substantial numbers of claimants to be moved off benefits and into work – 300,000 lone parents, a million people on incapacity benefits, and an increase of a million in the numbers of older people working (Department for Work and Pensions, 2006c: 3, para. 9). The strategy should also be viewed in the context of the pension reforms being hammered out at the same time by the Department in response to the Pensions Commission's 2005 Report, with its identification of the long-term decline in the ratio of workers to non-workers as a threat to the future viability of pensions provision (see Chapter 17). The Green Paper's concern with increasing the number of older workers is particularly relevant here (Department for Work and Pensions, 2006c: 3, para. 7) The government has proclaimed the effective abolition of youth unemployment, implying a shift of attention towards other groups (Timmins, 2007f).

The Department for Work and Pensions commissioned an independent review of Welfare to Work provision by the banker David Freud. (Such policy reviews by 'independent' outsiders, often drawn from the business world, have become something of a habit for this government; the Wanless review of NHS finance in 2001–02 and the Pensions Commission review, chaired by Adair Turner, of pensions policy in 2002–06 are other examples. In fact they had also been a trademark of the Thatcher style of policy-making.) Freud's main conclusion was that the private sector should play a much larger role in getting people off benefits and into work, and be paid by results for doing so (Freud, 2007).

In the wake of the Freud Report, the Department published a Green Paper, entitled *In Work, Better Off – the Next Steps to Full Employment*, as part of its welfare reform strategy in July 2007, essentially a follow-up to the 2006 Green Paper. This, partly a response to Freud, was mainly concerned with establishing appropriate roles for the public and private sectors in delivering the new Welfare to Work strategy (Timmins, 2007e). In a subsequent newspaper interview, Peter Hain, the newly appointed Secretary of State, announced a 'crusade' for the achievement of 'full employment in our generation'. He also seemed to hint at a more restricted role for the private sector than had been envisaged by his predecessor (Timmins, 2007c). Hain claimed, however, in a later speech, to have been misrepresented on this, denying that he had 'cooled' on private sector involvement and stating that '. . . there will be a greater role for private contractors' (Barker, 2007).

Conclusion

This chapter has explored various dimensions of employment policy, and traced its connections with social policy and social welfare. We have identified links between employment policy and economic policy and suggested that there is a connection between economic policy and social welfare. The contrasting experiences of post-war unemployment, before and since the 1970s, have been noted. Historically low rates of unemployment in the post-war period gave way to much higher levels subsequently, as a result of industrial restructuring brought about by globalisation and domestic economic policies. We have also glanced briefly at the employment experience of particular social groups, such as women and ethnic minorities. We have examined the impact of the policies of the Thatcher and Major governments of the 1980s and 1990s on unemployment, noting the discontinuity between these and previous post-war governments. We have discussed in some detail the labour market activation policies of recent governments, devoting particular attention to the New Deals of the Labour governments since 1997, and drawing attention to the way in which Labour policies have been influenced by those of their predecessors. Employment and other policy responses to the unemployment crisis can be seen to have evolved from 'passive' to 'active', and from an initial concern with youth unemployment to a concern with the longer-term unemployed. We have examined the prevailing philosophy that work is a source of welfare, noting that Labour have emphasised the 'welfare' and 'social justice' aspects of this relationship to a greater extent than their predecessors. We have noted the way that the goals of employment policy have been subtly reinterpreted, in that an unemployment target has been replaced by an employment target. We have also noted in passing the important connections that exist between employment policy and other areas of social policy, such as education and training policy, family policy, pensions policy and even (with the recent shift in policy towards 'harder to help' groups of the unemployed, such as those on incapacity benefits) health policy.

In this chapter you have been introduced to:

- the nature and purposes of employment policy, and the role of employment policy in relation to the pursuit of social welfare;
- the relation between employment policy and other areas of social and public policy;
- an exploration of trends in the British labour market since the 1970s;
- the development of in-work benefits and the partial integration of the tax and benefits system that has taken place since 1997 with the introduction of tax credits for the working poor.

Annotated further reading

There is a good chapter on employment policy in Rodney Lowe's *The Welfare State in Britain since 1945* (Lowe, 2005: Ch. 5). Two useful short books on unemployment and unemployment policy which deal with the subject historically are Sean Glynn's *No Alternative? Unemployment in Britain* (Glynn, 1991) and Noel Whiteside's *Bad Times: Unemployment in British social and political history* (Whiteside, 1991). There are good individual chapters on various aspects of employment policy in various edited collections, by Bailey (2006), Bryson (2003), Cressey (1999), Finn (2003), McKnight (2005), Robert Taylor (1994, 2001, 2005) and Whiteside (1998).

The Work Foundation, a left-of-centre think-tank, has published useful, critical, but sympathetic, evaluations of the first 10 years of Labour's employment policies in two reports by Coats (2007) and Brinkley *et al.* (2007). Brinkley *et al.* also provide (Ch. 2) a valuable survey of changes in the British labour market since the mid-1980s. These reports can be downloaded from the Work Foundation's website. The House of Commons Work and Pensions Committee has published a useful recent report on the government's most recent phase of employment policy (House of Commons Work and Pensions Committee, 2007), downloadable from the House of Commons website.

Finally, for those wanting some economic policy background to employment policy, there are some useful and accessible articles in edited collections by economic journalists such as Samuel Brittan (1989), Peter Jay (1994), Philip Stephens (2001) and David Smith (2005). Smith, the *Sunday Times*'s economics correspondent, also provides easy-to-read, balanced accounts of economic policy in the 1980s in *The Rise and Fall of Monetarism* and *From Boom to Bust* (Smith, 1987, 1993), as does Christopher Johnson in *The Economy under Mrs Thatcher 1979–1990* (Johnson, 1991). *The Observer*'s William Keegan does something similar for the 1990s and 2000s in *The Prudence of Mr Gordon Brown* (Keegan, 2004).

Chapter 17

Pensions policy

Objectives

- To introduce you to the main features of the UK pensions system.

- To provide an introduction to basic pension concepts and issues, and criteria for evaluating pensions systems.

- To examine the evolution of the present UK system.

- To explore some of the problems of the present UK system, in relation to issues of adequacy, equity and sustainability.

- To explore the recent evolution of pensions policy under New Labour.

- To examine reform initiatives associated with the work of the Pensions Commission and the government's response to this.

Introduction

Why should we study pensions policy? For many of you, pensions may seem a remote, relatively specialised and perhaps uninteresting topic. It is the aim, and hope, of this chapter to persuade you that it is otherwise. After all, at the very least, pensions are something that we all hope to enjoy one day. The present chapter is intended to be a case study of a particular, important, area of social provision. There are a number of reasons why such a study is worthwhile.

- Pensions policy is a major area of public policy and of public spending, in terms of the number of people affected by it, and the volume of financial resources devoted to it.

- It is an area of public policy which some people think is in crisis, at any rate in the United Kingdom; in this sense, it is a classic 'welfare state crisis' issue, and a policy area experiencing substantial reform at the present time.

- It is a policy area which in the United Kingdom exemplifies the idea of a 'mixed economy of welfare', or 'welfare pluralism', in which the private sector as well as the public sector are important.

- Pensions is a policy area which touches on other policy issues – ageing, ageism and discrimination, gender, the labour market and employment policy. 'Ageism' in this context might refer not only to the idea that the elderly retired are losers or excluded in various ways, but also to the idea that they are or might be relatively privileged in relation to younger groups – the idea of a 'conflict of generations' which has figured in some recent discussions.

- It is a policy area with interesting characteristics. The effects and consequences of pensions policy are temporally remote, being long-term rather than short-term; policy makers must think and plan many decades ahead. In this way pensions policy is, with its distant time horizons, rather like environmental policy.

- Finally, it is an area which affects all of us as beneficiaries or as contributors; we will, if we are lucky, live long enough to retire from full-time work and receive a pension, and in any case those of us who are or will be in full-time employment are involved in contributing, in one way or another, to the pensions of those who are now retired. None of us can escape involvement in pensions issues and policy.

Concepts and definitions

At its simplest, a pension is an income paid to someone who has withdrawn from full-time involvement in the labour market and paid work. It is invariably age-related and associated with *retirement*. In Britain, for example, the minimum age at which one can claim the basic state retirement pension is 65 for a man and 60 for a woman, although the ages will be equalised at 65 by 2020. Individuals can defer claiming a pension until 70 and there are financial advantages in doing this.

Pensions may be viewed as a form of *deferred income*. A worker pays in to a pension scheme during their working life, foregoing current income, and in return establishes a future claim on resources.

Alternatively, one can view it as a form of *insurance* against the risk of eventually being unable to work. It involves a pooling of risks, either at the level of a whole society as with state pensions schemes, or at the level of an individual enterprise, pension fund or insurance company with private schemes.

Pensions can be viewed as a form of *redistribution*, in which an individual redistributes income over his or her lifetime, from a period in which the individual is working to that in which the individual is no longer working. Redistribution is also involved in the transfer of resources from the working to the non-working, since retirement incomes and the current consumption of the retired must be paid for by the current production of those in work. The current generation of workers foregoes income which is used to support the current generation of retired persons.

Historical development

The concept of 'retirement' – full or partial withdrawal from paid work or remunerative occupation – is a comparatively recent one in Western societies, as is the development of pensions and pension systems as forms of income maintenance for the retired. Prior to this, people had tended to work until they were no longer able to, and there was no idea of a fixed age of retirement. Such 'learned professions' as law, medicine, the Church and university teaching, for example, were considered to be lifetime careers, and owners of businesses did not necessarily expect to have to retire at a particular age (Hill, 2007, Ch. 5).

Before the development of various public and private pension schemes, individuals who withdrew from the labour market and full-time employment might expect to be supported by the sale of assets, such as land, farms or businesses, or by their families, if without assets. Charitable support might also be available from religious and other organisations. In many countries, including England, poor law systems evolved in the early modern period to support the destitute elderly, those unable to work or lacking family support. The English Poor Law dates from 1601. Such locally funded and administered support might take the form of 'outdoor relief', a cash payment, in other words a form of social security, but might also be provided 'in kind', in the form of residential accommodation in poor houses or workhouses. From the mid-nineteenth century in Britain, especially after the amendment of the Poor Law in 1834, the latter was the preferred form of relief on the part of policy makers, but never succeeded in wholly supplanting outdoor cash relief. Poor Law outdoor relief, when it was available, was never generous. The policy emphasis in Britain before the twentieth century was on the encouragement of 'self-help' in various forms, which could include membership in and support from mutual aid organisations such as friendly societies, voluntary saving, and support from family members.

The inadequacy of the Poor Law, as far as the elderly poor were concerned, was increasingly recognised by the late nineteenth century, recognition that was assisted by the researches of social investigators such as Charles Booth. The development of a pensions agenda was the outcome of several decades of public debate and agitation over the issue of old age poverty, influenced by among other things, increasing life expectancy in the late nineteenth century, the desire of employers to get rid of older workers and to attract and retain younger workers, and the growth of democracy (Hill, 2007: 6–7).

A variety of private institutions, such as friendly societies, commercial insurance companies and building societies, were established, grew and expanded in coverage during the nineteenth century to provide savings opportunities and a degree of collective insurance against risks. These broadly exemplified a 'self-help' approach. Coverage was, however, mostly limited to those, such as the middle classes and skilled manual workers, in full-time regular employment. For that substantial proportion of the Victorian workforce whose employment was casual and irregular and earnings low, private schemes had little to offer.

The first public non-Poor Law financial support for elderly retired people in the UK, the Old Age Pension, was introduced in 1908, a measure passed by a reforming Liberal government (Macnicol, 1998: Ch. 6, 155–163). The pension was non-contributory, in that it was financed out of general taxation, was only available from the age of 70, was means-tested and only available to persons of 'good character' – the 'deserving', in other words. It was also, at a rate of 5s (25p) per week for a single person when introduced in 1909, below subsistence level.

Legislation in 1925 by a Conservative government saw the introduction of a state National Insurance-based retirement pension for limited classes of beneficiaries, funded by National Insurance contributions paid by employees and employers and a small Exchequer subsidy (widows' pensions were also introduced as part of the same measure). This was an 'add on' to the National Insurance employment and sickness benefit schemes introduced by the Liberals in 1911. This supplemented, rather than replaced, the 1908 scheme (Gilbert, 1970: Ch. 5, 235–351; Macnicol, 1998: Ch. 9).

Important legislation took place in 1946, when a Labour government enacted most of the proposals of the Beveridge Report. Beveridge envisaged what was essentially an extension of the 1925 scheme so that it became universal and ongoing rather than age-limited, and abolition of the 1908 scheme. It was underpinned by the basic Beveridge principles of flat-rate contributions for flat-rate benefits (although with additions for dependants) and universality, and exemplified the British version of the social insurance model (Harris, 1997, 2006). With modifications, this has survived to the present day. The Beveridge Report and the legislation based upon it embodied assumptions about the family and gender roles which have largely ceased to apply. The family was treated as a unit, men were assumed to be the only or major income provider, and married women were treated as homemakers and assumed to be dependent (Thane, 2006b: 82–85).

The government chose to implement the pension provisions of the 1946 National Insurance Act immediately, rejecting Beveridge's proposed 20-year build-up and accumulation of contributions. The system therefore became a 'pay as you go' scheme, rather than a funded one; the contributions of the current generation of workers paid for the pensions of the current generation of pensioners. Another problem with the 1946 scheme was the meagre level of benefits, well below subsistence level (and contrary to Beveridge's intentions). The flat-rate principle meant that benefit levels had to be low, since contribution levels had to be low enough for the lowest-paid worker to be able to afford them. Beveridge himself had never aimed at providing a generous state pension that would bring the beneficiary above subsistence level. He believed that individuals should, if they wished, supplement their basic state pension with their own voluntary forms of pension saving. British pension arrangements may be contrasted with developments in many other countries, including the United States, which established earnings-related public pension systems in this period.

Another component of the Beveridge–Labour approach of the 1940s was the retention of means-tested, non-contributory tax-financed social assistance, providing a cash benefit which would bring beneficiaries up to a specified level of weekly income, if their income and resources were below this, and would include an allowance for housing costs, something that the National Insurance state retirement pension failed to do. It was envisaged at the time that this would be a residual element, of decreasing importance, in the income support package for retired people. This means-tested benefit, which has undergone numerous changes of name in the last 60 years and is now known as Pension Credit, did not fade away into insignificance as envisaged. The reason for this has been the inadequacy of the basic National Insurance state pension, which has always been below the level of means-tested assistance which itself constitutes an unofficial poverty line – so anyone with only the state pension to depend on has had to apply for means-tested supplementation in order to make ends meet.

The subsequent history of public pensions is mainly a history of *ad hoc* piecemeal tinkering with the system established in the 1940s. Important changes were introduced in the 1970s, however, by another Labour government, which introduced an additional pension, or earnings-related supplement to the basic pension, called the State Earnings-Related Pension (SERPS).

By the 1970s the idea of married women as non-working dependants was coming under attack, and some changes in policy reflected the impact of changing views. The married women's option to pay a reduced National Insurance contribution which had existed since 1948 and enabled a married woman to claim a pension as her husband's dependant – was phased out in 1977. In 1978 a Home Responsibilities Credit was introduced which enabled married women with a contribution record to credit years spent out of the labour market engaged in family and caring responsibilities and thereby improve their contribution record and eventually claim a larger pension.

Conservative governments under Margaret Thatcher and John Major from 1979 to 1997 carried out some limited reforms of pensions policy. Their priority was to reduce pension spending commitments by attempting to limit the generosity of state pensions, but they did not fundamentally alter the structure of public pension provision. The basic state pension became subject to uprating in line with prices rather than earnings after 1980, which helped to limit cost increases, but entailed a reduction in quality, since earnings increases consistently outstripped price increases in this period and subsequently (by contrast with the 1970s). SERPS – the National Insurance-based earnings-related 'top-up' pension – was reformed and made less generous in 1986, as part of the Fowler review of social security, to reduce its future cost. The government succeeded in limiting the long-run rise in pension costs, but did not otherwise deal with underlying problems of the system.

The Conservatives saw occupational pension schemes as inflexible and as inhibiting labour mobility. Workers were, it was believed, less willing to change jobs and employers, given that pension transfers were sometimes difficult or impossible and, where possible, the terms were sometimes ungenerous. The Conservatives for this reason encouraged membership of personal pensions. These allowed for 'portability' and easy transfer. In 1987 the government extended the right to contract-out from SERPS, already in existence for occupational pensions, by permitting contracting-out into either a group or individual Approved Personal Pension.

Pension policy since 1997 is discussed in the section below on New Labour pensions policy.

Structure of UK pension provision

The pensions system 'model' embodied in UK arrangements is a three-tier model and approximately conforms to the OECD classification of pensions systems in terms of 'tiers' (or 'pillars', the term preferred by the World Bank in its 1994 Report) (World Bank, 1994; OECD, 2005; Hill, 2007: Ch. 4). There is a *first tier* consisting of universal means-tested coverage, now known as the Pension Credit, which aims at achieving at least subsistence level income. In the UK context this either tops up the state or other pension, or substitutes for these completely where these do not exist. There is a *second tier* constituted by the basic State Retirement Pension (BSP) and by the State Second Pension (S2P), and by the State Earnings

Related Pension Scheme (SERPS), the predecessor to S2P. There is, finally, a *third tier* of private occupational or personal provision, which is voluntary; this will often or usually substitute for the second-tier SERPS or S2P.

There are, therefore, up to three components to the first- and second-tier state pension system, but of course not everyone will receive or be entitled to all three. There is in principle universal entitlement to all three, but only the BSP is effectively universal, in that virtually all persons who have been in full-time employment for a minimum qualifying period, even the very rich, will receive it. Entitlement to BSP, S2P and its predecessor SERPS are earned through making contributions to the National Insurance (NI) scheme; it is therefore employment-related. Pension Credit, by contrast, is tax-financed. In principle, full entitlement to BSP and SERPS or S2P should take a recipient of these benefits above the threshold for Pension Credit, but it is not clear that it does so (Evandrou and Falkingham, 2005: 183–184).

Pensioners may also be able to claim additional benefits such as Housing Benefit and Council Tax Benefit. Retired persons also enjoy a range of subsidised consumption benefits or earmarked extra payments such as winter fuel allowance, free television licences from the age of 75 and subsidised travel by public transport.

'Private' or voluntary provision: occupational and personal pensions

Occupational pensions may be viewed as a component of an employee's total rewards package, along with other components of pay and conditions (in this sense a pension may be regarded as 'deferred pay'). Occupational pension coverage grew extensively after the war amongst manual as well as white-collar occupations, often as a result of collective bargaining between trade unions and employers.

The state's S2P is an alternative to voluntary provision. The state does not compel firms to provide pension schemes for their workforces, but where such schemes exist they are subject to a degree of state oversight and regulation and are subsidised. A firm which provides an occupational pensions scheme for its workforce providing benefits at least as good as those from S2P may opt out of the latter; in this case, the employer receives a rebate of the NI contributions paid which subsidise investment in the employers' own occupational scheme. Subsidy is also available in the form of tax relief on pension contributions. The amounts involved are substantial – around £12 billion in tax reliefs and £7 billion in NI rebates in 2004–05 (Pensions Commission, 2005: 25–26).

Private sector occupational pensions, provided by employers for their workforces, are of two types, '*defined benefit*' (DB) and '*defined contribution*' (DC). These are usually 'group' (as opposed to personal or individual) schemes and both types are what are called 'funded', as opposed to 'pay as you go' (PAYG), schemes. In recent years DB schemes have been in decline, while the number of DC schemes has been growing. DC schemes offer advantages to employers by comparison with DB schemes, because they do not involve an open-ended commitment to fund a particular level of retirement income for employees.

DB pension schemes, also called 'final salary' schemes, guarantee a pension which is a proportion of an employer's final salary, usually calculated on the basis of the number of years the employee has been in the scheme. A DC scheme (also known as a 'money purchase' scheme), on the other hand, offers no such guarantee. Pension contributions are deducted at a defined rate as a percentage of salary and invested, as with DB schemes, in a fund provided by an independent fund manager but, unlike DB schemes, the value of the pension actually paid out will depend purely on the size of the pension 'pot' thus accumulated, which will in turn depend firstly on the contribution rate and secondly on the performance of the assets – varying proportions of shares, bonds, property and cash – in which the fund invests. The fund management industry in the UK is a large and diversified one, with many institutions providing a variety of pension-related services, including investment management and annuities (see below). These are commercial organisations, which charge for their services, and the costs involved in setting up and managing pension schemes can be significant.

Public sector occupational pensions are mainly (local government and pre-1992 university schemes are exceptions) unfunded 'pay as you go' (PAYG) schemes, paid for ultimately out of taxation. There is a simple transfer, in which the current generation of workers pays for the pensions of the current generation of beneficiaries through taxes and National Insurance contributions (Pensions Commission, 2004: 12). Public sector occupational schemes are invariably of the DB type.

Personal pensions

Personal pensions are pension schemes for individuals. One of the supposed advantages of these is greater 'portability' – a personal pension is in some sense the property of the individual and can be taken with him or her when changing jobs. Personal pensions must necessarily be of the funded, DC type. Although private, these schemes are regulated and subsidised by the government via tax reliefs and NI rebates. One problem with most personal pension schemes is that of costs – annual management charges – which are typically much higher than those of the large group policies operated by employers.

Annuities

In DC schemes the lump sum or pension 'pot' accumulated must by law be converted into an income stream by purchasing what is called an annuity from a pension provider, such as an insurance company. A lump sum is thereby exchanged for a regular, usually monthly, payment. The annuity is funded by the purchase of long-dated bonds or 'gilts', government debt, which pays a high rate of interest. Annuities are of different kinds; they may be 'flat', that is, un-indexed and stay the same over the recipient's lifetime, or they may be indexed so that they increase year-on-year. They may or may not include provision for surviving partners.

Pension expenditure

Figures for pension spending vary considerably, depending on the assumptions used. The OECD gives what at first glance appears to be a high figure for total state pension spending in the UK of just over 8% of GDP. The Pension Commission gives an apparently lower overall figure of 4.8% of GDP in 2002, 6.1% if council tax and housing benefits are included, or 6.9% if unfunded public sector pensions are included, these figures all referring to normal-age retirees. If pensions and lump sums paid to public-sector early retirees are included, the overall figure for public spending amounts to 7.6%, a figure closer to the OECD total for state spending. The OECD figure appears a little higher because it includes all pension and disability benefits paid to claimants at all ages, not just to the over-65 population. Private pension spending adds between 3% and 4% of GDP (Pensions Commission, 2004: 25, Appendix D, page 105; Hill, 2007: 90, Table 4.2). These figures may be compared with those for expenditure in other OECD countries, with due regard for the difficulties of comparing (see Figure 17.1 reproduced from the Pension Commission's 2004 Report, which describes them as 'very imperfect estimates'). Compared with such countries as France, Germany and Italy, a higher proportion of UK spending is private, although UK private pension spending is smaller as a proportion of GDP than that in the US, Canada, Australia and the Netherlands. The UK's system clearly exhibits features of a 'mixed economy of welfare' or a higher degree of 'welfare pluralism' in comparison with continental European systems.

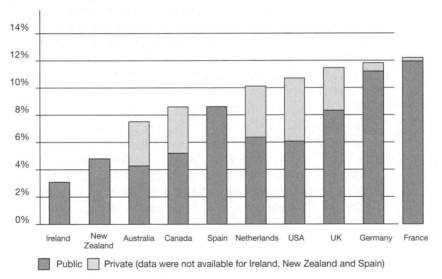

Public ▪   Private ▫ (data were not available for Ireland, New Zealand and Spain)

Note: The figures from the OECD for the UK differ from those used in the report because all pension transfers are included, not just to the population aged over 65, and because disability benefits paid at all ages are included.

Figure 17.1   Total pension expenditure as a percentage of GDP (according to the source, very imperfect estimates)
Source: OECD (2004) Social Expenditure Database, 1980–2001.

Evaluating pension provision: coverage, adequacy and inequality

There are a number of criteria for evaluating systems of pension provision. Systems may be evaluated in terms of *coverage*; in terms of the extent of *income replacement*; and in terms of *poverty prevention*, *inequality* or standard of living *adequacy*

(Hill, 2007: Ch. 3). 'Coverage' means the proportion of the population covered by pension schemes, as both contributors and recipients. The 'income replacement rate' is the ratio of a recipient's pension income to income from past earnings, in other words the proportion of earnings, given as a percentage, that pension income replaces. 'Poverty prevention' means the extent to which the system raises the incomes of people to or above an agreed standard of poverty. For example, in the European Union, the 'poverty level' is an income level of 60% of median income. In the following sections we shall examine the British pension system in the light of some of these criteria.

Coverage

Table 17.1 provides information about pension coverage in the UK. It shows that pension coverage is almost universal; 98% of persons of retirement age have a pension of some sort. 31% have only state pension benefits – Basic State Pension, SERPS, Minimum Income Guarantee (MIG) or Pension Credit (PC). 67% have some kind of 'private' pension, occupational or personal ('private' in this context includes public sector occupational pensions). Of course, most people in this group will also have one or more state pensions, since in addition to the Basic State Pension they may also be receiving MIG/PC, if their private occupational or personal pension is insufficient to take them above the eligibility threshold for this means-tested benefit.

There are, however, exclusions even from state pension coverage, principally among those on low earnings and working part-time. It was estimated that in 2002/03 around 5 million people were not accruing rights to any state pension (Evandrou and Falkingham, 2005: 184).

Private pension coverage is, unfortunately, far from universal and has been declining for several decades. Occupational pension scheme membership peaked in 1967 and contributions to such schemes as a share of GDP peaked in 1981 (Hills, 2006: 186). The problem with this state of affairs is, of course, that those excluded from private coverage tend to be people on low and interrupted earnings.

Income replacement

The British *state* pension system is, however, one of the least generous in the OECD group of countries – the 'developed' countries – in terms of 'replacement rate'. It delivers a lower level of pension income, relative to earnings, than those of continental Europe and even the USA. Most of the former provide a retirement level of income of at least 70% of working life earnings. At average earnings, the UK state system delivers a 37% earnings replacement rate, compared with 70% in the Netherlands, 76% in Sweden, 71% in France and 45% in the USA. At twice average earnings, the UK state system delivers 24%, the Netherlands 70%, Sweden 72%, France 54% and the USA 33% (Pensions Commission, 2004: 58). (The UK percentages assume full SERPS/S2P entitlement, in addition to the basic state pension.) The UK belongs with a group of countries – Ireland, Canada and New Zealand – whose state pension systems are aimed at poverty prevention rather than income replacement. Some observers have celebrated this state of affairs, contending that the UK system is therefore more fiscally sustainable in the long run than these foreign systems. The UK is predicted, given a

Table 17.1 Pension receipt (percentage): by type of pensioner unit, Great Britain, 2003/04[1,2]

	Pensioner couples	Single male pensioners	Single female pensioners	All pensioners
Includes retirement pension/minimum income guarantee/pension credit only	17	28	44	31
Plus				
Occupational, but not personal pension	64	58	50	57
Personal, but not occupational pension	9	9	2	6
Both occupational and personal pension	8	3	2	4
All including state pension	99	98	98	98
Other combinations, no retirement pension /minimum income guarantee/pension credit[3]	0	1	0	0
None	1	1	2	1
All people	100	100	100	100

1 A pensioner unit is defined as either a single person over state pension age (60 for women, 65 for men), or a couple where the man is over state pension age.

2 Data are consistent with Pensioners' Incomes Series methodology.

3 People receiving some combination of an occupational or personal pension only.

Source: Office for National Statistics (2006a) *Social Trends 36*, Table 8.8, p. 119, London: ONS. Crown copyright material is reproduced with the permission of the Controller of HMSO and the Queen's Printer for Scotland under the terms of the Click-Use Licence. *Original source*: Family Resources Survey, Department for Work and Pensions.

continuation of current pension policies, to spend a smaller proportion of GDP in 2050 than it does now, the only member of the EU15 group of countries in this position (Pensions Commission, 2004: 61, Table 3.1). Many other EU countries will require substantial increases in taxation or social insurance contributions in the coming decades to fund higher levels of pension spending. Private provision makes the difference in the UK pension system, making it more comparable to other countries in terms of the volume of resources directed towards the retired population, but private pension resources are unequally distributed, the better-off gaining most.

Poverty prevention and inequality

In relation to the third criterion, that of pensioners' living standards, poverty prevention and inequality, there has been an improvement overall in the standard of living of pensioners in the UK in recent decades. Between 1979 and 1996/97 average gross incomes of pensioner households increased by 62%, compared with an increase in real average earnings of 38% over the same period. This increase was unequally distributed, however; incomes for the richest fifth increased three times faster than for the poorest fifth of the population, and the increase of 31% for the lowest fifth between 1979 and 1996/97 was below the increase in average earnings (Evandrou and Falkingham, 2005: 168). To that extent, the degree of relative deprivation for this group increased during the period.

Although pensioners are more likely to be poor than the general population, their position relative to younger age groups has, it has been claimed, improved (Miles, 2002: 46). Old age is no longer invariably characterised by poverty for the mass of the population. Inequality in pensioners' incomes and standards of living mirrors that among the population at large. Women in old age are more likely to be poor than men, however, and women are more likely to experience more years of low-income poverty than men, as they live longer.

A rather gloomier picture of pensioner poverty is painted by the authors of the Poverty and Social Exclusion Survey, whose findings suggest that, depending on the measures used and the type of pensioner household considered, between 32% and 62% of pensioner households are in poverty (Patsios, 2006: 433, Table 15.1). Even compared with MIG benefit levels, between 7% and 46% of pensioner households are in poverty (MIG levels are for 2001 and MIG has since 2003 been replaced by Pension Credit). These results are, however, based on a survey carried out in 1999, with additional information from the 2001 census, so may not fairly reflect the present situation.

The claim that those pensioners living on state benefits have seen a particular improvement in their standard of living since 1997 is made in the government's 2006 White Paper on pension reform (it is repeated in Tony Blair's prime ministerial foreword to the White Paper) (Department for Work and Pensions, 2006a). The claim has been challenged by pressure groups such as Help the Aged, who deny Ministerial claims that 2 million pensioners have been lifted out of poverty since 1997 and argue that the proportion of pensioners living below the poverty line – 20% – is the same as in 1997. Further, the claim that pensioners' incomes have improved faster than the general rate of increase in incomes is false, and overlooks the differences among pensioners – the recently retired have larger incomes than older pensioners (Kohler, 2006, letter).

These comments are not entirely fair, since the DWP make it clear in the White Paper that they distinguish between absolute and relative poverty, and the 2 million figure refers to changes in absolute poverty. For relative poverty the figure is a moderately respectable 1 million. (The DWP poverty standard is 60% of median income.) The DWP figures suggest that there has been a fall from around 27% of pensioners in relative poverty to around 17% between 1996/97 and 2004/05 (Department for Work and Pensions, 2006a: 3–4).

Table 17.2 provides information about persistent low income among pensioner households by comparison with other groups. ('Persistent' is defined as three years out of four below 60% of median income, the poverty line used by the EU.) It shows that the incidence of persistent low income is higher for pensioners and that their position has changed little from the period 1996–99 to 2000–03, slightly improving for single pensioners. This contrasts with the position for singles and couples with children, which has shown some improvement over the same period, although not a dramatic one.

An issue that is a particular cause for concern, for the Pensions Commission and the authors of the British Academy study, for example, is the position of women (Pensions Commission, 2004: Ch. 8; Ginn, 2006; Thane, 2006b). Among those recently retiring, 85% of men have entitlement to a full basic state pension, compared to 30% of women (Department for Work and Pensions, 2006a: 12). Table 17.1 shows that a higher proportion of single female pensioners is wholly dependent on state benefits than is the case with men, and that male pensioners are more likely to have occupational and personal pensions.

There are a number of explanations for this. The inequalities experienced by older women are partly a reflection of the inequalities experienced by women earlier in life.

Table 17.2 Persistent low income (percentage): by family type, Great Britain, 1991–2003[1]

	3 out of 4 years below 60% of median income[2]			Entry rate into persistent low income[3] 1991–2003	Exit rate from persistent low income[3] 1991–2003
	1991–94	1996–99	2000–03		
Pensioner couple	13	17	17	2	9
Single pensioner	21	23	21	3	10
Couple with children	13	11	10	1	17
Couple without children	3	3	4	1	21
Single with children	40	27	23	3	16
Single without children	5	7	7	1	34
All individuals	12	11	11	1	16

1 Families are classified according to their type in the first year of the relevant period.
2 Equivalised contemporary household disposable income before housing costs. See Appendix, Part 5: Households Below Average Income, and Equivalisation scales.
3 Persistent low income is defined as experiencing low income for at least three consecutive years. An entry occurs during the first year of a persistent low income period, following a period of two years not in low income. An exit occurs as the first year of two not in low income, following a persistent low income period.
Source: Office for National Statistics (2006a) *Social Trends 36*, Table 5.20, p. 82, London: ONS. Crown copyright material is reproduced with the permission of the Controller of HMSO and the Queen's Printer for Scotland under the terms of the Click-Use Licence. *Original source:* Department for Work and Pensions from the British Household Panel Survey, Institute for Social and Economic Research.

The current generation of older women is less likely to have worked and to have experienced longer periods of interruption of work and earning because of caring responsibilities. Women's pension contribution histories are more likely to have been disrupted, and their ability to establish claims and entitlements providing them with adequate incomes thereby compromised. Another important factor is that of marriage break-up, divorce, and the increase in numbers of lone-parent households. In the UK lone parenthood has been associated with fewer opportunities for full-time employment. Women are more likely to work part-time, although, counterbalancing this, they are more likely to work in public-sector occupations such as teaching, nursing and care provision, which generally have a better record of retirement provision for part-timers.

Table 17.3 Ownership of occupational and personal pensions (percentage): working-age adults, by sex and age at last birthday, Great Britain, 2003/04

	16–24	25–34	35–44	45–54	55–59	60–64	All aged 16–59/64
Men							
Personal pension	2	12	20	20	21	11	15
Occupational pension	9	36	44	42	29	13	33
Any non-state pension	11	46	61	59	48	23	46
Women							
Personal pension	2	7	9	10	9		8
Occupational pension	11	35	37	38	27		32
Any non-state pension	13	41	44	46	35		38

Source: Office for National Statistics (2006a) *Social Trends 36*, Table 5.23, p. 84, London: ONS. Crown copyright material is reproduced with the permission of the Controller of HMSO and the Queen's Printer for Scotland under the terms of the Click-Use Licence. *Original source*: Family Resources Survey, Department for Work and Pensions.

Present trends in women's employment are helping to overcome some of these problems as women enter higher-paid and professional occupations in greater numbers and experience longer periods of full-time employment. Table 17.3 suggests that there is less gender inequality in occupational and personal pension ownership among younger age cohorts.

A pension 'crisis'?

As recently as the 1990s it was complacently assumed that the UK possessed a basically satisfactory pension system, conforming closely to the three-pillar pension ideal advocated by the World Bank in the 1990s (World Bank, 1994). In recent years the otherwise upbeat mood has dissipated, and the term 'crisis' has come to be applied to pension systems in the UK, as it has to those in some other countries (Parker, 2006).

Some analysts deny, however, that there is a *general* UK pensions crisis, in the sense of a deficiency of aggregate pension savings (Pemberton *et al.*, 2006c: 2). Nor is there a crisis of affordability in the public system in the UK, not simply because UK public pension expenditure is low by international standards, but because governments can always meet their pension obligations, whatever they are, by raising taxes or contributions. There is no question of resources failing to match obligations in a public PAYG system.

It does seem clear, however, that the fabric of the British system has undergone a degree of unravelling since the 1990s, and has been adversely affected by a number of events: the decline in occupational pensions; the fall in share prices associated with the bear market of 2000–03 and the collapse of the 'dot com' boom, which seriously reduced the value of most pension fund assets; the introduction of an increase in pension fund tax liability by the government in 1997 which has cost the fund management industry £5bn per year; the move to greater transparency in company accounting as a result of changes in reporting rules, which require a company's pension liabilities to be identified clearly on the company's balance sheet; and falls in annuity rates since the 1990s which mean that a pension 'pot' of a given size will, other things being equal, now buy a smaller pension.

A number of social and demographic changes have also been important in compromising the integrity of the British pension system. The British population, like others, is ageing, at around two years per decade on average. Estimates of future population ageing have had to be revised upwards, to the consternation of private pension providers. Ageing adds to pension costs, and has helped to undermine the assumptions on which occupational final-salary (DB) schemes have operated. Another factor is the trend towards earlier retirement that has spread in Britain and other European countries since the 1970s. A high proportion of men between the ages of 60 and 65 have withdrawn from full-time work, and the average age of retirement has gone down. There has, finally, been the decline in the British birth rate since the 'baby boom' that lasted from the 1940s to the 1960s. The 'dependency ratio' has fallen – the ratio of the working to the dependent population – implying that fewer workers are becoming available to finance the pensions of the retired with their contributions. Such trends have implications for the future funding of pensions and the maintenance of pensioners' living standards (Hill, 2007: Ch. 6).

Accompanying these developments have been trends and developments in state provision. One of these is the continuing decline in the value of the basic state pension as a proportion of average earnings as a result of its being indexed to prices rather than earnings since 1982, a state of affairs not reversed by Labour after 1997. Coupled with this is the gradual spread of means-testing with the introduction of the Minimum Income Guarantee, and its consolidation as the Pension Credit (PC). While not in itself constitutive of a 'crisis', the spread of means-testing is widely felt to be unacceptable (it has been estimated that as many as 70% of the retired population might be eligible for the Pension Credit by 2050).

There has been a loss of public confidence in the pension system in recent years, for which a number of factors are responsible. One is the pension mis-selling scandal of the late 1980s and 1990s, in which, encouraged by government policy, individuals were induced to leave perfectly good occupational schemes and take out personal pensions which were sometimes inferior in quality. Another confidence-undermining event was the plundering of the Mirror Group Newspapers pension fund by the Group's owner, the tycoon Robert Maxwell, in the late 1980s. This demonstrated that members of pension funds had less protection from the unscrupulous than had been believed. A third was the Equitable Life scandal, in which an insurance company apparently defaulted on its pension promises to policy holders.

One interpretation of the problem of the British pension system is that it is a simple one of inadequate spending and saving. More money needs to be spent and, by implication, saved. Britons are saving too little, both individually and collectively (Glennerster, 2006: 64). People are, it may be argued, too short-sighted to think and save for the long-term future. This has led to suggestions for a degree of compulsion in pension saving. An alternative view would be that the overall volume of pension saving and spending is not inadequate. What is problematic is its distribution. There are too many gaps in coverage and too great a degree of inequality, primarily in earnings (Miles, 2002: 50).

Complexity makes it very difficult for individuals to make rational pension planning decisions. The array of benefits, public and private, and their interactions, make such planning difficult. The existence of the earnings-indexed Pension Credit, for example, would seem to make it less worthwhile for individuals to save or make private pension provision, since the value of this will, if price-indexed, be overtaken by that of the Pension Credit, and in any case the value of such private savings and pensions the individual might have will be set against Pension Credit entitlements. Similarly, the shift from DB to DC occupational schemes has had the effect of making it much more difficult for the individual to calculate the future value of pension benefits, or indeed how much needs to be saved to provide a decent income in retirement.

Policy developments under New Labour

A 'New' Labour government with Tony Blair as Prime Minister was elected in 1997 and a Green Paper on pensions was published the following year (Department of Social Security, 1998). Labour's first priority was, however, in line with historical practice, not to think about large-scale reform of the system but to improve the incomes and living standards of pensioners dependent on state benefits immediately. 'Getting current pensioners cash has always been given preference over long-term reconstruction' (Glennerster, 2006: 72). This meant raising benefit rates and encouraging take-up. The new government refused, however, contrary to presumed commitments made while in opposition, to return to uprating the basic state pension in line with earnings rather than prices. A revamped system of means-tested support was, initially, the means of achieving improvements. The means-tested element of public provision, now known as Pension Credit, has been uprated annually in line with average earnings, unlike the basic state pension, which continues to be uprated in line with prices. In other words, eligibility for this benefit is growing and will continue to grow. The government also modified the earnings-related 'top-up' to the basic pension, replacing SERPS with the State Second Pension (S2P), which is more generous to lower earners.

The 1998 Green Paper endorsed the 'mixed economy' approach of all post-war governments and proposed an even larger role for the private sector, which, it was envisaged, should eventually account for 60% of all pension provision, as opposed to the then current 40% (Department of Social Security, 1998). This looked like classic New Labour 'Third Way'-ism. The government introduced so-called 'stakeholder' pensions – essentially a low-cost, private, personal pension – by private pension providers.

The government's approach could be interpreted as representing a shift away from universalism and towards selectivity, or targeting resources on the poorest, comparable with, for example, the shift in child support away from universal child benefit to the new tax credits: another example of 'Third Way'-ism, perhaps. The Secretary of State for Work and Pensions, John Hutton, appeared to acknowledge this in a ministerial statement in June 2006 when he said, in response to criticism on this point,

> ... we could have restored the link between the state pension and earnings, as many people were urging us to do, but if that had been our policy, 1.5 million more pensioners would be below the poverty line today. Instead, since 1997, we have spent three times as much on pensioners as it would have cost to restore the earnings link. We have targeted the bulk of that extra investment on the poorest pensioners, which was entirely right. (Hansard 2006, Col. 141)

The Pension Credit has certainly been successful in channelling more money to many older people and raising their standard of living, but there are problems with it as a major pillar of retirement income. One is that of the less than 100% take-up, an inevitable problem with means-tested benefits, which always involve disincentives of this kind, due either to ignorance or to dislike of the stigmatising aspects of seeking means-tested help. Another is the disincentive effect to private saving or pension investing, since unless this is high enough to take the pensioner above PC entitlement altogether, they lose a proportion of PC income with any increase in private pension or investment income, a problem with any means-tested benefit. At present this amounts to 40% loss of PC with increments in other sources of income (an improvement on MIG where it was 100%). There is also the interaction of PC with other means-tested, income-related benefits, notably Housing Benefit and Council Tax Benefit.

Perceptions of crisis in relation to the private, occupational sector continued to grow, particularly after 2002. In some cases, firms which became insolvent, or transferred ownership, left their workforces stranded and without pensions. The government responded to this in a piecemeal way, trying to improve security for occupational scheme members by creating a Pension Protection Fund in 2005 to assist beneficiaries whose occupational schemes had collapsed and a Pensions Regulator in the same year to oversee the private occupational sector. The government was, however, censured for its inadequate oversight and regulation of occupational pensions during the later 1990s and early 2000s by the Parliamentary Commissioner for Administration in a damning report published in March 2006. The Department for Work and Pensions was found guilty of maladministration in relation to the cases of between 85,000 and 110,000 occupational pensioners whose schemes had collapsed and who ought to be compensated, a claim denied by the government, which suggested that the compensation bill could be as high as £15 billion (Hall and Cohen, 2006).

New Labour's policies have proved modestly successful. They have assisted in reducing pensioner poverty to some extent. The desired shift from public to private, however, did not materialise, perhaps because of the growing crisis in the private pension sector. 'Stakeholder' pensions failed to catch on and were much less successful than hoped. The government has also sought to outlaw age discrimination and promote employment opportunities for older people. Some more fundamental rethinking of the current state of pensions was, however, evidently required, as the then Secretary of State for Work and Pensions, David Blunkett, acknowledged in an interview in 2005 (Hall and Timmins, 2005). In fact, rethinking had already begun.

The Pensions Commission

In 2002 the government announced the establishment of a three-person Pensions Commission, under the chairmanship of Adair Turner, whose task was to provide an in-depth review of contemporary pensions issues, and to make recommendations. A series of reports followed between 2004 and 2006 (Pensions Commission, 2004, 2005, 2006). The Commission's task was to engage in long-term thinking, not to provide short-term responses to immediate and pressing problems such as the collapse of occupational pensions, pensioners' living standards and gaps in coverage and entitlement. The work of Turner and his fellow commissioners represents a significant contribution to contemporary social policy-making.

Discuss and do

Why do you think the government set up a special commission to look at the pensions issue? What advantages might such an approach have for the government?

The first, 2004, report was diagnosis; the second, in 2005, was prescription. The Commission's analysis concluded that existing policy was inadequate because it was based on the assumption that the state would play a reduced role and the private sector a larger one in pensions provision, but private sector provision was in decline

(Pensions Commission, 2005: 2). There was a drift away from providing occu-pational pensions by many employers; the closing of many occupational schemes to new employees; and the conversion of many defined benefit (DB) schemes to osten-sibly less generous defined contribution (DC) schemes, which often involve a lower level of contributions by employers (Pensions Commission, 2004: 84–85, 88).

Employers' attitudes towards pension provision had changed, and it was no longer worthwhile, as it had once been, for self-interested reasons, to provide pen-sions. There were significant cost barriers for individuals and small firms in providing pensions coverage, given the annual management charges of most schemes (Pensions Commission, 2005: 3).

In 2002–03, 11.3 million people in work were not contributing to any private scheme and 8.8 million of these did not have a partner contributing to private schemes. Degree of involvement in private pension arrangements is correlated with such factors as employment status (i.e., whether employed or self-employed), size of firm, whether employed in the public or private sectors, income level, gender and ethnicity (Pensions Commission, 2004: 62–67). Workers in small firms, workers in the private sector, the self-employed, those on lower incomes, women and ethnic minorities are all less likely to be members of private pension schemes.

Pension adequacy was not simply about the total volume of spending on pen-sions; it was also about fairness, between generations, for example. The Commission stressed the importance of generational fairness, arguing that average pension ages should rise in proportion to rising life expectancy; each generation should face the same proportion of adult life contributing to and receiving a state pension (Pensions Commission, 2005: 4).

The Commission set out a number of options. These included allowing the living standards of pensioners to decline by reducing the quality of pension benefits (through lower uprating); requiring people to save more through higher public and private contribution and savings rates; or raising the age of pension entitlement. The solution eventually proposed was a combination of the second and third; the first course was rejected (Pensions Commission, 2004).

The main recommendations came in the second report in 2005. A new pension settlement was required which would deal with gaps in the state system, overcome barriers deterring voluntary private provision, maintain employer involvement in pensions provision, prevent the spread of means-testing, be sustainable in the face of rising longevity, be less complex, and maintain the improvements in pensioners' relative standard of living which the present means-tested approach had achieved (Pensions Commission, 2005: 4–6). Its key recommendations were as follows:

- 'The creation of a low cost, national funded pension savings scheme into which individuals will be automatically enrolled, but with the right to opt out, with a modest level of compulsory matching employer contributions, and delivering the opportunity to save for a pension at a low Annual Management Charge.'
- 'Reforms to make the state system less means-tested and closer to universal than it would be if current indexation arrangements were continued indefinitely. . . . In the long-term this implies some mix of both an increase in taxes devoted to pensions expenditure and an increase in State Pension Ages.' (Pensions Commission, 2005: 6)

The Commission recognised that the purely voluntary approach was no longer adequate. Its proposed National Pensions Savings Scheme (NPSS) would require employees to be automatically enrolled. Inertia would, it was hoped, ensure that people would choose to stay enrolled and thereby build up an adequate volume of pension savings. There were objections to compulsory enrolment in the scheme, because this would fail to allow for the diversity of individual preferences about saving for retirement.

Employees would be required to contribute 4% of salary, employers 3% and the Treasury, in the form of tax relief, 1%. These contributions would be collected by a national agency and invested in pension fund assets managed to keep the costs as low as possible. The Commission estimated that costs as low as 0.3% should be achievable. The scheme should contribute an extra 0.7% of GDP to pensioner incomes by 2050, helping to offset the decline in private occupational pensions (Pensions Commission, 2005: 7–8).

The Commission's other main proposal concerned the future of the state pension schemes. S2P, the Commission concluded, should cease to be earnings-related and become flat-rate, in order to concentrate resources on a more generous non-means-tested pension. Accruals of BSP rights via contributions should cease, and entitlement should become individual and universal, based on residence. This would be a way of dealing with the incomplete coverage of groups such as women. An immediate move in this direction would be to make the BSP universal from a particular age, such as 75 (Pensions Commission, 2005: 10). In this sense, the BSP would become, effectively, a 'citizen's pension'.

There should be a gradual rise in the age at which people became entitled to claim both the BSP and S2P; the Commission suggested that the State Pension Age (SPA) should rise to 66 in 2030, 67 in 2040 and eventually 68 in 2050 (Pensions Commission, 2005: 14). This would result in a substantial saving in pension expenditure. Beyond 2045, as the system adjusts to the long-term fall in fertility, public expenditure as a percentage of GDP should remain constant. This would be in accordance with the principle of fairness between generations. Such a policy had also to be linked to policies to tackle age discrimination in employment and employers' preference for retiring older workers. The report also proposed re-linking the BSP once more to average earnings, from 2010 or 2011.

The Commission had been explicitly asked by the government to look at the issue of people with incomplete work records, principally women and carers. The Commission's response was to claim that its proposals were consistent with the principle of individualised pension rights, for example the proposed reduction in means-tested support – the Pension Credit is calculated on the basis of household rather than individual entitlement – and changes to the BSP (Pensions Commission, 2005: 21). Another issue considered by the Commission was that of people on lower incomes, an important issue given the proposed rise in pension ages, higher levels of unemployment among older manual workers and the persistence of class-related health inequalities. The Commission pointed to the importance of public policy interventions in other areas for example, anti-discrimination legislation to ensure that there were job opportunities for older workers, and interventions to tackle health inequalities. State pension entitlement should also be more flexible. People should be able to claim part of their state pension, while continuing to work part-time, as is the case in Sweden (Pensions Commission, 2005: 22).

The Commission noted that state support for private pensions is poorly focused; half the benefits of tax relief flow to higher-rate taxpayers. Contracting-out from

S2P and the associated NI rebates should be phased out for defined contribution schemes and eventually for defined benefit schemes (Pensions Commission 2005: 25–26).

The Commission's 2005 report and its recommendations were broadly welcomed and became the focus of some public debate (Barr, 2006). The political reaction was interesting. The then Prime Minister, Tony Blair, and the Secretary of State for Work and Pensions, John Hutton, were in favour of the proposals (Timmins, 2006i), while Gordon Brown, then Chancellor of the Exchequer, and the Treasury seem to have been initially hostile and, it is claimed, sought to bury the report. As the chief architect of New Labour's pension policy after 1997, Brown perhaps felt that he had a particular stake in the arrangements – the Pension Credit – that the Commission was seeking to replace, but more important, probably, was a traditional Treasury concern with affordability.

Private fund management industry representatives were divided in their response, some favouring the report, others seeking to safeguard their members' interests as private pension fund and annuity providers. The National Association of Pension Funds (NAPF), for example, was hostile, denouncing the Pensions Commission recommendations as 'Stalinist', and alleging that they amounted to a plan for a state take-over of pensions saving (Timmins, 2006f). These criticisms were vigorously countered by Turner, and there was a lively debate in the media (Timmins, 2006i).

Responding to Turner: the government's White Papers

The government eventually produced a two-stage response to the Commission's proposals, publishing a White Paper in May 2006 and a second one on Personal Accounts the following December (Department for Work and Pensions, 2006a, 2006b). As late as March 2006 such newspaper headlines as 'Pensions revamp in jeopardy' pointed to disagreements between the Treasury and the then Chancellor, Gordon Brown, on the one hand, and the Prime Minister and Secretary of State on the other, about the nature and scope of the reforms (Timmins and Hall, 2006), but by May these had been resolved in favour of the latter (Blitz, 2006; Hall and Timmins, 2006). The proposals embodied broad acceptance of the Commission's ideas.

The age of entitlement to the basic state pension is to be raised, from 65 to 66 over a two-year period from 2024, to 67 over a two-year period from 2034, and to 68 over a two-year period from 2044, rather faster than envisaged by the Pensions Commission. This is obviously helpful from the point of view of reducing spending. The link with earnings would be restored but from 2012, or at the latest by the end of the next Parliament, i.e. 2015, rather than 2010 or 2011 as the Commission had recommended. The White Paper follows through on the Pensions Commission's proposals for universalising the basic state pension, although not precisely in the recommended form. The contributory principle is to be radically reformed and the number of years of contributions required for a full pension reduced from 39 to 30, enabling women to build a full pension with fewer years of paid work. A new weekly credit will be introduced for those caring for children and a credit for those caring for severely disabled people for more than 20 hours per week (Department for Work and Pensions, 2006a: 17–18).

The second White paper, on Personal Accounts, is concerned with the Pensions Commission's other main proposal, that for a national pensions savings scheme (Department for Work and Pensions, 2006b). This broadly follows the Commission's recommendations. There will be a system of personal pension savings accounts. The overall rate of contribution will be 8%. Employees will contribute 4% of salary within a band between £5,000 and £33,500 per year. There will be 1% tax relief (equal to the amount now offered on private pension saving). Employers will contribute 3%. There will be 'soft compulsion' in the form of automatic enrolment of employees, but with the right to opt out. The scheme will begin operation by 2012 (Department for Work and Pensions, 2006b: 143). There will be between 6 and 10 million scheme members. The White Paper devotes considerable attention to the implementation aspects of the new scheme. An arms-length governance structure for the scheme, involving a personal accounts delivery authority, will be established (Department for Work and Pensions, 2006b: 81). Powers to create this body were incorporated in the 2007 Pensions Act.

Discuss and Do

What do you think of the Turner Commission's, and the government's, idea of automatic enrolment of employees in the new pensions savings scheme? Should employees be able to 'opt in', rather than have to 'opt out'? Alternatively, should people be *compelled* to contribute to the scheme, whether they like it or not, as they will still have to do with the basic state pension?

The White Papers attracted mixed reviews. On the whole, there was acceptance of broad principles but disquiet about some of the details (Hall, 2006a). Some observers argued that its proposals would do little to solve the system's underlying problems (Pemberton *et al.*, 2006b; Thane, 2006a). Others pointed to the apparently perverse distributive consequences of earnings-linking the basic state pension. The winners will be the better-off elderly; poorer pensioners, dependent on means-tested benefits, will see no benefit from this change (Hall, 2006a). NAPF, the pensions industry representative body, worried about the threat to existing occupational schemes, and argued that employers currently contributing to occupational schemes might contribute less (Timmins, 2006h).

A wide-ranging debate in Parliament in June 2006 suggested that there was broad cross-party consensus on the essentials of the government's pensions reform programme (*Hansard*, 2006: Cols 138–147; Timmins, 2006e). The Opposition's response is of some importance because pension policy requires long-term views and commitments and a coherent and credible policy is one that has to outlast a particular government.

The second White Paper, on the new pensions saving scheme, was applauded by Lord Turner, who suggested that it was '99 percent' in line with his Commission's recommendations, Employers' organisations complained about the absence of help for small employers in meeting the cost of compulsory contributions but were supportive of other aspects of the White Paper, notably measures to protect existing occupational pensions saving and prevent employers' 'levelling down' to the scheme's 3% contribution level. Pensions industry representatives such as the ABI also felt that they had got something out of the White Paper (Timmins, 2006g).

The government's proposals were legislatively enacted in the 2006–07 Parliamentary session, with the passing of the Pensions Act 2007, forming the centrepiece of a welfare reform package in that session.

Stop and Think

What do the government's pension proposals tell you about the government's attitude towards the private sector in welfare, and about its relationship with the state sector?

Pensions policy-making

Pensions policy-making is interesting for a number of reasons. One is the challenge to 'rational' policy-making in a context where policy-makers have short time horizons, perhaps no more than the four or five years between general elections. Some commentators have suggested, therefore, the need for a different style of pensions policy-making, one that focuses on long-term sustainability and the achievement of inter-party consensus. It has been suggested, for example, that Sweden's pension reforms of the 1990s are exemplary here. Sweden reformed its pension system in the 1990s, employing a consensus-building and consensus-maintaining approach which has won plaudits from foreign observers (Hinrichs, 2006; Pemberton *et al.*, 2006c: 21).

The Labour government's most recent approach to pensions policy-making perhaps embodies some of these concerns. The Pensions Commission, not perhaps quite as an expert group but at any rate as a non-governmental group of the great and the good, can be viewed as an attempt to achieve broad agreement about the nature of the pensions problem and possible solutions to it. An underlying purpose of the Commission was to seek a consensus, as far as possible, on the issues with which it sought to deal and, in a sense, take the issue 'out of politics'. Pensions should not be, as they had been, a political football, subject to the short-term electoral considerations of political parties; policy should focus on the long term, important given the lengthy time horizons of the issue. The creation of the Pensions Commission can be regarded as 'arms-length' policy thinking; the government always had the option of repudiating the Commission's findings and pursuing some other strategy.

Stop and Think

Should pensions be 'taken out of politics'? *Could* they be taken out of politics?

Pension policy: a case of 'path dependency'?

Some policy analysts have suggested that pensions are a policy area characterised by 'path dependency'. 'Path dependency' (or 'dependence') is the idea that policy possibilities and choices are constrained by past decisions and the web of rules, institutions and interests which have been created by earlier policies, making it difficult to strike out on a completely new policy path. Institutional arrangements become 'locked-in' and harder to reform (Myles and Pierson, 2001: 312). Path dependency implies that any government will have relatively limited room for manoeuvre in reforming its pension system, given many decades of policy development and the accumulation of interests, incentives and 'stakes' inherent in a complex institutional structure that has been assembled in a piecemeal way over a long period of time. A 'clean sweep' and a fresh start become progressively more difficult to achieve. Some writers are, however, sceptical about the extent of pension policy 'lock-in' in the British system, arguing that policy change over the years has been too substantial to warrant application of the term (Pemberton, 2006: 41–42).

Conclusion

This chapter has sought to provide an overview of current pension issues and recent reform initiatives in the UK, with some sideways glances at experience in other countries. It has tried to identify pensions policy as a distinctive area of social policy with its own dynamic, as well as providing you with an account of the nuts and bolts of the present system and of some of the problems facing it, and how some of these problems might be overcome.

This chapter has:

- given you an understanding of the main features of the UK pensions system;
- introduced you to basic pension concepts and issues, and criteria for evaluating pensions systems;
- given you outline knowledge of the evolution of the present UK system;
- given you an overview of the problems of the present UK system, in relation to issues of adequacy, equity and sustainability;
- enabled you to trace the recent evolution of pensions policy under New Labour;
- given you an understanding of reform initiatives associated with the work of the Pensions Commission and the government's response to this.

Annotated further reading

A good, brief, readable and up-to-date examination of pensions policy is Michael Hill's *Pensions* (Hill, 2007). *Britain's Pensions Crisis: History and policy* is an outstanding collection of essays, the proceedings of a conference organised by the British Academy (Pemberton *et al.*, 2006a). For valuable historical background on the UK pension system, see John Macnicol's *The Politics of Retirement in Britain 1878–1948* (Macnicol, 1998), the relevant chapters of Pat Thane's *Old Age in English History* (Thane, 2000) and chapters by Harris and Pemberton in *Britain's Pensions Crisis* (Harris, 2006; Pemberton, 2006).

The two main reports of the Pensions Commission – *Pensions: Challenges and Choices* (2004) and *A New Pension Settlement for the Twenty-First Century* (2005)

– are a goldmine of accessible data and analysis on British pension issues, as well as, in the second report, putting forward influential policy recommendations. The government's response to the Commission's work are the two White Papers from the Department of Work and Pensions (2006a, 2006b): *Security in Retirement: Towards a new pensions system* (Cm 6841) and *Personal Accounts: A new way to save* (Cm 6975). The House of Commons Work and Pensions Select Committee has published a useful report on pensions reform: *Pension Reform*, Volume I (HC 1068–I). Volume II (HC 1068–II) is a valuable collection of verbal and printed minutes of evidence to the Committee on the issues from a wide range of organisations and individuals, including pension industry representatives such as NAPF and ABI, and pressure groups such as Which?, Age Concern, Help the Aged and the Pensions Reform Group. All Commission, DWP and Parliamentary Select Committee material is downloadable from the relevant websites.

Academic research on poverty, inequality and social exclusion among pensioners is reported on in articles by Patsios (2006) and by Evandrou and Falkingham (2005). Finally, *The Handbook of West European Pension Politics* is a major study of the comparative politics of pension systems (Immergut and Anderson, 2007).

Chapter 18

Family policy

Objectives

- To introduce and examine the concept of 'family policy'.

- To locate family policy in the context of UK social policy.

- To examine the changing relationship between the state and the family in the twentieth century.

- To identify and examine various policy areas which have an impact on the family.

- To examine in some detail specific family policies of Labour governments since 1997, including those for children, 'work–life balance' and 'family-friendly employment'.

Introduction

Family policy is of interest to students of social policy for many reasons. One is that it is a multidimensional, cross-cutting issue, potentially involving many different policy areas – employment, social security, education, community care and equality policies, amongst others. In fact, policy for the family might be regarded as a classic 'joined-up governance' issue, so important for Labour governments since 1997 (for more on 'joined-up' governance, see Chapter 6). Another is that family policy in the UK has, by comparison with that in other welfare states, such as France, rarely been explicitly formulated in detail (Pedersen, 1993). It therefore provides interesting opportunities for comparative lesson-drawing. Another interesting point about the family in the context of social policy is that it is both 'subject' and 'object' of policy; the family as a 'site' for welfare intervention both gives and receives.

In terms of 'giving', the family is a vital welfare agency in the UK, as it is in all countries. The family is a producer and provider of 'informal' welfare, and it is of course the most important welfare provider. It is a health care agency, a provider of education services and a social care agency, among others (Pahl, 2003: 172–180). The policy of social 'care in the community', for example, promoted by all UK governments since the 1970s, has been predicated on the existence of an informal, mainly female, labour force willing to provide care for family members. Such policy initiatives by the present Labour government as those to do with the promotion of 'work–life balance' may also be viewed as attempts to enhance the family's role in caring for children.

Politics and the family

The family has grown in importance in British politics during the course of the last 100 years. An appeal to the family and family values has now become an irresistible one for political parties, left and right. The Labour Party's 1997 election manifesto, for example, contained a section on family policy entitled 'We will strengthen family life' (Labour Party, 1997: 24–27), and the 2005 manifesto also included a chapter on the subject (Labour Party, 2005: Ch. 6). The Conservatives similarly emphasised their commitment to supporting the family (Conservative Party, 1997: 13–20). It will be remembered that one of Margaret Thatcher's more memorable (or infamous) remarks – 'There is no such thing as society' – was also a comment on the family; she went on to say 'there are individual men and women, and there are families' (see Chapter 10) (Thatcher, 1993: 628).

What is a family? Family and household change in the UK

The study of the family as a social institution has an extensive history, beginning with the work of nineteenth-century European sociologists such as Le Play and Westermarck, and Marxists such as Friedrich Engels, and continuing with work of twentieth-century writers such as the anthropologist Bronislaw Malinowski and the American sociologist William J. Goode (Therborn, 2004). In recent decades the study of the family and its evolution in past times has been significantly advanced by the work of a number of social historians (Anderson, 1980; Laslett, 1983).

The *household* is an important unit for social policy and demographic purposes, distinct from the family. Means-tested social security benefits, for example, are calculated on a household basis. A household is officially defined as '. . . a person living alone or a group of people who have the address as their only or main residence and who either share one meal a day or share the living accommodation' (Office for National Statistics, 2007: 202).

A *family* is officially defined as 'a married or cohabiting couple, either with or without their never-married child or children (of any age), including couples with no children or a lone parent together with his or her never-married child or children provided they have no children of their own. A family could also consist of a grandparent(s) with their grandchild or grandchildren if the parents of the grandchild or grandchildren are not usually resident in the household' (Office for National Statistics, 2007: 202). The Census definition of a *lone-parent family* is 'a father or mother together with his or her never-married child or children'. In fact, official definitions of households, families and lone-parent families vary slightly between the various official surveys sponsored by the government – the Census, the Labour Force Survey and the General Household Survey (Office for National Statistics, 2007: 202).

Contemporary comment and research on the family emphasises the diversity of family forms, both historically and comparatively, as well as in present-day Western societies, where cohabiting, unmarried parenthood, lone parenthood, step-families and same-sex relationships have become more common (Pahl, 2003: 160–162).

Single-person households have also become much more common. The traditional 'nuclear' family of Western European and North American societies, it is argued, is in decline, if indeed it was ever really dominant as a family form.

Tables 18.1, 18.2 and 183, derived from data provided by the Office for National Statistics in *Social Trends*, provide different ways of illustrating changing family and household structures in Britain (note: Great Britain, not the United Kingdom – in other words, Northern Ireland is excluded). Table 18.1 adopts a household approach. It will be seen that the number of one-person households has increased substantially between 1971 and 2006, from 18% to 28% of all households. The proportion of 'standard' couple family households with one or two children, which at 26% of all households in 1971 was not large, has shrunk as a proportion to 18% of the total. (Note that the partners in couple families may be married or cohabiting.) The proportion of lone-parent family households with dependent children has more than doubled over the period, from 3% to 7%. A striking trend revealed in this table is the overall increase in the number of households between the two selected dates, from around 18 million in 1971 to around 24 million in 2006, an increase of nearly a third. These trends obviously have important implications for housing policy, amongst others.

Household size

Household size varies by ethnic group, with some groups having larger families and being more likely to live in extended families. Indian, Pakistani and Bangladeshi

Table 18.1 Households[1] in Great Britain by type of household and family

	1971(%)	2006(%)[2]
One person		
Under state pension age	6	14
Over state pension age	12	14
One-family households		
Couple[3]		
No children	27	28
1–2 dependent children[4]	26	18
3 or more dependent children[4]	9	4
Non-dependent children only	8	7
Lone parent[3]		
Dependent children[4]	3	7
Non-dependent children only	4	3
Two or more unrelated adults	4	3
Multi-family households	1	1
All households (= 100%) (millions)	18.6	24.2

[1]For definition of 'household', see text.

[2]Data are at Q2 each year. See Appendix, Part 4: Labour Force Survey.

[3]Other individuals who were not family members may also be included.

[4]May also include non-dependent children.

Source: Office for National Statistics (2007) *Social Trends 37*, Table 2.2, p. 14, London: ONS. Crown copyright material is reproduced with the permission of the Controller of HMSO and the Queen's Printer for Scotland under the terms of the Click-Use Licence.

families contain more members than other ethnic groups. According to the 2001 census, employing official definitions of ethnicity (Office for National Statistics, 2007: 201), Bangladeshi households were largest, with 4.5 people per household, followed by Pakistani (4.1) and Indian (3.3); White British and Black Caribbean had 2.3 persons per household, and White Irish had the smallest households, at 2.2 persons (Office for National Statistics, 2007: 15). To some extent these differences are related to age structure. Smaller households – White British, White Irish and Black Caribbean – have, on average, an older age structure and are more likely to be single-person households (Office for National Statistics, 2007: 14–15, Figure 2.3).

Table 18.2 looks at families from the perspective of people in households. It will be seen that the percentage of people living in single-person households has doubled between 1971 and 2006, from 6% to 12%. The percentage of those with dependent children has shrunk from 52% to 37% over the period, while the percentage of lone parents has trebled, from 4% to 12%. Lone parenthood varies by ethnic group. Around half of Black Caribbean households with dependent children were headed by a lone parent, as were about a third of Black African households with dependent children, compared with about a fifth of white households (Office for National Statistics, 2007: 15–16).

The main findings revealed by the data in these tables are a trend towards smaller families, the decline in numbers of couple families with two children, the increase in lone parenthood and the increase in the number of children living in lone-parent families.

Marriage, divorce, civil partnerships, cohabitation

Other significant trends may be noted in marriage and divorce. Marriage is still the main form of partnership for men and women: 70% of the 17.1 million families in the United Kingdom in 2006 contained a married couple. There has, however, been

Table 18.2 People in households[1] in Great Britain by type of household and family

	1971 (%)	2006[2] (%)
One person	6	12
One-family households		
Couple		
No children	19	25
Dependent children[3]	52	37
Non-dependent children only	10	8
Lone parent[4]	4	12
Other households	9	5
All people in private households (= 100%) (millions)	53.4	57.1

[1]For definition of 'household', see text.
[2]Data are at spring each year.
[3]May also include non-dependent children.
[4]Includes those with dependent children only, non-dependent children only, and those with both dependent and non-dependent children.
Source: Office for National Statistics (2007) *Social Trends 37*, Table 2.3, p. 15, London: ONS. Crown copyright material is reproduced with the permission of the Controller of HMSO and the Queen's Printer for Scotland under the terms of the Click-Use Licence.

a steady decline in the number of marriages in the UK since the post-war peak in the early 1970s, and a rise in the number of divorces. In 2005 there were 283,700 marriages, compared with 480,000 in 1972. The fall in the marriage rate is due to a combination of factors – the fall in numbers of marriageable people, with the passing of the post-war 'baby boom' generation, and, probably, the rise in the age of marriage, accompanying the increase in rates of cohabitation.

There were 155,000 divorces in 2005, a slight fall from a peak reached in 1993. The sharp spike in the number of divorces in the early 1970s shown in Figure 18.1 is due to the Divorce Reform Act of 1969, implemented in 1971. There has also been a significant rise in the age of marriage. In 1971, in England and Wales the age of first marriage was 25 for men and 23 for women. By 2005 this had increased to 32 for men and 29 for women. Similar trends in age of first marriage are observable in most other European countries (Office for National Statistics, 2007: 19).

The Civil Partnership Act 2004, implemented in December 2005, permitted the formation of same-sex unions, with rights and responsibilities identical to those of civil marriage (see Chapter 19). During the first year of operation of the Act, 15,700 civil partnerships were formed (Office for National Statistics, 2007: 18).

There has been a substantial increase in cohabitation rates since the 1980s. Since 1986 the proportion of men under 60 cohabiting has more than doubled, from 11% to 24% in 2005, and for women it has nearly doubled over the same period, from 13% to 24%. The rise in cohabitation may be linked to the rise in the age of marriage (Office for National Statistics, 2007: 19). Table 18.3 overleaf shows the proportions of different categories of non-married people who are cohabiting.

With higher divorce rates, the environment in which children are brought up has

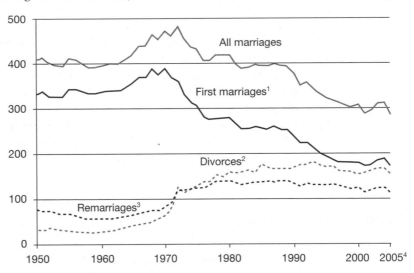

1 For both partners.
2 Includes annulments. Data for 1950 to 1970 for Great Britain only. Divorce was permitted in Northern Ireland from 1969.
3 For one or both partners.
4 Data for 2005 are provisional. Final figures are likely to be higher.

Figure 18.1   Marriages and divorces in the UK (thousands)
Source: Office for National Statistics (2007) *Social Trends 37*, Figure 2.9, p. 18, London: ONS. Crown copyright material is reproduced with the permission of the Controller of HMSO and the Queen's Printer for Scotland under the terms of the Click-Use Licence.

Table 18.3 Non-married people[1] cohabiting in Great Britain: by marital status and sex, 2005[2]

	Men (%)	Women (%)
Single	23	28
Widowed	14	6
Divorced	36	29
Separated	22	11

[1]Aged 16 to 59. Includes those who described themselves as separated but were, in a legal sense, still married.
[2]Data for 2005 include last quarter of 2004/05 due to survey change from financial year to calendar year. See Appendix, Part 2: General Household Survey.
Source: Office for National Statistics (2007) *Social Trends 37*, Table 2.12, p. 19, London: ONS. Crown copyright material is reproduced with the permission of the Controller of HMSO and the Queen's Printer for Scotland under the terms of the Click-Use Licence.

changed, with the growth of lone-parent families and stepfamilies. More than 10% of families with dependent children were stepfamilies in 2005. The great majority of these – 86% – consisted of a natural mother with a stepfather (Office for National Statistics, 2007: 20).

Fertility rates

Figure 18.2 and Table 18.4 provide information about trends in fertility in recent decades in the United Kingdom. They show a continuation in long-standing trends towards lower birth rates and smaller families. Rates of childlessness have risen, and the age of first birth has also steadily risen. Explanations for these trends include later ages of marriage and cohabitation and greater involvement by women in education and the labour market. Table 18.4 demonstrates the decline in fertility of women aged below 30 and the rise in that of women over 30. There has also been a rise in the proportion of births occurring outside marriage since the 1960s. By 2005, 43% of all births occurred outside marriage, testifying to the rise in cohabitation. By this time, most extramarital births were registered by both parents, and most by parents living at the same address.

The family under scrutiny

The family has always been an object of intense critical scrutiny for observers of diverse ideological standpoints. From both right-wing and left-wing political perspectives, the 'death of the family' has been regularly forecast, and celebrated or deplored according to taste. For the radical or 'anti-psychiatry' movement of the 1960s, for example, exemplified by the work of R.D. Laing and his followers, the family was a site of psychological oppression in which individuals might be driven mad (Laing, 1967: Ch. 3). Anthropologists such as Edmund Leach claimed to find no basis in history or ethnography for the contemporary Western family, asserting that 'Far from being the basis of the good society, the family, with its narrow

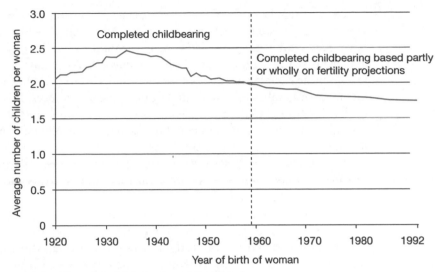

Figure 18.2 Completed family size in the UK

Source: Office for National Statistics (2007) *Social Trends 37*, Figure 2.15, p. 21, London: ONS. Crown copyright material is reproduced with the permission of the Controller of HMSO and the Queen's Printer for Scotland under the terms of the Click-Use Licence.

Table 18.4 UK Fertility rates (live births per 1,000 women) by age of mother at childbirth

Age of mother	1971	2005
Under 20[1]	50.0	26.2
20–24	154.4	70.5
25–29	154.6	98.3
30–34	79.4	100.7
35–39	34.3	50.0
40 and over	9.2	10.6
Total fertility rate[2]	2.41	1.79
Total births[3] (thousands)	901.6	722.5

[1]Live births per 1,000 women aged 15 to 19.

[2]Number of children that would be born to a woman if current patterns of fertility persisted throughout her childbearing life. For 1981 onwards, this is based on fertility rates for each single year of age, but for 1971 it is based on the rates for each five year age group.

[3]Total live births per 1,000 women aged 15 to 44.

Source: Office for National Statistics (2007) *Social Trends 37*, Table 2.16, p. 21, London: ONS. Crown copyright material is reproduced with the permission of the Controller of HMSO and the Queen's Printer for Scotland under the terms of the Click-Use Licence.

privacy and tawdry secrets, is the source of all discontents' (Leach, 1968: 44). For many utopian radicals, communists, anarchists and egalitarians from Plato to the present day, the family is naturally an object of suspicion, as the primary means for reproducing and transmitting class-based privilege and inequality from generation to generation through various forms of cultural and non-cultural capital. Radical utopians, viewing the family as selfish, inward-looking and antithetical to republican virtue, citizenship or society-wide communal attachments, have often proposed the abolition of the family and its replacement by collective forms of child rearing and care-provision (Marx and Engels, 1968: 49–51; Mount, 1982: Ch. 9).

For most feminists, the family is an agency for reproducing patriarchal power and women's oppression. It belongs to that 'private' realm to which, historically, women have been confined, to be distinguished from the 'public' realm inhabited by men and from which women have been excluded. It is a realm of concealed violence; most physical violence towards women and children is that carried out by male members of families towards female and younger members. It is also socially unjust, in that it is predicated on an unequal division of labour and an unequal division of resources, at any rate in the single-breadwinner, typically male-headed family. Most feminists are, however, probably not opposed to the family as such, but to particular family forms existing in patriarchal societies. Naturally these various ideological standpoints are not all distinct and individual critics of the family might hold to more than one of them.

The 'traditional' family also has its defenders, not all of them ideologically conservative (or Conservative, in the UK context). For the Conservative commentator and novelist Ferdinand Mount, the family is a 'subversive' institution, undermining the pretensions of an all-powerful State or Church and offering individuals some protection against them. Contemporary feminism of a radical or utopian variety is, in Mount's view, just one more manifestation of the same kind of phenomenon (Mount, 1982: 242–245).

For many conservatives, the family is an institution under threat from contemporary social changes, which may include easier divorce, the rise of lone parenthood, the apparent decline in the popularity of marriage and the accompanying rise in that of cohabitation, the movement of married women into paid work, and permissive attitudes to same-sex relationships and to abortion (Murray, 1990; Morgan, 1998). Not all conservatives would identify all these changes as equally problematical, some dismissing worry on this score as groundless or exaggerated (Mount, 1982: 218; Willetts 1989: 262–265).

Contemporary socialists of a social-democratic persuasion have long since made their peace with the 'traditional' family, as the recent Labour Party election manifestos cited in an earlier section demonstrate. The traditional two-parent family continues to have its defenders on the left, such as Norman Dennis and A.H. Halsey, who are critical of the rise of alternative family forms and particularly of lone parenthood, seen as responsible for growing poverty and criminality (Dennis, 1993; Dennis and Erdos, 1993).

Human rights and the family

Article 16(1) of the United Nations' 1948 Universal Declaration of Human Rights explicitly enunciated the right of men and women to marry and found a family as a basic human right (Sieghart, 1985: 120–121, 174). Article 16(1) also states that 'They are entitled to equal rights as to marriage, during marriage and at its dissolution'. Article 16(2) goes on to state that 'Marriage shall be entered into only with the free and full consent of the intending spouses'. Article 16(3) states that 'The family is the natural and fundamental group unit of society and is entitled to protection by society and the state' (Sieghart, 1985: 120–121, 174). These provisions on the family are echoed in all other human rights declarations, and articulated at

Discuss and Do **The family: here today, yesterday and tomorrow?**

Some people might say that we are now living in a 'golden age' of the family. Families are much smaller than in the past, with fewer dependents; standards of living are much higher; family relationships are more egalitarian and 'democratic' than they were in the past; there is greater tolerance of diversity in family types.

Would you agree, or do you think that family life is 'under threat' in contemporary societies? If so, what, in your opinion, are the main threats to family life at present:

- family break-up?
- the imperatives of work for both partners in a relationship?
- the decline in good-quality parenting?
- permissive acceptance of different kinds of family?

Or would you, on the other hand, agree with a writer like Mount, who seems to be saying that the family is a robust institution which hasn't really changed as much in its essentials as people think?

considerably greater length in some, such as the European Social Charter, adopted in 1961.

Severe restrictions on marriage and family life existed in virtually all societies until the late twentieth century, and still continue in some (Mount, 1982: 32–33). China, for example, imposed a minimum marriage age of 25, and a 'one child' policy, in 1980. In some countries, until comparatively recently, there were prohibitions on interracial marriage, and in many, if not most, countries, women are far from enjoying equal rights in relation to marriage and family life, 'free and full consent' to marriage may not exist and women may be treated as chattels.

More recently, a human rights perspective has been applied to the status and interests of children (Hewitt and Leach, 1993: 1–6). The UK ratified the United Nations Convention on the Rights of the Child in 1991. UK policy is obliged to conform, or appear to conform, to its provisions.

Stop and Think

How far do you think the state should intervene in family life to control or limit marriage and child-bearing? Would you, for example, regard China's 'one child' policy, and minimum marriage age, as a violation of human rights? Or is it a reasonable response to China's population 'problem'?

What is family policy?

Talking about the family (whatever the family may be) involves aggregating individuals and their interests. Recent and not-so-recent discussion has drawn attention to some of the anomalies and deficiencies involved in this. Feminists from the time of Eleanor Rathbone onwards have drawn attention to the absurdity of assuming that, for example, a male breadwinner's earnings are always shared equally within the family unit on the basis of need (for more on Rathbone and 'family endowment', see Chapter 10).

Broader and narrower definitions of family policy are possible. Family policy could be defined broadly as any policy directly or indirectly affecting the family. On this basis it would be hard to exclude any social policy from the definition. This, however, would be too broad a definition to be useful.

One approach to this might be to focus on what governments actually do when they are doing something which they claim to be 'family policy'. This is more difficult for the UK than for other countries, because British governments have been shy about employing the concept of family policy.

Kamerman and Kahn distinguish between what they called 'explicit' and 'implicit' family policy and, employing this distinction, classified a number of countries in terms of their policies for and towards the family (Kamerman and Kahn, 1978: 3). Some countries, such as France, have 'explicit' family policies; others, such as the UK, have only or mostly 'implicit' family policies. In France, much social policy is deliberately directed at the family; in the UK, policy is usually only indirectly concerned with it.

Family policy is not necessarily 'progressive' social policy. In many countries the pursuit of explicit family policies has been bound up with a 'pro-natalist' and state-building view of the family – the need, for example, to boost birth rates and population growth, depleted in some cases by the losses of war, as in France after the First World War, or the pursuit of aggressive foreign policy, in the cases of Nazi Germany and the Soviet Union (Pedersen, 1993). National strength has been seen as depending on high population numbers. The liberal, breadwinner-focused UK state, viewing the family as the private business of its citizens, has never been pro-natalist in this sense, even if pro-natalist sentiments have informed, if not determined, the views of some policy makers, as they did to some extent in the case of Beveridge's views on children's allowances (Beveridge, 1942: 154, para. 413).

Discuss and Do

Question for discussion: Do we need something called family policy? We can all think of ways in which existing social policies affect individual family members in some way – child protection legislation, education services, housing, social security which recognises family responsibilities through allowances for dependents – but do we need any more than this? What about, for example, the law governing marriage, such as that regulating same-sex unions or marriages? Is this an example of 'family policy'?

Historical background: the development of family policy in the UK

In the UK the family has been regarded as a private institution, into which the state should intrude in only limited ways, although the family has been subject to state regulation in relation to, for example, marriage and divorce (Glennerster, 2007: 153). Welfare policy has been circumscribed by such views, and also by the political salience of social class as a social division. The labour movement in the UK, for example, agitated for much of the twentieth century not for family benefits but for a 'living' or 'family' wage, to be gained through trade union collective bargaining and, failing that, through minimum wages in particular industrial sectors.

Some of the first state welfare interventions outside the ambit of the Poor Law, such as school feeding and school medical inspection, introduced by a Liberal government in 1906 and 1907, related to children. Another was the introduction of tax allowances for children for income tax payers in 1909 by the same government.

The development of health services in the UK in the twentieth century also exhibits a 'breadwinner' focus; the National Health Insurance scheme introduced in 1911, for example, although not formally exclusionary, assumed that the breadwinner's (effectively, the man's) health was of most importance and insured only the breadwinner, not the breadwinner's family. Children's health was taken care of, if at all, through maternal and infant health services provided by local authorities, as was that of women. Women's health was a matter of public concern largely in relation to their role as mothers until the 1940s. Women's and children's access to GP and hospital-provided health care would depend until then on their ability to pay or on the possibility of obtaining means-tested fee exemptions.

William Beveridge took for granted, in formulating his plans for post-war social security in his famous Report of 1942, the continuance of the 'conventional' nuclear family, based on a separation of male and female roles, the concept of the male breadwinner and the dependent housewife (see Chapter 10). In this he was merely conforming to prevailing norms about desirable family forms, not least those of the labour movement. Beveridge's assumptions, although in tune with contemporary opinion, turned out to be unsound.

The period of the 1940s, dominated by war and post-war reconstruction, can in some respects be regarded as a major era of family policy, implicit if not explicit, and also of the sanctification of the 'traditional' family, implied in Beveridge's views cited above. Such policies as food subsidies and food rationing, major components of social policy at the time, improved the diets of the mass of British working-class families (it had been estimated that half of British children in the inter-war period were malnourished), while the creation of a universal health service improved women's access to health care. The Family Allowance – a weekly flat-rate cash benefit payable for the second and subsequent children – was legislated by the wartime coalition government in 1945, and introduced the following year. The Labour government's reforms of social security, inspired by Beveridge, introduced new cash benefits for maternity – a cash lump sum together with weekly benefits, payable to the mother. The expansion of educational opportunities initiated in the 1940s was also eventually to have a significant impact on the lives of women, as well as working-class children.

The 1950s was the decade of the classic 'traditional' nuclear family, with a strong division of labour between wage-working male breadwinner on the one hand and home-based housewife and mother on the other. This was, however, to prove a temporary state of affairs. The relatively successful performance of the post-war British economy, generating jobs and strong demand for labour, drew women into paid work in increasing numbers, just as, of course, it drew in increasing numbers of migrants from abroad. This was also an era of increasing educational opportunity, involving developments in particularly secondary schooling and higher education, which was eventually to benefit girls as much as, or more than, boys.

From the 1950s onwards, women's contribution to family and household income gradually became indispensable, as a 'reasonable' standard of living became defined in relation to that available to a two-earner household. The single-earner household would be, from now on, subject to an increased risk of poverty, defined in relative deprivation terms. Women's earnings not only boosted family incomes and standards of living, but enabled them to achieve a degree of independence and autonomy, as did other changes in the period, such as improved opportunities to control fertility and limit family size.

Few of the trends and tendencies so far described, policy and other, were promoted or introduced or came about with the intention of liberating or empowering women; they were not the product of feminist ideology or movements, for these as yet hardly existed. Such liberation as was to take place was a largely unintended consequence of policy and broader social and economic changes and changes in technology, as in the case of contraception.

Social change in the 1960s: the 'permissive society' and equal opportunities

Important changes took place in the 1960s in the area of the regulation of sexual behaviour. These include the introduction of the contraceptive pill in 1961, which gave women easier control of their own fertility; homosexual law reform in 1967, in the shape of the Sexual Offences Act, which decriminalised sexual acts between consenting males over the age of 21; the age of consent was lowered to 18 in the 1990s (prohibition had never applied to females); reform of the abortion laws with the passing of the Abortion Act, also in 1967; and easier divorce with the passage of legislation in 1969 (Glennerster, 2007: Ch. 7). These measures, added to those economic and social changes described in the previous section, were to have significant implications for conventional views of the family and family life.

Public policy after the 1960s began to recognise the importance of women's employment, beginning with the passage of the Equal Pay Act in 1970 and the Sex Discrimination Act in 1975, both Labour measures. The 1975 Employment Protection Act established maternity provision for working women in the form of a maximum of 40 weeks' maternity leave, with maternity pay and the right to return to work similar in nature. The lack of affordable child care, however, continued to deter women from returning to work (Glennerster, 2007: 149–151).

Family policy issues in the 1970s and after

In this section we look at a number of family policy issues which became salient in this period – social security, the tax treatment of the family and domestic violence.

Social security and the family

Social security policy, like other public policy, makes assumptions about 'appropriate' family structures. These assumptions, of course, no longer hold good. In this model, the male breadwinner was seen as the primary claimant and beneficiary, and other family members as dependents, mirroring the economic dependency of working life. Non-contributory means-tested benefits such as the non-contributory version of Jobseekers' Allowance (there is also a contributory, National Insurance version of this), Income Support and Pension Credit are assessed on a household, rather than an individual, basis, as were their predecessors.

Feminist writers in the 1970s and later were particularly concerned by certain features of the social security system, such as the notorious 'cohabitation' rule, which prevents a lone parent claiming means-tested benefits such as Income Support in her own right if she is 'cohabiting', that is, living with a man (who is self-supporting) (Wilson, 1974: 20). Feminists have criticised the rule for appearing to make a lone female parent dependent for her upkeep and that of her children on a man, thereby upholding and enforcing a particular model of conventional family life (Pateman, 1988: 248). The rule is, however, merely an application of the general principle that means-tested benefits such as Income Support and its predecessors are, and always have been, assessed on a household basis. Couples' needs are aggregated for benefit purposes. The non-working partner of a working man or woman in a 'conventional' family relationship, living in a single household, whether married or not, and caring for children, has never been able to claim Income Support in his or her own right.

Contrary, furthermore, to the assertions of some feminists, the cohabitation rule does not discourage women from forming new relationships, although it might require them to be circumspect about doing so, nor does it prevent women being financially supported by men who remain non-resident (Pascall, 1986). There is also something inconsistent in criticising the rule for apparently upholding a conventional model of the family, and at the same time criticising it for discouraging women from entering into new family relationships.

What most people found objectionable about the cohabitation rule was the policing and surveillance of intimate relationships that were involved as part of the fraud-prevention activities of the social security agencies. Of course, media and public opinion was to some extent inconsistent about this, concerned as it was at the same time about the evils of benefit fraud.

Other feminists have recognised that the benefits system is not quite as morally conservative, in relation to lone parents, as some critics have thought. Income Support and its means-tested predecessors supported lone-parent claimants without stigma and without a requirement to work, a position presumably derived from 'traditional' assumptions that children are better off being looked after at home by their mothers, and also to the fact that Income Support was a universal benefit claimed by all – unemployed, disabled, pensioners (until the introduction of similar but separate benefits such as MIG, later Pension Credit, for pensioners – see Chapter 17) – who satisfy the income and needs criteria. One feminist commentator observed that 'modern welfare policies have permitted the transformation of traditional family forms and the formation of autonomous households by lone mothers while at the same time attempting to enforce assumptions about men's obligation to maintain – a Janus-faced [policy]' (Lewis, 2000: 82, cited by Glennerster, 2007: 30).

There is a range of different cash benefits for people in financial need. Means-tested, non-contributory benefits for families with children – such as Income Support (IS) and Jobseekers' Allowance (JSA) – may include additional payments for carers and children, in the latter case, for claims made before April 2004. Since that date, financial needs of children have been met by the Child Tax Credit, also available for low-earning working parents. Since the mid-1980s it has been possible for either adult in a couple to be the named claimant for IS and JSA. However, in the overwhelming majority of cases it remains the man who is named as the head of household and who receives the benefit (Pascall, 1997).

The 'fiscal welfare state': the tax system

Richard Titmuss, in his important article on the social division of welfare, pointed to the importance of the tax system in affecting welfare, arguing that it constituted a welfare system in its own right, complementary to that of the statutory services (Titmuss, 1958: Ch. 2). The state in the UK has long recognised some aspects of family life through the medium of the tax system. Tax allowances for children were introduced by Lloyd George, then Chancellor of the Exchequer in a Liberal government, in 1909. These constituted a recognition of the costs of children for middle-class tax-paying families. A tax allowance – an offset against tax – is effectively a subsidy (for more on tax allowances, see Chapter 8). These tax allowances survived until the 1970s, when they and the Family Allowance were amalgamated to create a single cash benefit, Child Benefit.

Until 1989 a woman's income was treated for tax purposes as if it were her husband's. Incomes were aggregated and the man received a tax allowance, supposedly to reflect the costs of being married, regardless of whether his wife was wholly dependent on him. A married man therefore received more net pay per pound earned than a working woman (Glennerster, 2007: 211). This appeared to fall foul of the spirit, if not the letter, of equal pay law, and was attacked by feminist critics and by the Equal Opportunities Commission as being discriminatory. In 1989 the married man's allowance became the 'married couple's allowance', claimable by either partner. Couples could also opt for separate assessment of tax liability. This is now automatic; the Married Couple's Allowance was abolished in 2000 for people below retirement age, although in fact the value of the allowance had been allowed to decline under the Conservatives (Lewis, 2001: 496).

Domestic violence

A degree of physical chastisement of wives by their husbands had long been officially tolerated as something acceptable, although the degree of violence permissible was circumscribed. In the 1970s recognition began to dawn that domestic violence was a 'problem'. The response to it was hesitant and fragmented, and from the beginning involved, and continues to involve, a strong voluntary element. The issue of domestic violence, which includes wife-battering, child abuse, marital rape and elder abuse, exhibited the ambivalence of official attitudes and policy towards the family; on the one hand, some recognition and acknowledgement of what are essentially human rights violations, and, on the other, belief that the family is a private sphere which should not be subject to much in the way of state control or monitoring. The establishment of the Chiswick Women's Refuge in the early 1970s helped to publicise the issue of marital violence and led to the creation of a number of other refuges and to something of a voluntary movement organised around the issue. Changes in the law followed in 1976 and 1978 which made it easier for women to obtain non-molestation orders and exclusion injunctions, which could involve arrest, against abusive partners. Although far from perfect, this represented an improvement in the protection available to women, and subsequent case law has gone further in developing this. The enforcement of the law necessarily required a more sensitive and responsive approach from the police, whose handling of domestic violence issues was deemed inadequate (Glennerster, 2007: 164–166). The 1996 Family Law Act further extended the powers of courts and police in relation to arrest and remand. More collaboration between different agencies, including the police, women's refuges and social services, has been encouraged since the 1990s in order to respond appropriately to the issue.

Conservative family policy 1979–97

> Welfare benefits, distributed with little or no consideration of their effects on behaviour, encouraged illegitimacy, facilitated the breakdown of families, and replaced incentives favouring work and self-reliance with perverse encouragement for idleness and cheating. (Thatcher, 1993: 8)

The foregoing quote from Margaret Thatcher's first volume of memoirs suggests an attitude of strong support for the family on her and her party's part, as well as a belief that the family is easily undermined by over-generous state financial provision. Her notorious remarks on the relative importance of family and society, made in 1987 (in an interview with a woman's magazine), have been quoted earlier in this chapter (Thatcher, 1987, 1993: 628). On the one hand, the Conservatives claimed to be the party of the family, and to be committed to family values; on the other, they pursued policies whose effects in some sense undermined the family.

It was argued by their left-wing opponents that these governments pursued child-*un*friendly policies, and that the side-effects of many Conservative policies were harmful to children. High levels of unemployment and a stringent approach to the uprating of cash benefits led to the emergence of high levels of child poverty in the UK, the highest in Europe, by the mid-1990s.

The Conservatives were actually open to attack regarding their family (non)policy, not only from the socialist left but also from the 'New Right', and also, paradoxically, from conservative-inclined leftist writers like Dennis and Halsey, on the grounds that the drift of policy in the 1980s – *de facto* support for lone parents via the social security system – undermined the two-parent family and led to the growth of lone parenthood (Dennis, 1993; Dennis and Erdos, 1993; Lewis, 2001: 492).

It is also possible to exaggerate the child-unfriendliness of Conservative policies. Conservative income support policies for working families, such as the Family

Income Supplement, introduced in the 1970s, and its successor Family Credit, introduced in 1988, were foundations on which subsequent Labour governments have been able to build since 1997 and are forerunners of the present tax credit schemes.

The Conservatives, lone motherhood and child support

The Conservatives struggled, and largely failed, to deal with what was perceived to be the problem of lone motherhood, which grew substantially in the 1980s. By the 1990s there were a million lone parents, making up 14% of all parents with dependent children. Two-thirds of these were dependent on Income Support. Numbers on Income Support had more than doubled from 330,000 in 1980 to 770,000 in 1989. A third of these had never married; 7% were widowed and the remainder were divorced (Glennerster, 2007: 215).

The Conservative response to what Peter Lilley, the Conservative Social Security minister, called 'the inadvertent nationalisation of fatherhood' (Lewis, 2001: 496) was to introduce a more rigorous approach to child maintenance, attempting to compel absent fathers to support their children, both in order to reduce public spending on Income Support and to deter men from leaving their families. The policy took the form of the Child Support Act 1991, a deeply unpopular measure, possibly the most hated of any passed by the Thatcher and Major governments. Effectively this involved the state taking over responsibilities for the pursuit of maintenance from individuals and from the courts. The principle was widely supported, the practice much less so. A body, the Child Support Agency, was set up to administer the law. The failure of the legislation was largely due to the determination of the Treasury, apparently against the advice of the Department of Social Security, to claw back as much money as possible from absent fathers, even those who had already made individual settlements through the courts, and its refusal to allow any money clawed back to be disregarded in calculating Income Support entitlement (Glennerster, 2007: 216). This substantially reduced support for the measure both from the general public, from targeted absent parents and from lone-parent claimants, who stood to gain nothing by cooperating with the agency.

The Conservatives and nursery provision

A significant policy development in the 1990s was the expansion of mostly private-sector nursery provision for those workers with young children. State-funded nursery provision declined markedly as central government restrictions on local authority funding caused the closure of many nurseries, while the reprioritisation of education around the demands of the national curriculum led schools away from the provision of nursery places. The private sector responded with an increase in the numbers of both private nurseries and work-based nursery facilities. Such moves were, somewhat belatedly, recognised by the Conservative government with its introduction of nursery vouchers in 1996, which gave parents some help in meeting nursery costs which they could then choose to 'top-up'. Although this scheme was short-lived, being abolished by the new government in 1997, it did at least begin to officially recognise this sea-change in the nature of employment. Similarly, one of the last acts of the Conservative governments was to extend social security benefits (Income Support and Family Credit) to allow parents with low incomes greater access to nursery provision.

Discuss and Do

What do trends in women's employment, divorce, lone parenthood, family size and other changes in family life during the period of Conservative government (1979–97), highlighted statistically in an earlier section, tell you about the impact of policy on the family? Do they suggest that officially proclaimed views and policies have a large impact, or a small one, on people's decisions about family life?

'New' Labour and families

The Conservatives, led by John Major, were heavily defeated by 'New' Labour, led by Tony Blair, in 1997. Labour claims to have reprioritised the family as a focus of policy, thereby distinguishing itself from its Conservative predecessors. There is probably more continuity between Conservative and Labour policies on the family than the present government would wish to acknowledge. Labour has, nevertheless, made a difference. Labour, for example, appointed a Minister of State for Children, Young People and Families, the first such post in British government.

New policy thinking about the family and gender relations made up a significant element of the Labour Party's 'modernisation' of its structures and doctrines that began after the disaster of the 1983 election. The Commission on Social Justice proposed some sweeping policy changes: renegotiation of the relationships between mothers, fathers and children; new demands for flexible work patterns, support for child care and other measures to accommodate caring work within the home; and reviews of the social security system, childcare and social services (Commission on Social Justice, 1994: 79–80). Much of this analysis was not new and was derived from a decade and more of discussion among feminists both inside and outside the Labour Party.

A more distinctive aspect of the Commission's discussion was its stress on social 'investment' and its linking of economic policy and social policy, economic success and social success. 'Welfare to work' was part of this; so too was work–life balance, as was the need to 'build strong families', encourage good-quality parenting and support the unpaid work of parents and other carers (Commission on Social Justice, 1994: 104–105). 'Labour-market and family policy go together; the social revolution in women's life chances demands a reappraisal of the role of men as workers and fathers as well as that of women as employees and mothers' (Commission on Social Justice, 1994: 223).

This analysis was echoed by New Labour's principal 'guru' in the 1990s, the sociologist Anthony Giddens, in his various writings on the 'Third Way' and in his 1999 Reith Lectures (Giddens, 1998: 89–98; Giddens, 1999: Ch. 4). A unifying concept in Labour's approach to social policy and to the family was to be that of 'social exclusion' (see Chapter 10). This was to play a role in Labour's policy for deprived families and children.

Family policy began in a rather incoherent and contradictory way, with cuts in lone parents' benefits a deeply unpopular move among Labour backbenchers. Labour leaders were impressed by the public relations implications of appearing to reward lone parenthood. On the other hand, lone parents were to be beneficiaries of Labour policies in other ways in subsequent years, notably through general improvements in benefits, such as Income Support, for those with children.

The consultation paper *Supporting Families* claimed that marriage was the appropriate basis for raising children (Home Office, 1998; Glennerster, 2007: 229). It proposed the promotion of good parenting and easing the strains of divorce for children, and a National Family and Parenting Institute was set up to give effect to this view (Glennerster, 2007: 229). The Labour leadership – Tony Blair and Jack Straw, for example – appeared to be ambivalent about the family: more tolerant than the Conservatives about diversity in family forms, but also apparently committed to the traditional model of the married couple family (Lewis, 2001: 490).

An important initiative was Tony Blair's commitment in 1999 to ending child poverty in 20 years, a major initiative given the size of the problem (4.4 million children in poverty) and the range of policies – employment, tax and social security – needed to address it (Lewis, 2001: 490). One parental obligation is, of course, the obligation to work and be self-supporting, an obligation which now seems to apply to both parents; it is assumed that all adults are in the labour market. It has been observed that '. . . there is a tension (at best) in Labour's obvious preference for the traditional family and willingness to talk about it in moral terms, while pursuing a determined policy to ensure that all adults, male and female, are in the workforce' (Lewis, 2001: 491).

Child care

Labour established a National Childcare Strategy in 1998, placing the provision of child care for working parents at the centre of employment policy. The government sought to extend nursery provision to every four-year-old and to address a longer-term objective of employment policy, that which aims to improve educational standards. The 1998 proposals included plans to fund part-time 'early years learning' for three- and four-year-olds, as well as the Sure Start programme, an area-based programme to tackle disadvantage by bringing together care, health and education services for young children. Money was also provided for child care initiatives at local level. Free nursery care was made available in 1998, providing 12.5 hours per week, to be increased to 15 hours per week by 2010. A 'mixed economy' approach to care provision, involving private and voluntary providers, was adopted, representing some continuity with the previous Conservative approach. The 2006 Childcare Act went on to give local authorities a statutory duty to ensure that there is enough child care provision for those who want it. Funding for child care services remains demand-led, via the Childcare Tax Credit, another area of continuity with the Conservatives (the Conservatives' Family Credit – predecessor of Labour's various Tax Credits – included a child care disregard). The level of subsidy for low-earning parents is, however, now much greater, having increased from £46 million in 1998 to £884 million by 2004 (Lewis and Campbell, 2007: 373).

Parental, maternity and paternity leave

Statutory maternity leave had been established by a Labour government in the 1970s. 'New' Labour implemented early on the European Directive on Parental Leave, required by its decision to adopt the European Social Chapter. Parents of children under five who had worked for their employers for one year could take 13 weeks leave, in blocks of from one to four weeks a year. Take-up was low. The right to leave was extended from April 2003 to cover paternity and adoption leaves, with paternity leave, of two weeks, to be paid at the level of flat-rate maternity leave. By 2005 93% of fathers took leave. The 2006 Work and Families Act will permit fathers, by 2010, to take over maternity leave from 20 weeks after the birth if the mother returns to work, but the value of this change will be limited by the low level of maternity pay, below the level of most men's earnings. However, maternity leave and pay have been transformed in the last 10 years. Paid maternity leave is planned to extend to 52 weeks by 2010, while maternity pay has been substantially increased. The number of mothers eligible for statutory maternity pay increased from 90,000 in 1997 to 300,000 in 2001 (Lewis and Campbell, 2007: 374). There have been increases in the number of recipients of maternity allowance, from 12,000 in 1997 to an estimated 54,000 in 2007. Government expenditure on statutory maternity pay and maternity allowance has risen from £500 million (SMP) and £36 million (MA) in 1997–98 to £1.6 billion and £280 million in 2007–08.

Working hours

British fathers work some of the longest hours in Europe, reducing their commitment to care work and their partners' involvement in paid work. Labour committed itself to 'fairness at work' in 1997, stating that employees should not be forced to work more than 48 hours a week. Labour did not, however, reverse the Conservatives' negotiation of an individual's right to opt out of the 1993 EU Working Time Directive. Labour has since sought to promote 'flexibility' in working arrangements. In 2001 the government established an individual's right to request flexible working patterns for the parents of children under six. The 2006 Work and Families legislation extended this right to the carers of adults, although not to those of older children. Labour has laid stress, as did the Conservatives, on the idea of 'individual choice' (Lewis and Campbell, 2007: 374–375).

It has been suggested that Labour's work–life balance policies are as much about promoting economic policy goals as they are about promoting social goals and values. The government has always sought to present its family measures as being business-friendly as well as family-friendly. In this way Labour's policies might be seen as continuous with those of the Conservatives. An important difference between the parties is, however, the issue of voluntarism and the extent to which employers should be coerced into family-friendliness. The Conservatives, although not necessarily opposed to family-friendly policies, were, and always had been, opposed to prescriptive legislation and to creating a rights-based culture (Glennerster, 2007: 214; Lewis and Campbell, 2007: 376–377). Labour has been prepared to pursue this to some extent.

Children, child protection and children's services

An important aspect of family policy is that relating to child protection – protection of children from abuse and neglect (see Chapter 13). Much policy development in this area has been driven by a series of scandals over the years involving the deaths of children, often killed by a step-parent, and where relevant statutory agencies, usually local authority social services but also including the NHS and police, have failed to act. The most recent phase of Labour policy in this area is that associated with the 'Every Child Matters' strategy, launched in 2003 in the wake of the Victoria Climbié tragedy and the subsequent Laming Report on this (H.M. Treasury, 2003). Victoria Climbié was an eight-year-old child from the Ivory Coast, taken by foster-parents to London, who died in 2000 after months of abuse and neglect. Lord Laming's report revealed shortcomings on the part of official agencies – local authority social services, the NHS and the police – which at various times had dealings with Victoria during her few months of life in the UK (Department of Health/Home Office, 2003).

Most recently an ambitious and comprehensive strategy for children has been launched by the Secretary of State for Children, Schools and Families, Ed Balls, in December 2007 (Department for Children, Schools and Families, 2007). This proposes an all-embracing Children's Plan, covering a full range of interventions and services, including education and early-years learning, as well as health (including mothers' ante-natal health), children's safety, play and leisure – an example of 'joined-up governance'. It builds on existing, long-standing initiatives, including those for Sure Start Children's Centres, the promotion of work–life balance and the commitment to eliminating child poverty. The underlying rationales for all this are those of New Labour's policies from the beginning – a mixture of 'social investment' and equal opportunities.

Conclusion

In this chapter we have tried to provide you with a highly selective overview of a large and complex field. We have suggested that family policy in the UK now seems to have become an important area. At the same time, there is some ambiguity about the nature of government commitment to the family. On the one hand, 'policing' the family seems to have become an aspect of policy: the government has promoted the idea that parents have responsibilities – to work, to be good parents and so on. This is associated both with a 'social investment' strategy – enhancing the quality of 'human capital' in a context of globalisation and the need for economic competitiveness – and with a law and order approach. On the other hand, the government has displayed and encouraged a tolerant attitude to diversity in family forms; has directed more resources towards families with dependents, especially working families, as part of a programme for eliminating child poverty, a policy which has, however, been only partly successful; and has tried to induce employers, business and workforces to adopt a new approach to the balance between work and family life.

Some of the explicit, proffered rationales for policy change might be, to some extent, window-dressing, or coexist with other rationales that are hidden or that governments are shy about advertising. In many respects, despite supposed 'modernisation', Labour remains an old-fashioned social democratic party, committed to public-sector values, public spending and some measure of equality, but open to new influences, trends and electoral opportunities (see Chapters 8 and 10). At least some of Labour's family programme since 1997 could be viewed as a gender equality strategy, or at least the beginnings of one (see Chapter 19). Women have an equal right and obligation to work; that implies an equal obligation on men to care, and to share equally in other household responsibilities. These goals are far from being attained. As an election-winning strategy, however, it has something to be said for it, as the Conservative Party under David Cameron is now realising.

There is, finally, some ambiguity about women's involvement in the world of work as far as gender equality is concerned. Women are much more likely to work part-time, are more likely to be lower-paid, and are more likely to work in particular occupations and sectors – the public sector and the 'caring' industries, which include teaching as well as health care (nursing and a range of ancillary health occupations) and social care. These are in fact occupations and activities that women traditionally carried out unpaid within the family, or as paid domestic servants and governesses for the families of others. One way of viewing the recent expansion of women's employment is as the 'commodification' of family tasks and activities, something called for by utopians of an earlier age, as well as by some contemporary feminists (Lewis, 2001: 491). Women are now carrying out much the same tasks that they have always done but now, or to a greater extent, as part of the formal economy, and being paid for doing so. Whether the achievement, on this basis, of levels of female involvement in paid work comparable with men's represents real gender equality is an interesting question.

In this chapter, you have

- examined the concept of 'family policy';
- located family policy in the context of UK social policy;
- examined the changing relationship between the state and the family in the twentieth century;
- identified and examined various policy areas which have an impact on the family;
- examined in some detail specific family policies of Labour governments since 1997, including those for children, 'work–life balance' and 'family-friendly employment'.

Annotated further reading

An outstanding recent sociological study of the family, both historical and comparative, and remarkably wide-ranging, is that by the Swedish sociologist Goran Therborn (Therborn, 2004).

There are useful brief introductory accounts of family policy in social policy texts by Jane Millar (Millar, 2003) and Jan Pahl (Pahl, 2003). Howard Glennerster's excellent history of post-war British social policy, now in its third edition, is good on the family (Glennerster, 2007). Susan Pedersen has provided a valuable historical and comparative account of the twentieth-century emergence of family policy in the

UK and France (Pedersen, 1993). Much writing about family policy is really about gender and social policy, so it is worth consulting texts on this subject, such as Gillian Pascall's (Pascall, 1986, 1997).

There is a useful book chapter surveying developments since 1997 by Jane Millar in an edited collection (Millar and Ridge, 2002). Other useful chapters in edited collections providing overviews of recent developments include those by Ruth Lister (Lister, 1994), Fiona Williams (Williams, 2005) and Jane Lewis, who is a prolific and distinguished writer on family and gender (Lewis, 2001).

Pessimistic conservative views about the family have been contributed to by a number of writers, not all of them describable as 'conservative', including Charles Murray, Amitai Etzioni, Patricia Morgan, Norman Dennis and George Erdos (Dennis and Etzioni would object to the label 'conservative' – the former is an old-fashioned social democrat but conservative on the family, the latter a 'communitarian') (Murray, 1990; Dennis, 1993, 1997; Dennis and Erdos, 1993; Etzioni, 1994: Ch. 2, 1997; Morgan, 1998). Two examples of optimistic conservative views are a book by Ferdinand Mount, which is lively and readable, and a book chapter by David Willetts (Mount, 1982; Willetts, 1989).

Chapter 19

Social divisions and equal opportunities policies

by Mary Knyspel and Guy Daly

Objectives

- To explore what is meant by the term 'social divisions'.

- To examine the debates associated with equality.

- To describe Britain's equal opportunities and anti-discrimination policies in relation to: ethnicity, gender, disability, sexual orientation and age.

- To review the Labour government's approach to promoting equality.

Introduction

A social divisions perspective in social policy challenges inequality, discrimination and social injustice faced by groups in society. As can be seen from the newspaper article, reproduced in Box 19.1, wage inequalities between men and women persist to this day. However, it is just one example of what can be argued are the many social inequalities that exist between various groups in society to which we all belong. This chapter has as its focus, therefore, an exploration of some of the social divisions that persist between groups in British society along with an explanation of the state's response in terms of social policy initiatives. This chapter will start by defining the concept of social divisions and showing how this approach differs from other sociological perspectives on the structure of society. The concepts of equality and social justice will be explained. Then, the extent to which the state intervenes to combat inequality will be examined, paying particular attention to equal opportunities and anti-discrimination legislation. Evidence of discrimination, inequality and social injustice faced by groups, or social divisions, in Britain will be presented, followed by an examination of existing legislation. The social divisions explored in this chapter are race, gender, disability, sexual orientation and age. To some commentators, not least Marxist and socialist ones, the most fundamental social division is social class. Certainly, class is a powerful determinant of life chances.

Box 19.1

Councils face £2.8bn bill for equal pay

Wage discrimination claims leave black hole in local authority finances

Polly Curtis, education editor, *The Guardian* Wednesday 2 January 2008

Council bosses across England are having to remortgage their town halls and raid reserves to meet a £2.8bn bill to pay back a generation of women who have been discriminated against, the Guardian can reveal.

Schools are to be told to find up to a third of the bill out of their reserves to compensate classroom assistants and cleaners who have been systematically underpaid. There are fears they could be forced to lay off other workers to pay women back.

... New research by the councils' organisation Local Government Employers (LGE), seen by the Guardian, identifies a bill of £1bn for back pay and £1.4bn a year to meet the higher pay costs. Another £400m needs to be found to protect the wages of men who face pay cuts to rectify past positive discrimination in their favour.

... Jan Parkinson, managing director of LGE, said that a £2.8bn bill, even in the context of councils' £85bn annual budget, would hit some services.

'The schools hold their own budgets and can ignore employment recommendations made by councils. In the circumstances, it seems a fair balance of responsibilities if councils take care of the legal and industrial relations issues and schools pay for back pay from their considerable reserves,' she said.

Reprinted with permission.

However, an examination of class inequality and associated policy responses has been excluded from this chapter, since there are no anti-discrimination laws associated with class *per se* in the same way as, for example, disability and race. However, that is not to say that Britain does not have social policies that have the expressed intention of addressing class inequality in various ways, whether that is in relation to alleviating poverty, poor housing, health inequalities, education inequalities or social exclusion more generally. These policies are discussed in the chapters that precede this one. Other divisions such as religion and national identity are mentioned only briefly in this chapter. Further reading on these divisions is identified at the end of the chapter. However, before proceeding to discuss various examples of social divisions and some of the associated social policies, the chapter starts with an exploration of what is meant by social divisions.

What are social divisions

As individuals, we are able to identify ourselves using several classification systems. For example, we can identify ourselves in terms of gender, ethnicity and age. Researchers and providers of services often ask us to identify ourselves using these and other categories. We are also able to describe other people with similar labels and create groups of people. Empirical studies using a range of indicators such as health, wealth, well-being and power show that some groups or divisions of people consistently fare better than others. Conversely, certain groups face much higher levels of inequality and discrimination. A social divisions perspective has a systematic concern with division, inequality and social injustice. As Payne (2000: 249–253) has stated:

> ... a social divisions approach represents a distinctive concern with division, inequality and social justice... [While d]ivisions are the normal state of society, [i]t is the persistence of their associated disadvantages that is the problem, with extremely unequal access to the desirable things in life continually impinging on the same categories of people.

This approach therefore emphasises the *multiplicity* of social divisions. Divisions are a normal part of society; diversity and difference are to be celebrated. However, it is the inequality, discrimination and disadvantage associated with these divisions that is challenged. A social division is a relatively fixed, socially constructed, social group which consistently demonstrates an imbalance of power, resources and opportunities between categories. Payne (2000) identified nine core characteristics to which a social division conforms:

- A social division contains two or more interrelated, socially sanctioned, materially and culturally different categories.
- It tends to be long-lasting and sustained by dominant cultural beliefs and practices.
- A social division is socially constructed.
- The categories are hierarchical with unequal opportunities and resources.
- Movement across the divides is rare or achieved slowly.
- Category membership produces shared identities.
- All members of society fit in one or other category.
- Empirical methods examine life chances and life styles.
- The principle of social divisions is a universal systematic feature of human society.

Examples of social divisions include class, race, gender, disability, sexual orientation, age, religion and national identity. Clearly, one's identity and position arise from the interplay of multiple divisions. Anthias (1998) suggests that the multiple labels are like different layers of clothing which can be worn in a different order at different times, revealing our position in society and affecting our life chances. So, the relative importance of each division in terms of life chances varies according to situation and across time, with multiple categories having the potential to cancel out or compound disadvantage. For example, the underperformance of black boys at school has been a major area of concern for some time, recently prompting the Mayor of London, Ken Livingstone, to call for more black teachers (*The Independent*, 2004), and Trevor Phillips, the then Chair of the Commission for Racial Equality, to suggest that black boys be taught separately (BBC, *Inside Out*, 7 March 2005). However, the situation for middle-class black boys, particularly those at public school, is different.

Here is a complex interrelationship between gender, ethnicity, class and outcome. A number of writers have used the term 'triple jeopardy' to highlight the problems compounded by multiple divisions: *Triple Jeopardy: Growing Old in a Second Homeland* (Norman, 1985); *Triple Jeopardy: African American Women with Disabilities* (ODDC, 2003); *Triple Jeopardy: Muslim Women's Experience of Discrimination* (Hamdani, 2005).

A social divisions perspective is distinct from other approaches to inequality in society (Anthias, 1998, 2001; Payne, 2000). It differs from structural functionalist approaches in its challenge to the status quo. The individualism and relativism of postmodernism does not explain the consistent and deeply entrenched inequalities revealed by empirical studies. Marxist and feminist analyses address key issues, but may be too narrow in focus to engage fully with the complexity of multiple divisions. The celebration of diversity and difference in multiculturalism challenges traditional identity hierarchies but does not sufficiently address the underlying causes of inequality.

Before going on to examine British social policies in relation to combating social inequalities, it would be useful to remind ourselves briefly of the major debates associated with equality. Advocates of *equality of outcome* believe that everyone should obtain an equal share of society's resources, that is, income or other material benefits. This form of equality is often thought of as being unworkable, or even unjust, as it does not reward talent or effort. Advocates of *equality of opportunity* believe that everyone should have an equal opportunity or access to the best paid jobs, positions of power and material benefits. This type of equality is criticised because it does not eliminate inequality. Inequality remains: new élitist and privileged groups emerge based on merit or occupation, rather than inheritance or social divisions. British social policy tends to aim to achieve equality of opportunity by outlawing discrimination. Indeed, New Labour's approach to social policy has been depicted very much as one that seeks to promote equality of opportunity rather than equality of outcome (Williams, 2005). Very much related to New Labour's approach has been a discourse of social justice which is another concept associated with the debates on equality. In a world of scarce resources, who should get what? One of the most influential debates on this topic is that between Rawls and Nozick. (See Chapters 9 and 10 for discussions of their ideas.)

Combating inequality

Most advanced welfare states have in place policies to combat inequality and outlaw discrimination (which are not one and the same thing), although the extent to which the state intervenes varies enormously – between nations and within nations depending upon the ideological disposition of the government of the day. Welfare states pursue different conceptions of equality. As is explored in greater detail in Chapter 22, Esping-Andersen (1996) identifies the social democratic Scandinavian states as the most egalitarian with regard to outcome. In comparison, the social insurance model found in many Western European states emphasises equity over redistribution. Conversely, liberal welfare states such as the United States target welfare narrowly and, therefore, perform badly in terms of poverty eradication and the promotion of equality of outcome.

The European Union introduced the Racial Equality Directive and Employment Equality Directive (2000) to tackle the threat to the economic and social cohesion of the Union posed by discrimination. This directive prompted EU member states 'to introduce legislation prohibiting direct and indirect discrimination at work on grounds of age, sexuality, religion and disability' (Macnicol, 2006: 251) and was arguably the prompt and precursor to some of the swathe of 'equalities' legislation enacted in the UK over the last few years, including the following:

• Race Relations (Amendment) Act 2000
• Disability Discrimination Act 2005
• Employment Equality (Sexual Orientation) Regulations 2003
• Employment Equality (Age) Regulations 2006
• Equality Act 2006.

In the UK, the government's Women and Equality Unit (2005) website states that: 'The Government has a vision for a modern Britain: A vision of equality and opportunity for all.' An examination of policies in Britain to combat inequality for the social divisions of race, gender, disability, sexual orientation and age follows. Evidence of discrimination, inequality and social injustice faced by these groups will be presented. The extent to which the state in the UK intervenes to combat inequality and the effectiveness of its equality policies will be assessed. Reference will also be made to policies from other nations where appropriate.

Ethnicity

A precise definition of 'race' or ethnicity is difficult to achieve as these terms are highly contested. However, the two terms are not synonymous. Indeed, the term 'race' is considered particularly problematic, being based on a mythical and imagined creation, such that many writers avoid its use (Mason, 2000a: 93) or place it in inverted commas (Law, 1996; Ratcliffe, 2004). However, in practice 'race' and ethnicity tend to be deployed extremely loosely to imply commonalities of language, religion, identity, national origins and/or even skin colour (Ratcliffe, 2004). The 1976 Race Relations Act defined discrimination on racial grounds as meaning any of the following: race, colour, ethnic or national origins, and nationality or citizenship (Blakemore and Drake, 1996). In Britain, the categories of ethnicity used by the Office of National Statistics have been expanded with time. Table 19.1 shows an expansion in the number of categories in the UK population census from 1991 to 2001. The 2001 census included 'Mixed' ethnic groups and had a separate question on religion, thus arguably allowing for a more sophisticated analysis of ethnicity.

Table 19.1 Definitions of 'race' and ethnicity in the UK population census 1991 and 2001

1991 UK Census	2001 UK Census White
Black Caribbean	White British
Black African	White Irish
Black Other (*Please specify*)	White Other (*Please specify*)
Indian	Mixed – White and Black Caribbean
Bangladeshi	Mixed – White and Black African
Pakistani	Mixed – White and Asian
Chinese	Mixed – Other (*Please specify*)
Other (*Please specify*)	Asian or Asian British – Indian
	Asian or Asian British – Pakistani
	Asian or Asian British – Bangladeshi
	Asian or Asian British – Other (*Please specify*)
	Black or Black British – Caribbean
	Black or Black British – African
	Black or Black British – Other (*Please specify*)
	Chinese
	Other Ethnic Group (*Please specify*)

There is substantial evidence to suggest that there is significant and persistent discrimination and inequality for minority ethnic groups in the UK. For example, people from minority ethnic groups are more likely to experience unemployment than white people (Jones, 1993; Blakemore and Drake, 1996; Modood, 1997; Mason, 2000b, 2003). Since the early 1990s the gap has narrowed, but in the early part of this century it remains 10–15% higher for Bangladeshi, Pakistani and Black-Caribbean people than for white people (Ratcliffe, 2004). In addition, there are differences in employment rates between men and women from minority ethnic groups. African-Caribbean women have similar employment rates to white people, but significantly higher rates than Pakistani and Bangladeshi women (Ratcliffe, 2004).

In addition to employment inequalities, inequality is experienced by black and minority ethnic groups in most if not all other areas of life. In housing, black and minority ethnic people are more likely to become homeless, are four times as likely to be in areas of high concentrations of deprivation, have their mobility constrained by local authority allocation processes, and are under-represented in relation to participation in housing management. In education, as we have seen above, the under-achievement of black boys in school is an area of major concern in the UK. In matters of policing and the criminal justice system, the 'culture' of policing and the actions of individual officers have been shown to be discriminatory (Ratcliffe, 2004). Indeed, until recently, the police and criminal justice system were excluded form the provisions of anti-discrimination legislation. However, the murder of Stephen Lawrence and the subsequent MacPherson Enquiry resulted in changes in the legislation with the enactment of the Race Relations Amendment Act 2000.

Of late, a particularly emotive issue sometimes associated with 'race' relations is the topic of asylum and immigration. Refugees, asylum seekers and illegal immigrants are being portrayed as a major social problem by the media and politicians alike. Indeed, this became a central issue in the 2005 General Election in Britain. Negative attitudes came to the fore. In many respects, hostility to asylum seekers, refugees and other minorities such as travellers is not restricted to Britain in the 2000s; it has occurred and continues to occur across Europe and beyond. For example, the Annual Report of the European Monitoring Centre on Racism and Xenophobia (EUMC, 2004) showed that racism against the Roma community continues. According to the EUMC, vulnerable groups to racial violence include (in alphabetical order): ethnic minorities, illegal immigrants, Jews, Muslims, North Africans, people from the former Yugoslavia, refugees/asylum seekers, and 'gypsies'/Romi/Sinti. The majority of the perpetrators of such violence are seen to be young men, sometimes but not always associated with far right groups (EUMC, 2005).

Table 19.2 overleaf shows that Britain has a long, if somewhat inconsistent or contradictory, history of legislation associated with nationality, immigration and 'race' relations. The first Race Relations Act of 1965 outlawed discrimination in public places. The 1968 Commonwealth Immigrants Act extended the provision to the 'private' sphere and included housing, employment and service provision in its anti-discrimination legislation. The Race Relations Act (1976) applied to indirect as well as direct indiscrimination. As mentioned above, the MacPherson Report (1999), an inquiry into the death of Stephen Lawrence, was highly critical of the police. The subsequent Race Relations (Amendment) Act of 2000 brought the police and other public bodies into the provisions of the legislation. It also imposed a new Statutory Duty on public authorities and associated agencies to promote equality. These positive duties are proactive rather than reactive and mark a change in the direction of equality legislation.

However, before the first Race Relations Act in 1965 was set up, Britain had already reduced rights of entry with the introduction of a work voucher system to Commonwealth migrants. Immigration control has become increasingly more restrictive since the 1960s. All governments since this time have claimed that successful race relations require careful immigration controls. However, these controls are often perceived to be racist. In the 1990s there was an increased use of welfare measures to control, monitor and marginalise asylum seekers (Lewis, 2003). The 1999 Act saw the dispersal of refugees and a stigmatising voucher system was introduced.

It is more than 30 years since the 1976 Race Relations Act came into force, yet 'racial' inequality is still a problem in Britain today. While there have been some improvements in the lives of some individuals, there remains much to be done to ensure that everyone from an ethnic minority has an equal opportunity to succeed. Speaking at the Clement Attlee Lecture in April 2004, the then Chair of the Commission for Racial Equality, Trevor Phillips (2005), stated:

> [C]oming from a minority ethnic community still appears to carry added disadvantages . . .. Whatever class you belong to, your race is an obstacle all by itself – for example African Caribbean men and Pakistani men, when compared with white men of similar qualifications, will on average be earning between £5,000 and £6,500 less each year. And the impact of race on people's life chances is not reducing with time. Rather the opposite – our race seems more likely than ever to trap us in the place into which we were born. Babies of mothers born in

Table 19.2 Summary of nationality, asylum, immigration and race relations legislation

Legislation	Main features
Aliens Act 1905	Immigration control bureau with the power of expulsion established
Aliens Restriction Act 1914	Home Office control over movement of aliens
Aliens Restriction (Amendment) Act 1919	Extended the terms of the previous Act to peacetime
British Nationality Act 1948	Commonwealth citizens were given the right to work, settle and bring families to the United Kingdom
Commonwealth Immigrants Act 1962	Restricted admission to settlers from the Commonwealth to people issued with employment vouchers
White Paper on Immigration from the Commonwealth 1965	Employment vouchers limited to 8,500 per annum
Race Relations Act 1965	Discrimination in public places outlawed. Race Relations Board and National Committee for Commonwealth Immigrants established
Commonwealth Immigrant Act 1968	Housing, employment and service provision included in anti-discrimination legislation
Immigration Act 1971	Partiality grandfather clause introduced
Race Relations Act 1976	Commission for Racial Equality created
British Nationality Act 1981	Three categories of citizenship established: British Citizenship; Citizenship of British Dependent Territories: British Overseas Citizenship
Immigration Act 1988	Amended British Nationality Act to incorporate 'free movement' provision of EC law
British Nationality (Hong Kong) Act 1990	Restrictions set up for immigrants from Hong Kong
Asylum and Immigration Act 1993	Application for asylum process updated. Provision for fingerprinting asylum seekers introduced
Immigration and Asylum Act 1999	Introduction of policies for vouchers for food and clothes, restrictions on illegal employment and dispersal of asylum seekers
Human Rights Act 1999	European Convention on Human Rights brought into legislature
Race Relations (Amendment Act) 2000	Earlier Act amended to include the police. Duty placed on public authorities to actively promote race equality
Racial and Religious Hatred Act 2006	Created an offence of inciting hatred against a person on the grounds of their religion
Equality Act 2006	Made it illegal to discriminate on religious or belief grounds in the provision of education and training and goods and services

Source: Adapted from Race for Racial Justice (2005) and Lewis (2003).

Pakistan are on average twice as likely to die before their first birthday. I can also tell you with statistical certainty that an African Caribbean boy just as able as I was has twice as much chance of seeing the inside of a jail as he has of taking a university degree .... A Muslim man or woman who goes for a job is a third as likely as a non-Muslim to get it .... This is not just about the poor. Of the 17,000 doctors on the grade just below consultant, earning at least twice the average wage, 12,000 of them are from ethnic minorities. They could consider themselves well-off were it not for the fact that they have little prospect of the advancement likely for their white colleagues.

Gender

Gender inequality can also be seen to pervade almost every aspect of life. For example, if one starts by an examination of the composition of the House of Commons itself, one sees that there are substantially fewer women Members of Parliament (MPs) than men. The 2005 General Election in Britain returned 128 women MPs (19.6%) compared to 517 men to the House of Commons (UK Parliament, 2005). A survey by the Equal Opportunities Commission (2005) showed that women are still significantly under-represented in positions of influence in business, the police, media and the senior judiciary, despite the fact that women make up over half Britain's population and nearly half the workforce. One of the reasons put forward by the EOC for this was that women find it difficult to combine work with family responsibilities in a culture of long hours, especially at senior levels. Women 'pay' for their caring role in terms of progression and promotion. Focusing on informal caring of a sick, disabled or elderly person, Evandrou and Glaser (2003) showed that there is also a pension cost of caring too.

Women still earn less than men; the weekly median total individual income for all men in 2003/04 was almost twice that for all women (Women and Equality Unit, 2005). Figure 19.1 shows that women's pay starts to fall dramatically at child-rearing age and never really picks up again. The drop in pay can be explained to some extent by a higher proportion of women working part-time or reduced hours during this period.

Lifespan lower pay can also be explained by the horizontal and vertical segregation. Horizontal segregation results in lower pay for women because proportionately more women work in the low-paid service sector while proportionately more men work in higher-paid jobs in manufacturing and construction. This is an international problem, as even Scandinavian nations, renowned for gender

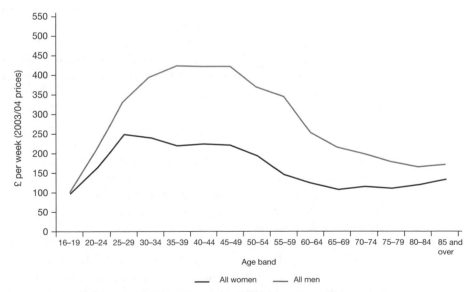

Figure 19.1 Median total individual income by age band, all women and all men, 2003/04
Source: Women and Equality Unit (2005) *Individual Income 1996/97 – 2003/04*. London: Department of Trade and Industry. Crown copyright material is reproduced with the permission of the Controller of HMSO and the Queen's Printer for Scotland under the terms of the Click-Use Licence.

equality in the workplace, exhibit occupational gender segregation. Indeed, sex segregation is on average higher in Nordic nations than in other OECD nations because of the high number of public sector service jobs. So, Scandinavian welfare corporatism has reconstituted patriarchy in male-dominated corporate institutions (Hearnes, 1987) and institutionalised women's dual roles as mothers and workers (Borchorst and Siim, 1987). This may not necessarily impede gender equality, as pay differentials are relatively low in Nordic countries. Vertical segregation, or the 'glass ceiling' (see Box 19.2), means that proportionately more men than women are in high-status supervisory or management positions. Only 9% of the top business leaders and national newspaper editors are women, yet women make up 45% of that workforce (Equal Opportunities Commission, 2004).

The United Kingdom has had legislation that makes discrimination on the grounds of gender in the workplace unlawful for over 30 years. The Equal Pay Act 1970 made it unlawful for employers to discriminate between men and women in terms of their pay and contractual conditions. The Sex Discrimination Act 1975 (SDA) applies to both men and women and makes sex discrimination unlawful in employment and vocational training, education, the provision and sale of goods, facilities and services and premises. In employment and vocational training, it is also unlawful to discriminate against someone on the grounds of being married. The Sex Discrimination (Gender Reassignment) Regulations of 1999 have made it illegal to be discriminated against on the grounds of gender reassignment. The Employment Equality (Sexual Orientation) Regulations of 2003 has outlawed discrimination on the grounds of sexual orientation. New laws came into effect in 2003 resulting in a number of changes to the maternity and paternity leave rights for parents and adopted parents. The new laws also allow parents of disabled children or non-disabled children under the age of six the right to apply to work flexibly on a permanent basis.

However, despite over 30 years of legislation, gender inequality in the workplace persists. There remains much to be done for greater equality to be achieved. In 2004, the Women and Work Commission was created to examine the problem of the gender pay gap and other issues affecting women's employment, with a particular focus on how men's and women's education and skills affected which jobs they could obtain, promotion and career progression (the 'glass ceiling'), women's experiences in the job market before and after having children, and the different experiences of women working full-time and part-time.

This issue of child care is clearly something that needs to be addressed if the occupational inequality gap is to decrease markedly. That said, there have been some major developments in Britain's child care strategy over the last 10–20 years, initially under the last period of the Conservatives' rule under John Major but particularly under New Labour since its election into government in 1997. One significant development of employment policy in the 1990s was the expansion of nursery provision and pre-school education provision for those workers with young children. There has been an expansion of both private and state provision (Department for Education and Skills, 2007). Such moves were encouraged by the introduction of nursery vouchers in 1996. The 1997 Budget took these developments further, declaring the advent of a National Childcare Strategy, which would place the provision of child care for working parents at the centre of employment policy in the future. Nursery provision is offered to every four-year-old and Britain

Box 19.2

Glass ceiling still blocks women from executive floor

David Teather, *The Guardian*, Monday 2 October 2006

The number of women in Britain's boardrooms has fallen sharply, wiping out the small but steady gains made over the past few years. At the end of the most recent financial year there were only 12 women holding executive director roles at FTSE 100 companies, compared with 20 a year ago. Women occupied 112 non-executive seats in the boardroom this year, dropping from 122 in the previous survey.

It is so far unclear whether the figures are an aberration after a cluster of high-profile departures or a reversal of long-term trends. In the Guardian's annual survey in 2003, there were 15 female executive directors, rising to 17 in 2004 and 20 last year.

Jenny Watson, chairwoman of the Equal Opportunities Commission, said previous data had suggested that with the slow pace of change it would take 40 years to get as many women into Britain's boardrooms as there were men. 'These figures show that possibly things are stalling,' she said. 'There is an argument that there are more women going to university and working and that they will come through but this says to me that argument isn't holding water.' Ms Watson said that while some employers were improving attitudes to flexible working, they tended not to apply the same principles to very senior jobs.

A broader survey of the FTSE 350 published today by the accountancy firm Deloitte supports the gloomy view of women's progress in the boardroom. Deloitte said the number of executive director jobs held by women had stuck at only 3% last year.

Reprinted with permission.

Discuss and Do

The 'glass ceiling' is a phrase used to describe the invisible barrier that stops women (and other disadvantaged groups) from progressing further in their careers, for example by being blocked from promotion to more senior positions in an organisation:

[the] impermeable barrier that blocks the vertical movement of women; below this barrier, women are able to get promoted; beyond this barrier, they are not. (Baxter and Wright, 2000: 276)

Can you think of some of the overt and covert barriers that might exist or be employed to block women's progression within organisations?

has seen an expansion of after-school clubs (though many also operate as before-school clubs) and homework clubs. Furthermore, the current system of Working Families' Tax Credits is arguably an attempt to take into account the often prohibitive cost of child care. In addition, working parents have had their rights extended over the last 10 years with, for example, New Labour since its election introducing paid paternity and adoption leave, extended maternity leave and increased maternity pay, and a new right to request flexible working for parents of young and disabled children and carers of adults. All of this, it is claimed, helps to combat gender inequality in work. (See Chapter 16 for further discussion of this area.)

Research by the OECD (2004) shows that in countries with relatively well-developed systems of work/family reconciliation policies, women tend to have higher employment rates in their thirties. Both formal child-care and paid maternity leave are important factors, as is employers' flexibility in connection with work/family balance. In an evaluation of EU legislation, Neilson (1998) concluded that women are disadvantaged because of their lower level of qualifications, the shortage of adequate child care provision, their restricted mobility and the continuing prejudices shown by employers. Clearly, equal opportunities legislation has done much for women, but this alone is not enough for gender equality in the workplace to be achieved. However, for the most part, the initiatives implemented in the UK over the last decade have been more about providing equality of opportunity rather than equality of outcome. Overall, inequalities in pay, pensions and care responsibilities, while they might have diminished, continue to persist (Rake, 2001; Williams, 2005).

Disability

A social model of disability emphasises the society as the cause of disability rather than the individual, unlike the medical model that focuses on an individual's impairment (Oliver, 1990). That is, it is economic, social and physical barriers that need to addressed in order for equality to be achieved. The newspaper article in Box 19.3 about Jodee Mundy and her family shows that being disabled or being brought up in a family whose members are disabled (in Jodee Mundy's situation due to the deafness of her parents and siblings) is disabling because of society's response to such circumstances. As Shakespeare (2000: 56) explains:

> People are disabled by society, not by their bodies. It is the social and environmental barriers, prejudicial attitudes and other exclusionary processes which make living with an impairment so hard for disabled people and their families.

Social barriers and discriminatory practice pervade all areas of life including the political process, access to buildings and services, the mass media and leisure (Barnes, 1990). The economic disadvantage faced by disabled people compared to the non-disabled is well documented (Martin and White, 1988; Berthoud et al., 1993; Hyde, 2000). Disabled people are more likely to be unemployed or in part-time work, receive lower pay and are at higher risk of poverty than non-disabled people (Disability Rights Commission, 2007). Not only are incomes low, but a disability often incurs extra cost.

One of the greatest problems experienced by disabled people is the attitudes of others, and not only the 'uneducated'. Social policy analyses, particularly feminist analyses of caring, have been criticised for focusing on dependency and neglecting the view of disabled people (Morris, 1991, 1992; Oliver and Barnes, 1998; Shakespeare, 2000). Morris (1992) suggests that such an approach is detrimental to the validity of the research and to the civil rights of disabled people. Research from Norway (Grue and Lœrum, 2002) shows that disabled mothers experience negative attitudes and live out their motherhood within a discourse of disability.

Medicine and technology, while offering vast improvements to the lives of disabled people, can also be the source of discrimination. For example, there are members of the deaf community who are proud of their deaf identity and therefore reject the attempt made to 'cure' deafness through genetic research or cochlear implants. Indeed, as Jodee Mundy and her family's story shows, it is society rather than deaf people which needs attention (Box 19.3).

As yet, legislation put in place to combat inequality has had mixed results. One can go back at least to the Second World War to review the modern welfare state's response to disability. The Disabled Persons (Employment) Act of 1944 offered reserved occupations in workplaces employing more than 20 people. However, it did little to address discrimination at work and completely neglected other areas of

---

Box 19.3

Everyone in Jodee Mundy's family is deaf – except for her

After growing up straddling two worlds, she is convinced that, far from being a problem, deafness is the glue that binds them together

Rebecca Atkinson, *The Guardian*, Saturday 29 December 2007

Jodee Mundy is the only person in her immediate family who can hear. Her mother and father are both deaf. Her two elder brothers, Shane and Gavin, are deaf. So too are her two sisters-in-law (one of whom comes from a family with three generations of deafness) and her two nieces and nephew (one other nephew, Oskar, can hear). Cast the net wider and Jodee's family includes a deaf aunt, uncle, two great-great-aunts and a succession of deaf cats.

'I remember when I first realised my family were deaf,' says Jodee. 'I was five. Mum and I were in a shop looking at the Barbies. Mum signed to me that it was time to go. I was so absorbed in the dolls that when I looked around she'd gone. I was lost. So I ran to the front desk and the woman there made an announcement on the Tannoy: "Gillian Mundy, your daughter is waiting for you at the front desk." She kept repeating it, but Mum didn't come. I had this anxiety that she would never come back. Then Mum appeared through the clothing racks and signed to me, "Where have you been? I've been so worried." And I said, "But the lady made an announcement." And Mum just looked at me and said, "I'm deaf, you know that." And it just hit me, what that actually meant – that she couldn't hear.'

This was the pivotal moment when she realised that her mum's normality was everyone else's abnormality.

'Suddenly I was different. I remember walking away with Mum to the car park and we were signing and people were looking at us, and I'd never noticed it before. From that day on I realised how society was treating my family.' The main pressures, Jodee argues, don't come from within the family, but from outside. 'We would be out somewhere and people would stare. I would often over-hear people saying things like, "Oh, it's so sad they are deaf and dumb", or they would mock us for signing.'

'The fact that most people think talking is the only way to communicate is so narrow-minded because hearing people are the ones who can't communicate when they are on a bus and there is someone outside waving goodbye. They are the ones who can't communicate under water if they are scuba diving. They are the ones that can't communicate across the street or in a loud night-club. It's deaf people who can. I wish people would see the richness and the wealth of the deaf world.'

Reprinted with permission.

life. The Disability Discrimination Act of 1995 (DDA) granted legal rights to disabled people in employment, access to services, education, transport and housing. The Disability Rights Commission Act of 1999 established a Disability Rights Commission (DRC) which in October 2007, was subsumed within the Commission for Equality and Human Rights. In September 2002 the law was extended to cover access to education for all disabled people. New regulations brought into effect in October 2004 made significant technical detailed changes to the Disability Discrimination Act 1995. New employment rights and rights of access became law, changes were made to the meaning of discrimination and harassment, and the small employers exemption was removed. The Disability Discrimination Act of 2005 put into place the remaining measures arising from the recommendations of the Disability Rights Task Force.

The DDA 2005 has been criticised from some quarters for using vague terms like 'reasonable adjustments'. In practice, the government did continue initially to rely on a policy of voluntary compliance and persuasion (Hyde, 2000). Research has shown that willingness to comply with the DDA is dependent on both knowledge of the DDA and attitudes to disabled people (Jackson *et al.*, 2000). Therefore, while the Disability Discrimination Act is a step forward, disabled people continue to experience prejudice and discrimination. According to the outgoing Disability Rights Commission (2007) certain advances have been gained, including there being more disabled people in employment than a decade ago, improvements to housing, the built environment and transport to make them more accessible, and a greater number of disabled children and young people gaining educational qualifications and progressing into further and higher education. However, after more than 10 years of the Disability Discrimination Act 1995 and further legislation under New Labour, disabled people continue to face significant inequalities. Some of the stark inequalities that still persist include:

- the disproportionately high numbers of unqualified disabled people, comprising 33% of all unqualified people;
- the disproportionately high numbers of unemployed disabled people, comprising 40% of all unemployed people;
- that the proportion of disabled people living in relative poverty has increased over the last 10 years;
- that of all children living in poverty, 33% have at least one disabled parent;
- that amongst working people, disabled workers still tend to earn 10% less than non-disabled workers;
- that disabled people have disproportionately poorer morbidity and mortality rates;
- that disabled people continue to have to rely on poor and inaccessible transport;
- that disabled people continue to suffer harassment and abuse. (Jolly *et al.*, 2006; Breakthrough, 2007; Disability Rights Commission, 2007)

Sexual orientation

This section will focus on equality for gay men and lesbian women. Historically in Britain, gay men and lesbian women have not enjoyed the same civil rights as heterosexual individuals. Homosexual activity between men was illegal until the late 1960s. The Sexual Offences Act (1967) came into force in England and Wales and decriminalised homosexual acts between two men over 21 years of age and 'in private'. Lesbianism has never been legally prohibited, but it has been considered to be unnatural. The *Diagnostic and Statistical Manual of Mental Disorders* classified homosexuality as a mental disorder until it was removed in the third edition in 1980. Only ego-dystonic homosexuality remained as a disorder, and this was removed from the DSM III-R in 1987. However, in some countries homosexual acts still carry the death penalty.

Gay men and lesbian women experience discrimination and inequality in many areas of life, including work, parenthood, pensions and inheritance. They are subject to verbal abuse and physical violence. Gay and lesbian relationships have not (until very recently with the advent of Civil Partnerships) been recognised in law, affecting inheritance, benefits and pensions and parental responsibility. Gay and lesbian partners were not allowed to register the death of their partner, nor were they eligible for bereavement benefits or compensation. Lesbian mothers had lost custody of their children on the grounds of their sexual orientation. However, New Labour's period of government has witnessed a swathe of civil rights legislation in relation to gay men and lesbian women, an approach that Williams for one has described as recognising the diversity of partnership relationships and a 'waning influence of a "morality from above"' (Williams, 2005: 300) in relation to these matters at least. Accordingly, the new millennium has seen a raft of legislation to afford rights to gay men and lesbian women. In 2001, the age of consent for gay men was equalised with that for heterosexuals. In 2003 the government repealed Section 28 of the 1988 Local Government Act. (This legislation had been advocated by proponents of the New Right under Margaret Thatcher's premiership. Section 28 had meant that a local authority was neither permitted intentionally to promote homosexuality, nor to publish material with the intention of promoting homosexuality, nor to allow in its schools any teaching that promoted the acceptability of homosexuality as a normal form of family relationship.) In employment, the 2003 Employment Equality (Sexual Orientation) Regulations outlawed discrimination (direct discrimination, indirect discrimination, harassment and victimisation) in employment and vocational training on the grounds of sexual orientation. In addition, the right to apply for flexible working within the 2002 Employment Act was extended to the same-sex partner of a biological parent.

The Civil Partnership Act of 2004, allowing same-sex couples aged 16 and over to obtain legal recognition of their relationship by forming a civil partnership, came into force on 5 December 2005 in the UK. Same-sex couples may do this by registering as civil partners of each other, provided they are of the same sex, they are not already in a civil partnership or lawfully married, they are not within the prohibited degrees of relationship, and they are both aged 16 or over (and, if either of them is under 18 and the registration is to take place in England and Wales or Northern Ireland, the consent of the appropriate people or bodies has been obtained). In the first 13 months following the passing of the law, that is up until the end of

December 2006, there were 18,059 civil partnerships formed in the UK (see Figure 19.2). The Act also sets out the legal consequences of forming a civil partnership. Rights and responsibilities include joint treatment for income-related benefits and pensions, parental responsibilities, inheritance and next-of-kin recognition. There would also be a formal court-based process for dissolution of the partnership. The Children Act of 2002, implemented in 2004, gives same-sex couples the right to be able to apply to adopt jointly.

When one makes international comparisons, one notes that the rights of gay and lesbian people vary enormously across nations. Denmark introduced the first civil partnership scheme in 1989. Gay marriage has been allowed in the Netherlands since 2000 and in Belgium since 2003. In 2005, the Spanish government backed a bill to allow marriage and the adoption of children to gay couples. In America views on gay marriage are extremely polarised. In 2004, the then US President George W. Bush defended traditional conservative values and called for a constitutional amendment to protect 'marriage' as a union between a man and a woman as husband and wife. Whilst it is probably too early to evaluate the effectiveness of British anti-discrimination legislation for gay and lesbian people, there have been significant changes since the election of the Labour government in 1997.

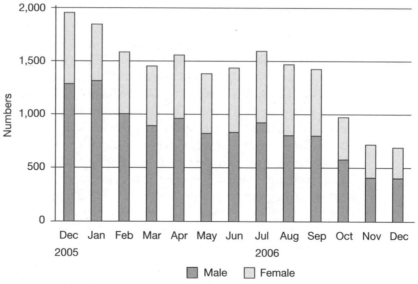

Figure 19.2 Civil partnerships
Source: National Statistics website,
http://www.statistics.gov.uk/cci/nugget.asp?id=1685&pos=&colrank=1&rank=374 (last accessed 6 February 2008). Crown copyright material is reproduced with the permission of the Controller of HMSO and the Queen's Printer for Scotland under the terms of the Click-Use Licence.

Age

This section deals with age as a social division and, specifically, age in relation to older people. Age is arguably a different type of 'social division' from some of the others considered in this chapter, for example 'race' and gender, in that it is a social phenomenon that we all experience; being younger (and hopefully older) is something that we will all experience, whereas 'race' and gender are immutable concepts in that we cannot easily change our sex or 'race' (Macnicol, 2006). As mentioned above, age and older people will be the focus of this section, since children and young people and the socio-political responses to those phenomena are dealt with in the preceding section on gender as well as in Chapter 13 on social care and Chapter 15 on education.

As we can see from the newspaper article (Box 19.4) written by Cherie Booth QC, barrister and wife of the then Prime Minister, Tony Blair, while discrimination on the grounds of sex, 'race' and gender had all been outlawed by 2005, age discrimination remained within the law until 2006.

Box 19.4

Future perfect

Cherie Booth, *The Guardian*, Saturday 17 December 2005

Five years ago, I made a speech, which I called 'discrimination, domesticity and diversity', which attempted to predict how employment law across Europe would look in 2005. I anticipated some changes (and advocated others) to combat discrimination against women and gay people, and to promote work/life balance. The end of 2005 is a good time to take stock and look forward to the next years.

... I have no doubt that the hottest topic over the next few years in employment law will be age discrimination. By 2007, discrimination on the grounds of age will [have been] outlawed, as it is now on the grounds of sex, race and disability. Age discrimination, with its easy and misleading generalisations, remains a widespread and, to a large degree, accepted part of British working life. As a nation, we simply can no longer afford to restrict the employment opportunities available to older individuals or lose their experience and skills.

Discuss and Do

Bill Bytheway has offered the following definition of ageism: 'Ageism can be seen as a process of systematic stereotyping of and discrimination against us when we are considered old' (in Vincent, 2000: 149).

Age discrimination only became unlawful in 2006 whereas discrimination on the grounds of 'race' and sex had been in existence for the three preceding decades and discrimination on the grounds of disability was legislated for in 1995.

Why do you think it took so long for the UK to legislate against age discrimination?

Even so, ageism is now recognised as one of the forms of prejudice and discrimination experienced by people in the UK. Age discrimination law currently applies in employment and vocational training where an individual has been treated less favourably on the basis of their age without justification. Such discrimination can occur to younger or older people. The Employment Equality (Age) Regulations 2006 brought in legislation effective from October 2006 which meant age discrimination was no longer lawful, particularly in relation to recruitment, promotion or training. In addition to this, employers of people aged 65+ had now to consider permitting them to carry on working after the age of 65 years. In certain circumstances, age discrimination may be lawful, but there must be an 'objective justification' in every case. An objective justification allows an employer to discriminate both directly and indirectly on the basis of age. They must, however, show that this discrimination is 'proportionate' and contributes to a 'legitimate' aim. At the time of writing this chapter, age discrimination law does not apply to goods and services (though human rights law may give some protection in these areas) – something which Help the Aged has campaigned to have changed (Help the Aged, 2007). However, it is not just in relation to employment or even the 'receiving of goods and services' where older people experience inequality. Such inequality may well permeate all aspects of an older person's life.

Even so, the experience of being an older person is arguably changing in modern Western societies, with people no longer having children by a certain age, retiring at a fixed point (traditionally 65 years of age for men and 60 years of age for women, though this is to be equalised by 2020) or arguably having to live their lives in an age-defined expected way. Some older people retire earlier than the state retirement age, while others continue long after they could have retired. Indeed, as mentioned above, in the UK it is no longer necessary to retire at 65 years of age. Older people are also increasingly engaging in pursuits that traditionally would not be seen to be ones associated with older people. Also, people are generally living longer, that is more people are now living into their late seventies and early eighties. This, along with the impact of people having fewer children, is meaning that the UK is an ageing population. Indeed, the ratio of the 65+ years groups as against the 20–64-year-olds is currently 27% but is predicted to increase to 50% by 2050 (Phillipson, 2006). Relatedly, the profile of the working population is changing, that is, it is becoming a workforce whose average age is increasing, whereby the proportion of the workforce aged between 50 and 65 years has increased from 21% in 1992 to 25% in 2004 and is predicted to increase to 32% in 2021 (Phillipson, 2006).

However, old age is of course not experienced uniformly. Older women have different experiences from older men; older people from minority ethnic groups are generally in very different circumstances from those of many from the majority ethnic population. For example, women live longer than men, have traditionally retired earlier, are less likely to have an occupational or state pension, and are more likely to be living in residential care when they reach 85 years of age (see Vincent, 2000). In addition, the experience of living as an older person in the UK is very much shaped by material circumstances which are themselves shaped by income such as pension provision and other state benefits.

Under the Conservative governments, the gap between rich and poor pensioners widened substantially such that when New Labour was returned to government in 1997 more than 25% of pensioners were living in poverty (Evandrou and Falkingham, 2004). Part of the reason for the increase in the numbers of pensioners living in relative poverty by 1997 was due to the policy changes in relation to pensions enacted by the Conservatives, not least the removal of the link between increases in the state pension and increases in earnings. The Conservatives broke this link and instead increased the state pension in line with inflation. (See Chapter 17 for a fuller discussion.) This had a significant impact on the value of the pension. Since returning to power, New Labour has failed to re-establish the link between earnings and pensions. However, since 1997 the Labour government has bolstered the incomes of older people in a number of other ways including winter fuel payments, free eye tests for people over 60 years of age, and free television licences for people over 75 years of age. In addition, significant changes to the benefits regime (see Chapter 17) have included the establishment of a minimum income guarantee for all pensioners which has gone some way to addressing pensioner poverty. However, New Labour's approach is based on a targeted benefits regime instead of a universalist increase in the basic state pension (see Evandrou and Falkingham, 2004).

Overall, then, policy changes have been made over the last decade in combating the social inequalities faced by older people, particularly in relation to employment discrimination and, to a lesser extent, pensioner poverty (Evandrou and Falkingham, 2004). However, one does need to remember that, as with the other social divisions covered in this chapter, older people are not a uniform, homogeneous group. As Vincent has said (2000: 150–151)

> The systematic circumstances and life chances of people of different age do not arise because people's hair gets greyer, [or because] they slip into a prepared social box labelled 'old, poor, useless'. Rather, in the struggle for a decent standard of living and a modicum of social esteem, the life courses of some people offer them a greater chance of success than others. Some kinds of people collectively reach old age in times and circumstances in which their personal history and changing social circumstances lead to a relative lack of social and economic power; it is this that constitutes the real basis of social division.

Other social divisions

The divisions discussed above are not exhaustive. People also face discrimination because of their class, religion or national identity. As mentioned at the beginning of the chapter, the matter of class inequalities is dealt with in other chapters. In terms of religion or national identity, one observes examples of religious intolerance such as a rise in Islamophobia in Britain, stretching back at least to incidents following the Gulf War, '9/11' and more recently the War in Iraq. Hate crimes against Arabs and Muslims in the United States increased by 1,700% in 2001 according to FBI crime statistics (BBC News, 2002).

In Britain, there is legislation to address religion and age discrimination. The 1989 Fair Employment (Northern Ireland) Act aimed to bring about equitable employment opportunities between Catholic and Protestant communities. In Britain, the Employment Equality (Religion or Belief) Regulations came into force from December 2003, making it unlawful to discriminate against workers because of religion or similar beliefs unless there is a genuine occupational requirement, such as a teacher in a faith school. The regulations have outlawed direct discrimination, indirect discrimination and harassment on the grounds of religion or belief. Furthermore, employers must make allowances for religious observance in the workplace. The Equality Act 2006 also made it illegal to discriminate on religious or belief grounds in the provision of education and training and goods and services. However, there are some exceptions to the law, for example, as mentioned above, discrimination may be lawful on religious or belief grounds where it is deemed that a certain religion or belief is necessary for a particular role.

Conflicting discourses

There are many overlaps between the experiences, policy responses and theoretical discourses associated with each of the social divisions examined above. There is much empirical evidence that demonstrates that inequality still persists for each of these groups. However, balanced against this, one can argue that for each of these groups the law is being used more and more to prevent discrimination and promote equality of opportunity. In Britain, anti-discrimination legislation has been set up and amended since the late 1960s and early 1970s with regard to race and gender. Recent Acts have made discrimination illegal on the grounds of age, sexual orientation, disability and religious belief. The obvious commonalities prompted the government to establish a single equal rights body, the Equality and Human Rights Commission, in 2007. In Europe, the Racial Equality Directive and the Employment Equality Directive, introduced by the European Community in 2000, afford EU citizens a common minimum level of protection against discrimination. The European Union has established a common framework with Member States to tackle unfair discrimination on six grounds: gender, ethnicity/race, disability, sexual orientation, religion/belief and age. This surge of new legal activity in combating discrimination has arguably precipitated the swathe of activity in the UK in relation to equality law.

Similarities can also be found in the experiences of different groups. For example, both homosexuals and disabled people experience high levels of violence and intolerance and negative attitudes with regard to the rights to sexual relationships and parenthood (Sherry, 2004). Advocates of equal rights for both groups challenge pathologisation, demand inclusion and oppose hegemonic normality. As such, both Disability Studies and Queer Theory owe a debt to feminism (Sherry, 2004). Indeed, a social constructionist approach to the structure of society is used by equal rights campaigners for women and for gay, lesbian, older and disabled people.

However, there are fundamental contradictions between social divisions too. Familial isolation is higher among gay and disabled people because they are less likely to have the support of role-models within the family and community that exist for women or black people (Shakespeare, 1996; Sherry, 2004). Sharp and Earle (2002) suggest that there are irreconcilable differences between feminists and disability rights advocates on the issue of post-24 weeks abortion. Both parties oppose the 24-week rule but their motives are fundamentally different, with feminists arguing for a woman's right to choose compared to disability rights activists' opposition to what they argue are disablist practices. Social policy analyses, particularly feminist analyses of caring, have been seen to exclude and marginalise disabled people with their focus on dependency (Morris, 1991, 1992; Oliver and Barnes, 1998; Shakespeare, 2000).

A social divisions perspective embraces the quest for equality for all affected groups. Much can be learnt by students of social policy from the discourses from the various groups. However, there are distinctions and contradictions between the groups and neither students nor practitioners should overlook these. Indeed, the state's commitment to equal opportunities for all is not accepted by everyone. There are several reasons for this. One reason relates to the most fundamental debates of relativism versus absolutism. Put simply, relativism is the belief that there are multiple truths: social reality is socially constructed. In absolutism, there is only one truth. This is not a new debate: Plato opposed relativism over 2,000 years ago. The new Pope denounced relativism and associated 'isms' shortly before his selection. The reproductive technologies such as abortion and contraception, so greatly welcomed by feminists, are considered 'immoral' by the Roman Catholic church. The proposal that there should be equal rights for gay and lesbian women in relation to marriage is rejected by many religious and conservative groups.

There are also fundamental differences between the parties on the right and left in terms of equality. Support for equal rights increases as one travels from right to left in the political spectrum. In countries with perceived high levels of immigration there has been an increase in membership of extreme right parties such as the British National Front and Le Pen's Front National in France. In the 1970s and 1980s the derogatory term 'the Looney Left' was used by the media and politicians to describe groups advocating equality. This has moved on to debates about 'political correctness'. In America, the term 'the Moral Majority' has been used to describe the predominantly white, heterosexual citizens who believe that welfare reform has gone too far.

Conclusions

This chapter has focused on the role of the state in combating inequalities faced by various social divisions. It has shown that the UK, along with other countries' welfare regimes, has introduced legislation to combat inequality and to eliminate discrimination initially in relation to 'race' and gender. Latterly, this legislation has been amended and expanded over the past couple of decades to plug omissions in relation to disability, age, sexual orientation, religion and belief. However, the legislative changes of the last decade or so have been predicated on a philosophy of equality of opportunity rather than equality of outcome (Williams, 2005). To summarise these policy changes, there now exists legislation to combat the discrimination and prejudice faced by social groups, whether based on 'race' or ethnicity, gender, disability, sexual orientation, age, religion or belief. The Labour government believes its approach has been one that has created a new framework to challenge persistent patterns of discrimination and inequality, and promote and protect diversity, good relations and human rights. New Labour's approach is one which it believes promotes 'respect for the dignity and worth of every individual, . . . and opportunities for everyone to achieve their potential and to participate in society, ... [in which] there is mutual respect between groups based on understanding and valuing diversity and on shared respect for equality and human rights' (Meg Munn (2006), the then Minister for Women and Equality).

However, the approach adopted by New Labour is one very much focused on promoting equality of opportunity, and whilst equal opportunities legislation is a useful tool to combat inequality of opportunity, it remains debatable that such an approach is sufficient to combat the inequalities of outcome that persist. As Williams has observed, New Labour's approach to combating the inequalities and social injustices faced by the various social divisions explored in this chapter is one which does not

> ... provide a complex reflection of how inequalities operate across class, gender, age ethnicity and disability. The main social justice issue [for New Labour] is poverty, with education and employment the main vehicles for tackling it. Policies tend to position [social groups] in terms of their access to educational qualifications and employment rather than the meanings that these give to their lives and the social networks of which they are a part. While of great political importance, the target–investment–outcome approach it has generated tends to occlude a vocabulary and an analysis of cultural practices and injustices, and the way they are both part of, and distinct from, economic deprivation. (Williams, 2005: 299)

Web resources

There are several organisations, governmental and non-governmental, national and international, that provide useful information to people who have an interest in equal opportunities (see below). Employers and employees, researchers and equal rights activists can use these sites to keep up-to-date with legislation, research and publications, find examples of good practice, seek advice, and take part in campaigns.

- The **Equality and Human Rights Commission** was set up on 1 October 2007, merging the Commission for Racial Equality (CRE), the Disability Rights Commission (DRC) and the Equal Opportunities Commission (EOC). www.equalityhumanrights.com

- **Equal** is a European Commission initiative, funded through the European Social Fund. It tests and promotes new means of combating all forms of discrimination and inequalities in the labour market, both for those in work and for those seeking work, through transnational cooperation. www.equality-online.org.uk

- The **Women and Equality Unit** is a government unit within the Department of Trade and Industry, set up to oversee the issue of equality in Britain. The Ministers for Women, supported by the Women and Equality Unit (WEU), are responsible for promoting and realising the benefits of diversity in the economy and more widely. www.womenandequalityunit.gov.uk

- **Disability** is the website of the UK government's Disability Policy Division, a part of the Department for Work and Pensions (DWP). This site provides information on rights, policies and legislation for disabled people. www.disability.gov.uk

- **Stonewall** aims to achieve equality and justice for lesbians, gay men and bisexual people by challenging the underlying cultural and attitudinal values that allow discrimination to flourish. It is a professional lobbying group set up in 1989 by women and men who had been active in the struggle against Section 28 of the

Local Government Act. It lobbies for legal change, works with policy makers from a range of organisations, and provides information and examples of good practice. www.stonewall.org.uk

Annotated further reading

Payne (2006) provide a good overview of the concept of social divisions and an examination of class, gender, race and many other social divisions, including some of those omitted from this chapter. Blakemore and Drake's (1996) *Understanding Equal Opportunity Policies* gives a good introduction to the study of equal opportunities. Ratcliffe (2004), Mason (2000a, 2003) and Blackstone *et al.* (1998) are excellent sources for the issues and debates associated with ethnicity and 'race'. Further reading on gender inequality includes books by Daly (2000), Pascall (1999) and Scott and Jackson (2000). Jackson (1999) and Jackson *et al.* (2000) also provide useful reading on sexuality. Barnes (1990) provides a good overview of the issues associated with disability. Shakespeare's critical analyses (1996, 1998, 2000) challenge society's attitudes and treatment of disabled people. For those interested in a comparative analysis, Ginsburg's (1992) book compares four welfare states from a social divisions perspective, although this is a little dated now. Sainsbury's (1996) *Gender, Equality and Welfare States* examines comparative social policy from a gender perspective. There are several journals that are particularly useful for further reading: *Critical Social Policy, Disability and Society, Race and Class* and the *Feminist Review*.

Chapter 20

Crime and criminal justice

by Tony Colombo and Helen Poole

Objectives

- To understand what crime is.

- To analyse who are the criminals.

- To provide an overview of the the English and Welsh system of criminal justice.

- To understand the explanations of why society chooses to punish offenders.

Introduction

The Code of Hammurabi (1792–1750 BC) is believed to form the basis of one of the earliest surviving criminal justice systems and was originally developed by the Babylonians in a province of the Middle East that is now known as Iraq (Langer, 1987), ironically, one of the most lawless regions in the world today. The Code still exists and has been preserved on basalt rock columns. Within its scribe the concept of crime is recognised along with methods of trial and a series of punishments, which appear to be based on the Old Testament retaliatory principle of *lex talionis* (an eye for an eye). Our modern system of administering criminal justice is undoubtedly more complex and varied as it attempts to address a myriad of issues which seem to be in a constant state of flux, including the integration of human rights legislation, the influence of European Union policy, the management of cross-border crimes resulting from globalisation and terrorism, and the impact of new technologies such as the Internet and DNA profiling on crime investigations and criminal justice management (Davies *et al.*, 2005). Yet, in many respects, both systems are essentially the same in the sense that each appears to be organised around four principal elements:

1. A series of substantive laws which define what forms of behaviour are to be criminalised and so subject to control.

2. A process for responding to crime in terms of capturing, convicting and punishing offenders.

3. A dominant mode of thinking that helps guide policy makers in terms of how they should interpret notions of justice.

4. An established justification for punishment along with a series of sentences that reflect the leading penal philosophy.

A further issue linking the Code of Hammurabi to modern systems of criminal justice is that despite almost 4,000 years of administrative effort we have still not succeeded in managing and controlling crime. In fact, recent research has shown that the public has lost patience with our current criminal justice system, believing that sentences are 'too lenient', that judges are 'out of touch' with popular views on matters of law and order, and that the prison and probation services were doing a 'poor job' at managing offenders (Home Office, 2000). Many scholars are equally disillusioned, with some asserting that the official response to crime has become such a 'complete failure' that if our own domestic heating systems worked as inefficiently as our criminal justice system we would have all frozen to death by now (Wilson and Ashton, 2001).

The aim of this chapter is to critically introduce a range of issues significant to understanding the nature of criminal justice policy and practice, and why it has proved difficult to resolve the central problem of crime. In particular, our discussion will be organised around four highly divisive questions which emanate from each of the principal criminal justice elements mentioned earlier, namely:

- What is crime?
- Who are the criminals?
- How can we start to make sense of our system of criminal justice?
- Why do we punish offenders?

What is crime?

Stop and Think

What do you think are criminal acts? Lists a few and say why they are crimes.

The legal and social construction of crime

An important starting point for any system of criminal justice is to define the forms of behaviour that are to be regulated. This is achieved through the criminal law: 'a body of specific rules regarding human conduct which have been promulgated (written down and distributed) by political authority, which apply uniformly to all members of the classes to which the rules refer (equally to everyone in society), and which are enforced by punishment administered by the state' (Sutherland and Cressey, 1970: 8). The two main sources of criminal law in England and Wales, and countries of the British Commonwealth, are common law (case law) and statutory law (Ormerod, 2005). Scotland, the United States and the countries of Continental Europe operate through a slightly different approach to creating laws, namely, an established codified constitution.

Thus, one response to the question 'what is crime?' seems self-evident: 'Crime is any intentional act in violation of the criminal law (statutory or common law) committed without defence or excuse and penalised by the state as an indictable or summary offence' (Tappan, 2001: 31). Such a legalistic approach has the advantage of precision as it provides a formal definition of most indictable (serious) criminal acts and judicial guidance on the maximum penalty that can be administered for each offence. For example, S. 1 (2) of the Theft Act 1968 clearly states that a person is guilty of theft if he or she: 'Dishonestly appropriates [takes] property belonging to another with the intention of permanently depriving the other of it'. Moreover, section 7 of the Act goes on to state that a person convicted of theft can be sentenced to prison for up to seven years.

However, it is important to note that there is nothing about the specific nature of an act itself that makes it inherently criminal. In other words, the types of behaviour defined as deviant by the criminal law do not represent naturally distinct categories of conduct which possess a series of characteristics that make them identifiable as crimes. Instead, crime should be understood as a socially constructed phenomenon which is shaped and defined by the legal rules that any given society or culture decides to set for itself (Henry and Lanier, 2001).

Once deviance is understood in these terms, it becomes apparent that there exists no objective reality from which to make judgements about what constitutes the right or wrong way to behave. Nor does there appear to be a consensus either within or across societies about which forms of conduct should be criminalised (Sellin, 1938). For example, some people might consider the use of drugs such as cannabis as unhealthy, dangerous and immoral, while others may view them as beneficial and a normal part of their leisure activity. The point is that the activity of cannabis use itself has no natural value status outside the subjective opinions of other people. In other words, what you do is not as important as the social context within which your actions take place and the kind of popular reaction they receive (Becker, 1963). For example, even the meaning attributed to the act of taking the life of another person against their will is dependent on the social circumstances. Thus, although we usually define such conduct as murder, this outcome is not inevitable: during wartime the military may be labelled as *heroes* for killing the enemy; the state provides itself with the legitimate power to execute some offenders in the name of *punishment*; and we explain and legally justify other forms of taking human life by using various labels such as *accidents*, *self-defence*, *infanticide*, *suicide* and in some countries such as Switzerland, *euthanasia*. Once you start to recognise that deviance can only be conceptualised as a social phenomenon, it soon becomes apparent why criminal justice systems throughout the world have never succeeded in resolving the problem of crime.

The relative nature of crime

An immediate difficulty stems from the fact that because there is no social consensus on what forms of conduct should be criminalised, all notions of crime are by definition relative in the sense that the use of such deviant labels can be applied to different forms of behaviour, at different times and in different places. As a result, agencies within the criminal justice system often appear as though they are engaged in a perpetual process of chasing shadows. For example, a range of behaviours once criminalised, and so subject to control by criminal justice agencies such as the police and judiciary, have since been made lawful, including holding gold in the house, writing a cheque for less than one dollar, printing books (Rock, 1973), suicide (Suicide Act, 1961), abortion (Sexual offences Act, 1967) and homosexual conduct between consenting adults over the age of 16 (Sexual Offences (Amendment) Act, 2000). Even people whose ideas were at one time condemned by their society as criminal have subsequently come to be regarded as heroes. For example, Nelson Mandela (who spoke out against apartheid in South Africa) and Vaclav Havel (whose plays and speeches were critical of the communist regime within the Czech Republic) were both arrested and imprisoned for their views before eventually emerging to become the democratically elected presidents of their respective countries.

The process, however, is not one-way and new crimes are also being created, particularly in the areas of technology (credit card fraud, video piracy, computer hacking), public health (banning of smoking in public places, accurate labelling of packaged food), sexual conduct (stalking, rape within marriage), the environment (control over levels of toxic emissions in the atmosphere), and public protection (gun control, anti-terrorist legislation). In fact, it would appear that the scope of criminality is actually expanding, which implies that more resources will be needed to ensure that the criminal justice process is able to effectively manage and control the range of behaviours that are continually being redefined as crimes. For example, it has been observed that there currently exist around 8,000 different crimes within Britain and that approximately 140 new crimes are being created each year, a trend which the government anticipates is likely to continue indefinitely (Faulkner, 2000).

On the basis of this evidence it could also be argued that the criminal justice system itself constitutes a social problem, as it seems to be caught up in a bizarre form of circular logic in which the mechanisms of criminal justice are responsible for both defining crime and then responding to crime (Taylor *et al.*, 1973). Conversely, from a social constructionist perspective, it would appear that the only way to resolve the problem of crime is to abolish the criminal law, as its power to label particular forms of conduct as deviant suggests that the law itself is the formal cause of crime. Actually, this reasoning is not as bizarre as it seems, for all that is required is for society to reconceptualise the way in which it understands deviance. Thus, we might decide to medicalise rather than criminalise particular forms of conduct and so transfer responsibility to, say, mental health rather than criminal justice practitioners (Timmermans and Gabe, 2004).

The influence of power on crime

Because crime does not exist as an objectively verifiable phenomenon, questions about which forms of conduct should be defined by the criminal law as unacceptable or wrong must be resolved at either the societal or cultural level. Once we understand the nature of crime in these terms it becomes essential to ask: Why, or for what purpose, was the criminal law created in the first place? And who gets to decide which types of behaviour should be labelled as crime under the criminal law? Such questions raise broader social and political concerns about the nature of the criminal justice system, and encourage policy makers and professionals alike to step back from the process and consider which groups within society are likely to benefit most from our current approach to defining and managing the crime 'problem'.

According to conflict theorists such as Taylor *et al.* (1973) the criminal justice system serves the interests of those who own the most material wealth and political power. This is achieved by using the criminal law, along with its associated mechanisms for enforcing criminal 'justice', as a weapon in order to criminalise and harshly punish any actions that threaten the dominant economic, political and social groups within any given society. Thus, within most Western societies the forms of conduct most likely to be defined as unlawful are those which threaten to undermine the traditional capitalist, patriarchal, white, Christian way of life. For example, it is claimed that the criminal justice system upholds the interests of the ruling élite within society by placing a disproportionate amount of its time and effort on policing, prosecuting and punishing *crimes of the streets* such as assault, robbery, burglary, vandalism and some sexual offences, which are disproportionately carried out by socially and economically disadvantaged groups, relative to *crimes of the suites*, including fraud, tax evasion, insider trading, unlawful working practices and environmental pollution, which tend to be carried out by large, economically powerful corporations (Nelken, 2002). This disparity occurs despite the fact that the unlawful behaviour of businesses can often result in more social harm.

Moreover, it is not just economic interests that are protected. According to feminist scholars such as Smart (1990), the criminal justice system always works in the interests of maintaining a patriarchal society. Thus, socially (through popular reactions to crime), politically (through criminal justice policy) and professionally (through the deployment of criminal justice resources and crime prevention advice) considerable emphasis is placed on informing everyone about the potential dangers of street crimes (especially violent offences such as: murder, rape and robbery), and women in particular are told to be aware of *stranger danger*. Yet, research suggests that women are often more vulnerable to attack while in their own home and from someone they know (Stanko, 2001).

Thus, the criminal law may well be used to uphold moral values, but the question that should concern policy makers is: whose moral values and political interests is the criminal law being used to uphold? For example, how comfortable would you feel living in a society with a criminal justice system designed to enforce the moral and political values of the former Nazi regime within Germany, or to uphold the discriminatory practices underlying the former apartheid regime of South Africa?

Who are the criminals?

Most criminological research attempts to understand the causes of crime by engaging in a game of 'spot the difference' between offenders and non-offenders (Coleman and Norris, 2000). If it can be shown that criminals possess biological, psychological or social characteristics not typically found among the law-abiding population, then criminal justice policy and practice can be formulated in an effort to account for any such differences. For example, because we now know that some offenders commit crime as a result of severe mental health difficulties, a series of initiatives have been developed in order to divert mentally disordered offenders away from the punitive aspects of the criminal justice process and into care by health and social services (Department of Health and Home Office, 1992).

An immediate difficulty for researchers and policy makers, however, is in trying to establish who should be classified as a criminal for the purpose of criminological study. One possible approach might be to state that if crime is any behaviour in violation of the criminal law, then the criminal can be defined as any person who behaves in ways that are prohibited by the criminal law (Tappan, 2001). Unfortunately, while such a definition may seem obvious, it is not sufficiently discerning, as most (if not all) of us have broken the law at some point in our lives even if we would consider our actions to constitute only minor indiscretions, such as driving above the speed limit or not returning items taken from our place of work.

In an effort to resolve this problem, Tappan (2001) responded to such claims by asserting that convicted offenders represent the closest possible approximation to those who have violated the criminal law. His argument is that while this population is not representative of all offenders, the fact that they have been formally identified as criminal through the selective processes of detection, prosecution and punishment makes them sufficiently distinct for the purposes of research. Furthermore, Tappan argues that it would be morally wrong to identify someone as a criminal unless they had been formally convicted of a crime in accordance with the due process of the law.

However, such an approach significantly reduces the size of the population that could potentially be defined as criminal. For example, according to the official statistics, it is estimated that around 10,850,000 offences were committed during the year 2004/05, yet only 181,000 offenders were convicted by the courts and received either a custodial or a non-custodial sentence (Home Office, 2005). One reason for such disparity in these figures is because as offenders move through the various stages of the criminal justice process there exist a comprehensive range of sieves and filters which may result in a resolution to their case prior to it being fully adjudicated within the criminal courts.

Thus, criminals are not always caught, convicted and punished for their offences. In this section we discuss the key stages suspected offenders must go through within the criminal justice process, and consider the various ways in which they can be diverted away from experiencing the full force of the criminal law. In fact, control theorists (see next section) would probably liken any discussion concerning these various diversionary sieves and filters as akin to a guide on *how to get out of jail free!*

The 'dark figure' of crime

You may be interested to learn that in the case of the majority of criminal offences committed each year, the various agencies of the criminal justice system never respond. In fact, it is widely acknowledged that the Official Criminal Statistics, which are reported annually and aggregate crime data obtained from the 43 police forces in England and Wales, tell us about less than half the volume of crime that actually takes place. The remainder constitute the 'dark figure' of crime which goes unreported to the police (Coleman and Moynihan, 2000).

Since the 1980s, the British Crime Survey (BCS) has, amongst other things, been used in order to try to gain a clearer understanding of this 'dark figure' by asking people about their experiences as victims of crime. For example, data from the BCS

for 2004/05 estimates that around 5,250,000 crimes went unreported in this particular year (Home Office, 2005). It is also interesting to note that respondents
provided a range of reasons why offences are not reported, including lack of faith
in the police's ability to solve the crime, fear of reprisals from the offender, or
because the offence amounted to a victimless event such as substance abuse
(Coleman and Moynihan, 2000).

Once a suspected crime has been reported and the police consider the allegation
as significant enough to officially record, the formal process of investigation begins.
During the annual period 2004/05, the police in England and Wales recorded over
5.5 million offences.

The police

The police represent the front-line agency within the criminal justice process and
spend around 85% of their time patrolling the streets investigating offences and
dealing with traffic management issues, all in an effort to protect the public and
keep the peace (Bayley, 2005). Because of their daily contact with the public, the
actions of the police are high profile and so tend to have a significant impact on
popular perceptions of the criminal justice system in general (Home Office, 2000).
As an agency, they are divided into 43 separate forces across England and Wales,
which inevitably leads to variations in policing practice as they respond to particular
geographic (rural/urban) and socio-cultural needs of the communities they serve.
The police are also afforded a great deal of legitimate discretion in terms of how
they do their job, which inadvertently means that their actions can have a significant
impact on the execution of justice. For example, the Macpherson report (also
referred to as the Stephen Lawrence inquiry) concluded that the police had made a
catalogue of errors during the course of investigating the death of Stephen
Lawrence, a black victim who was attacked and stabbed to death by a group of
youths. A particularly significant conclusion in this report was that because of racist
attitudes, believed to be institutional within the police force, they were too slow in
responding to the crime, which might have resulted in the loss of important evidence
(Macpherson, 1999). As a result, no one has ever been convicted of Stephen
Lawrence's murder.

Actually, during the annual period 2004/05, of the 5.5 million crimes recorded by
the police, they managed to detect an offence, i.e. identify the person believed to be
responsible, in only about 1.4 million cases. In other words, on average, the police
'clear up' only about 26% of crime, or one in four recorded offences. This rate
varies for different offences, so for murder the detection rate is around 90%, while
it might be as low as 10% for theft. However, in surveys the public consistently
overestimates the amount of crime that is actually solved by the police (Home
Office, 2000).

Once someone has been detected for an offence, there are a number of legitimate
courses of action available other than charging the accused and sending them to
court. The police can choose to take no further action (NFA) where, for example,
the victim and police do not feel it would be appropriate to continue. Moreover, in
cases which involve young offenders or people suffering from drug, alcohol, mental
health or other specific problems, there are a number of 'diversionary' measures that

can be employed whereby the accused is offered professional help via health and social services.

A traditional form of disposal employed by the police is the formal caution. For an offender to receive a caution there must be sufficient evidence to prove guilt and they must admit to the offence. The caution is then placed on their record. More recently, under the Crime and Disorder Act 1998, the use of cautions has been replaced by introducing a system of pre-court reprimands and final warnings for young offenders. During the annual period 2004/05 only 4% of offenders were given a formal caution, while 9% of cases were filtered in other ways such as through NFAs or diversion to a mental health unit. Thus, out of the 26% of detected offences, only 13% of offenders were actually formally charged with an offence.

The Crown Prosecution Service

At this stage, all information pertaining to the criminal charge is forwarded to an independent agency known as the Crown Prosecution Service (CPS). This agency, which is essentially made up of lawyers, came into existence following the Prosecution of Offences Act, 1985. Their remit is to operate independently of the police, and provide advice on the quality and nature of the evidence obtained during the course of the criminal investigation process.

If the CPS is satisfied that sufficient evidence has been obtained to warrant prosecution, the case will be allowed to proceed to the court adjudication phase of the criminal justice process. However, in order to help guide their decisions, the CPS must be cognisant of the public interest element concerning each particular criminal case. For example, if the accused had severe learning difficulties to the extent that they would find it impossible to either understand or appreciate the nature and purpose of the trial process, then little public advantage would be gained by continuing with the prosecution. Ultimately, if the CPS decide that the police do not have enough evidence to obtain a conviction, they may order a 'discontinuance of proceedings', which effectively means that all charges against the suspected offender are dropped.

The magistrates' court and crown court

Criminal cases are tried in either the magistrates' court, before three Justices of the Peace (JPs) or a professional District Judge, or in front of a circuit judge and jury in the crown court. The decision as to where a particular criminal case is heard depends on whether the offence is classified as indictable, summary or triable either way.

Indictable offences include all serious crimes such as murder, rape, arson and robbery, and are tried in the crown court. Less serious crimes are referred to as summary offences and include road traffic violations, being drunk and disorderly, and not paying your television licence. These lesser offences account for the vast majority of criminal cases in England and Wales, about 95% of all crimes, and are tried in the magistrates' court. Some offences such as burglary are considered as triable either way and in such cases the accused, who is referred to as the defendant in court, can usually elect in which court they wish their case to be tried. Their decision will usually be based on whether they feel lay magistrates or a jury would be more sympathetic to their case.

During the annual period 2004/05 the vast majority of cases heard in the magistrates' court, about 250,000, resulted in a conviction, of which 90% pleaded guilty from the outset of the trial. In the same year, 78,000 defendants were committed for trial in the crown court, of which 58,000 or 75% were found guilty. If a defendant is found not guilty they will be acquitted and released. However, under the Criminal Justice Act 2003 any defendant may be tried again for the same offence if substantial new evidence comes to light, overturning a long-established rule protecting against 'double-jeopardy'. The first conviction under this law was achieved in 2006 when Billy Dunlop, acquitted of murdering his girlfriend 15 years earlier, was found guilty following a second trial (BBC News, 11/9/2006).

Once a guilty verdict has been returned there are a variety of sentencing options available to both the magistrates' and crown courts.

Custodial and non-custodial sentences

The menu of disposals or punishments that are available to both criminal courts has grown rapidly in the past decade or so. However, sentencing is still based on the principles that were introduced under the Criminal Justice Act 1991, which established that custody (imprisonment) should be reserved for the most serious indictable offences and repeat offenders. Conversely, offenders who were convicted of committing less serious offences should be dealt with through non-custodial means such as fines and community-based punishments.

The aim of providing such a range of disposals is to afford judges with options so that they can choose sentences that best fit the severity of the crime and also suit the particular circumstances of the offender. However, it has been argued that the range of sentencing options is also politically motivated by a need to better manage the penal system. In particular, it is hoped that by providing acceptable alternatives to imprisonment this will help relieve the prison overcrowding crisis (Cavadino and Dignan, 2002).

How can we start to make sense of our system of criminal justice?

Whenever anyone writes anything about the criminal justice system it soon becomes a retrospective. Trying to keep up with the scope, scale, pace and persistence of change, in terms of new legislative reforms, policy initiatives, new agency formations and reformulations, review and report proceedings, etc., is at times overwhelming. For example, at the time of writing the administration of justice in England and Wales is experiencing significant change: a new Ministry of Justice has been established in order to take charge of crime-related matters which have traditionally been the responsibility of the Home Office; the administration of punishment is being streamlined through merging the National Probation Service and the Prison Service into one agency, now known as the National Offender Management Service (NOMS); and the series of wide-ranging reforms introduced by the Criminal Justice Act 2003 continue to have a significant impact on the criminal courts, judiciary, criminal procedures, and the administration of justice. Many of the reforms consolidated in the 2003 Act originate from the government White Paper, *Justice for All* (Home Office, 2002). At the heart of these reforms is the political intention to create a criminal justice system that on the one hand commands the respect of the public by delivering faster and more effective justice for victims, while on the other follows the principles of due process in order to safeguards the rights of the accused (Home Office, 2002).

For many scholars, however, this approach to the administration of justice is fundamentally flawed because its goals originate from two diametrically opposed perspectives on how the criminal justice system should operate, namely the *due process* and the *crime control* models of criminal justice (Packer, 1968; King, 1981).

The due process model

Justitia, the blind goddess of justice, situated outside the 'Old Bailey' Crown Court in London, symbolises the key principles underlying the due process model of criminal justice. The sword in the right hand represents punishment and the scales in the left hand signify the importance of determining who should be punished after making a rational and balanced consideration of all the evidence. Justitia is blindfolded to denote impartiality under the rule of law; that everyone, regardless of who they are or what crimes they may have committed, should be treated equally, fairly and dispassionately. A principle that should also be exercised in accordance with the due process of law is the accused's right to be tried by a jury of their peers and to the presumption of innocence before the criminal law.

Generally, supporters of this approach, such as the organisations Liberty and the National Council for Civil Liberties, believe that a primary concern of the due process model should be to inject justice into the criminal process through establishing policies and procedures which create impartiality – a fair and equitable balance between the rights of the accused and the power of the state. In other words, due process advocates would argue that in order to safeguard against potential 'miscarriages of justice', the criminal justice system should be likened to an obstacle course in which the procedures governing each successive stage act as a 'formidable impediment' to carrying the accused any further along the process towards conviction (Packer, 1968).

A good example of such a procedural safeguard is the Police and Criminal Evidence Act, 1984 (PACE) which, along with its associated Code of Practice, tries to create a balance between the powers of the police and the rights of the accused. Among other things, the PACE Act 1984 places limits on the length of time a suspect can be held for questioning, requires the police to notify the suspect of their right to legal advice, sets out conditions for the admissibility of evidence, requires that all interviews are recorded, and ensures that the accused is notified of their right to remain silent from which no adverse inferences can be drawn about their level of involvement in the offence.

However, some due process advocates argue that this legislation does not go far enough and cite several post-PACE miscarriages of justice to support their case, including revelations concerning the West Midlands Serious Crime Squad whose unlawful practices led to the wrongful conviction and eventual release in 1993 of 14 people.

Alternatively, they suggest that rather than tinker around at the edges a more fundamental overhaul of our legal system is required. In particular, it is claimed that because Britain lacks a written constitution like France or North America, there are no entrenched rights and principles governing the operation of the criminal justice system. The Human Rights Act 1998, which for the first time ensures that domestic law does not contravene the European Convention on Human Rights, may go some way towards protecting the interests of suspected offenders. However, in general we still rely on parliamentary legislation and common law rights created by judges which can easily be redefined or repealed altogether (Padfield, 2000).

Another important safeguard afforded to suspects within the criminal process, which is also central to the due process model, is the *presumption of innocence*. Essentially, there are two aspects to such a presumption. First, this long-held principle stipulates that it is the duty of the state to prove that the defendant has broken the criminal law (Sankey LC in *Woolmington* v *DPP*, 1935). Thus, the police cannot simply go out and arrest on the basis of a hunch and then demand that the suspect prove their innocence. Secondly, the standard of proof required in order to establish guilt is higher on a criminal charge, where the case against the accused must be proven 'beyond reasonable doubt', than for a civil charge, where it is only necessary to prove guilt on 'a balance of probabilities' (Padfield, 2000).

The requirement of such a high standard of proof in criminal cases not only helps guard against wrongful convictions but more fundamentally symbolises the acknowledgement of an important due process philosophy officially remarked upon as long ago as 1823 by Holroyd in the *Hobson case*, namely: 'it is a maxim of English law that ten guilty men should escape rather than one innocent man should suffer'. The question that remains unresolved, however, is precisely how high should this evidential threshold be? If the criminal courts employed the lower standard of proof as applied in civil cases, i.e. by determining each case on a balance of probabilities, then obviously many more factually guilty suspects could be successfully prosecuted. For due process supporters, however, the unacceptable corollary is that it would also be easier for many more factually innocent people to slip through the net and be convicted. Alternatively, the demand of due process for a suspect's presumption of innocence, which could only be challenged through strictly proving their guilt beyond any doubt at all, would certainly protect the innocent but suffer from the corollary of rarely achieving a successful prosecution. With regard to this point, it is interesting to note that Holroyd did not suggest that it was better that 100 or indeed 1,000 guilty men should be set free in order to protect against a single innocent conviction.

Finally, the due process model also believes that the best way to uphold moral standards within society and to encourage law-abiding behaviour is to lead by example. Thus, due process advocates insist that the legal system should never benefit from its own illegalities, such as through the use of unlawfully obtained evidence. However, such a strict level of concern for the abuse of power could lead to inefficiencies within the system. For example, if the police obtained evidence showing beyond any doubt that a suspect had committed an offence, but it was also discovered that the evidence had been obtained unlawfully, then due process thinking would insist that the suspect be released because of this procedural irregularity. Their justification for such an action would be based on the premise that to accept such procedural irregularities would encourage future abuses of power to take place, which in the longer term would be far more damaging to society than releasing a few culpable offenders.

The crime control model

In direct contrast to the due process model, a pure crime control perspective views the repression of all criminal conduct, regardless of the consequences to people's civil rights, as the most significant function to be performed by the criminal justice system. Without this degree of control, it is envisaged that disrespect for the criminal law would develop, resulting in the collapse of public order, creating fear and anxiety among law-abiding citizens.

In order to avoid such an infringement of our social freedom, a high rate of detection and conviction of suspects must be upheld and this can only be effectively achieved through minimising the opportunities for a case to be challenged. Thus, according to the crime control perspective, the criminal justice system should function much like a conveyor belt, where the police are given extensive powers and freedom to act on their own professional assumptions in order to establish the facts necessary to differentiate the innocent from the guilty. This then leaves the remaining stages of the criminal process with the task of swiftly trying and sentencing the offender.

Earlier it was noted that under the PACE Act 1984 a number of due process safeguards were introduced in an attempt to redress the 'balance' between the power of the state and the rights of the individual. However, a closer look at the way the criminal process actually operates in practice reveals the presence of a number of features highly characteristic of the crime control model. Focusing specifically on the PACE Act 1984, the Philips Commission 1981 advocated giving greater powers to the police so that they could be more effective at repressing crime. Thus, many of the operational rules that were once informally used by the police have now been legitimised. For example, before 1984 many suspects were induced to come to the police station without being charged on the basis that they were 'helping the police with their inquiries'. The PACE Act 1984 now formalises this practice by allowing for pre-charge detention. Hence, popular crime control lines such as 'the police are forced to break the law in order to get results' have in some cases been removed: 'police and court officials need not abuse the law in order to subvert the principles of justice; they need only use it' (McBarnet, 1983: 156).

Advocates of the crime control paradigm would also assert that the judicial 'conveyor-belt' process of dealing with offenders could be made significantly quicker and simpler if those accused of a crime could simply be persuaded to admit their offence at the outset and so enter a guilty plea, thus leap-frogging the trial phase altogether and moving directly on to sentencing.

Reading in the area of criminal law and policy for the first time, one might understandably be forgiven for thinking that the adoption of such an approach is more akin to a game of Monopoly – move directly to jail – rather than a fair and equitable system of criminal justice. In reality, however, such an approach is a typical feature of the criminal process. In both England and North America a large majority of defendants plead guilty and forgo their right to an adversarial trial (Baldwin and McConville, 1977), not least because of the operation of 'plea-bargaining' and inducements in terms of reduced sentences for early guilty pleas. Thus, the alleged evidence against them is never heard, the reliability of witness statements is not cross-examined and the all-important 'beyond reasonable doubt' presumption is never tested.

Supporters of the crime control perspective, therefore, clearly envisage a criminal justice system which is primarily managed and controlled by the police. Generally, it is accepted that 'a few' mistakes may possibly be made during the police's efforts to try to differentiate the probably guilty from the probably innocent. However, it is also argued that such mistakes should be tolerated as they are insignificant relative to the larger goal of repressing crime. Ideally, of course, the aim would be to secure as many guilty pleas as possible before the trial stage, thus eliminating the possibility for any potential errors to be uncovered, which might be interpreted as weaknesses in the system and so consequently reduce respect for the law.

If the system did show signs of weakness, perhaps through revealing that guilty defendants were being released or that too many innocent defendants were being convicted, then the introduction of some degree of due process safeguard into the system would be tolerated. However, only those rules which may make fact finding more reliable, such as preventing coercive interrogation practices, would be acceptable. However, to suggest, as do due process supporters, that illegally obtained evidence should be deemed inadmissible or that a conviction relying on such evidence should be quashed is viewed by crime control advocates as ridiculous: why should perfectly credible evidence be ruled as inadmissible simply because the methods used to obtain it were improper?

The due process and crime control models create a constant tension within the criminal justice system, essentially between the rights of the accused and those of the victim. This tension is made more complicated by the fact that these two perspectives cannot be separated from one another like oil and water. Instead, the pure form of each tends to be diluted by aspects of the other, ultimately forming a new hybrid paradigm. In the future it is likely that greater emphasis will be placed on formulating an evidence-based system of criminal justice that is organised around a combination of due process and crime control policies which have been shown to 'work' in terms of their ability to manage and reduce the risk of crime (Farrington, 2002).

Why do we punish offenders?

Punishment may be broadly defined as 'the deliberate use of public power to inflict pain on offenders' (Andrews, 2003: 128). According to the classical philosophers Cesare Beccaria and Jeremy Bentham, punishment is essentially an evil process which must be justified if societies are to avoid their actions being denounced as primitive and barbaric (Beccaria, 1764, in Bellamy, 1995). In this respect, attempts should be made to link the use of punitive sanctions such as imprisonment with a desired outcome (Cavadino and Dignan, 2002). To date, however, moral philosophers have been unable to agree on precisely what is being achieved by the infliction of pain and hardship on known offenders (Walker, 1991). Our aim in the final section of this chapter is to critically introduce a number of possible justifications for the use of punishment.

Reductivism

A traditional moral justification for the use of punishment is based on the philosophical notion of *reductivism*, a utilitarian principle which asserts that the use of punitive methods such as imprisonment will help prevent future incidents of crime (Walker, 1991). Towards this goal, the key reductivist strategies include deterrence, incapacitation and rehabilitation.

Deterrence

This approach starts from the assumption that people are rational beings who are able to calculate the costs and benefits associated with committing crime (Cavadino and Dignan, 2002). Thus, it is believed that punishment is justified on the grounds that potential offenders will be deterred from their actions because they fear the unpleasant consequences that may result if they are caught. Punishment may act as either a specific or a general deterrent to crime. The former seeks to influence the future behaviour of an individual offender, while the latter attempts to control the future conduct of society in general.

Specific deterrence may be delivered in a variety of ways. For example, a severe sanction may be imposed in the hope that the offender finds the experience so unpleasant that they stop offending through fear of having to experience more of the same or worse punishment the next time. Indeterminate imprisonment may also be given in which decisions about release are based on clear evidence that the offender's behaviour has changed. In the case of general deterrence, punishments are designed to send a broad message of discouragement to all would-be offenders. For example, prior to the eighteenth century use of the death penalty and public executions were common even for the most minor of crimes (Emsley, 2005).

The problem with the notion of deterrence, however, is that it is only likely to work effectively when extreme sanctions are imposed, and even then the research evidence is inconclusive. For example, during the 1980s the Conservative government introduced the 'short, sharp shock' treatment for young offenders, though crime continued to rise, suggesting that this approach had failed as a deterrent (Muncie, 1990). West (1982) also showed that after experiencing severe punishment, inmates were actually more likely to reoffend as they developed a grudge against the system and aimed to 'get their own back'. In fact, West concluded that the best way to stop recidivism is not to catch the offender in the first place, as crime naturally stops as offenders get older.

Even if punishment did operate as an individual deterrent, other social factors such as the stigma associated with being labelled an 'ex-offender' may obscure its effect by denying them access to legitimate opportunities such as work, which in turn increases the likelihood that they might return to crime. Moreover, the logic behind the notion of punishment operating as an effective general deterrence suggests that it would only be necessary to lock up a few people who would serve as an example to the rest of society. However, the UK prison population as of June 2007 stands at 80,205 an increase of around 20,000 from just a decade ago (National Offender Management Service, 2007). Moreover, we put more people in prison than any other country in Western Europe (Cavadino and Dignan, 2002). Finally, using deterrence as a moral justification offers no rights to the accused. For example, if punishing one person may be viewed as likely to benefit the majority, then what is wrong with punishing the innocent? As a general deterrence, the fact that you may be innocent is not so important relative to the wider utilitarian objective of controlling future levels of crime.

Incapacitation

The aim of incapacitating offenders is to protect society from the actions of criminals. It can take various forms: imprisonment, which physically removes the offender from society; injunctions, which prevent the offender from entering areas where they are likely to offend, thus a paedophile may be prevented from going near schools or playgrounds; and disqualification such as from driving in order to prevent motoring offences. The logic of incapacitation as a justifiable form of punishment appears to make sense; if you are denied the opportunity for offending, then future levels of crime will be reduced.

Consequently, it has been argued that imprisoning more offenders and for longer periods of time will have a significant impact on levels of crime (Wilson, 1975). However, the evidence supporting such an assertion is inconclusive. For example, Tarling (1993), using official criminal statistics, has noted that a 25% increase in the prison population would only lead to a 1% drop in crime, which questions the economic viability of such an initiative. Furthermore, he argues that a 40% drop in the prison population would only lead to a 1.6% increase in the overall level of offending (Brody and Tarling, 1980).

Some scholars argue that the recent political willingness to embrace incapacitation as a solution to crime has started to have a fundamental impact on how we understand the nature of punishment itself. In particular, it is argued that a new form of penology is starting to emerge which has little concern for the moral justification of punitive sanctions. Instead, criminal justice agencies and legislators are starting to place a greater emphasis on managerialism – the ability to identify, manage, contain and control groups of people who are assessed, via risk measures, as a potential danger to society (Feeley and Simon, 1992). These scholars go on to argue that traditionally understood terms such as guilt, recidivism and rehabilitation are becoming less important relative to the specialist language of risk, prediction and management. Ultimately, the underlying logic of incapacitation is that it helps make crime levels more tolerable by locking up those who are deemed by criminal justice experts to constitute a social threat.

Rehabilitation

This is another approach to reducing future levels of crime. Punishment is inflicted in an attempt to change the personal values and behaviour of offenders. Such an approach was particularly popular prior to the 1960s when it was believed that scientific developments in areas such as biology, psychology and social work would be able to resolve many social problems such as crime (Coleman and Norris, 2000). This line of thinking is also associated with the positivist paradigm which tried to understand crime and criminal behaviour as analogous to an illness in which the underlying disease causing dysfunctional conduct could be treated through various forms of behavioural modification programmes. However, during the 1970s much of this work was discredited on the basis that nothing seemed to work (Martinson, 1974), though the methodological nature of this research was itself later criticised and its results dismissed (Martinson, 1979).

Today, there has been a small revival in the rehabilitative approach. Therapeutic programmes now make the more modest claim that their goal is to 'facilitate change' rather than 'coerce a cure'. The essential aim of such programmes is to try to encourage offenders to understand the consequences (unacceptable nature) of their own behaviour in the hope that they will decide to change. A good example of such an approach is referred to as restorative justice. This focuses on resolving the dispute, conflict or trouble (formally known as crime) between the victims, the offender and the wider community. Within this context crime is viewed not as an abstract violation of the law, but as a form of interpersonal harm (Hughes, 2001). One such restorative process is referred to as 'reintegrative shaming' (Braithwaite, 1989). It involves the victim and offender meeting in order to discuss the offence that has taken place. In particular, the aim is to provide the victim with an opportunity to explain to the offender how the crime has affected them. In this way, it is hoped that the offender will come to understand and feel remorse for the consequences of their actions, and in turn decide to change their future conduct. Such an approach may well work in cases involving property crime, such as theft or burglary, but it is questionable whether offences against the person such as rape and violence could be effectively managed in this way.

Retributivism

Retributivism is backward-looking in the sense that punishment is justified because it penalises criminal behaviour that has already taken place. In other words, it is not concerned with future conduct as was the case with the reductivist approach. Instead, offenders are punished on the basis of what they deserve for their unlawful conduct – their 'just deserts'. Thus, the use of pain and violence by the state is legitimised on the basis that society is perceived as entitled to seek revenge against those who commit crime (Lacey, 2003). An immediate difficulty with such an approach is that the use of state violence legitimises the use of social violence and as a solution to problematic situations. It also ignores the collateral impact that punitive sanctions may have on the relatives of offenders.

A further retributivist justification for punishment is that it acts as a mechanism for restoring social harmony and balance. The logic here is based on the theoretical idea that we are all bound to one another under an implicit social contract which protects each of us from any harm to ourselves or our property. This social contract is made explicit by the criminal law which applies equally to all members within any given society. Thus, if someone were to break the law then this social contract would be disrupted and the offender is viewed as having gained an unfair advantage over the law-abiding community. In such cases punishment is administered in an attempt to adjust for any advantage gained through crime by taking away the gains from their offending behaviour. For example, the Proceeds of Crime Act 2002 established the Assets Recovery Agency whose job it is to recover the proceeds gained from unlawful acts.

In the broadest of terms the retributivist approach is akin to the biblical principle of *lex talionis*. However, the classical thinker Beccaria was not in favour of extreme punishments such as the death penalty, as he believed this would lead to irrational practices and disrespect for the criminal law. Instead, he argued that punishment should be no harsher than was necessary. This 'softer' approach is more palatable within modern Western societies and has encouraged the emergence of a 'new retributivism' (Hudson, 2003), the key principles of which are that more emphasis be placed on the offence committed rather than the circumstances of the offender; that punishment is administered in proportion to the seriousness of the offence; and that punishment (as opposed to rehabilitation) should be the main aim of the penal system (Von Hirsch, 1976). Furthermore, in order for punishment to be proportionate to the seriousness of the offence, Von Hirsch argues that it is necessary to develop a tariff system that provides a fixed penalty for every type of crime, which is set out in advance so that everyone is clear about what punitive sanctions they could expect to receive for particular forms of unlawful conduct.

Our current system of punishment is designed around the idea of the 'just deserts' approach developed by Von Hirsch (1976), which has several advantages over reductivist philosophies:

- Firstly, offenders are afforded more rights, as the punishment must fit the crime. One of the aims of reductivism is to use punishment as a general deterrent and so courts are free to give arbitrary sentences as a symbolic message to the wider society. Such sentences, however, may be disproportionate to the seriousness of the offender's actions and so unacceptable within a 'just deserts' model.

- Secondly, through the notion of the social contract, all members within society are treated equally and as rational human beings who are able to make choices and are entitled to be treated with dignity and respect – unlike some treatment and rehabilitation orders which assume that offenders are sick and not able to control their own conduct.

- Finally, because the approach is backward-looking, offenders are punished for what they have done, and not for what they *may do* in the future.

However, both retributivism in general and the 'just deserts' approach in particular face a number of problems which have proved difficult to reconcile:

- Firstly, even 'new retributivism' is still based on the principle of *lex talionis* which raises the questions: is it morally right to exchange one form of evil (crime) for another (punishment)?; can two actions which instinctively seem 'wrong' ever make things right? Perhaps our feelings of revenge, of 'getting our own back', of inflicting pain on offenders for pain's sake rather than to rehabilitate offenders should be curbed and not indulged.

- Secondly, the theoretical idea that the law applies equally to all members of society under some implicit notional social contract is less evident in reality

(Hudson, 2003). Many detected offenders are socially and economically disadvantaged and so are under a greater degree of pressure to obey the law. Furthermore, punishment for their crime is likely to increase the offender's position of inequality rather than restore it, as both the offender and their family become stigmatised and more economically disadvantaged due to imprisonment and the subsequent problems associated with getting housing, jobs, friends, etc. as an ex-offender.

- Finally, in terms of the 'just deserts' tariff, is it possible to develop a system which offers proportionality between offences? For example, it might be argued that a punishment proportionate to the offence of murder is execution (which itself is a morally problematic sanction), but what penal measure would be equivalent to offences such as assault, burglary, rape, shoplifting, insider-share dealing, environmental pollution, etc.? The current penal system uses prison sentences as the basis for such a tariff system, though, as we mentioned earlier, there is much popular disagreement as to what should amount to an offender's 'just deserts' (Home Office, 2000).

Conclusion

This chapter has been consciously 'painted with a broad brush' in the hope of providing as wide a context of understanding about crime and criminal justice matters as possible in the space permitted. It is hoped that some of the ideas presented here will encourage you to explore aspects of the subject yourself, especially in terms of helping you to evaluate the various debates concerning criminal justice policy and practice that are frequently discussed by the media and politicians.

Annotated further reading

Perhaps the most useful text for trying to understand the nature of crime is Henry and Lanier (2001), *What is Crime: Controversies over the nature of crime and what to do about it*. A good overview of the criminal justice system and related policy matters is provided by Davies, Croall and Tyrer (2005), *Criminal Justice: An introduction to the criminal justice system of England and Wales* (3rd edition). For a general discussion of prison issues, refer to Cavadino and Dignan (2002), *The Penal System: An introduction*, while a clear yet controversial viewpoint of prison policy can be found in Murray (1997), *Does Prison Work?* Finally, a good starting point for understanding the various philosophies associated with punishment itself is Hudson (2003), *Understanding Justice*.

Chapter 21

The living environment

Objectives

- To provide an introduction to 'green thinking' and its relationship to social policy.

- To provide an overview of green thinking.

- To provide an account of green social policy.

- To explore what the implications of green social policy are for food production and consumption, transport and work.

Introduction

At first sight the two subjects of social policy and the environment appear to have little in common. It is true to say that they share a common interest in promoting social welfare, although the meanings of social welfare for the two strands of thought are quite different from one another. Indeed, environmental thinking could suggest that traditional social policy, far from being to do with the promotion of welfare, is in fact part of the 'problem' of welfare. However, in recent years much debate and comment has attempted to argue the case for the development of a sustainable social policy. At the core of this argument is the notion that planet Earth possesses a finite stock of (physical) resources and that the use, or overuse, of those resources is going to present very real challenges for the development and delivery of social policies and the promotion of social justice within society. This chapter will not focus on the details of the scientific arguments about environmental change, global warming and the climate but instead will concentrate on the potential impact of such environmental change upon our social welfare and the development of social policy.

An overview of green thinking and social policy

'Green' thought and ideas about human interaction with the living environment can be traced back for many hundreds of years. However, such ideas have only really begun to have an impact on policy and policy-making since the 1960s and 1970s (Fitzpatrick, 2001) with the development of an 'environmental movement'. This movement has as the basis for its thinking, and its critique of modern society, the notion that the Earth is a planet of finite (physical) resources yet apparently infinite demands on those resources. Humanity is using those resources at an unsustainable rate, i.e. we are using these resources faster than they can be replaced. At the same time, we are producing vast amounts of waste, which is often toxic and polluting, and further damages the planet's natural resources.

The green movement has argued, increasingly successfully, that the rate of growth pursued by Western economies, alongside increasing rates of production and consumption, is diminishing those resources at a faster rate than they can be replenished (see Dobson, 2000, for an accessible introduction to 'green' political theory). Furthermore, the western model of economic growth has been, in recent years, transplanted to developing nations as a model to tackle global poverty, and to former communist nations as a model to modernise and democratise those nations following the widespread collapse of communism. We can see this too in countries such as China that still profess their communist heritage but pursue a model of rapid economic growth. Indeed the two most dynamic economies in the current period, India and China, are both pursuing such an economic course. The adoption of an apparently global model of economic growth is, argues the green movement, deeply flawed and itself unsustainable.

Stop and Think

Should there be international limits to growth in order to address environmental change, even if that means that developing nations must slow their rate of economic growth and expansion?

Environmental thinking instead emphasises that there are 'limits to economic growth' which must be both recognised and observed. These limits are emphasised by five closely related factors (Dobson, 2000):

- that we have entered an age of accelerating industrialisation;
- the rapid and unsustainable growth of the global population;
- widespread malnutrition;
- the depletion of non-renewable natural resources;
- the deteriorating environment.

This has, however, led to something of a political impasse, since developing nations argue that to enforce such limits to growth at this time simply entrenches existing patterns of global poverty and maintains the positions of the wealthy Western economies. Thus, they argue that such poverty should be tackled by allowing those countries to modernise their economies by rapid economic growth, and that only once such countries are on a more level 'playing field' should they be committed to binding international environmental targets. In turn, countries of the West, often led by the United States, have argued that they themselves should only be bound by environmental targets, such as those set by the Kyoto Protocol, if all countries are to be bound by them. They further argue that Western economies are in a position to employ cleaner and greener technology and that the developing economies are in fact the greater polluters because of the technologies they use, for example the burning of large quantities of coal in China.

As a human society we have always used natural resources and created waste, but what is singularly different about our current situation is that the rate of use of resources, and the production of waste by-products, is so much faster than at any other point in human history. Furthermore, it is argued, the rate of resource deple- tion and waste production is higher and faster than that from which we can potentially recover. This is a general point but within this there are specifics of which we need to take account. In particular, we have seen a massive increase in the burning of (carbon-producing) fossil fuels (oil, coal, wood and natural gas) at an unsustainable rate. An argument raging in the scientific community and govern- ments, though now largely accepted since the publication of a large-scale study by the United Nations, is that this level of human activity and intervention in the natural world leads to the production of greenhouse gases which itself is a direct cause of climate change (IPCC, 2007). This is leading to a (rapid) warming of our planet, though the extent and impact of that warming is widely disputed, which in turn it is suggested will lead to dramatic changes in our weather patterns and physical geography.

The widespread flooding in the UK during the summer of 2007 may be such an example, as may the potential flooding of vast areas of coastal land if predicted sea level rises are accurate. This in turn will raise questions of human welfare and the response of governments. For example, how should the UK government respond to a more generalised and widespread threat of flooding and to the welfare needs of those people who live in houses built on flood plains?

Stop and Think

How should the UK government respond to the concerns of householders who have never before experienced flooding but now find that they are living in a flood risk area?

On a more global scale, many low-lying areas around the world, i.e. those most at risk of permanent flooding should sea levels rise significantly, are home to some of the most densely populated countries and poorest peoples of the world. The potential level of environmental displacement caused by global climate change is unclear, but an estimated 162 million people live in coastal areas threatened with flooding (Myers and Kent, 1995).

Stop and Think

Given current concerns about immigration in Europe and the UK, how should the government prepare for potential immigration increases resulting from climate change, the creation of 'environ- mental migrants'?

The green response to the threat of environmental disaster is firstly to acknowledge the limits on our physical resources and the damage caused by our over-consumption of those resources. The solution, though as we will see there are many shades of green in this debate, is for a radical change in our way of life, particularly in the wealthy West. In short, we have to rein in our consumption and change the ways in which we use resources in order both to conserve resources and to allow them to be replenished, but also to limit any further damage we cause to the environment.

On first assessing these arguments it is difficult to see the connection with social policy – or rather with welfare in its broadest sense. However, there are three areas we may wish to examine. Firstly, our current conception of welfare and welfare solutions to social problems is intrinsically part of the environmental problem. Secondly, if we accept the 'limits to growth' thesis put forward by environmental lobbyists, then society's overall welfare must begin, if it has not done so already, to diminish, at least in terms in which we traditionally understand welfare to be improved. Finally, the green solution(s) to the looming environmental crisis will fundamentally change the ways in which we regard welfare and social policy, i.e. we will have to redefine what we mean by social welfare. Each of these three areas:

- is 'welfare' part of the problem?
- will 'welfare' diminish?
- a new welfare settlement?

will now be examined in more detail.

Is 'welfare' part of the problem?

Greens argue that our current welfare settlement, often described as the Keynesian Welfare State (KWS) (Burrows and Loader, 1994), is designed to support the traditional capitalist productive economy, and to support consumption. Even the most basic social response to welfare, the question of poverty, has focused on patterns of consumption and has developed systems designed, for example, to provide some level of income replacement in order to maintain a 'standard of living'. For example, the system of income support that prevails in the United Kingdom is premised upon the maintenance of some, often implicit, level of income, and to fall below such a standard on a wide scale is a mark of a general social failing.

Many poverty surveys are therefore conducted with some reference to prevailing levels of consumption and expenditure and define poverty in reference to 'acceptable' social norms and standards. From the early poverty surveys conducted by people such as Booth in London and Rowntree in York at the end of the nineteenth century, to the most recent, 'basket of goods' approaches often adopted, it is suggested that to be without certain goods and services is a mark of poverty (Rowntree, 1901; Townsend, 1979; Mack and Lansley, 1985; Hills, 1998). In such surveys it is reasonable to suggest that in modern Britain to be without a television or washing machine indicates a measure of poverty because those goods are so commonplace. In taking this approach, it is difficult to make meaningful comparisons with the levels of genuine and absolute poverty experienced by the peoples of many developing nations. It may even be regarded as verging on the ridiculous to suggest that poverty is even an issue for wealthy Western economies when compared to those developing nations, though clearly deprivation does persist in these economies. But when poverty is measured in the relative terms defined by poverty surveys, then it is clear to see that welfare is being measured against a scale of the goods that an individual or family possesses and, as such, the welfare response is to provide a level of income commensurate with the accepted lifestyle of the surrounding society. For green theorists, however, this is clearly problematic, since as overall standards of consumption continue to rise in Western economies, then the welfare systems of those economies are designed to maintain the poor of that society in relation to overall standards. Systems of income support are therefore seen as contributing to the mentality of growth underpinning those economies and therefore contributing to wider environmental problems.

So it is with the wider welfare state in that the principal pillars of Western welfare – education, health and housing, as well as income support systems – are designed with the explicit intention of maintaining economic growth by the provision of a healthy and well-educated workforce. Welfare policies such as the New Deal, Sure Start or the National Minimum Wage are all providing support for the poor of Britain by putting individuals squarely in the way of work and keeping them there; support for those out of work is geared to returning individuals, as quickly as possible, to productive labour (Jordan, 1998). A core principle of the 'New Labour' welfare model has been that the best way to get someone out of poverty is through paid work, and we can see this model extending into policies adopted at an international level through agencies such as the European Union and the World Trade Organisation. For greens then, welfare defined in this way is clearly part of the environmental problem.

Will 'welfare' diminish?

Clearly a meaningful answer to this question will depend firstly on what one defines as 'welfare'. If we were to take the definition given to welfare implicit in the Western model of welfare provision, then we would have to conclude that the answer will be yes. If we accept that improved welfare is defined in some relation to levels of consumption and therefore of continuing increases in the levels of consumption enjoyed, then the limits-to-growth notion that is core to green thinking will see a reduction in levels of consumption.

One implication of the limits-to-growth thesis is that such limits to growth are soon going to be reached and therefore that the assumption we have made over the past 200 or so years, that our society will continue to grow, become more wealthy and improve the welfare of all, is mortally wounded. As resources become ever scarcer and begin to run out, they will tend to become the reserve of those who can afford them through the marketplace. Yet the notion that the ownership of a car and of independent car travel, or of foreign holidays, should become reserved for the very wealthy will be, at the least, highly contentious and most likely unacceptable to many. Governments may therefore have to leave the distribution of such resources less and less to the market and become more 'dictatorial' in their distribution. But that itself will be a highly contentious and fiercely resisted change.

We have already witnessed some of the potential areas of controversy and conflict implicit in the above argument. During the 1980s and 1990s government in Britain sought to reduce the role of the state in the provision of goods and services, seeking instead to use the market to deliver such goods. Government attempted to step back from involvement in the provision of traditional services such as water and sewerage services and domestic fuel supply which had for many years been regarded as public goods and therefore correctly provided by the state. Instead, the Conservative government in the 1980s and early 1990s tried to create a marketplace in which goods such as water, gas and electricity would be supplied on a commercial basis.

This has in turn led to the 'discovery' of new social problems such as fuel and water poverty, with some individuals and families finding that they could no longer afford to maintain a supply. Government attempted to regulate this market to ensure fairness in the supply of such essential services, but new concepts such as 'self-disconnection' have been introduced into the language of public policy. Where public authorities, as they were, found great difficulty in denying supply to those who could not or refused to pay, particularly where children or older people were present, the introduction of metering and prepayment systems has made the disconnection of supply much easier in the modern privatised world and government has been pressured into further regulating the marketplace to protect vulnerable groups.

We have thus witnessed the development of a much more hands-off approach from government and the development of a regulatory culture with the constitution of bodies such as the water regulator (Ofwat) and the electricity generation regulator (Ofgem). We could of course conceive of a much wider regulatory framework having to be invested and put in place to regulate the supply of resources that will become ever more 'essential' as their reserves diminish. But is it conceivable, for example, to have a government office for the regulation of the supply of (clean) air?

We must note that this premise of diminishing welfare is by no means accepted universally, or even widely. The approach to the green debate that is being adopted by governments around the world is one that sees possible technological solutions to the issues of environmental change that will at the very least mitigate many of the problems. Thus the approach embodied in Agenda 21, across much of Europe, has emphasised the creation of sustainable policies for both the economy and welfare. This has caused considerable growth in industries involved in the recycling of waste and the promotion of alternative technologies such as the generation of domestic power (solar and wind) and the development of alternative (bio) fuels for transport. The underlying principle here is that our existing way of life is to be preserved by developing ingenious solutions to our environmental problems so that our standard of living is neither compromised nor diminished.

The growth of such industries as recycling or green energy production, or the incorporation of such new technologies, for example, in the construction of new homes, in turn becomes part of the wider productive economy further prompting growth, employment and a greater standard of welfare in its traditional sense. There are still, however, questions of fairness or social justice to be addressed, since not every household will find the domestic generation of electricity by wind or solar power either practicable or affordable. And as others point out, the pursuit of a 'technological fix' does little to address the fundamental questions raised by a looming economic crisis and may even further harm our planet. Lovelock estimates, for example, that the production of sufficient biofuels to meet current, let alone future, demand would require a land area of several planet Earths (Lovelock, 2006).

A new welfare settlement?

If we accept the above two points, that welfare is indeed part of the problem because of its productivist focus, and that welfare as we currently conceive it will diminish in both its quantity and quality, then we must ask what the new welfare settlement will look like? Greens argue that we must first turn away from the traditional productivist models of welfare that have dominated the political arena of the past 150 years or so. They argue, however, that this will not mean that welfare will cease to grow, but that what we regard as welfare will change and that welfare as measured traditionally by reference to income and consumption will continue to grow, but that this growth will be slower and more sustainable. It also therefore implies, in a world that recognises limits to growth, that the West will reduce its share of the use of global resources in order to allow for a more even and equitable rate of development for the rest of the world. There is, thus, an implicit assumption that a 'green social policy' will be, by its very nature, a better model of social justice.

Many greens further argue that their conception of welfare will be a better form of welfare in that it will no longer focus simply on the material development of individuals, families and society. Instead they see welfare as including the emotional, social and psychological development of people, which they argue is severely damaged by the pursuit of economic growth above all else. This point also has gained a sympathetic response among some 'traditional' social theorists who perceive the damage being caused to social networks and social capital in modern Western societies (Putnam, 2000). This leads us to consider some very interesting questions in terms of how we will make use of and organise the fair or just distribution of a diminishing stock of natural resources, what our personal relation to wider society will be, how we will relate to one another, and what will be the nature of our political and welfare system. And perhaps one of the most interesting questions raised by this debate will be the notion of work and our individual and collective relationship to work in the future.

Stop and Think

What is meant by 'welfare' in the green view of society?

Green theory

Whilst it may appear that as the environment is so fundamentally important it must therefore be high on all political agendas, that is not the case and there is a great deal of debate both among politicians and within the green movement about the approach we need to adopt. Although, as we have already indicated, green thinking has a long history back at least to the beginnings of the industrial revolution, it has only been in recent years that those ideas have gained a wider acceptability and a place in policy-making. The now almost universal acceptance that a process of climate change is taking place and that human intervention is largely to blame for the extent and speed of that change has brought environmental politics firmly onto the political agenda. From the early 1990s and the debates at the Earth Summits held in Rio de Janeiro and Kyoto, the concept of 'sustainability' or sustainable development has become firmly established in our political dialogue and incorporated increasingly into policy instruments. The key to this idea of sustainability is an attempt to resolve the mismatch between our demands on the planet's resources and its capability to supply and maintain those resources.

Furthermore the concept also implies that we have to address questions of space and time in social policy. Many of the problems caused by environmental change are ignorant of national boundaries. Pollution, storms and flooding do not stop at national boundaries. Similarly, once a resource is used up, it is used up for everyone, not just the countries in which it is found. The question of time implies that, as caretakers of the planet, we have a responsibility to future generations to leave a planet that remains habitable. In the same way, we have an expectation that future generations too will maintain their environmental legacy (Fitzpatrick and Cahill, 2002).

The standard, if not classic, definition of sustainability has been noted as the ability to '... meet the needs of the present, without compromising the ability of future generations to meet their own needs' (Brundtland Commission, 1987). We might even argue that this notion of 'futurity', the preservation of resources for future generations, implies that the world itself is imbued with a concept of rights. Sustainability also implies a redistribution of resources away from the relatively affluent Western economies to the less developed world and that those relatively poorer countries be allowed to enjoy the same benefits and levels of welfare (see Dobson, 1998).

Stop and Think

Is it possible to talk about the 'rights' of the environment or even rights for plants or animals? And can such rights outweigh the rights of human beings?

However, despite the relative success that is suggested by the fact that the political mainstream has essentially adopted the rhetoric of sustainability, there remain different 'shades' of green within the environmental movement. There are, therefore, no clear and accepted ideas of how and which policies governments ought to be developing. Dobson (2000) suggests that at one end of the scale is the 'light greens' (or weak sustainability theory), who argue that the position we must reach is one in which demand for available resources matches supply and that we achieve a state of equilibrium. The 'dark greens', by contrast, argue for a much more radical approach, both towards the environment and human welfare more generally.

This light green approach is clearly popular politically. The approach broadly acknowledges the importance of the environment and environmental issues but suggests that improvements in technology and human ingenuity can overcome most, or even all, environmental problems presently facing the world. Most importantly, economic growth is still held to be the most important goal of society. The solutions that fall within the light green part of the political spectrum therefore seek to promote a society that will have both economic growth and environmental improvements.

From the perspective of the light greens, the anti-poverty approach which the more purist, or fundamentalist, green approach advocates, whereby there are immediate reductions in overall consumption, is seriously misguided. An absolutist environmentalism is a luxury afforded to the Western middle classes who can worry about resource usage because they have sufficient themselves. In contrast, developing countries must first be concerned about poverty and the general welfare of their populations which may lack even basic needs of food, clothing and shelter. Such countries are under enormous pressure to 'go for growth' as a way out of poverty and, it is argued, are in no position to reduce their use of resources and are arguably currently more sustainable and environmentally friendly since they do not waste the small amount of resources that they have.

The light green approach also emphasises a pro-business stance and argues that for most businesses a good environmental profile makes good business sense since it will both reduce costs and promote a strong image to customers. Business is also important for the development of a new generation of green entrepreneurs who are willing to develop both sustainable business practices and new businesses that promote economically viable solutions to the environmental problems we face. These new businesses will then themselves become part of a wider economic growth which, in turn, promotes greater social welfare – the founding of new businesses selling, for example, recycling services, green transport or energy production will create new jobs and wealth in the economy.

The 'dark greens' argue that the 'light green' approach is itself unsustainable as it does nothing to introduce the fundamental changes that are required (Dobson, 2000). In short, dark greens argue that we must adopt a more ecocentric or biocentric and less anthropocentric approach. In other words, we must prioritise nature over humankind and can no longer assume that the natural world is there simply for the use and exploitation of humanity. This involves attributing rights to both the animal and plant kingdoms. We can see some parallels here to debates surrounding imperialism or slavery in the eighteenth and nineteenth centuries, that is, that the empires and peoples dominated by European nations were regarded as lacking rights and therefore open for exploitation. At the core of a dark green approach is a rejection of human centredness.

For some dark greens the central problem is one of population growth; the world's population has already reached a point that is no longer sustainable and is continuing to grow at an unsustainable rate. Quite simply, the world must reduce its population in order to reduce the over-consumption of natural resources; we can thus see elements of eugenic arguments which suggest that natural selection be allowed to take its course. At one end of the scale, it could be suggested that nature itself be allowed a free hand and that disasters such as famine or AIDS are useful methods of regulating the population. At the other end, policies such as 'one child per family' as adopted in China might be more widely implemented in order to slow population growth.

Finally, dark greens see great virtue in an approach to the economy and society more generally, in which the mantra of 'small is beautiful' is widely adopted. They wish to see far greater degrees of local sustainability in which industry, business and human habitats are organised on a much smaller and more local scale than currently. Modern methods of organising national and international trade, far from being efficient and profitable, greatly contribute to our environmental woes. In the food industry, for example, how many miles might the average plate of food have travelled before it is eaten and how much processing has that food undergone before it is consumed? Much better, they argue, to source food locally where it can be produced in more sanitary conditions and in which it does not rely on over-processing. In perhaps its utopian vision, the dark greens see a society in which people live and work within their local communities and are much more self-sufficient than we are currently able to be.

Tony Fitzpatrick (2001) adopts a slightly different classification of the debate whereby he portrays three versions of environmentalism: free-market environmentalists, environmental pragmatists and environmental radicals. Firstly, he sees a group of 'free-market environmentalists' for whom the solution to many environmental problems, as for many other issues, is to be found in the market. Allowing the market to establish a price for the purchase and use of natural resources, they argue, will regulate more effectively than government will ever be able to do. Government might have a role in applying environmental taxes, such as fees for disposing of waste or congestion charging, but overall the market should determine the price and distribution of resources.

Stop and Think

Is the market an appropriate method of regulating the supply of scarce natural resources?

Secondly, Fitzpatrick identifies 'environmental pragmatists' who, he says, support the agenda of sustainable development and who attempt to address environmental concerns by pursuing economic growth which has been rendered environmentally harmless. The model for the development of sustainability involves a combination of local, national and international government initiatives working alongside the private sector.

Finally, Fitzpatrick sees a group he describes as 'environmental radicals' which includes eco-socialists, eco-feminists and eco-anarchists. In common with one another, they argue that 'wide-ranging institutional reform' is necessary and that tweaking existing structures is insufficient. Environmental radicals also pursue a more democratic approach, arguing in favour of a bottom-up approach and for far greater levels of 'horizontal democracy' than we currently enjoy. For eco-socialists, the focus is on levels of consumption and the inequalities that such levels produce and the ability (or inability) to consume. A more equal society would militate against further environmental problems since people would no longer seek to overconsume.

For eco-feminists, there is a pattern of men attempting to dominate nature just as in society women are dominated through patriarchy. Women, by contrast, are seen as having innate caring and nurturing qualities – thus feminist solutions to environmental issues would, by their nature, be less environmentally damaging. Eco-anarchists propose a more organically organised society, rejecting solutions offered by both governmental intervention and the marketplace. This group has certain elements of commonality with the dark greens described by Dobson, since they propose much greater local organisation of society. Though greatly simplified, each of these positions views society as inherently better at preserving its natural environment than the models which currently dominate contemporary political and social life. (For a much more thoroughgoing discussion of these positions see Fitzpatrick, 2001 and Dobson, 2000.)

Green social policy

Interest in the conjunction of social policy and the environment has grown substantially in recent years and it is suggested that 'social policy is central to discussions of sustainability because it is a major means by which governments provide a minimum level of support for the population' (Cahill, 2002). Cahill goes on to explain the ways in which environmental concerns impact upon our traditional thinking about social policy. He says we will need to be concerned with our rate of economic and industrial growth – that is, that the whole nature of consumer society is at the very least alien in a more ecological world. In short, we may have to break with the traditional notion that sees quality of life improvements only with economic growth and greater productivity. We will also need, according to Cahill, to be concerned with how decisions we take now will impact upon future generations whilst at the same time attempt to meet the basic needs of the poor both now and in the future.

We have briefly outlined above some of the principles behind green thinking about society, but how might this translate itself into social policy? Fundamental to developing green politics is a rejection of 'traditional' politics and policies since, as we have already suggested, they are built around the notion of productivism and ever greater consumption as a measure of social welfare. The traditional political parties are in short arguing about who is the better manager of capitalism without questioning the principles of that system. Furthermore green politics and policy imply a rejection of traditional 'big' politics with its focus on the national and international stage; much more relevant, they argue, is a local or community-level politics. We can identify three core elements that would make up the foundations of a green social policy:

- a Basic (Citizen's) Income;
- decentralised and deregulated communities;
- a redefining of freedom.

Firstly, at least in terms of welfare, is the establishment of some form of Basic (or Citizen's) Income (BI) that will meet basic needs for all people as of right. This would be an income not based upon our willingness to participate in work, or our work record, nor by a test of our means. Instead a BI would be paid on the basis of our 'citizenship' – that we are all citizens of a society and that as citizens we have a right to be able to meet our basic needs. Intrinsic to a basic income, however, is the notion of reciprocity – an idea that all citizens have an obligation to our wider society. Thus we might be required, as a condition of receiving our basic income, to engage in work that benefits the whole community (see Fitzpatrick, 2001, 2002).

Stop and Think

If a citizen's or basic income was introduced which adequately met basic needs, would anybody continue to work?

A second fundamental change would be the development of decentralised and deregulated communities. These communities would be small and self-governing, regulating their own economic and social activities within a wider social network. Work would be organised at a local level, reducing the need for the daily commute to work, and shopping would be done at a local level, particularly for food which would also be grown locally. Such communities would be democratically organised at a local level with people able to have much more direct control over the type and level of social services that are provided. An obvious danger here, however, might be degeneration into parochialism, with such small local communities rejecting outsiders such as immigrants, travellers or simply a visitor from an alternative nearby community. What is also not clear is how society overall might deal with a local community which collectively chose to reject green principles and opt out of the green society.

Finally we would see a redefinition of our principle of freedom. The classical view of political freedom embodies the 'harm principle' outlined by the philosopher John Stuart Mill (see Chapter 9). He argued that everyone should be allowed to enjoy and exercise freedom so long as this does not adversely affect (harm) others. For greens, society needs to extend this principle to include harm done by individuals and society to the wider environment, that is both to non-human species (animals and plants) and also to non-living aspects of the environment such as the landscape. The principle would then embody the right of human beings to enjoy a clean and sustainable ecosystem and the rights of animals to live a life free from cruelty (Fitzpatrick, 2002)

How would this wider green revolution in ideas and politics translate into the development of green social policies? In considering this question, we are going to examine three areas of particular concern:

- food
- transport
- work.

Food

At a global level perhaps the greatest concern in food policy is the ability of the planet to continue to feed its population. World population currently stands at around 6.65 billion and some estimates suggest that in the next 100 years that figure will have increased to around 11 billion. Even if we have not turned over all available agricultural land to the production of biofuels to run our cars, this is going to present an enormous problem. Population, it seems, is destined, in the very near future, to outstrip the ability of the planet to feed itself. UNICEF estimates that around 800 million children are undernourished while 2 billion have poor diets, and population growth is most rapid in those countries least able to feed themselves.

Solutions range from attempts to control population growth to the search for improved technological solutions to food production that will allow better and more reliable crops to be grown. Genetic modification of seeds (and animals) is one route being pursued in order to produce foods that offer greater resistance to pests and diseases and increase crop yields. Developing countries, however, continually find themselves caught in a dilemma. To address issues of poverty they want to generate foreign currency and grow their economies. This often means that they are forced to grow 'cash crops' in order to compete in world markets. Yet those cash crops are largely exported, so while these crops might provide an income for some members of the population they force a decline in the availability of land for the production of locally grown and sustainable food supplies (Lang *et al.*, 2002).

Food policy, however, is full of apparent contradictions. In the wealthy West we are able to overconsume food to such an extent that our health is continually damaged, whilst in less developed nations problems of starvation and malnutrition persist. In the West we appear to have a crisis of overproduction in which food is either destroyed if the international price is deemed too low, or else dumped on world markets which further undermines the economic efforts of less developed countries. Furthermore, in the West we have developed an enormous interest in food and 'lifestyle' yet continue to experience ever-decreasing standards of both diet and health.

The diet of the modern British citizen is high in fat, salt and sugar, often associated with the consumption of highly processed and convenience foods. Less cooking and communal eating of food takes place in British homes, partly due to longer working hours, dual-earner households and greater commuting to work. All of this in turn encourages ever greater consumption of convenience foods. This implies that we are becoming increasingly deskilled in both the growing and cooking of food. At the same time we take less exercise as a society than in previous years, despite the growth of gym membership, and appear to have less opportunity to engage in exercise.

Stop and Think

It is often said that the British diet during the years of rationing during and after the Second World War was better than modern diets. What reasons can we suggest for this?

Food poverty is persistently cited as a problem issue, despite overall falls in the cost of the food bill of an average family, with the lowest nutritional standards found among the poorest households. Poor households suffer from higher levels of diet-related disease (heart disease, stroke, some cancers, diabetes and dental decay) and higher levels of mortality and morbidity among children and babies (Department of Health, 1998c; Lang *et al.*, 2002). Food poverty, we can note, is highest among populations where the range of food consumed is relatively narrow and with particularly low intakes of fruit and vegetables. 'The less income people have, the narrower the range of foods they consume, the higher the proportion of their household expenditure is on food and the worse their diet related health is' (Lang *et al.*, 2002).

We also appear to be enduring a crisis in both our food production and its distribution. Intensive farming, made possible by the development of chemical fertilisers, pesticides and the hormonal and dietary supplements given to animals, has increased both the availability and yields of food but also increased food risk. Increasingly high levels of food-related disease appear to be becoming more likely. Intensive food production also introduces other environmental impacts such as decreased ecological diversity as natural habitats are removed and destroyed to make industrialised agriculture more possible.

Much of the money we spend on food is wasted. Cahill suggests that only 10% of the energy involved in food production actually goes into growing the food. The rest is expended in the transport, packaging, retailing and advertising of that food. Indeed, we might be spending upwards of £10 each week on packaging alone. Furthermore, we have undergone a further revolution in food production in that we no longer seem bound by traditional seasons. As such, we are able to enjoy the food we want at any time of the year, such as strawberries at Christmas. There is an environmental cost to this, however, since much of this food is produced overseas. The average Sunday dinner, for example, could have travelled up to 49,000 food miles from farm to plate (Soil Association). We have already alluded to the problems faced by farmers in developing countries where they are involved in agricultural production for export rather than local consumption. On top of this, we seem to be inventing ever more contradictions in our food policy such that the UK now imports some 60% of its apples and 80% of pears, both of which can be easily grown in the UK climate but the production of which has declined as orchards are torn out to make way for more profitable use of the land.

We have also witnessed a revolution in food retailing with the 'big 4' supermarkets (Asda/Wal-Mart, Tesco, Sainsbury and Morrisons) controlling some 85% of the food retail market. Increasingly, food is sold by the larger supermarkets in often out-of-town retail warehouses, for which transport is essential. This practice has also led to the creation of 'food deserts' (Lang *et al.*, 2002) whereby small local shops which can no longer compete are forced to close. While food in the supermarkets may be cheaper, it may not be so easily accessible, especially for poor households.

The local production and retailing of food advocated by a green social policy would address the issues raised here in a number of ways. These would include the reduction of food miles, pollution and transportation of food. Also, the issues of the chemicalisation of food production and the ability of developing nations to feed their populations would be addressed. Food policy and environmental concerns around food production have a clear impact on social policy with implications for a population's long-term health.

Transport

Transport itself is of great concern to environmentalists as well as to social policy more generally. The wide and increased availability of the motor car, certainly since the end of the Second World War, has arguably increased social inclusion. The ability of people to move about more freely, to enjoy leisure activities, to take employment that is often some considerable distance from where we live have all, arguably, promoted greater levels of social equality.

By transport, therefore, we mostly talk about road transport and in particular the car – over 90% of all travel in Britain is by road and over 80% of all vehicles on Britain's roads are cars. By the early 1990s in the UK people travelled 681 billion passenger kilometres annually, a threefold increase since 1952, and on average we spend 15 days each year travelling. Much of the travel in which we engage is work-related commuting or business travel or distribution of goods. Most of that travel is conducted by men. Women's travel is more likely to include a higher proportion related to home and family, including 'doing the school run' or shopping. Women are more likely to be users of public transport than men. By the end of the last century around 80% of men and 55% of women held driving licences (Huby, 1998). Yet, around 30% of all households lack access to a car. This figure is higher in urban areas and is concentrated among the elderly and poorer households. More generally, among those in professional and managerial employment, the ownership of two or more cars is most prevalent.

There is clearly then a gender and age dimension (and a disability one too – see Chapter 19) to transport. Transport policy itself raises both questions of social justice and environmental impact. Environmental questions can be raised about the impact and necessity of the rapid increase in journeys across the UK. The increase in journeys increases environmental pollution, but also has impacts in terms of the building of more roads to accommodate increased traffic, in terms of the health impacts of that pollution on the population and in terms of increases in deaths and injuries resulting from road accidents. There has also been a considerable impact in terms of increased crime involving the theft of vehicles and items from cars as well as increases in driving-related offences such as speeding.

Sea and air travel have also increased considerably over the last half-century with a rapid rise in air travel during the 1990s with the development of the budget airline industry. Walking and cycling have declined as regularly used forms of transport: cycling accounted for 21 billion kilometres in 1951, but only 4.4 billion kilometres in 1994. Cycling represents only 1% of road traffic and is most likely to be used for short journeys. Thus, although cycling and walking are the most environmentally sustainable forms of transport, they are continually relegated by our preference for the car, which we use to make around one third of all journeys of less than two miles (Huby, 1998).

Public transport accounts for around 6% of all journeys and is dominated by rail transport which is particularly important for commuting. The use of rail travel has remained fairly constant as a proportion of all journeys, although bus travel has declined despite campaigns in the mid-1980s by some local authorities to maintain low fares for using public transport, such as the Fares Fair campaign led by the Greater London Council.

The social problems associated with transport and car use include pollution, both the direct pollution of exhaust emissions but also secondary pollution when exhaust fumes react in the atmosphere and cause other health problems, for example respiratory problems caused by increased ozone levels. While carbon dioxide, a major part of exhaust emissions, is not itself a pollutant causing health problems, it is a major greenhouse gas thought to contribute to global warming and climate change. Pollution is also associated with the disposal of vehicles when they are scrapped as the vehicles themselves are constructed with toxic and polluting chemicals.

Another important social issue associated with road travel is the number of accidents involving vehicles. Some 30 million people are estimated to have died as a result of road traffic accidents worldwide. Many deaths involve non-vehicle users, pedestrians and cyclists for example, who are more vulnerable when involved in an accident with a vehicle. By contrast the vehicles themselves have been made much safer for their occupants with the introduction of a wide range of safety features such as seat belts and airbags. Although overall rates are falling, the majority of those killed or injured in road accidents are under 40 years of age and many are children (Cahill, 2002).

Stop and Think

Consider the exansion plans for airports in Britain, for example the suggested runway expansion for Heathrow. Without this development BAA suggests that the British economy will be damaged and fall behind that of our international competitors. What has been the 'green' response to the proposal?

Work

Work is perhaps the most critical area for an examination of social policy and the environment. As we have noted, green thinkers identify the core problem for the world as being an obsession with production and consumption. We have an economy and supporting welfare network that measure well-being in terms of our level of production and consumption. Green thinkers argue that we have an unhelpful definition of work and what it means and that this definition and our relationship to the world of work needs to be redefined.

> Imagine 15 women sitting in rocking chairs in a circle, each with her own baby on her lap. That is *not* work. Now imagine that an instruction is given: 'Hand your baby to the person to your left.' Now that *is* work.
>
> Something is wrong with that logic. This definition of work yields a strange and unwanted consequence. It leaves us with only one way in which child rearing can be considered to be productive work. Strangers must raise our children. Then it is work. (Cahn, 2000)

Cahn (2000) suggests that the current way in which we define 'real' work, as an activity done in return for market wages, is flawed. It ignores the vast contribution of the non-market economy and it devalues real work. How, for example, could the raising of the next generation not be considered a valuable and valued contribution to the economy? We are familiar in social policy literature with arguments around the feminisation of labour, that is, that much caring work for families, children and elderly relatives is done by women. It is also work that goes largely unrecognised and is 'expected' as part of normal family duties. We could suggest that this argument is extended to include work undertaken by the wider family, friends and neighbours. What would the cost be if all such work were accounted for economically? In terms of welfare policy we should note that the active employment policies pursued by many Western governments aim to achieve mass employment and to put as many people into paid jobs as is possible. In the UK under New Labour, single-parents, over 90% of whom are women, have thus been encouraged to take jobs once their children enter senior school at around 11 years of age. The message seems to be that paid employment is valued more highly than the task of caring for children.

Failing to give value to activities such as child raising and over-prioritising the pursuit of paid work could be argued to be misguided. It suggests that child raising is a private (family) activity and of no benefit to the wider community. Yet the UK's apparent obsession with 'yob culture' and the anti-social behaviour of some young people, by contrast, points to the inherent value and social benefits of child rearing, that it is a 'public good'.

Both Bill Jordan (1998) and Ruth Levitas (1998) have argued that the model for examining social exclusion, which has become the dominant orthodoxy in the United Kingdom, has been to suggest that the primary way to combat social exclusion is via paid work (Jordan, 1998; Levitas, 1998). For Jordan we have defined welfare almost exclusively in terms of its relation to the labour market and that any notion of 'rights' to welfare implies an obligation to work. It is a reflection back to the welfare of the Poor Law as claimants must seek to demonstrate their 'worthiness'.

For Jordan there are three elements to this orthodoxy. Firstly, prosperity is related to the skills of the workforce. Welfare systems must then emphasise the training and education of workers and ensure that individuals are flexible and adaptable in order to increase their employability. An educated and flexible workforce will improve welfare for themselves and their families because they are better placed to take higher-paid jobs. This then leads to a second point, that the workforce must be increasingly productive and prepared to work long hours in order to gain greater rewards. For greens this again emphasises the value of the formal labour market over the informal, and arguably damages individual and family welfare because of the long hours and pressure to be more productive. To support the formal labour market, the welfare system has to be configured firstly to promote paid work (welfare to work) and secondly to reward those who can no longer work in proportion to their employment record. Perceived free-riding is to be tackled and eliminated. As such, we undergo ever more strict and stringent tests to prove our eligibility and worth.

For green thinkers, this attitude to work is outdated and misguided. Firstly, it is inextricably linked to the productive economy in that we value work which allows us to produce more and consume more. Secondly, we give little or no value to unpaid work. There must be, it is argued, 'a reconceptualisation of the nature and value of work' (Dobson, 2000). Ruth Levitas reinforces this point when she argues that the discourse that has come to dominate political circles, what she calls the Social Integrationist Discourse, regards the route out of social exclusion as being via integration into the workplace.

The preoccupation with paid employment as the method best suited to improving individual and social welfare ignores the limits-to-growth thesis which forms the core of green thinking around welfare and the environment. In contrast, greens argue that, although we will not be working any less, the work we engage in will be more meaningful and rewarding, though the reward will not necessarily be monetary. An interesting viewpoint on this is put forward by André Gorz (1985) who suggests that in order to meet their own basic needs over a lifetime each person will need to engage in paid work for around 20,000 hours. This would translate to around 10 years of full-time or 20 years half-time work, in contrast to a working life of around 40–50 years that is currently the norm.

This does not mean, however, that we would be inactive for the rest of our lives. Gorz argues that we would engage in heteronomous and autonomous activities. Heteronomous activities are those in which we have a social duty to engage. This will include paid work producing the goods and services required by society but also work of a more social nature, such as caring duties. Autonomous activities include those which are for our own personal development and will include further education and training as well as leisure activities. In return every citizen would receive a basic or citizen's income at a level sufficient to meet their basic needs. Gorz attempts, by this definition, to give value to both paid and unpaid work in equal measure and to overcome the current difficulties we have in recognising and valuing unpaid work.

Stop and Think

How could society ensure that individuals engaged in socially necessary but unpaid work such as caring?

Conclusion

As we have seen, the basis of a green critique of welfare and social policy is founded in the fundamentals of a critique of the economic system. Welfare, it is argued, is part of and is core to an economic system that regards progress in terms of growth. Such an ideology of growth is at odds, say the greens, with both common sense and the realities of the world around us. Economic growth, and the pursuit of growth, is a key part of the problems which we now face. Growth as it has been conceived is responsible for the rapid diminution of natural resources around the globe and for the pollution of our planet. Greens suggest that we are rapidly nearing the point at which those resources that have powered the industrial revolution will themselves run out and at the same time the crucial environmental 'tipping points' when the damage caused to the Earth itself will become irreparable.

From a green perspective, social policy, as traditionally conceived is part of the overall problem because it is designed to support this damaging ideal of economic growth. This pursuit of growth will ultimately damage our welfare as resources run out and our environment becomes more uninhabitable. 'Green' social policy proposes that we need to give up the pursuit of growth and switch to using resources which are sustainable. This would imply a much greater local, rather than regional, national or international focus for employment and wider welfare services such as health and education, along with the introduction of new areas of social policy interest such as transport, travel and food production.

Critics argue that this approach is far too 'doom-laden' and harks back to an idealised pre-industrial world that it is simply not possible to recreate. The critique also suggests that the developments we have been able to enjoy as a result of the rapid industrial progress of the past 200 years will enable us to find solutions to many of the environmental issues that have been identified. Thus, the greater employment of technology in areas such as energy efficiency and the growth of new industries such as those around recycling will allow us both to tackle environmental problems and to continue to grow economically.

The whole debate presented by the emergence of an environmental social policy brings to light some potentially new and threatening social problems that we will have to develop new social policies to address. Issues such as the enforcement of recycling targets or the reduction in the number of miles we travel each year are highly controversial, particularly in the domestic arena. We also face new international welfare issues such as the threat of increased food poverty and famine. Similarly, mass migration as a result of the availability and access to food, medicines or other resources or as a result of environmental disaster is becoming an increased possibility. It appears, then, that whether or not we accept the green critique of social policy, a new social policy that incorporates a green agenda is inevitable.

Annotated further reading

The environment and the impact of environmental change on wider society is a vast area of research and writing currently and so it is only possible to highlight a few of the many available resources. The volumes published in 2002 by Michael Cahill (*The Environment and Social Policy*), Michael Cahill and Tony Fitzpatrick (*Environmental Issues and Social Welfare*) and Fitzpatrick and Cahill (*Environment and Welfare: Towards a green social policy*) all provide a wide-ranging and accessible introduction to the specific issues around the environment that might be of interest to anyone studying social policy. Also still of interest is the earlier volume by Meg Huby (*Social Policy and the Environment*, 1998).

The books by Andrew Dobson (*Fairness and Futurity*, 1998; *Green Political Thought*, 2000) give a broad introduction to the politics of the environment and to the ideological stance represented by the various strands of the green movement. The article by Tim Lang and colleagues, 'Food, social policy and the environment' (2002), is particularly instructive in relation to food policy and food poverty, while the volume by James Lovelock (*The Revenge of Gaia*, 2006) gives an interesting insight into the science behind many of the green arguments around the environment, and by implication welfare and social policy. The works by Robert Putnam (*Bowling Alone*, 2000) and Edgar Cahn (*No More Throw-away People*, 2000), while not claiming to be green critiques, do give a useful synthesis of what might be considered to be green thinking in practice.

Chapter 22

International social policy: globalisation and the European Union

by Harry Cowen

Objectives

- To consider the pertinence of the international dimension in studying social policy.

- To outline the developments of globalisation and their influences upon national policy making.

- To analyse the new global social policy structures, governance and institutions, and their impacts upon national social policies.

- To focus upon the European Union, a leading sub-global regional institution, and describe its genesis, its structures and the major economic and political issues.

- To chart the origins and assess the key features of the European Union's social policy.

Introduction

This chapter locates the subject of social policy in the context of the international arena. Social policies do not function in a hermetically sealed environment, and we need to understand not only the singular attributes of a particular nation's policies and institutional frameworks, but also the ways in which policy structures and strategies may resemble or diverge from those operating in other countries. Having viewed certain aspects of international social policy, the chapter moves on to investigate contemporary forces of globalisation which have rapidly transformed the environment in which national policy-makers must now work. The third main section of the chapter represents an enquiry into the key global institutions of the post-World War II period, responsible for shaping social policy at a trans-national level, reflecting a further tier of governance, and those hegemonic world financial institutions whose policies exert a profound impact upon national and regional social policy-making. In the fourth part, the chapter focuses upon what is indisputably the most comprehensive and relatively coherent example of sub-regional governance, in the form of the European Union, tracing its historical genesis, its institutional economic and political frameworks within which social policies are designed and debated, and the key issues exercising the participants of the EU as a whole. The fifth section analyses the specific features of the EU's social policy and social concerns arising out of the organisation's development. The sixth section inspects the political impact of the growth of the Union's membership, the consequential effects on the EU's constitution and decision-making processes, and the formulation of reforms to deal with the attendant anxieties. The final section of the chapter deals with the British response to the latest stage in the European Union's growth.

International social policy

It is clear that individual countries' social policies do not operate in isolation. For a number of years, there was a burgeoning literature which built up the field of comparative social policy, and which focused on separate nations. This included comparison of the economic growth rates, but also studied the distinct approaches between, e.g., Germany and the UK with regard to unemployment benefits or housing assistance (see Chapter 8). Hill (1995) looked across the range of social policies in different countries. Walker and Maltby (1997) looked at old age and pensions. Hantrais (2004) has investigated a whole range of social policies in European societies: family policy, employment, pensions, social security, poverty and education. Sykes and Alcock (1998) charted the differences in European social policy.

Evident problems arose, not least in the measurement of differences, and the various ways of recording information (in some cases, hardly at all!). Notwithstanding, Esping-Andersen's *The Three Worlds of Welfare Capitalism* (1990) was a path-breaking piece of work in the search for a set of explanations for the success and failure of economic and social policies from nation to nation. This study produced the concept of diverse welfare *regimes*. Data from 18 advanced industrial nations were collected and analysed to produce a three-part typology of welfare regimes: the social democratic state, the corporatist state and the liberal state. Into these 'ideal types' were slotted the pertinent countries most congruent with the appropriate form of regime. The archetype of the Social Democratic welfare state resembled Sweden and the other Nordic states. Germany was characterised as a Corporatist state; the USA, the UK and Ireland figured as typical Liberal states (see Chapter 9 for an articulation of theoretical principles underlying the liberal welfare state, and see also Chapter 10). Esping-Andersen's model continued through the 1990s and into the current century as the most dominant for differentiating welfare systems.

The cardinal criteria for distinguishing national welfare systems were as follows:

- the extent to which welfare protection was given by non-market providers (termed the measure of 'decommodification');
- the extent to which access to welfare was determined by social class (measuring the extent of stratification);
- the extent to which high levels of employment were achieved.

Esping-Andersen suggested that it was not possible for a modern economy to possess all three pre-requisites: a balanced budget, mediocre economic equality and high levels of employment. Hence, choices made by the individual nations to opt for one or two of the goals have produced divergent routes. Following on from Esping-Andersen, other analysts have suggested there is another type of welfare regime: the Mediterranean, comprising Spain, Portugal and Greece (Maurizio-Ferera cited in Giddens, 2007). Even a fifth type has been suggested by Giddens (2007), comprising the states of the former Communist bloc now striving to adapt their welfare states to the model of the Western industrialised nations.

The Esping-Andersen model, however, is posited on economies adopting different trajectories. As such, the assumptions have come under challenge. Hemerijck (2002) argues that no clear-cut distinctions really exist empirically between the different regimes, which adopt *combinations* of tax, public welfare and employment policies. A 'hybrid' model is more the case. Over the past 15–20 years a definite convergence of welfare states has occurred. Comprehensive aims have come to mirror each other's. Esping-Andersen himself noted in his *Welfare States in Transition* (1996) that the post-war period of sustained economic growth and full employment, simultaneously with greater equality, was no longer feasible for even the most social democratic of the European welfare states.

To summarise, then, in the face of pressures from trends in global capitalism, welfare states generally have had to considerably modify policies, not least in increasing unemployment levels and the numbers of people on social security (see Chapter 8). The economic climate has changed globally, and it is expedient to turn to a discussion of globalisation to fully comprehend the international context of social policies.

Globalisation

Less than two decades ago, economics, sociology and social policy texts paid scant attention to the global, in their respective analyses. Nowadays, the social sciences book market is flooded with publications on globalisation or those that contain the word global in their title. There are various definitions. George and Wilding's is helpful, in that it incorporates competing definitions:

> Globalization is the increasing inter-connectedness of the world through the compression of time and space brought about by advances in knowledge and technology as well as by political events and decisions. (George and Wilding, 2002: 19)

Below is another:

> [Globalization] is a two-way set of processes . . . Globalization – in its diverse forms – doesn't just come from the outside. Every time I switch on a computer, send an e-mail, look at information on the Internet, put on the television or radio, I actively contribute to globalization at the same time as I make use of it. (Giddens, 2007: 8)

The world is indeed a much smaller place: a message from Manchester to New York takes less than a second! As one might expect, given the multiplicity of articles and books on the subject, how one responds to the phenomenon depends on the political perspective adopted.

Political perspectives on globalisation

George and Wilding rather neatly package the range of positions into five over-arching views. *Technological enthusiasts* focus upon the perceived benefits of modern advanced technology driven by the market – an irresistible, positive force. *Marxisant pessimists* note the very logic of capitalism and its age-old, restless pursuit of profits: neo-liberalism widening wealth inequalities on a global scale. For *plural pragmatists*, the consequences of globalisation result in a melange: a mixed bag of neither all good nor all bad; globalisation possesses multiple elements, not merely economic or technological. The *sceptic internationalists* argue that the notion of neo-liberalism, market ideology and the power of the multinationals sweeping all before them is fallacious and exaggerated. The *political economy* approach favoured by George and Wilding (2002) regards the political and economic features of globalisation as both positive and negative, but as a phenomenon neo-liberalism seems to be driving the future.

The forces of neo-liberalism

There appears little doubt, regardless of any particular political stance taken, that at the beginning of the twenty-first century, boosted by the crumbling of the communist system in 1989, neo-liberalism is exerting a profound hold over nations across the globe. Witness the power of the multinational corporations (many with annual turnover exceeding that of the GDP of some smaller national states), the power of the Bretton Woods financial institutions, and the internationalisation of trade and finance. More specifically, neo-liberalism operates through the incessant privatising of public enterprises, huge tax cuts, rigid controls over trade unions, major reductions in public social expenditure, and removal of any controls over the movement of finance out of or into national economies (Steger, 2003).

As we shall see, all of these strongly influence the contours of social policy and the very processes of national governance and decision-making, arguably inducing a whole series of social problems which social policy is expected to solve. Such problems usually stem from factors like impacts upon work and unemployment, where multinationals like Ford threaten to relocate, weaken the trade unions and extract special concessions from government. Other impacts include the spread of disease from rapidly increasing travel and migration, or doctors and nurses leaving poor countries for the more affluent West (George and Wilding, 2002: Ch. 3).

Stop and Think

Which of the political perspectives do you think reflects globalisation today? What are your reasons?

Hence, globalisation, with its economic emphasis upon neo-liberal markets and competitiveness, has augured in new frames of reference for managing national economies and policies, refocusing attention on minimising costs of service provision and maximising national growth and competitiveness within the global economy (see Chapter 8). Health, education, employment and social security are all policy areas subjected to global factors. Globalisation has nurtured a series of global policy health networks. Health spending and cost containment issues have become politicised. The state more readily intervenes in local education matters, global education policy networks are expanding, as is the higher education sector in the face of intense international competition. Global pressures lie behind the restraints in a whole host of state social security systems and also the levels of social security provision and spending. State benefits are cut, state welfare policies retreat rather than advance, and responsibilities for maintenance of subsistence living standards are redirected onto the individual (George and Wilding, 2002).

To recap, globalisation implies something different from international developments. A range of ideological perspectives is available to evaluate the impacts of globalisation: the forces of neo-liberalism, however, cannot be underestimated. Having discussed the tendencies of globalisation and the ramifications of the global capitalist economy for national state strategies, the chapter now shifts attention to social policy actually formulated at global level.

Global social policy

Until the seminal work of Deacon with Stubbs and Hulse (1997) within the social policy discipline, few commentators were focusing on global social policy *per se*. The prime orientation was the comparative assessment of discrete national states. Deacon posited that a number of trends had made it circumspect to alter the direction of international social policy analysis, namely the break-up of the communist bloc, the growth of global economic competition, and thus the exacerbating burdens thrust upon the national states to perform; the growing challenges to global capitalism in the wake of corporate power; and the collapse of limpid national boundaries in the spheres of economics and policy-making.

Hence, new themes which no one national state is able to manage have emerged in the social policy arena: issues of social justice between states, the aim of a supranational citizenship and the tensions between the universal provision of social and welfare services on the one hand, and the need for diversity of provision suited to different groups and societies on the other. Further, regarding the governance of globalisation, one must be cognisant of the new types of agencies responsible for providing economic and social welfare: the major players now are the plethora of agencies of international governance. The outcomes of their actions, for Deacon, may be categorised in terms of the changing redistribution of resources across the globe, the regulation of those activities distinctly harmful in the epoch of a *laissez-faire* capitalism, and the features of global or supranational provision.

The global social policy institutions

How are these changes effected? Basically, through an impressive variety of international organisations, wielding a considerable authority over social policy. By the 1990s they numbered 1,000 (Yeates, 2001). The most prominent concerns of transnational cooperation include social policies in employment, migration, social security, education, health and social services.

Indisputably, the neo-liberal paradigm governing their multilateral trade rules has been to the detriment of social, health and environmental standards. International financial and development institutions adopt a high profile in enabling access for public projects in developing countries. Who, then, are the main players affecting social policy?

The International Monetary Fund (IMF), based in Washington, DC, drives *economic* growth through an explicitly (but now *possibly* weakening in the face of persistent criticisms) neo-liberal orientation. It has usually adopted a non-committal approach in the way of offering social policy advice. Yet in the wake of the fall of the Soviet Union, it was proactive in assisting the new Eastern European economies to construct their social security systems.

The World Bank, also based in Washington and founded as a result of the post-war Bretton Woods agreement, is engaged in assisting global economic development, but it adopts more of a social development stance in the endeavour to confront the vagaries of world poverty.

The Organisation for Economic Co-operation and Development (OECD), based in Paris again, comprises most of the world's affluent nations, and came into being for the encouragement of *European* economic growth. It is intent on supporting social and economic welfare, whilst matching social policy objectives to budgetary constraints.

The *European Union,* perhaps the globe's most significant sub-regional actor, is discussed in greater detail below.

The International Labour Organisation (ILO), based in Geneva, Switzerland, since the 1980s, is devoted to maintaining common international employment, labour and social standards, but has invariably come under serious challenge from the overtly neo-liberal global institutions (not least because of its long-term opposition to the privatisation of pensions and state social security schemes).

The World Health Organisation (WHO), a United Nations' agency based in Geneva, has been involved in global health initiatives such as child immunisation and combating malaria as well as developing anti-AIDS strategies.

Other United Nations (UN) agencies include the United Nations Children's Fund (UNICEF), the United Nations Development Programme (UNDP), and the series of summit conferences of the UN which debate strategies for facilitating social policies and social development at the global level.

Disagreement does exist between the key players: conflicting advice on the one hand, and clashes of ideological perspective on the other (especially between the US-dominated social 'liberal' strategies of the World Bank and the more socially inclined, protectionist policies of the ILO). Business-orientated individuals, too, wield considerable power and influence in the course of global social policy debates, as illustrated in Deacon's large-scale survey (Deacon with Stubbs and Hulse, 1997) into the role of the key global actors in post-1989 Eastern Europe. Resulting from his enquiry in the 1990s, Deacon produced his global governance reform agenda, highlighting the regulation of global competition; increased accountability for the Bretton Woods institutions; reforming the United Nations in the context of the USA's consistent avoidance of an appropriate financial contribution; the strengthening of global, political, legal and social rights to facilitate a system of global

---

| Box 22.1 | **Major global institutions** |

- The International Monetary Fund (IMF), based in Washington, DC, founded Bretton Woods: supports economic growth through an explicitly neo-liberal orientation. Offers social policy advice only.
- The World Bank, based in Washington, DC, founded Bretton Woods: assists global economic development. More of a social development stance in anti-world poverty strategy.
- The Organisation for Economic Co-operation and Development (OECD), based in Paris. Membership: most of the world's affluent nations. Supports social and economic welfare.
- The European Union, based in Brussells, Strasbourg and Luxembourg. Viewed as the globe's most significant sub-regional actor.
- The International Labour Organisation (ILO), based in Geneva. Aims at maintaining common international employment, labour and social standards. Opposes privatisation of pensions and state social security schemes.
- The World Health Organisation (WHO), based in Geneva. A United Nations agency. Involved in global health initiatives such as child immunisation and combating malaria, development of anti-AIDS strategies.
- The United Nations (UN).

Other agencies include United Nations Children's Fund (UNICEF), United Nations Educational, Scientific and Cultural Organisation (UNESCO), United Nations Development Programme (UNDP). Summit conferences debate global strategies re social policies and social development.

---

citizenship; and the empowering of international civil society. These were modified in Deacon's recent volume (2007) to reflect a slightly weakened confidence in the willingness of the Washington-based organisations to cooperate in a more equitable globe. He maintains that the winning over of international corporations to socially responsible practice will count, although debates within the anti-globalisation movement about what are the actual prospects for and policies of alternative globalisations will be important.

> But eventually success, if there is to be any, will depend on the construction of a global political alliance that embraces most of these actors and sites. (Deacon, 2007: 179)

However, such a reform agenda, in common with other advocacies of reform, is understandably subject to serious scrutiny and critique: does one readily accept that no alternative to neo-liberal economic structures exists? Ferguson and colleagues (2002) are sceptical of Deacon's seeming confidence (deriving from his 1990s study) that the OECD, WTO, IMF and other key international actors are able to perform their part in pursuing the politics of global social responsibility. Deacon's reformist belief 'that the leaders of global capital will willingly place the needs of the environment and the world's people above the drive for profit' must be seen as utopian, they contend (Ferguson *et al.*, 2002: 149).

Stop and Think

Does the concept of global governance possess too many pitfalls? What are they?

But is it the case that the individual states are left with no voice in charting the future of global social policies? Held's extensive work on global governance (Held and McGrew, 2002; Held, 2004) suggests not. Similarly, Yeates's investigation into whether international government agencies heap unavoidable pressures onto social policy agendas of subservient states, also supports this position. Individual governments *do* retain power. 'Globalisation' is not unstoppable. The G7 countries (unarguably the richest nations in the world) affect nations' interest rates and financial markets through the IMF. The General Agreement on Tariffs and Trade (GATT) and the World Trade Organisation (WTO) regulate international trade via negotiations between the key Western capitalist governments.

> The world political system is still inter-governmental and is premised on constitutionally sovereign states . . . International co-operation is, at the end of the day, the co-operation of sovereign states. (Yeates, 2001: 125)

International key actors do not necessarily succeed in overriding individual countries' domestic strategies. A further development gives the lie to the idea of global institutional hegemony, and that is the rise of an anti-globalisation movement, which the chapter now moves on to discuss.

Global social policy and the anti-globalisation movement

Since the late 1990s a range of protest groups and organisations have mobilised across the world against the human and social injustices of the policies of the powerful transnational bodies – the WTO, the EU, the G8 nations (G7 plus Russia), the World Bank – alongside the actions of the transnational corporations.

In the advanced capitalist countries mass protests outside the conference venues of these august bodies have exceeded 50,000 demonstrators since the early demonstration in Seattle, USA, in 1999. Official responses from the host nations have on occasions been brutal, including deaths or injuries of protesters in Gothenburg, Sweden (June 2001), in Genoa, Italy (July 2001) and in Brussels, Belgium, not to mention many unpublicised deaths in countries deemed 'peripheral'.

With respect to the impact of the movement on global social policy, the International Government Organisations (IGOs) have felt compelled to address some of the social, health and environmental implications of their policies, and multinational drug companies have made *some* adjustments to their pricing of AIDS drugs. But, in the last analysis, Yeates (2002) questions whether any progress on social policy has materialised at all. Deacon, too, in his more recent evaluation of current global social policy, concludes that in spite of the evidence of a greater concern with equity *vis-à-vis* social policy in the UN agencies, the World Bank still delivers minimal social provision and protection, and the WTO is accelerating the global market in private health, social care, education and insurance services (2007).

What the anti-globalisation movement *has* achieved is in validating the existence of mass public support for its arguments and in widening the reception of its ideas outside an exclusive group of cognoscenti (Yeates, 2002). Furthermore, social policy commentators have had to incorporate into their scenarios the effects of transnational monetary, environmental and trade policies upon economic, health and social welfare.

To summarise, the post-war creation of powerful economic and political global institutions, fuelled by Western capital, has transfigured the shape of economic and social policymaking. Seminal debates currently concern whether expectations of effective reform are realistic or whether radical change is the remaining alternative. They also entail the extent to which global governance threatens the continuation of national sovereignty. Assuredly, the rise of the anti-globalisation movement has raised general consciousness of the issues.

In the next section we look at the workings and policies of a major, and relatively successful sub-regional body whose structures and policies affect all populations across Europe: the European Union. The section outlines the history of the organisation and its current structures, and identifies the significance of its major treaties. Following this, the chapter will evaluate the progress of social policy inside the EU.

The European Union, its origins and structures

The European Union is the archetype of a sub-regional global institution. It is a mammoth international organisation with a number of member states who, in the spirit of international cooperation, delegate a part of their sovereignty to facilitate decisions of economic, social and political significance at the European level.

The historical origins of the Union may be traced back to the Second World War. The concept of European integration was forged as an antidote to the perpetuation of war and human and environmental devastation. Robert Schuman, France's Foreign Minister, delivered an inaugural speech on 9 May 1950, to create the European Community, initially a supranational institution with the task of regulating French and German coal and steel production. Since that time, the organisation has been subject to regular jostling between the major powers for political ascendancy to protect their own 'national interests'.

During the 1960s General de Gaulle, the French President, fought against the federal orientation of most of the other member states. His aim was the advancement of French power (Borchardt, 1995). As a consequence, his government vetoed for the second time Britain's application to join in 1967 (although, with the General gone, Britain had gained admission by the early 1970s). In the 1980s, Jacques Delors' presidency of the European Commission pushed the Union in a clear federalist direction, including the idea of a single market for Europe, a single currency (the euro) and institutional reform (Pinder, 2001). Over this same period, Margaret Thatcher, UK Prime Minister at the time, opposed the single currency and institutional reform. She was highly vocal over the size of the UK contribution to the European budget, considered too disproportionate to the anticipated national benefits (also see Chapter 16 for discussion of Thatcher's response to the EU and employment).

In 1951, the Treaty of Paris formally set up the European Coal and Steel Community (ECSC) and the European Atomic Energy Community (Euratom). The Treaty of Rome was signed in 1958 to mark the formation of the European Economic Community (EEC), which embraced only six European nations: Belgium, West Germany, France, Italy, Luxembourg and the Netherlands. It was fundamentally a trading bloc. The UK joined in 1973 along with Ireland and Denmark. In

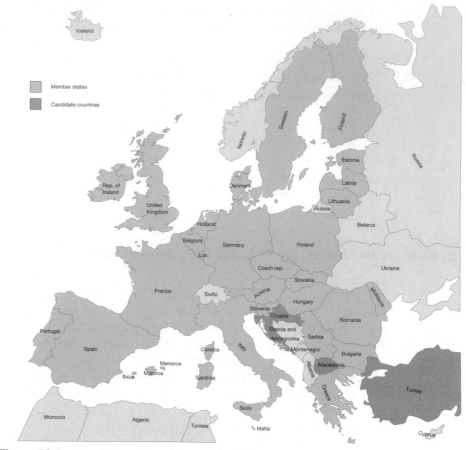

Figure 22.1 The 27 member states of the European Union

1981 Greece joined, followed by Portugal and Spain in 1986; Austria, Finland and Sweden acceded in 1995. A further 12 countries from Eastern and Central Europe joined in the decade of the new century (see Figure 22.1). Boxes 22.2 and 22.3 list the EU treaties and member states with their years of accession.

The Treaty of Maastricht in 1992 launched the current European Union, with the explicit purpose of deepening the economic and political ties between the countries of Europe. At the same time it established the framework for economic and monetary union in Europe, through the European Monetary Institute (EMI) which laid the ground for the new EU currency (the euro).

What of the main institutions in the present EU? These may be seen as five first-tier institutions, each one with a specific role to play of significance for social policy, given the importance of decision making and the structures of governance to the framing of directives and legislation bearing upon the policy area.

The European Commission

The Commission, based in Brussels, is the driving force and the executive body of the European Union. It is pivotal for European policy-making. It is made up

Box 22.2	**Treaties of the European Union**

1951 **Treaty of Paris**: set up of ECSC and Euratom.

1958 **Treaty of Rome**: formation of EEC.

1991 **Treaty of Maastrich**: launch of EU and beginnings of social policy; established economic and monetary union.

1997 **Treaty of Amsterdam**: enhanced the status of social policy and citizenship rights in the EU.

2001 **Treaty of Nice**: prepared the EU for further enlargement; extended Qualified Majority Voting.

2007 **Treaty of Lisbon ratified**: reforms earlier treaties appropriate to major enlargement of EU; sets out strategy for Union in context of globalisation.

Box 22.3	**Growth of the European Union**

1952 The founding members of the ECSC were Belgium, the Netherlands, Luxembourg, France, Italy and West Germany.

1973 The UK joined the EC with Denmark and Ireland.

1981 Greece joined the EC.

1986 Portugal and Spain joined the EC.

1995 Austria, Finland and Sweden acceded to the EU.

2004 Accession to the EU of Czech Republic, Estonia, Hungary, Latvia, Lithuania, Poland, Slovakia, Slovenia, Malta and Cyprus, bringing the size of the membership to 25.

2007 Bulgaria and Romania entered the Union.

of 20 commissioners, elected for five years by the respective governments of the member states. The more powerful states of Germany, Italy, Spain, France and the UK are each entitled to two commissioners. The latter are expected to act in the *collective* interests of the EU, not as their nation's promoters. Whereas its essential purpose is to advance new legislation, it has to consult with a range of civil society interest groups, such as employers and representatives of trade unions. The Commission is divided into a number of *Directorates General* (equivalent to Departments) which include 'Employment, Industrial Relations and Social Affairs' (DG V) and 'Education, Training and Youth' (DG XXII).

The Council of the European Union

This body represents the governments of the member states. Its meetings are held in Brussels, and set the agenda for EU policies, while the *Council of Ministers* meets in

Brussels and Luxembourg. The Council is chaired by the representative of the country holding the presidency of the EU at that time. The presidency is held for a period of six months (Portugal held it for the latter half of 2007).

More commonly termed the Council of Ministers, the Council formulates the EU political objectives, and attempts to achieve coordination of the respective national policies and facilitate integration into the EU's overarching objectives. Decisions are made by a system of unanimous or Qualified Majority Voting (QMV).

The European Parliament

This is democratically elected by the citizens of the member states, who elect their Members of the European Parliament (MEPs) to sit in Strasbourg (732 of them: the UK is entitled to 78). The MEPs serve for five years. The prime goal is to protect European citizens' interests, and hence it meticulously inspects the activities of both the Commission and the Council. But the precise democratic process contrasts with the British 'Westminster' model (see Chapter 6), in that the EU possesses minimal authority for the passing of laws; it also lacks substantial control over finances or the leverage to raise monies. Attempts to extend its legislative powers have usually been neutered by the member states. The Parliament is able to make decisions germane to social policy, on spending, liaising with the European Council in such fields as education and social programmes, and on exceptional occasions to reject the Budget *per se*.

The European Court of Justice

This sits in Luxembourg and is responsible for ensuring that the EU bodies respect fundamental rights; it possesses the jurisdiction to give rulings on matters relating to freedom, security and justice.

The European Court of Auditors

The Court controls and manages the EU budget, and sits in Luxembourg. It is empowered to bring actions before the Court of Justice, and its powers also extend to all who receive Union funds.

In addition, backing up the above are five other important bodies:

- Of direct relevance for social policy, the *European Economic and Social Committee (ESC)* represents the opinions of organised civil society on economic and social matters: it comprises representatives of workers' interest groups, employers and consumers' and environmental interest groups (known as the 'social partners'). Its key task is to deliberate upon new legislation and mediate between the assorted interest groups.

- The *Committee of the Regions* represents the positions of regional and local authorities; the *European Central Bank* deals with monetary policy and the management of the euro; the *European Ombudsman* handles citizens' complaints regarding maladministration by any EU institution or body; and the *European Investment Bank* is responsible for the financing of investment projects.

From the limited beginnings of a European Economic Community, then, the European Union is now the world's most cohesive economic and political international organisation, embracing 27 member states (Figure 22.1). And while the policies between the different member states have varied, ranging from totally pro-Europe to very hostile, the structure as described has remained very stable (Pinder, 2001: Ch. 2; European Commission, 2003). The next section looks at how the European Union approaches social policy, how it is gradually adopting 'corporate' policies, and what paramount issues have arisen.

European Union social policy

The European Union arguably boasts the most developed social policy of the sub-global institutions. Nevertheless, the interpretation of social policy has remained traditionally rather restrictive and the extent of European intervention in areas of social policy is invariably a controversial subject. Matters of social policy in the EU relating to employment and labour relations first took shape under the Maastricht Treaty. The earlier Treaty of Rome, preoccupied with economics and trade, had made no mention of a social policy.

European social policy focuses mostly upon:

- improvement of the working environment to protect workers' health and safety;
- working conditions;
- information and consultation of workers;
- equality between men and women at work;
- integration of people excluded from the labour market.

Although the structure of employment services varies from one member country to another according to the particular social and political culture (see Chapter 16 for an examination of Britain's labour markets and state strategies), one might only speculate as to the reams of EU documentation and codification accrued in the task of harmonising their policies, given their salience to the EU's single market, and thus preventing a deterioration of the higher standards experienced by employers in the more socially conscious welfare states. Despite this leaning towards labour policy, Threlfall (2002) articulates the gradual shifts that the EU has made towards a more inclusive social welfare policy.

In 1989, Jacques Delors encouraged a set of guiding social principles through the '*Community Charter of Fundamental Social Rights of Workers*' (the Social Charter) providing rights to social protection for people lacking the means of subsistence, people of retirement age and disabled persons, though a predominant issue was that the Mediterranean newcomers, generally poorer than the initial member states and thereby incurring lower labour costs, could gain unfair advantage over the latter states.

The Maastricht Treaty of 1991 proved pivotal in promoting the idea of a European social policy, in spite of barriers erected in the way of the policy-makers by the United Kingdom government. The new EU treaty implied the aims of a common approach to social policy arenas such as education and youth policy and public health. Further, the Maastricht agreements reaffirmed European citizenship rights. In the long run this led to the EU dealing with a host of social policy topics like housing and social security support for migrants, widening choices for university students, and access to health care.

The Treaty of Amsterdam 1997 also turned out to be iconic for the generic status of social policy in the Union: European citizenship rights were enhanced with its clarification that anybody, not simply workers, holds the right to reside in any country. Gender equality became a cardinal goal (European Commission, 1999).

In 2000, directives for addressing discrimination were advanced – first on racism (equal treatment regarding employment, irrespective of racial or ethnic origin) and second, for combating discrimination in employment on the basis of disability, belief, age or sexual orientation (Threlfall, 2002).

Generally, EU law and directives on social policy present a highly uneven picture. Yet actions and concerns about welfare do go beyond the technical legalities. For example, a long-standing concern has been the situations of poverty and special exclusion. Again, the European Commission pushed the Council to accept major objectives towards more secure income levels, social integration, sustainable pensions, and high quality sustainable health care.

The Charter of Fundamental Rights for social policies was not, on the one hand, actionable in law. But its principles act as a benchmark in countering poor social practices among member states. It is obvious that the EU acts as a sort of welfare state. Through the Open Method of Coordination (OMC), a whole set of structural dialogues on social exclusion, pensions and health care take place between the various nations and between them and the Commission: a more nuanced mode of joined-up social policy-making (Deacon, 2007).

With respect to some other specific social policy areas, the following are of interest.

Education and training

While the convergence of policies in this area has been notably absent (for instance, Germany's structured corporatist approach to training differs from that of the UK's pragmatism), substantial EU cooperation transpires in the design and delivery of vocational training systems (Hantrais, 2007).

Family policy

Family policy now has a much higher profile in the EU's social policy framework. The European Commission ('The social situation in the European Union', 2006, cited in Hantrais, 2007: 122), alerted to the widespread fall in fertility rates, produced a report on Europe's demographic trends, and called for greater support for families in the arena of caring. *The Charter of Fundamental Rights* now includes articles on 'rights of the child' and 'respect for private and family life'. Nevertheless, the national policy shifts in Europe have represented responses to family restructurings, rather than intrinsic acts of change. Unfortunately, the EU is reluctant to unify or harmonise discrete national family policies, so that member countries are still able to discriminate on grounds of sexual orientation (Hantrais, 2007).

Policy for older and disabled people

Given the trends in population decline, greater demographic ageing, and worrying imbalances between the generations, the EU social policy profile has matured. However, a sizable problem of coordination is the very unevenness of trends and impacts from one member state to another (see Chapter 13 for a discussion of trends in the British state).

An illustration of these disparities is that in the early part of the current decade, Austria, Germany, Greece and Italy were most affected by the situation of simultaneous population fall and ageing. The poorer Central and Eastern European economies were more disturbed by the population decline than by the ageing, due to their lower longevity (Hantrais, 2007).

Stop and Think

Why do you think social policy has been slow to develop in the Europenan Union?

It is a fact that European national variations in retirement age are minimal. But social tensions have arisen among the generations. Hence, EU documents now frequently concentrate on concerns with generational solidarity and the adequacy of pension levels in member states (see Chapter 17 and also the European Commission Report 'Adequate and sustainable pensions' cited in Hantrais, 2007: 178), albeit by dint of heightening awareness through reportage, continuous interaction, and sharpening the focus on practices such as abuse of elders.

To summarise, although the development of an EU social policy has been halting and unbalanced, visible progress has occurred in the setting of standards and principles that member states are expected to achieve. In the final section, the chapter surveys more recent trends in the EU's burgeoning membership and the crises over the formal constitution, each of which has a direct bearing upon decision-making on social policy issues and upon the future of European social policy *per se*.

Union enlargement, death of a constitution and the new EU reform treaty

As we have noted, in the relatively short history of the Union, the EU has grown from the original six members to one of 27 in the early twenty-first century (see Box 22.3). By the turn of the current century it was obvious that both the pace and scale of the EU's enlargement required institutional change and reform (Laursen, 2001). British MEP Andrew Duff, a specialist on the European Constitution, catalogues an

To what extent do you think global social organisations threaten national sovereignty? In illustrating your answer to this question, select the European Union and one other global social policy institution, and discuss its impact upon Britain in any one social policy area from the following:

- employment policy

- family policy

- education and training

- health policy

- policy for older and disabled people

- povery and social inclusion.

array of setbacks to the European Union's constitution, not least from the French and Dutch referenda's rejection of it, and argues for a whole renegotiation of the Constitution, with a set of reforms of a practical bent, to ensure its success, adding:

> The sudden prospect of having to renegotiate the Constitution in order to get it through the sceptical barrier of public opinion will appal many EU insiders. (Duff, 2005: 195)

Again, with a pro-European rallying call dramatically echoing the introduction to Marx and Engels' *1848 Communist Manifesto,* sociologists Ulrich Beck and Anthony Giddens (currently a Labour peer in the British House of Lords) proclaimed in an 'Open letter on the future of Europe' distributed to newspapers across Europe in June 2005:

> The proposed European Constitution is dead. The people of France and the Netherlands have spoken. (Giddens, 2007: 231)

Following a period when the future of the Union itself may have appeared to many in doubt, an EU Reform Treaty was eventually agreed in Lisbon in October 2007, another milestone treaty to reform the much enlarged 27-member bloc. The following section discusses the new treaty in finer detail.

Is a 27-member EU just too cumbersome to work efficiently and equitably?

The Lisbon EU reform treaty

This treaty was designed to replace the European Constitution rejected by the French and Dutch referenda in 2005. The Treaty will come into force in 2009, but was ratified in December 2007. A major aim was to speed up decision-making in the notably enlarged EU. What precisely does the treaty do? The agreed points are also of relevance to the social policy agenda. In the first place, the Lisbon Treaty amends, rather than replaces, the earlier treaties, after six years of prolonged inter-governmental tensions within the European Union, makes decision-making more effective for a 27-strong Union, and focuses more on effects of globalisation and international economic competition for the bloc as a whole than hitherto.

Second, it offers national parliaments an unprecedented involvement in the making of European laws. Parliaments may judge whether EU proposals conform to the principles of 'subsidiarity' (that the EU should only act where it adds value). Third, it institutes a new system of majority voting for national ministers in the Council, so that new legislation requires support of ministers representing at least 65% of the EU's population (this will be to the advantage of the UK). Fourth, the rules of 'enhanced cooperation' now make it easier for EU states to work closer together without implicating countries who prefer not to participate. Fifth, the Charter of Fundamental Rights is finally incorporated into EU law, and gathers together the rights already possessed by EU citizens, applicable to all member states. It is perhaps the Union's growing recognition of its situation globally that represents the keenest set of social policy issues for the future.

Globalisation and the Lisbon Treaty

The Lisbon Treaty expresses the disquiet with the wider developments of globalisation beyond the EU's boundaries, given that the carefully protected economic and political barriers through internal negotiations over the past decades have come under growing pressure from the generally easier movements of work and trade across borders in the first decade of the new millennium. Thus, the treaty beckons the European Union to look outwards.

The Commission President Jose Manuel Barroso in January 2006 expressed the EU's aims for becoming more globally proactive:

> Our ambition is clear. We are aiming for top-class universities, highly trained and educated workforces, strong social security and pensions systems, the most competitive industries and the cleanest environment. To those who say that it cannot be done I say, a decade or so ago who would have thought that Ireland would have become one of the most prosperous countries of the European Union? ... (Barroso, 2006)

And where does the British government stand on the Lisbon Treaty?

Britain and the new reform treaty

Britain played a leading role in the Lisbon meeting, intent on preserving its national rights of sovereignty. The new British Prime Minister Gordon Brown was acutely aware of the growing antagonisms towards the European constitution in the light of his repeated refusal to hold a referendum on the new treaty. The calls for a referendum continued after Lisbon, accompanied by campaigns from the right-wing *UK Independence Party* and the *Democracy Movement* for total withdrawal from the EU.

Such criticisms of the treaty included the ostensible loss of sovereignty, assuming that the EU will have obtained all the powers to complete a final European and political union. In a debate on BBC News on 24 July 2007 (reported in Centre for European Reform, 2007), Ruth Lea, Director of the 'Global Vision' think-tank and former Policy Director of the Institute of Directors, described the Reform Treaty as 'unique in leaving no more significant powers in the hands of the governments of member states'. On the pro-European side of the debate, Charles Grant, Director of the Centre for European Reform, argued that 'the Treaty provides the chance for the Union to deal with bigger global issues, and Britain needs the co-operation with others for tackling such'.

However, unsurprisingly, the 'Eurosceptic' mass media were unconvinced with the finalising of the agreement in Lisbon: 'The PM transformed the lavish banquet into a sordid Last Supper for Britain as an independent sovereign state.' (*The Sun*); 'The European reform treaty to be argued by Gordon Brown and fellow EU leaders in Lisbon today marks a profound shift from free market reform.' (*The Daily Telegraph*).

Conclusions

In this chapter you have been introduced to:

- the pertinence of the international dimension in studying social policy;
- the developments of globalisation and their influences upon national policy-making;
- analysis of the new global social policy structures, governance and institutions, and their impacts upon national social policies;
- the operations of the European Union, a leading sub-global regional institution, its genesis, structures and the major economic and political issues;
- the origins and key features of the European Union's social policy.

From our consideration of these topics, we may arrive at a set of conclusions. With the transformed economic climate in capitalist economies, national state strategies invariably converge because of intensifying global processes and enhanced power of global institutions, and in conjunction with the capitalist world's most powerful national states, driven by neo-liberal ideology. These economic trends directly affect welfare states' social policies. Furthermore, key global social policy actors are also tied to the neo-liberal demands of corporate capital. In turn, their activities narrow the options of national policy-makers through budgetary restrictions. Yet it is less certain that national sovereignty is substantially quashed. Global governance is notoriously difficult to achieve, and the relatively new anti-globalisation movement has already made its presence felt in opposing Washington's dominance. On the other hand, the European Union has demonstrated the potentialities of cooperation between nations for facilitating national and regional economic growth. The development of its overall social policy is less dramatic, given the frequent reluctance of the stronger national states to share their wealth and social advantages. Nevertheless, standards of social provision and social protection have increased and citizen rights have expanded. Debate over the future of European Union social policy will undoubtedly revolve around its current substantial enlargement and, ironically, the problems of competing in the wider global economy.

Annotated further reading

International social policy has become a fertile area of study over the past decade and even more so the topic of globalisation, the published output of which has proliferated alarmingly. An excellent text making the connection between human welfare and global theories is George and Wilding, *Globalization and Human Welfare* (2002). Bob Deacon's *Global Social Policy and Governance* (2007) is essential reading for gaining an overview of the prime global institutions and their impacts upon social policy. The journal *Global Social Policy* is a good source of contemporary data and commentary. Sykes *et al.* (eds), *Globalization and European Welfare States: Challenges and Change* (2001b) offers a useful set of contributions on the rapid shifts in the international social policy agenda. For a technical understanding of how the European Union operates the latest edition of Neil Nugent's *The Government and Politics of the European Union* (2006) is a most comprehensive text. In addition, the European Commission's Europa website (europa.eu) offers up-to-date information; the Commission's publications are also helpful. The third edition of Linda Hantrais' *Social Policy in the European Union* (2007) is a key text for keeping abreast of new developments in the field; the *Journal of European Social Policy* should also be consulted regularly.

Concluding comment to Part IV

The election of the first Labour government in almost 20 years in 1997 arguably saw a shift in emphasis in social policy in the UK. The party that had initially brought the welfare state into being has, under the Blair and Brown-led Labour administrations, revisited many of its first principles with a view to *modernising* the welfare state in line with twenty-first century aspirations and realities. In 1997 New Labour inherited a welfare state very different from that of the last time their party held the reins of power. Since their return to power, New Labour's decade of government has seemingly transpired both to consolidate aspects of the Conservatives' approach – consumerism, welfare markets, private sector provision – and to promote a new approach which has emphasised the importance of public sector investment and provision. As such, one can argue that we have seen the emergence of a new British welfare consensus, even a 'new Beveridge'.

A new Beveridge?

We use the term 'a new Beveridge' not so much in the sense that it became known in post-war Britain, as emblematic of a state-led, run and funded welfare system providing, in theoretical and rhetorical terms, cradle to grave provision, but as a return to welfare principles. The Labour Party in opposition in the late 1980s and early 1990s had made much of a return to principles of responsibility and social solidarity. Labour presented this as the antidote to what they perceived as the selfish individualism of the 1980s. Indeed, New Labour's mantra in the 1990s was 'the rights we enjoy reflect the duties we owe'. In redefining itself, 'New' Labour sought to gain, electorally, the ground occupied by the voters of 'middle England' and to shed its image as the party solely of the working class. Instead, New Labour adopted a 'one nation' approach to both politics and social policy.

The social principles New Labour espoused owe much to the works of communitarian thinkers (for example Etzioni and Hutton) and stress in particular the idea of duties incumbent upon anyone seeking to claim 'rights' in modern society – conditional citizenship. We have therefore seen in New Labour's social policy an emphasis on responsibilities as well as rights. For example, a citizen's duty to find and keep a job in return for a right to claim welfare benefits has formed the cornerstone of Labour's social policy and in many ways has sought to re-establish a link set at the heart of the Beveridge solution. The connection of Beveridge's welfare principles to the economic principles espoused by Keynes, in particular the maintenance of full employment as a counterpoint to the provisions of a welfare state, has much resonance with the rhetoric of New Labour. New Labour has, however, updated this principle. Rather than Beveridge's outdated and discredited idea of full male employment, New Labour's social policy is predicated on a notion of full employment opportunity. For New Labour everyone has the opportunity to work and is therefore expected to engage in paid employment. New Labour has extended this principle to the young unemployed, the long-term unemployed, lone parents and the disabled. Alongside the opportunity and duty to work, the government has introduced the National Minimum Wage. Under New Labour, benefits dependency is no longer an option. Indeed, the resurrection of the Poor Law principle of less eligibility is in part a signal that reliance on the welfare state is no longer the easy option.

But New Labour's back to basics message has not been confined to employment policy. Initiatives across a range of policy areas have attempted to promote values of community, responsibility and social solidarity. In education, New Labour – as part of its 'Education, Education, Education' agenda – has pursued its emphasis on literacy and numeracy. In addition, it has promoted the development and uptake of pre-school nursery and child care provision as well as wrap-around child care for school children, sometimes as part of its extended schools initiative. Parental duties have been further rein-forced by making parents take greater responsibility for the general behaviour and even the criminal activities of their children with the introduction of ASBOs and other requirements under the Crime and Disorder Act.

Health too has come centre stage under New Labour. Labour was elected in 1997 under a slogan of '24 hours to save the NHS'. Since 1997, and particularly in its second and third terms, we have wit-nessed significant increases to the funding of the NHS such that it now compares favourably with the levels of funding amongst other EU countries. However, alongside this investment has been significant restructuring of the NHS, a reinforcement of health quasi-markets, an encouragement of private and voluntary sector providers, and an emphasis on 'targets'. Even so, what is arguably different about Labour has been its emphasis on combating health inequalities and more interventionist state involvement, for example with the smoking ban in public places eventually implemented in all four countries in the UK. Other public health initiatives have included those on healthy eating and exercise, alongside an emphasis more generally on primary health care services. Indeed, behaviour in general was identified as a legitimate concern of government social policy, exemplified under New Labour by the activities of the Social Exclusion Unit to reduce the numbers of people sleeping rough and proposals to reduce the high rate of teenage pregnancy.

Whereas the Conservatives had emphasised individualism, compe-tition and the market, New Labour has championed 'partnership' whereby 'joined-up problems' require 'joined-up solutions'. 'Joined-up government' was to be the answer to the inability of different welfare services to be able to work together effectively, with indi-vidual citizens often on the receiving end of disjointed and unresponsive provision. This drive for coherent welfare delivery has led to the establishment of multi-professional and multi-disciplinary Children's Services and Adult Services departments in local authorities.

Perhaps, however, the underlying principle upon which much of New Labour's social policy is founded is that of social inclusion. The rise of the 'underclass' debate in British social policy in the decade before Labour's election victory struck a chord with senior politicians. In particular the work of Charles Murray had stressed the lack of attachment to more widely accepted social norms and values as vital to the identification of an underclass – values such as the work ethic and values of family and community support. These ideas found resonance in the writing of the Labour MP Frank Field, briefly Minister for Welfare Reform, and the commentator Will Hutton who outlined a scenario of a 30:30:40 society where there was an increasing level of detachment for large numbers of Britain's population. It is with such issues firmly in mind that New Labour insisted that the job of a modern welfare state should be to 'provide a hand up, not a hand out'. In other words the task of welfare policy into the twenty-first century is to help people to help themselves – to create the economic climate for job creation and prosperity – wherein people are both able and duty bound to work. As we have seen, New Labour's solution to social exclusion, inequality and poverty is education and work.

A new welfare consensus?

Aspects of the rhetoric of New Labour echo some of the themes of the New Right Conservatives: individualism, choice, personal responsibility, the effectiveness of the market and quasi-markets. However, New Labour has arguably also shifted the consensus (back) to a belief in the place of the state in the provision of welfare: state involvement in tackling welfare problems and providing welfare services based on a notion of collective duty and the necessity of public goods.

Although Labour was quick to distance itself from the operation of the internal market in the National Health Service, it replaced it with commissioning and an even more hands-on involvement in the running of the NHS. In housing, Labour has continued with the promotion of home ownership as the preferred form of housing tenure and continued to residualise the role of local authorities in the provision of housing. In education, not only have we seen an emphasis on literacy and numeracy, we have also seen a continuation of testing, league tables and inspection. In addition, Labour has pursued the promotion of City Academies as a solution to 'failing' schools. In higher education, Labour has gone further than the Conservatives as far as student tuition fees are concerned, introducing top-up fees of £3,000 in 2006. This was deemed necessary in order to help pay for New Labour's desired expansion of higher education to one where 50 per cent of eighteen-year-olds would go on to higher education. Labour has espoused a future based on a 'knowledge-based economy', whereby success for individuals and the UK would be based on a highly educated and highly skilled workforce. New Labour has seen its role as being to create the economic conditions for that success – by establishing and sustaining a low-interest, high-productivity, low-cost economy. (As we have seen, this emphasis on economic growth is questioned by environmentalists.) It would appear that Labour has managed to adopt a new economic orthodoxy and to rid itself of some of its own economic and welfare sacred cows.

There are two aspects of New Labour's social policy which are particularly distinct from the previous Conservative administration: constitutional reform and civil liberties. New Labour has implemented significant constitutional reform that signals both looser political ties at home and closer ties to a more powerful European Union. The creation of a devolved Scottish Parliament and Welsh Assembly and the re-establishment of political power at Stormont in Northern Ireland have arguably precipitated radical differences in social policy within the four countries of the UK. In contrast, the policies implemented via the EU continue to influence the development of UK social policy, arguably promoting a convergence of the UK's social policy with that of other EU countries. One significant area of influence of the EU during New Labour's rule has been in civil liberties. New Labour has implemented significant equal opportunities legislation, in part precipitated by the European Equality Directive and the Racial Equality Directive, including in relation to 'race' and ethnicity, gender, disability, sexual orientation and age. This agenda is in stark contrast to the policies of the Conservatives, the apotheosis of which was probably Section 28 of the 1988 Local Government Act. All of this would suggest that there are significant differences between New Labour and the New Right but also significant continuities. Thus we are arguably witnessing the building of a new welfare consensus around a renewed belief in proactive state involvement and the promotion of and investment in public services to tackle issues of social welfare.

Future directions

We would suggest that the tendencies outlined above are set to continue, probably irrespective of which political party finds itself in government following Gordon Brown's first term of office. Government's role in the provision and funding of welfare has, over the last decade, seen significant investment and general renewal. At the same time, an increased emphasis on the individual – via the discourse of choice, personalisation and responsibility – in welfare provision is set to continue. The welfare state, as it developed in the years following the end of the Second World War, is no more (it probably never was). The role of government continues to develop as both regulator and monitor of social policy – a regulator both of the vast range of welfare providers within the different quasi-markets that have formed and also of the behaviour of individuals as citizens and welfare recipients. How well government is able to respond to such a vast and widespread regulatory task will continue to be the subject of discussion in social policy texts and wider circles, as will the on-going assessment of where the welfare consensus lies in the future.

References

Ackers, L. and Abbott, P. (1996) *Social Policy for Nurses and the Caring Professions*. Buckingham: Open University Press.

Adams, C. (2006) 'Blair warned on effects of "biting" health reforms'. *Financial Times*, 13 April.

Adams, J. and Schmuecker, K. (2006) 'Divergence in priorities, perceived policy failure and pressure for convergence', in Adams, J. and Schmuecker, K. (eds), *Devolution in Practice 2006: Public Policy Differences within the UK*. Newcastle-upon-Tyne: IPPR North.

Addison, P. (1975) *The Road to 1945*. London: Quartet.

Addison, P. (1992) *Churchill on the Home Front*. London: Jonathan Cape.

Alcock, P. (1997) 'The discipline of social policy', in Alcock, P., Erskine, A. and May, M. (eds), *The Student's Companion to Social Policy*. Oxford: Blackwell.

Alcock, P., Erskine, A. and May, M. (eds) (1997) *The Student's Companion to Social Policy*. Oxford: Blackwell.

Alford, R.R. (1975) *Health Care Politics*. Chicago: University of Chicago Press.

Allardt, E. (1986) 'The civic conception of the welfare state in Scandinavia', in Rose, R. and Shiratori, R. (eds), *The Welfare State East and West*. New York: Oxford University Press.

Allsop, J. and Baggott, R. (2004) 'The NHS in England: from modernisation to marketisation?', in Ellison, N., Bauld, L. and Powell, M. (eds), *Social Policy Review 16*. Bristol: Policy Press.

Anderson, M. (1980) *Approaches to the History of the Western Family 1500–1914*. Basingstoke: Macmillan.

Andrews, M. (2003) 'Punishment, markets and the American model: an essay on a new American dilemma', in McConville, S. (ed.), *The Use of Punishment*. Cullompton, Devon: Willan Publishing.

Annesley, C. (2003) 'Americanised and Europeanised: UK social policy since 1997'. *British Journal of Politics and International Relations* 5(2): 143–165.

Anthias, F. (1998) 'Rethinking social divisions: some notes towards a theoretical framework'. *Sociological Review* 46(3): 505–535.

Anthias, F. (2001) 'The concept of "social division" and theorising social stratification: looking at ethnicity and class'. *Sociology* 35(4): 835–854.

Archer, L., Hutchings, M. and Ross, A. (2003) *Higher Education and Social Class: Issues of Exclusion and Inclusion*. London: Routledge.

Armstrong, H. (1997) 'Five sides to a new leaf'. *Municipal Journal*, 4 July, pp. 18–19.

Atkinson, A.B. and Micklewright, J. (1989) 'Turning the screw: benefits for the unemployed, 1979–1988', in Atkinson, A.B. (ed.), *Poverty and Social Security*. Hemel Hempstead: Harvester Wheatsheaf.

Atkinson, R. (2007) 'Everyone in Jodee Mundy's family is deaf – except for her'. *The Guardian*, 29 December.

Audit Commission (1986) *Making a Reality of Community Care*. London: HMSO.

Audit Commission (1998) *A Fruitful Partnership. Effective Partnership Working*. London: Audit Commission.

Bacon, R. and Eltis, W. (1978) *Britain's Economic Problem: Too Few Producers* (2nd edn). London: Macmillan.

Bacon, R. and Eltis, W. (1996) *Britain's Economic Problem Revisited*. Basingstoke: Macmillan.

Bagehout, W. (2001) *The English Constitution*. Oxford: Oxford Paperbacks / Oxford World's Classics.

Baggott, R. (2004) *Health and Health Care in Britain* (3rd edn). Basingstoke: Palgrave.

Bailey, N. (2006) 'Does work pay? Employment, poverty and exclusion from social relations', in Pantazis, C., Gordon, D. and Levitas, R. (eds), *Poverty and Social Exclusion in Britain: The Millennium Survey*. Bristol: Policy Press.

Baker, M. (2005) 'Which is the fairest path of all?' *Times Educational Supplement*, 21 October.

Baldwin, J. and McConville, M. (1977) *Negotiated Justice*. London: Martin Robertson.

Ball, S. (2003) *Class Strategies in the Education Market: The Middle Classes and Social Advantage*. London: RoutledgeFalmer.

Ball, S. (2007) 'Going further? Tony Blair and New Labour education policies', in Clarke, K., Maltby, T. and Kennett, P. (eds), *Social Policy Review 19*. Bristol: Policy Press.

Barker, A. (2007) 'Hain changes welfare-to-work tone'. *Financial Times*, 13 September.

Barker, K. (2004) *Review of Housing Supply: Final Report*. London: H.M. Treasury.

Barker, P. (ed.) (1984) *Founders of the Welfare State*. London: Heinemann.

Barker, R. (1997) *Political Ideas in Modern Britain*. London: Routledge.

Barnardo's (2006) 'Failed by the system – Barnardo's reveals what you really need to know about the 2006 GCSE results'. Press release, 23 August.

Barnes, C. (1990) *Disabled People in Britain and Discrimination: A Case for Anti-discriminatory Legislation*. London: Hurst.

Barnes, M. (1999) 'Researching public participation'. *Local Government Studies* **25**(4): 60–75.

Barnett, J. (1982) *Inside the Treasury*. London: André Deutsch.

Barr, N. (2004) *The Economics of the Welfare State*. Oxford: Oxford University Press.

Barr, N. (2006) 'Turner gets it right on pensions'. *Prospect*, January, pp. 48–50.

Barroso, J. (2006) 'Globalisation: voices from the debate'. Foreign and Commonwealth Office, fco.gov.uk, January.

Barry, B. (2001) 'The muddles of multiculturalism'. *New Left Review* (8): 49–71.

Batty, D. (2001) 'Timeline for the Climbié case'. *The Guardian*, 24 September.

Bauld, L., Judge, K., Barnes, M., Benzeval, M., Mackenzie, M. and Sullivan, H. (2005) 'Promoting social change: the experience of Health Action Zones in England'. *Journal of Social Policy* **34**(3): 427–445.

Baxter, J. and Wright, E.O. (2000) 'The glass ceiling hypothesis: a comparative study of the United States, Sweden and Australia'. *Gender and Society* **14**(2): 275–294.

Bayley, D. (2005) 'What do the police do?', in Newburn, T. (ed.), *Policing: Key Readings*. Cullompton, Devon: Willan Publishing.

BBC, *Inside Out* (7/3/2005) http://www.bbc.co.uk/london/insideldn/insideout/index.shtml, accessed 24 May 2007.

BBC News (19/11/2002) www.bbc.co.uk/1/hi/world/americas/2488829.stm, accessed 10 June 2005.

BBC News (11/11/2005) 'Girl, 15, hurt in school stabbing'. http://news.bbc.co.uk/1/hi/england/southern_counties/4426594.stm

BBC News (11/9/2006) 'Double jeopardy man admits guilt'. http://news.bbc.co.uk/1/hi/england/5144722.stm

BBC News (27/11/2007) 'Crisis warning over house prices'. http://news.bbc.co.uk/1/hi/england/london/7114397.stm

Beccaria, C. (1764) 'On crimes and punishment and other writings', in Bellamy, R. (ed.) (1995) *A Short Selection of Beccaria's Original Writings*. Cambridge: Cambridge University Press.

Becker, H. (1963) *Outsiders*. New York: Free Press.

Becker, S. and Bryman, A. (2004) *Understanding Research for Social Policy and Practice: Themes, Methods and Approaches*. Bristol: Policy Press.

Bell, D. (1996) *The Cultural Contradictions of Capitalism*. New York: Basic Books.

Bellamy, R. (1992) *Liberalism and Modern Society*. Cambridge: Polity.

Berger, P. (1963) *Invitation to Sociology*. New York: Anchor Books.

Berlin, I. (1969) *Four Essays on Liberty*. Oxford: Oxford University Press.

Berthoud, R., Lakey, J. and McKay, S. (1993) *The Economic Problems of Disabled People*. London: Policy Studies Institute.

Beveridge, W. (1942) *Social Insurance and Allied Services* (Cmd 6404). London: HMSO.

Blackstone, T., Parekh, B. and Sanders, P. (eds) (1998) *Race Relations in Britain: A Developing Agenda*. London: Routledge.

Blair, T. (1993) 'Why crime is a socialist issue'. *New Statesman*, 29 January, pp. 27–28.

Blair, T. (1998) *The Third Way: New Politics for a New Century*. Fabian Society Pamphlet no. 558, London: The Fabian Society.

Blair, T. (1999) 'Full speech to Labour Party Conference'. *The Guardian*, 28 September.

Blair, T. (2004) 'What we have achieved means we fight on territory laid out by us'. *The Guardian*, 24 June.

Blake, A. (1985) *The Conservative Party from Peel to Thatcher*. London: Fontana.

Blakemore, K. and Drake, R. (1996) *Understanding Equal Opportunities Policies*. Hemel Hempstead: Prentice Hall.

Blank, R.H. and Burau, V. (2004) *Comparative Health Policy*. Basingstoke: Palgrave.

Blitz, J. (2006) 'Pragmatic pair pull a bumpy and bloody deal out of the den'. *Financial Times*, 26 May.

Boone, J. (2005) 'Still a twist or two left in Twizzler controversy'. *Financial Times*, 12 March.

Boone, J. (2007) 'Private school tax breaks at risk'. *Financial Times*, 7 March.

Booth, C. (1892) *Life and Labour of the People in London*, Vol. I. London: Macmillan.

Booth, C. (2005) 'Future perfect'. *The Guardian*, 17 December.

Booth, R. (2007) 'ITN man once interviewed the influential, now he sleeps rough'. *The Guardian*, 15 December.

Borchardt, K.-D. (1995) *European Integration: The Origins and Growth of the European Union* (4th edn). Luxembourg: European Commission.

Borchorst, A. and Siim, B. (1987) 'Women and the advanced welfare state – a new kind of patriarchal power?' in Showstack Sassoon, A. (ed.), *Women and the State: The Shifting Boundaries of Public and Private*. London: Hutchinson.

Boyson, R. (1971) *Down with the Poor*. London: Churchill Press.

Braithwaite, J. (1989) *Crime, Shame and Reintegration*. Oxford: Oxford University Press.

Bramley, G. (1994) 'An affordability crisis in British housing: dimensions, causes and policy impact'. *Housing Studies*, **9**(1): 103–124.

Branigan, T. (2007) 'We must have a soul, new leader tells party. Speech combines rhetoric on values with first glimpses of policy detail'. *The Guardian*, 25 June.

Braye, S. (2000) 'Participation and involvement in social care: an overview', in Kemschall, H. and Littlechild, R. (eds), *User Involvement and Participation in Social Care*. London: Jessica Kingsley Publishers.

Breakthrough (2007) *Response to Office for Disability Issues Consultation – Equality for Disabled People*. Manchester: Breakthrough Ltd.

Briggs, A. (1961) 'The welfare state in historical perspective'. *European Journal of Sociology* **2**(2): 221–258.

Briggs, A. (1983) *A Social History of England*. London: Weidenfeld & Nicolson.

Brighouse, H. (2004) *Justice*. Cambridge: Polity.

Brinkley, I., Coats, D. and Overell, S. (2007) *7 out of 10: Labour under Labour 1997–2007*. London: Work Foundation.

Brittan, S. (1975) 'The economic contradictions of democracy'. *British Journal of Political Science* **5**(2): 129–159.

Brittan, S. (1976) 'The economic contradictions of democracy', in King, A. (ed.), *Why is Britain Becoming Harder to Govern?* London: BBC.

Brittan, S. (1989) 'The Thatcher government's economic policy', in Kavanagh, D. and Seldon, A. (eds), *The Thatcher Effect: A Decade of Change*. Oxford: Oxford University Press.

Brody, S.R. and Tarling, R. (1980) *Taking Offenders Out of Circulation*. Home Office Research Study no. 64. London: HMSO.

Brown, G. (2003) 'State and market: towards a public interest test'. *Political Quarterly* **74**(3): 266–284.

Brundtland Commission (1987) *Our Common Future*. Oxford: Oxford University Press.

Bryman, A. (2008) *Social Research Methods* (3rd edn). Oxford: Oxford University Press.

Bryson, A. (2003) 'From welfare to workfare', in Millar, J. (ed.), *Understanding Social Security: Issues for Policy and Practice*. Bristol: Policy Press.

Buiter, W.H. (2006) 'Minimum wage does not correct a distortion: It is a distortion'. *Financial Times*, 28 March: letter.

Bullock, A. (1967) *The Life and Times of Ernest Bevin*. London: Heinemann.

Bulmer, M. and Rees, A.M. (eds) (1996) *Citizenship Today: The Contemporary Relevance of T.H. Marshall*. London: UCL Press.

Burgess, R. (1984) *In the Field*. London: Allen and Unwin.

Burrows, R. and Loader, B. (1994) *Towards a Post-Fordist Welfare State?*. London: Routledge.

Butcher, T. (1995) *Delivering Welfare: The Governance of the Social Services in the 1990s*. Buckingham: Open University Press.

Butler, D. and Stokes, D. (1974) *Political Change in Britain*. London: Macmillan.

Cabinet Office (1999) White Paper: *Modernising Government* (Cmnd 4310). London: The Stationery Office.

Cahill, M. (1994) *The New Social Policy*. Oxford: Blackwell.

Cahill, M. (2002) *The Environment and Social Policy*. London: Routledge.

Cahill, M. and Fitzpatrick, T. (2002) *Environmental Issues and Social Welfare*. Oxford: Blackwell.

Cahn, E. (2000) *No More Throw-away People: The Co-production Imperative*. Washington, DC: Essential Books.

Carter, J. (ed.) (1998) *Postmodernity and the Fragmentation of Welfare*. London: Routledge.

Carter, N. (1989) 'Performance indicators: "backstreet driving" or "hands off" control?'. *Policy and Politics* **17**(2): 131–138.

Carter, N., Klein, K. and Day, P. (1992) *How Organisations Measure Success: The Use of Performance Indicators in Government*. London: Routledge.

Castles, F.G. (2004) *The Future of the Welfare State: Crisis Myths and Crisis Realities*. Oxford: Oxford University Press.

Cavadino, M. and Dignan, J. (2002) *The Penal System: An Introduction*. London: Sage.

Centre for European Reform (CER) (2007) 'For and against the new EU Treaty'. BBC News, 24 July, www.cer.org.uk/articles/article_bbc_grant_24july2007.html

Chaney, P. and Drakeford, M. (2004) 'The primacy of ideology: social policy and the first term of the National Assembly for Wales', in Ellison, N., Bauld, L. and Powell, M. (eds), *Social Policy Review 16*. Bristol: Policy Press.

Chapman, J. (2007) 'Fury over Cameron plan to silence Scottish MPs'. *Daily Mail*, 29 October.

Chen, S. (2003) 'The Wanless Report: financing future health care needs'. *Political Quarterly* **74**(1): 118–122.

Chitty, C. (1989) *Towards a New Education System: The Victory of the New Right?* London: Routledge.

Chitty, C. (2004) *Education Policy in Britain*. Basingstoke: Palgrave Macmillan.

Churchill, H. (2007) 'Children's services in 2006', in Clarke, K., Maltby, T. and Kennett, P. (eds), *Social Policy Review 19*. Bristol: Policy Press.

Clarke, J. and Newman, J. (1997) *The Managerialist State*. London: Sage.

Clarke, J., Cochrane, A. and Smart, C. (1987) *Ideologies of Welfare: From Dreams to Disillusion*. London: Hutchinson.

Clarke, J., Cochrane, A. and Smart, C. (1992) *Ideologies of Welfare: From Dreams to Disillusion* (new edn). London: Routledge.

Clarke, J., Cochrane, A. and McLaughlin, E. (1994) *Managing Social Policy*. London: Sage.

Clarke, J., Gewirtz, S. and McLaughlin, E. (2000) 'Reinventing the welfare state', in Clarke, J., Gewirtz, S. and McLaughlin, E. (eds), *New Managerialism, New Welfare?* London: Sage.

Clarke, J., Smith, N. and Vidler, E. (2005) 'Consumerism and the reform of public services: inequalities and instabilities', in Powell, M., Bauld, L. and Clarke, K. (eds), *Social Policy Review 17*. Bristol: Policy Press.

Clarke, M. and Stewart, J. (1999) *Community Governance, Community Leadership and the New Local Government*. York: Joseph Rowntree Foundation.

Coats, D. (2007) *The National Minimum Wage. Retrospect and Prospect*. London: Work Foundation.

Cockett, R. (1994) *Thinking the Unthinkable: Think-Tanks and the Economic Counter-Revolution, 1931–1983*. London: HarperCollins.

Cole, I. and Furbey, R. (1994) *The Eclipse of Council Housing*. London: Routledge.

Coleman, C. and Moynihan, J. (2000) *Understanding Crime Data: Haunted by the Dark Figure*. Milton Keynes: Open University Press.

Coleman, C. and Norris, C. (2000) *Introducing Criminology*. Cullompton, Devon: Willan Publishing.

Collinson, P. (2007) 'Hackney predicted to be a winner before the games. House price growth in UK towns and cities'. *The Guardian*, 29 December.

Commission on the NHS (2000) *New Life for Health*. Inquiry chaired by Will Hutton. London: Vintage.

Commission on Social Justice (1993) *The Justice Gap*. London: Viking.

Commission on Social Justice (1994) *Social Justice: Strategies for National Renewal* (Borrie Commission Report). London: Viking.

Commission on Taxation and Citizenship (2000) *Paying for Progress: A New Politics of Tax for Public Spending*. London: Fabian Society.

Conservative Party (1997) *You Can Only Be Sure with the Conservatives: the Conservative Manifesto 1997*. London: Conservative Central Office.

Cox, C. and Boyson, R. (eds) (1975) *Black Paper 1975*. London: The Critical Quarterly Society.

Crace, J. (2007) 'Sats under the microscope – Key stage 2 test results are here again, and they're as controversial as ever'. *The Guardian*, 6 December.

Cressey, P. (1999) 'New Labour and employment, training and employee relations', in Powell, M. (ed.), *New Labour, New Welfare State?* Bristol: Policy Press.

Crosland, A. (1956) *The Future of Socialism*. London: Jonathan Cape.

Crosland, C.A.R. (1964) *The Future of Socialism*. London: Jonathan Cape.

Crosland, S. (1982) *Tony Crosland*. London: Jonathan Cape.

Crossman, R. (1979) *The Crossman Diaries*. London: Hamish Hamilton and Jonathan Cape.

Crouch, C. (2004) *Post-Democracy*. Cambridge: Polity.

Curtis, P. (2007a) 'Test results for third of primary students wrong, says study'. *The Guardian*, 2 November.

Curtis, P. (2007b) 'Cash prize for new tests "could tempt teachers to cheat" '. *The Guardian*, 15 December.

Curtis, P. (2008) 'Councils face £2.8bn bill for equal pay'. *The Guardian*, 2 January.

Dahrendorf, R. (1998) 'The new labour market', in Stevenson, W. (ed.), *Equality and the Modern Economy*. Little Missenden, Bucks: Smith Institute.

Dalley, G. (1999) 'Care, costs and containment: the social policy of long-term care'. *Policy and Politics* 27(4): 533–540.

Daly, G. (2001) 'Citizenship, public accountability and older people: user involvement in community care provision'. *Education and Ageing* 16(1): 55–76.

Daly, G. and Davis, H. (2004) 'From community government to communitarian partnership? Approaches to devolution in Birmingham'. *Local Government Studies* 30(2): 182–195.

Daly, G. and Davis, H. (2008) 'Local government and local governance', in Alcock, P., Erskine, A. and May, M. (eds), *The Student's Companion to Social Policy* (3rd edn). Oxford: Blackwell.

Daly, G., Mooney, G., Poole, L. and Davis, H. (2005) 'Housing stock transfer in Birmingham and Glasgow: the contrasting experiences of two UK cities'. *European Journal of Housing Policy* 5(3): 327–341.

Daly, M. (2000) *The Gender Division of Welfare: The Impact of the British and German Welfare States*. Cambridge: Cambridge University Press.

Daly, M. (2003) 'Governance and social policy'. *Journal of Social Policy* 31(1): 113–128.

Davies, G. and Piachaud, D. (1985) 'Public expenditure on the social services: the economic and political constraints', in Klein, R. and O'Higgins, M. (eds), *The Future of Welfare*. Oxford: Blackwell.

Davies, H. (ed.) (2006) *The Chancellor's Tales: Managing the British Economy*. Cambridge: Polity.

Davies, M., Croall, H. and Tyrer, J. (2005) *Criminal Justice: An Introduction to the Criminal Justice System of England and Wales* (3rd edn). Harlow: Pearson Education.

Davis, E. (1998) *Public Spending*. Harmondsworth: Penguin.

De Swaan, A. (1988) *In Care of the State: Health Care, Education and Welfare in Europe and the USA in the Modern Era*. Cambridge: Polity.

Deacon, A. (1997) Editor's Introduction, in Deacon, A. (ed.), *From Welfare to Work: Lessons from America*. London: Institute of Economic Affairs.

Deacon, B. (2007) *Global Social Policy and Governance*. London: Sage.

Deacon, B., with Stubbs, P. and Hulse, M. (1997) *International Organisations and the Future of Welfare*. London: Sage.

Deakin, N. (1987) *The Politics of Welfare*. London: Methuen.

Deakin, N. (1994) *The Politics of Welfare: Continuities and Change*. Hemel Hempstead: Harvester Wheatsheaf.

Deakin, N. and Parry, R. (2000) *The Treasury and Social Policy: The Contest for Control of Welfare Strategy*. Basingstoke: Macmillan.

Dennis, N. (1993) *Rising Crime and the Dismembered Family*. London: IEA Health and Welfare Unit.

Dennis, N. (1997) *The Invention of Permanent Poverty*. London: IEA Health and Welfare Unit.

Dennis, N. and Erdos, G. (1993) *Families without Fatherhood*. London: IEA Health and Welfare Unit.

Department for Children, Schools and Families (DCSF) (2007) *The Children's Plan: Building Brighter Futures* (Cm 7280). London: The Stationery Office.

Department for Communities and Local Government (DCLG) (2007) Green Paper: *Homes for the Future: More Affordable, More Sustainable*. London: The Stationery Office.

Department for Education and Skills (DfES) (2001a) Green Paper: *Schools: Building on Success*. London: The Stationery Office.

Department for Education and Skills (DfES) (2001b) White Paper: *Schools Achieving Success*. London: The Stationery Office.

Department for Education and Skills (DfES) (2003) Green Paper: *Every Child Matters*. London: The Stationery Office.

Department for Education and Skills (DfES) (2006a) Green Paper: *Care Matters: Transforming the Lives of Children and Young People in Care*. London: The Stationery Office.

Department for Education and Skills (DfES) (2006b) 'Education and Inspections Bill: higher standards, better schools for all'. Press release, 28 February.

Department for Education and Skills (DfES) (2007) *Provision for Children Under Five Years of Age in England*. London: DfES.

Department for Transport, Local Government and the Regions (DTLR) (2001) White Paper: *Strong Local Leadership – Quality Public Services*. London: The Stationery Office.

Department for Work and Pensions (DWP) (2001) *United Kingdom National Action Plan on Social Inclusion 2001–2003*. London: DWP.

Department for Work and Pensions (DWP) (2005) *Five Year Strategy: Opportunity and Security Throughout Life* (Cm 6447). London: The Stationery Office.

Department for Work and Pensions (DWP) (2006a) White Paper: *Security in Retirement: Towards a New Pensions System* (Cm 6841). London: The Stationery Office.

Department for Work and Pensions (DWP) (2006b) White Paper: *Personal Accounts: A New Way to Save* (Cm 6975). London: The Stationery Office.

Department for Work and Pensions (DWP) (2006c) Green Paper: *A New Deal for Welfare: Empowering People to Work* (Cm 6730). London: The Stationery Office.

Department for Work and Pensions (DWP) (2007) Green Paper: *In Work, Better Off: Next Steps to Full Employment* (Cm 7130). London: The Stationery Office.

Department of Education and Science (DES) (1987) *Meeting the Challenge*. London: HMSO.

Department of the Environment, Transport and the Regions (DETR) (2000) Green Paper: *Quality and Choice – A Decent Home for All*. London: DETR.

Department of Health (DH) (1989a) White Paper: *Working for Patients* (Cm 555). London: HMSO.

Department of Health (DH) (1989b) White Paper: *Caring for People: Community Care in the Next Decade and Beyond* (Cm 849). London: HMSO.

Department of Health (DH) (1992) White Paper: *The Health of the Nation: A Strategy for Health in England* (Cm 1986). London: HMSO.

Department of Health (DH) (1997) White Paper: *The New NHS*. London: HMSO.

Department of Health (DH) (1998a) White Paper: *Modernising Social Services: Promoting Independence, Improving Protection, Raising Standards*. London: The Stationery Office.

Department of Health (DH) (1998b) *Modernising Mental Health Services: Safe, Sound and Supportive*. London: The Stationery Office.

Department of Health (DH) (1998c) *The Independent Inquiry into Inequalities in Health* (Acheson Report). London: HMSO.

Department of Health (DH) (2000) *The NHS Plan: A Plan for Investment, A Plan for Reform*. London: The Stationery Office.

Department of Health (DH) (2001) *The Carers and Disabled Children's Act – Policy Guidance*. London: The Stationery Office.

Department of Health (DH) (2002) *Delivering the NHS Plan: Next Steps on Investment, Next Steps on Reform* (Cm 5503). London: The Stationery Office.

Department of Health (DH) (2005) Green Paper: *Independence, Well-being and Choice – Our Vision for the Future of Social Care for Adults in England*. London: The Stationery Office.

Department of Health (DH) (2006) *Our Health, Our Care, Our Say: A New Direction for Community Services – Health and Social Care in Partnership*. London: The Stationery Office.

Department of Health (DH) (2007) *Our NHS, Our Future: NHS Next Stage Review*. Interim report by Professor Lord Darzi. London: Department of Health.

Department of Health/Home Office (1992) *Review of Health and Social Services for Mentally Disordered Offenders and Others Requiring Similar Services* (Cmnd 2088) (Chairman Dr John Reed, CB). London: HMSO.

Department of Health/Home Office (2003) *The Victoria Climbié Inquiry. Report of an Inquiry by Lord Laming* (Cm 5730). London: The Stationery Office.

Department of Health and Social Security (DHSS) (1983) *NHS Management Inquiry* (Griffiths Report). London: DHSS.

Department of Social Security (DSS) (1998) *A New Contract for Welfare: Partnership in Pensions* (Cm 4179). London: The Stationery Office.

Diamond, P. and Giddens, A. (2005) 'The new egalitarianism: economic inequality in the UK', in Giddens, A. and Diamond, P. (eds), *The New Egalitarianism*. Cambridge: Polity.

Disability Rights Commission (DRC) (2007) *Creating an Alternative Future*. London: DRC.

Dixon, A., Le Grand, J., Henderson, J., Murray, R. and Poteliakhoff, A. (2003) *Is the NHS Equitable? A Review of the Evidence*. LSE Health and Social Care Discussion Paper no. 11. London: LSE Health and Social Care.

Dobson, A. (ed.) (1998) *Fairness and Futurity: Essays on Environmental Sustainability and Social Justice*. Oxford: Oxford University Press.

Dobson, A. (2000) *Green Political Thought*. London: Routledge.

Doling, J. (1993) 'British housing policy: 1984–1993'. *Regional Studies*, **27**(6): 583–588.

Doyal, L. (1994) 'Challenging medicine? Gender and the politics of health care', in Gabe, J., Kelleher, D. and Williams, G. (eds), *Challenging Medicine*. London: Routledge.

Drake, R.F. (2001) *The Principles of Social Policy*. New York: Palgrave.

Driver, S. (2005) 'Welfare after Thatcher: New Labour and social democratic politics', in Powell, M., Bauld, L. and Clarke, K. (eds), *Social Policy Review 17*. Bristol: Policy Press.

Driver, S. and Martell, L. (2002) *Blair's Britain*. Cambridge: Polity.

Duff, A. (2005) *The Struggle for Europe's Constitution*. Brussels: Federal Trust.

Dunleavy, P. and Hood, C. (1994) 'From old public administration to new public management'. *Public Money and Management* **14**(3): 9–16.

Durkheim, E. (1964, original 1893) *The Rules of Sociological Method*. New York: Free Press.

Dworkin, R. (1981) 'What is equality? Part 1: Equality of welfare. Part 2: Equality of resources'. *Philosophy and Public Affairs* **10**(3): 185–246; **10**(4): 283–345.

Dyson, A., Kerr, K. and Ainscow, M. (2006) 'A "pivotal moment"? Education policy in England, 2005', in Bauld, L., Clarke, K. and Maltby, T. (eds), *Social Policy Review 18*. Bristol: Policy Press.

Easton, D. (1965) *A Framework for Political Analysis*. Englewood Cliffs, NJ: Prentice-Hall.

Editorial (2005) 'Gruel in schools'. *Financial Times*, 12 March.

Elcock, H. (1994) *Local Government: Policy and Management in Local Authorities* (3rd edn). London: Routledge.

Ellison, N. (2006) *The Transformation of Welfare States?* London: Routledge.

Elston, M.A. (1991) 'The politics of professional power: medicine in a changing health service', in Gabe, J., Calnan, M. and Bury, M. (eds), *The Sociology of the Health Service*. London: Routledge.

Emsley, C. (2005) *Crime and Society in England 1750–1900*. Harlow: Pearson Education.

English, R. and Kenny, M. (eds) (2000) *Rethinking British Decline*. Basingstoke: Macmillan.

Equal Opportunities Commission (EOC) (2004) *Sex and Power: Who Runs Britain? 2004*. London: EOC.

Equal Opportunities Commission (EOC) (2005) *Sex and Power: Who Runs Britain? 2005*. London: EOC.

Erikson, R. (1993) 'Descriptions of inequality: the Swedish approach to welfare research', in Nussbaum, M.C. and Sen, A. (eds), *The Quality of Life*. Oxford: Clarendon Press.

Erikson, R. and Åberg, R. (eds) (1987) *Welfare in Transition: A Survey of Living Conditions in Sweden 1968–1981*. Oxford: Clarendon Press.

Erskine, A. (1997) 'The approaches and methods of social policy', in Alcock, P., Erskine, A. and May, M. (eds), *The Student's Companion to Social Policy*. Oxford: Blackwell.

Esping-Andersen, G. (1990) *The Three Worlds of Welfare Capitalism*. Cambridge: Polity.

Esping-Andersen, G. (ed.) (1996) *Welfare States in Transition: National Adaptations in Global Economies*. London: Sage.

Esping-Andersen, G. (ed.) (2002) *Why We Need a New Welfare State*. Oxford: Oxford University Press.

Etzioni, A. (1994) *The Spirit of Community: Rights, Responsibilities and the Communitarian Agenda*. New York: Crown.

Etzioni, A. (1997) 'The parenting deficit', in Mulgan, G. (ed.), *Life After Politics*. London: Fontana.

EUMC (2004) *The Annual Report of the European Monitoring Centre on Racism and Xenophobia*. Vienna: European Monitoring Centre on Racism and Xenophobia.

EUMC (2005) *Racist Violence in 15 EU Member States. A Comparative Overview of Findings from the RAXEN National Focal Points Reports 2001–2004*. Vienna: European Monitoring Centre on Racism and Xenophobia.

European Commission (1999) *Treaty of Amsterdam: What has Changed in Europe*. Luxembourg: European Commission.

European Commission (2003) *How the European Union Works: A Citizen's Guide to the EU Institutions*. Brussels: European Commission.

Evandrou, M. and Falkingham, J. (2004) 'How have older people fared under New Labour?', in *Simulating Social Policy for an Ageing Society*. London: LSE.

Evandrou, M. and Falkingham, J. (2005) 'A secure retirement for all? Older people and New Labour', in Hills, J. and Stewart, K. (eds), *A More Equal Society? New Labour, Poverty, Inequality and Exclusion*. Bristol: Policy Press.

Evandrou, M. and Glaser, K. (2003) 'Combining work and family life: the pension penalty of caring'. *Ageing and Society* 23(5): 583–601.

Farrington, D. (2002) 'Developmental criminology and risk-focused prevention', in Maguire, M., Morgan, R. and Reiner, R. (eds), *The Oxford Handbook of Criminology*. Oxford: Oxford University Press.

Faulkner, D. (2000) *Crime, State and Citizen*. Winchester: Waterside Press.

Feeley, M.M. and Simon, J. (1992) 'The new penology: notes on the emerging strategy of corrections and its implications'. *Criminology* 30(4): 452–474.

Ferguson, I., Lavalette, M. and Mooney, G. (2002) *Rethinking Welfare: A Critical Perspective*. London: Sage.

Fergusson, R. (1994) 'Managerialism in education', in Clarke, J., Cochrane, A. and McLaughlin, E. (eds) (1994) *Managing Social Policy*. London: Sage.

Finer, S.E. (1952) *The Life and Times of Sir Edwin Chadwick*. London: Methuen.

Finlayson, G. (1994) *Citizen, State and Social Welfare in Britain 1830–1990*. Oxford: Oxford University Press.

Finn, D. (2003) 'Employment policy', in Ellison, N. and Pierson, C. (eds), *Developments in British Social Policy 2*. Basingstoke: Palgrave Macmillan.

Fitzpatrick, T. (2001) *Welfare Theory: An Introduction*. London: Palgrave.

Fitzpatrick, T. (2002) 'Green democracy and ecosocial welfare', in Fitzpatrick, T. and Cahill, M. (eds), *Environment and Welfare: Towards a Green Social Policy.* London: Palgrave.

Fitzpatrick, T. (2003) *After the New Social Democracy: Social Welfare for the Twenty-First Century.* Manchester: Manchester University Press.

Fitzpatrick. T. (2005) *New Theories of Welfare.* Basingstoke: Palgrave Macmillan.

Fitzpatrick, T. and Cahill, M. (2002) *Environment and Welfare: Towards a Green Social Policy.* London: Palgrave.

Flynn, N. (1997) *Public Sector Management.* Hemel Hempstead: Prentice-Hall/Harvester Wheatsheaf.

Foot, M. (1983) *Loyalists and Loners.* London: Collins.

Foster, C.D. and Plowden, F.J. (1996) *The State Under Stress.* Buckingham: Open University Press.

Fraser, D. (ed.) (1976) *The New Poor Law in the Nineteenth Century.* London: Macmillan.

Fraser, D. (2003) *The Evolution of the British Welfare State* (3rd edn). Basingstoke: Palgrave Macmillan.

Freeden, M. (1996) *Ideologies and Political Theory: A Conceptual Approach.* Oxford: Clarendon Press.

Freeman, R. (2000) *The Politics of Health in Europe.* Manchester: Manchester University Press.

Freud, D. (2007) 'Reducing dependency, increasing opportunity: options for the future of welfare to work'. An independent report to the Department for Work and Pensions. Leeds: CDS.

Friedman, M. (1962) *Capitalism and Freedom.* Chicago: University of Chicago Press.

Gamble, A. (1981) *An Introduction to Modern Social and Political Thought.* Basingstoke: Macmillan.

Gamble, A. (1985) *Britain in Decline* (2nd edn). Basingstoke: Macmillan.

Gamble, A. (1987) *The Free Economy and the Strong State: The Politics of Thatcherism.* London: Macmillan.

Gamble, A. (1988) *The Free Economy and the Strong State: The Politics of Thatcherism.* London: Macmillan.

George, V. and Wilding, P. (1985) *Ideology and Social Welfare* (2nd edn). London: Routledge.

George, V. and Wilding, P. (1994) *Welfare and Ideology.* Brighton: Harvester.

George, V. and Wilding, P. (2002) *Globalization and Human Welfare.* Basingstoke: Palgrave.

Giddens, A. (1998) *The Third Way: The Renewal of Social Democracy.* Cambridge: Polity.

Giddens, A. (1999) *Runaway World: How Globalisation is Reshaping Our Lives*. London: Profile Books.

Giddens, A. (2000) *The Third Way and its Critics*. Cambridge: Polity.

Giddens, A. (2007) *Europe in the Global Age*. Cambridge: Polity.

Gilbert, B.B. (1970) *British Social Policy 1914–1939*. London: Batsford.

Gillborn, D. and Mirza, H. (2000) *Educational Inequality: Mapping Race, Class and Gender. A Synthesis of Research Evidence*. London: Ofsted.

Ginn, J. (2006) 'Gender inequalities: sidelined in British pension policy', in Pemberton, H., Thane, P. and Whiteside, N. (eds), *Britain's Pensions Crisis: History and Policy*. Oxford: British Academy/Oxford University Press.

Ginsburg, N. (1992) *Divisions of Welfare: A Critical Introduction to Comparative Social Policy*. London: Sage.

Glasby, J. and Littlechild, R. (2002) *Social Work and Direct Payments*. Bristol: Policy Press.

Glasby, J. and Littlechild, R. (2004) *The Health and Social Care Divide: The Experiences of Older People* (2nd edn). Bristol: Policy Press.

Glendinning, C., Powell, M. and Rummery, K. (eds) (2002) *Partnerships: A Third Way Approach to Delivering Welfare*. Bristol: Policy Press.

Glennerster, H. (1995) *British Social Policy since 1945*. Oxford: Blackwell.

Glennerster, H. (2001) 'Social policy', in Seldon, A. (ed.), *The Blair Effect: The Blair Government 1997–2001*. London: Little, Brown.

Glennerster, H. (2003) *Understanding the Finance of Welfare: What Welfare Costs and How to Pay for It*. Bristol: Policy Press.

Glennerster, H. (2006) 'Why so different? Why so bad a future?', in Pemberton, H., Thane, P. and Whiteside, N. (eds), *Britain's Pensions Crisis: History and Policy*. Oxford: British Academy/Oxford University Press.

Glennerster, H. (2007) *British Social Policy: 1945 to the Present*. Oxford: Blackwell.

Glennerster, H. and Hills, J. (eds) (1998) *The State of Welfare: The Economics of Social Spending* (2nd edn). Oxford: Oxford University Press.

Glennerster, H. and Low, W. (1991) 'Education and the welfare state: does it add up?', in Hills, J. (ed.), *The State of Welfare – The Welfare State in Britain since 1974*. Oxford: Clarendon Press.

Glennerster, H., Power, A. and Travers, T. (1991) 'A new era for social policy: a new enlightenment or a new leviathan?' *Journal of Social Policy* 20(3): 389–414.

Glennerster, H., Hills, J., Travers, T. and Hendry, R. (2000) *Paying for Health, Education and Housing: How Does the Centre Pull the Purse Strings?* Oxford: Oxford University Press.

Glynn, S. (1991) *No Alternative? Unemployment in Britain*. London: Faber.

Goddard, A. (1999) 'Costs thwart broader access'. *Times Higher Education Supplement*, 8 October.

Goes, E. (2004) 'The Third Way and the politics of community', in Hale, S., Leggett, W. and Martell, L. (eds), *The Third Way and Beyond*. Manchester: Manchester University Press.

Goffman, E. (1963) *Stigma: Notes on the Management of Spoiled Identity*. Englewood Cliffs, NJ: Prentice-Hall.

Goldsmith, M. and Gladstone, D. (2005) *Road Map to Reform: Health*. London: Adam Smith Institute.

Goldson, B., Lavalette, M. and McKechnie, J. (eds) (2002) *Children, Welfare and the State*. London: Sage.

Goodin, R.E. (1982) 'Freedom and the welfare state: theoretical foundations'. *Journal of Social Policy* 11: 149–176.

Goodin, R.E. (1988) *Reasons for Welfare*. Princeton, NJ: Princeton University Press.

Goodman, A. and Sibeta, L. (2006) 'Public spending on education in the UK'. Paper prepared for the Education and Skills Select Committee, July 2006, Institute of Fiscal Studies Briefing Note no. 71. London: Institute of Fiscal Studies.

Gorz, A. (1985) *Paths to Paradise: On the Liberation from Work*. London: Pluto Press.

Gough, I. (1979) *The Political Economy of Welfare*. London: Macmillan.

Gray, J. (1986) *Liberalism*. Milton Keynes: Open University Press.

Gray, J. (1994) *The Undoing of Conservatism*. London: Social Market Foundation.

Green, T.H. (1991) 'Liberal legislation and freedom of contract', in Miller, D. (ed.), *Liberty*. Oxford: Oxford University Press.

Greenleaf, W.H. (1983) *The British Political Tradition. Vol. 3: A Much Governed Nation*. London: Methuen.

Greer, S. (2003) 'Policy divergence: will it change something in Greenock?', in Hazell, R. (ed.), *The State of the Nations 2003: The Third Year of Devolution in the United Kingdom*. London: UCL Constitution Unit; Exeter: Imprint Academic.

Greer, S. (2005) *Territorial Politics and Health Policy*. Manchester: Manchester University Press.

Greer, S. (2006) 'The politics of health-policy divergence', in Adams, J. and Schmuecker, K. (eds), *Devolution in Practice 2006: Public Policy Differences within the UK*. Newcastle-upon-Tyne: IPPR North.

Griffiths, R. (1988) *Community Care: Agenda for Action. A Report to the Secretary of State for Social Services* (the Griffiths Report). London: HMSO.

Grue, L. and Lœrum, K.T. (2002) '"Doing motherhood": some experiences of mothers with physical disabilities'. *Disability and Society* 17(6): 671–683.

Habermas, J. (1976) *Legitimation Crisis*. London: Heinemann.

Hale, S., Leggett, W. and Martell, L. (eds) (2004) *The Third Way and Beyond*. Manchester: Manchester University Press.

Hall, B. (2006a) 'Critics accept broad thrust but worry about the details'. *Financial Times*, 26 May.

Hall, B. (2006b) 'Half-baked NHS reforms could harm patients, says think-tank'. *Financial Times*, 5 June.

Hall, B. and Cohen, N. (2006) 'Pensions report urges redress for victims'. *Financial Times*, 15 March.

Hall, B. and Taylor, A. (2006) 'Ministers set targets to reduce welfare claimants'. *Financial Times*, 24 January.

Hall, B. and Timmins, N. (2005) 'Search for consensus on way to overhaul pensions'. *Financial Times*, 15 June.

Hall, B. and Timmins, N. (2006) 'Mess with Turner at your peril, says Hutton'. *Financial Times*, 9 March.

Hall, P., Land, H., Parker, R. and Webb, A. (1975) *Change, Choice and Conflict in Social Policy*. London: Heinemann.

Ham, C. (1992) *Health Policy in Britain* (3rd edn). London: Macmillan.

Ham, C. (2004) *Health Policy in Britain* (5th edn). Basingstoke: Palgrave.

Ham, C. and Hill, M. (1993) *The Policy Process in the Modern Capitalist State*. Hemel Hempstead: Harvester Wheatsheaf.

Ham, C. and Pickard, S. (1998) *Tragic Choices in Health Care*. London: King's Fund.

Ham, C., Robinson, R. and Benzeval, M. (1990) *Health Check*. London: King's Fund Institute.

Hamdani, D. (2005) *Triple Jeopardy: Muslim Women's Experience of Discrimination*. Gananoque, Ont.: Canadian Council of Muslim Women.

Hammersley, M. and Atkinson, P. (1995) *Ethnography: Principles and Practice* (2nd edn). London: Routledge.

Hansard (2006) http://www.publications.parliament.uk/pa/cm200506/cmhansrd/cm060627/debindx/60627-x.htm, 27 June.

Hansen, R. (2000) 'British citizenship after Empire: a defence'. *Political Quarterly* **71**(1): 42–49.

Hantrais, L. (2004) *Family Policy Matters: Responding to Family Change in Europe*. Bristol: Policy Press.

Hantrais, L. (2007) *Social Policy in the European Union* (3rd edn). Basingstoke: Palgrave.

Harloe, M. (1995) *The People's Home? Social Rented Housing in Europe and America*. Oxford: Blackwell.

Harris, B. (2004) *The Origins of the British Welfare State: Social Welfare in England and Wales 1800–1945*. Basingstoke: Palgrave Macmillan.

Harris, J. (1972) *Unemployment and Politics: A Study in English Social Policy 1886–1914*. Oxford: Clarendon Press.

Harris, J. (1981) 'Social policy making in Britain during the Second World War', in Mommsen, W. (ed.), *The Emergence of the Welfare State in Britain and Germany*. London: Croom Helm.

Harris, J. (1984) 'The Webbs', in Barker, P. (ed.), *Founders of the Welfare State*. London: Heinemann.

Harris, J. (1990) 'Society and the state in twentieth-century Britain', in Thompson, F.M.L. (ed.), *The Cambridge Social History of Britain 1750–1950. Vol. 3: Social Agencies and Institutions*. Cambridge: Cambridge University Press.

Harris, J. (1997) *William Beveridge: A Biography* (2nd edn). Oxford: Oxford University Press.

Harris, J. (2006) 'The roots of public pensions provision: social insurance and the Beveridge plan', in Pemberton, H., Thane, P. and Whiteside, N. (eds), *Britain's Pensions Crisis: History and Policy*. Oxford: British Academy/Oxford University Press.

Hassan, G. and Warhurst, C. (2001) 'New Scotland? Policy, parties and institutions'. *Political Quarterly* 72(2): 213–226.

Hatcher, R. (2005) 'Transforming the school system through privatisation and sponsorship'. *Radical Education Journal* no. 2, February, pp. 6–7.

Hatcher, R. (2006) 'Privatisation and sponsorship: the re-agenting of the school system in England'. *Journal of Education Policy* 21(5): 599–619.

Hay, J.R. (1975) *The Origins of the Liberal Welfare Reforms 1906–1914*. Basingstoke: Macmillan.

Hayek, F.A. (1944) *The Road to Serfdom*. London: Routledge.

Hayek, F.A. (1960) *The Constitution of Liberty*. London: Routledge & Kegan Paul.

Hayek, F.A. (1976) *The Road to Serfdom*. London: Routledge & Kegan Paul.

Hayek, F.A. (1982) *Law, Legislation and Liberty*. London: Routledge & Kegan Paul.

Hazell, R. (ed.) (2003) *The State of the Nations 2003: The Third Year of Devolution in the United Kingdom*. London: UCL Constitutional Unit; Exeter: Imprint Academic.

Heald, D. (1983) *Public Expenditure*. Oxford: Martin Robertson.

Hearnes, H.M. (1987) 'Women and the welfare state: the transition from private to public dependence', in Showstack Sassoon, A. (ed.), *Women and the State: The Shifting Boundaries of Public and Private*. London: Hutchinson.

Heclo, H. (1981) 'Toward a new welfare state?', in Flora, P. and Heidenheimer,

A.J. (eds), *The Development of Welfare States in Europe and America*. New Brunswick, NJ: Transaction Books.

Heclo, H. and Wildavsky, A. (1981) *The Private Government of Public Money*. Basingstoke: Macmillan.

Held, D. (ed.) (1991) *Political Theory Today*. Cambridge: Polity.

Held, D. (2004) *Global Covenant: The Social Democratic Alternative to the Washington Consensus*. Cambridge: Polity.

Held, D. and McGrew, A. (2002) *Governing Globalization*. Cambridge: Polity.

Helm, D. (ed.) (1989) *The Economic Borders of the State*. Oxford: Oxford University Press.

Help the Aged (2007) *Age Discrimination in Goods, Facilities and Services*. London: Help the Aged.

Hemerijck, A. (2002) 'The self-transformation of the European social model(s)', in Esping-Andersen, G. (ed.), *Welfare States in Transition*. London: Sage.

Hendrick, H. (ed.) (2005) *Child Welfare and Social Policy: An Essential Reader*. Bristol: Policy Press.

Hennessy, P. (1988) *Whitehall*. London: Secker & Warburg.

Hennessy, P. (1996) *The Hidden Wiring: Unearthing the British Constitution*. London: Indigo/Cassell Group.

Henriques, U.R.Q. (1979) *Before the Welfare State: Social Administration in Early Industrial Britain*. London: Longman.

Henry, S. and Lanier, M. (2001) *What is Crime? Controversies over the Nature of Crime and What to Do About It*. Lanham, MD: Rowman and Littlefield.

Hewitt, P. and Leach, P. (1993) *Social Justice, Children and Families. Commission on Social Justice Issue Paper 4*. London: Institute for Public Policy Research.

Hewson, C., Yule, P., Laurent, D. and Vogel, C. (2003) *Internet Research Methods: A Practical Guide for the Social and Behavioural Sciences*. London: Sage.

Hill, D. (1994) *Citizens and Cities: Urban Policy in the 1990s*. London: Harvester Wheatsheaf.

Hill, M. (1993a) *The Welfare State in Britain: A Political History since 1945*. Aldershot: Edward Elgar.

Hill, M. (1993b) *The Policy Process: A Reader*. Hemel Hempstead: Harvester Wheatsheaf.

Hill, M. (1995) *Social Policy: A Comparative Analysis*. Hemel Hempstead: Prentice Hall / Harvester Wheatsheaf.

Hill, M. (1997) *The Policy Process in the Modern State*. Hemel Hempstead: Harvester Wheatsheaf.

Hill, M. (2003) *Understanding Social Policy* (7th edn). Oxford: Blackwell.

Hill, M. (2007) *Pensions*. Bristol: Policy Press.

Hills, J. (1997) *The Future of Welfare: A Guide to the Debate* (2nd edn). York: Joseph Rowntree Foundation.

Hills, J. (1998) *Income and Wealth: The Latest Evidence*. York: Joseph Rowntree Foundation.

Hills, J. (2004) *Inequality and the State*. Oxford: Oxford University Press.

Hills, J. (2006) 'Financing UK pensions', in Pemberton, H., Thane, P. and Whiteside, N. (eds), *Britain's Pensions Crisis: History and Policy*. Oxford: British Academy/Oxford University Press.

Hills, J. (2007) *Ends and Means: The Future Roles of Social Housing in England*. London: LSE.

Hills, J. and Stewart, K. (eds) (2005) *A More Equal Society? New Labour, Poverty, Inequality and Exclusion*. Bristol: Policy Press.

Hinrichs, K. (2006) 'Reforming pensions in Germany and Sweden: new pathways to a better future?', in Pemberton, H., Thane, P. and Whiteside, N. (eds), *Britain's Pensions Crisis: History and Policy*. Oxford: British Academy/Oxford University Press.

Hirschman, A.O. (1970) *Exit, Voice and Loyalty: Responses to Decline in Firms, Organizations and States*. Cambridge, MA: Harvard University Press.

H.M. Treasury (2002) *Securing our Future Health: Taking a Long-Term View. Final Report* (the Wanless Report). London: H.M. Treasury.

H.M. Treasury (2003) *Every Child Matters* (Cm 5860). London: The Stationery Office.

H.M. Treasury (2006a) *Public Expenditure Statistical Analyses* (Cm 6811). London: The Stationery Office.

H.M. Treasury (2006b) *Prosperity for All in the Global Economy – World Class Skills. Final Report* (Leitch Review of Skills). London: The Stationery Office.

H.M. Treasury (2007) *Meeting the Aspirations of the British People: Pre-Budget Report and Comprehensive Spending Review* (Cm 7227). London: The Stationery Office.

Hobsbawm, E.J. (1968) *Industry and Empire: An Economic History of Britain since 1750*. London: Weidenfeld & Nicolson.

Hobsbawm, E.J. and Rudé, G. (1969) *Captain Swing*. London: Lawrence & Wishart.

Home Office (1998) *Supporting Families*. London: The Stationery Office.

Home Office (2000) *Attitudes to Crime and Criminal Justice: Findings from the 1998 British Crime Survey*. Home Office Research Study 200. London: Home Office.

Home Office (2002) *Justice for All*. London: Home Office.

Home Office (2003) *Respect and Responsibility: Taking a Stand against Anti-social Behaviour*. London: The Stationery Office.

Home Office (2005) *Criminal Statistics: England and Wales*. London: The Stationery Office.

Home Office (2006) *Respect Agenda*.

Houlder, V. (2006a) 'Experts to review advances in tax system'. *Financial Times*, 4 September.

Houlder, V. (2006b) 'Poorest households pay higher share of tax and get lower proportion of benefits'. *Financial Times*, 4 September.

House of Commons Health Committee (2002) *First Report. The Role of the Private Sector in the NHS*. Vol. I, HC 308-I: *Report and Proceedings of the Committee*. Vol. II, HC 308-II: *Minutes of Evidence and Appendices*. London: The Stationery Office.

House of Commons Treasury Committee (2007) *Comprehensive Spending Review: Prospects and Processes. Sixth Report of Session 2006–07*. HC 279. London: The Stationery Office.

House of Commons Work and Pensions Committee (2007) *The Government's Employment Strategy. Third Report of Session 2006–07*. HC 63-I. London: The Stationery Office. www.parliament.uk/parliamentary_committees/work_and_pensions_committee.cfm

Huby, M. (1998) *Social Policy and the Environment*. Buckingham: Open University Press.

Hudson, B. (2003) *Understanding Justice*. Buckingham: Open University Press.

Hughes, G. (2001) 'Restorative justice', in McLaughlin, E. and Muncie, J. (eds), *The Sage Dictionary of Criminology*. London: Sage.

Hughes, G. and Lewis, G. (eds) (1998) *Unsettling Welfare*. London: Routledge/Open University.

Hulme, R. and Hulme, M. (2005) 'New Labour's education policy: innovation or reinvention?', in Powell, M., Bauld, L. and Clarke, K. (eds), *Social Policy Review 17*. Bristol: Policy Press.

Hyde, M. (2000) 'Disability', in Payne, G. (ed.), *Social Divisions*. Basingstoke: Palgrave.

Immergut, E.M. and Anderson, K.M. (eds) (2007) *The Handbook of West European Pension Politics*. Oxford: Oxford University Press.

Inman, K. (1999) 'Changing roles'. *Community Care*, 3–9 June, pp. 20–21.

Inman, P. (2002) 'Elderly to get free care in Scotland'. *The Guardian*, 9 February.

IPCC (2007) *Climate Change 2007: The Physical Science Basis*. Contribution of Working Group I to the Fourth Assessment Report of the Intergovernmental Panel on Climate Change. Geneva: United Nations.

Jack, A. (2006) 'Decision on Herceptin to come "within six months"'. *Financial Times*, 16 February.

Jack, A. and Timmins, N. (2006) 'Alzheimer's decision a test for ministers'. *Financial Times*, 24 January.

Jackson, C.J., Furnham, A. and Willen, K. (2000) 'Employer willingness to comply with the Disability Discrimination Act regarding staff selection in the UK'. *Journal of Occupational and Organizational Psychology* 73(1): 119–129.

Jackson, S. (1999) *Heterosexuality in Question*. London: Sage.

James, S. (1997) *British Government: A Reader in Policy Making*. London: Routledge.

Jay, P. (1976) *Employment, Inflation and Politics*. London: Institute of Economic Affairs.

Jay, P. (1994) 'The economy 1990–94', in Kavanagh, D. and Seldon, A. (eds), *The Major Effect*. London: Macmillan.

Jenkins, P. (1989) *Mrs Thatcher's Revolution* (2nd edn). London: Pan Books.

Jenkins, S. (1995) *Accountable to None: the Tory Nationalization of Britain*. London: Hamish Hamilton.

Johnson, C. (1991) *The Economy under Mrs Thatcher 1979–1990*. Harmondsworth: Penguin.

Johnson, N. (2001) 'The personal social services', in Savage, P. and Atkinson, R. (eds), *Public Policy under Blair*. Basingstoke: Palgrave.

Johnson, P. (1985a) *Saving and Spending: The Working-class Economy in Britain 1870–1939*. Oxford: Oxford University Press.

Johnson, P. (1985b) *The Historical Dimensions of the Welfare State Crisis*. London: Suntory-Toyota International Centre for Research in Economic and Related Disciplines.

Jolly, D., Priestley, M. and Matthews, B. (2006) 'Secondary analysis of existing data on disabled people's use and experiences of public transport in Great Britain'. A research report for the Disability Rights Commission.

Jones, B., Kavanagh, D., Moran, M. and Norton, P. (2006) *Politics UK* (6th edn). Harlow: Longman.

Jones, C. and Novak, T. (1980) 'The welfare state', in Corrigan, P. (ed.), *Capitalism, State Formation and Marxist Theory*. London: Quartet.

Jones, C. and Novak, T. (1999) *Poverty, Welfare and the Disciplinary State*. London: Routledge.

Jones, H. (1994) *Health and Society in Twentieth-Century Britain*. London: Longman.

Jones, K. (1991) *The Making of Social Policy in Britain, 1830–1990*. London: Athlone Press.

Jones, P. and Cullis, J. (2000) '"Individual failure" and the analytics of social policy'. *Journal of Social Policy* 29(1): 73–93.

Jones, T. (1993) *Britain's Ethnic Minorities*. London: Policy Studies Institute.

Jordan, B. (1998) *The New Politics of Welfare*. London: Sage.

Joseph, K. (1977) *Monetarism is Not Enough*. London: Centre for Policy Studies.

Joseph, K. and Sumption, J. (1979) *Equality*. London: John Murray.

Judge, K. (ed.) (1980) *Pricing the Social Services*. Basingstoke: Macmillan.

Judge, K. (1982) 'The growth and decline of social expenditure', in Walker, A. (ed.), *Public Expenditure and Social Policy*. London: Heinemann.

Judge, K. and Matthews, J. (1980) *Charging for Social Care: A Study of Consumer Charges and the Personal Social Services*. London: Allen & Unwin.

Jupp, V. (2006) *The Sage Dictionary of Social Research Methods*. London: Sage.

Kamerman, S.B. and Kahn, A.J. (eds) (1978) *Family Policy: Government and Families in Fourteen Countries*. New York: Columbia University Press.

Kavanagh, D. (1987) *Thatcherism and British Politics: The End of Consensus?* Oxford: Oxford University Press.

Kavanagh, D. (1997) *The Reordering of British Politics: Politics after Thatcher*. Oxford: Oxford University Press.

Keating, M. (2002) 'Devolution: what difference has it made? Interim findings from the ESRC programme on devolution and constitutional change', www.devolution.ac.uk

Keating, M. (2005) 'Devolution briefings: policy making and policy divergence in Scotland after devolution'. ESRC Research Programme on Devolution and Constitutional Change.

Keegan, W. (1989) *Mr Lawson's Gamble*. London: Hodder and Stoughton.

Keegan, W. (2004) *The Prudence of Mr Gordon Brown*. Chichester: Wiley.

Kelleher, D. (1994) 'Self-help groups and their relationship to medicine', in Gabe, J., Kelleher, D. and Williams, G. (eds), *Challenging Medicine*. London: Routledge.

Kincaid, J. (1984) 'Richard Titmuss', in Barker, P. (ed.), *Founders of the Welfare State*. London: Heinemann.

King, A. (ed.) (1976) *Why is Britain Becoming Harder to Govern?* London: BBC.

King, D. and Wickham-Jones, M. (1999) 'Bridging the Atlantic: the Democratic (Party) origins of Welfare to Work', in Powell, M. (ed.), *New Labour, New Welfare State?* Bristol: Policy Press.

King, D.S. (1999) *In the Name of Liberalism: Illiberal Social Policy in the United States and Britain*. Oxford: Oxford University Press.

King, M. (1981) *The Framework of Criminal Justice*. London: Croom Helm.

Kjær, A.M. (2004) *Governance*. Cambridge: Polity Press.

Klein, R. (1973) *Complaints Against Doctors – A Study in Professional Accountability*. London: Charles Knight.

Klein, R. (1980a) 'The welfare state: a self-inflicted crisis?', *Political Quarterly* 51(1): 24–34.

Klein, R. (1980b) 'The social policy man: priest or pragmatist?', *Times Higher Education Supplement*, 15 February.

Klein, R. (1989) *The Politics of the NHS*. London: Longman.

Klein, R. (1990) 'The state and the profession: the politics of the double bed'. *British Medical Journal*, 3 October.

Klein, R. (1993) 'O'Goffe's tale, or, what can we learn from the success of the capitalist welfare states?', in Jones, C. (ed.), *New Perspectives on the Welfare State in Europe*. London: Routledge.

Klein, R. (1996a) 'The welfare state: a self-inflicted crisis?', in Day, P. (ed.), *Only Dissect: Rudolf Klein on Politics and Society*. Oxford: Blackwell.

Klein, R. (1996b) 'The social policy man: priest or pragmatist?', *ibid*.

Klein, R. (1996c) 'O'Goffe's tale, or, what can we learn from the success of the capitalist welfare states?', *ibid*.

Klein, R. (1996d) 'The state and the profession: the politics of the double bed', *ibid*.

Klein, R. (2005) 'Transforming the NHS: the story in 2004', in Powell, M., Bauld, L. and Clarke, K. (eds), *Social Policy Review 17*. Bristol: Policy Press.

Klein, R. (2006) *The New Politics of the NHS: From Creation to Reinvention*. Abingdon: Radcliffe Publishing.

Klein, R., Day, P. and Redmayne, S. (1996) *Managing Scarcity: Priority-Setting and Rationing in the National Health Service*. Buckingham: Open University Press.

Kohler, M. (2006) 'Pension reform must not be sold on the back of bogus statistics'. *Financial Times*, 30 June.

Kooiman, J. (ed.) (1993) *Modern Governance – Government–Society Interactions*. London: Sage.

Kooiman, J. (2000) 'Levels of governing: interactions as a central concept', in Pierre, J. (ed.), *Debating Governance*. Oxford: Oxford University Press.

Kvale, S. (1996) *Interviews: An Introduction to Qualitative Research Interviews*. London: Sage.

Kymlicka, W. (2002) *Contemporary Political Philosophy: An Introduction* (2nd edn). Oxford: Oxford University Press.

Labour Party (1997) *New Labour: Because Britain Deserves Better*. General Election Manifesto. London: Labour Party.

Labour Party (2001) *New Ambitions for our Country*. General Election Manifesto. London: Labour Party.

Labour Party (2005) *The Labour Party Manifesto 2005: Britain Forward Not Back*. London: Labour Party.

Lacey, N. (2003) 'Penal theory and penal practice: a communitarian approach', in McConville, S. (ed.), *The Use of Punishment*. Cullompton. Devon: Willan Publishing.

Laing, R.D. (1967) *The Politics of Experience and the Birds of Paradise*. Harmondsworth: Penguin.

Lal, D. (1995) *The Minimum Wage: No Way to Help the Poor*. London: Institute of Economic Affairs.

Laming, Lord (2003) *The Victoria Climbié Inquiry: Report of an Inquiry*. London: The Stationery Office.

Lang, T., Barling, D. and Caraher, M. (2002) 'Food, social policy and the environment: towards a new model'. *Social Policy and Administration* 35(5): 538–558.

Langan, M. (2000) 'Social services: managing the third way', in Clarke, J., Gewirtz, S. and McLaughlin, E. (eds), *New Managerialism, New Welfare?* London: Sage.

Langan, M. and Clarke, J. (1993) 'The British welfare state: foundation and modernization', in Cochrane, A. and Clarke, J. (eds), *Comparing Welfare States: Britain in International Context*. London: Sage.

Langer, W.L. (1987) *An Encyclopedia of World History*. London: Harrap.

Laslett, P. (1983) *The World We Have Lost: Further Explored*. London: Routledge.

Laursen, F. (2001) 'EU enlargement: interests, issues and the need for institutional reform', in Andersen, S.S. and Eliasen, K.A. (eds), *Making Policy in Europe* (2nd edn). London: Sage.

Laville, S. and Kumi, A. (2006) 'Four-month-old son of Gordon and Sarah Brown diagnosed with cystic fibrosis'. *The Guardian*, 30 November.

Laville, S. and Smithers, R. (2007) 'War over school boundaries divides Brighton. Council brings in lottery for sought-after places. Parents in old catchment area threaten court action', *The Guardian*, 1 March.

Law, I. (1996) *Racism, Ethnicity and Social Policy*. Hemel Hempstead: Prentice Hall.

Lawson, N. (1992) *The View from No. 11: Memoirs of a Tory Radical*. London: Bantam.

Le Grand, J. (1982) *The Strategy of Equality*. London: Allen & Unwin.

Le Grand, J. and Bartlett, W. (eds) (1993) *Quasi-Markets and Social Policy*. Basingstoke: Macmillan.

Le Grand, J. and Vizard, P. (1998) 'The National Health Service: crisis, change or continuity?', in Glennerster, H. and Hills, J. (eds), *The State of Welfare: The Economics of Social Spending*. Oxford: Oxford University Press.

Le Grand, J., Mays, N. and Mulligan, J.-A. (eds) (1998) *Learning from the NHS Internal Market: A Review of the Evidence*. London: King's Fund.

Leach, E.R. (1968) *A Runaway World*. London: BBC.

Leach, S. and Wingfield, M. (1999) 'Public participation and the democratic renewal agenda: prioritisation or marginalisation?'. *Local Government Studies* 25(4): 46–59.

Lee, D. and Newby, H. (1983) *The Problem of Sociology*. London: Hutchinson.

Lee, J. (2005) 'Academies unproven, say MPs'. *Times Educational Supplement*, 18 March.

Lee, S. (1986) *Law and Morals: Warnock, Gillick and Beyond*. Oxford: Oxford University Press.

Levin, P. (1997) *Making Social Policy – The Mechanisms of Government and Politics, and How to Investigate Them*. Buckingham: Open University Press.

Levitas, R. (1998) *The Inclusive Society? Social Exclusion and New Labour*. Basingstoke: Macmillan.

Levitas, R. (2005) *The Inclusive Society? Social Exclusion and New Labour* (2nd edn). Basingstoke: Palgrave Macmillan.

Lewis, G. (2003) 'Migrants', in Alcock, P., Erskine, A. and May, M. (eds) *The Student's Companion to Social Policy* (2nd edn). Oxford: Blackwell.

Lewis, J. (2000) 'Family policy in the post-war period', in Katz, S., Eekelaar, J. and Maclean, M. (eds), *Cross-Currents: Family Law and Policy in the US and England*. Oxford: Oxford University Press.

Lewis, J. (2001) 'Women, men and the family', in Seldon, A. (ed.), *The Blair Effect: The Blair Government 1997–2001*. London: Little, Brown.

Lewis, J. and Campbell, M. (2007) 'Work/family balance policies in the UK since 1997: a new departure?' *Journal of Social Policy* 36(3): 365–381.

Lewis, J. and Glennerster, H. (1996) *Implementing the New Community Care*. Buckingham: Open University Press.

Leys, C. (2001) *Market-Driven Politics: Neoliberal Democracy and the Public Interest*. London: Verso.

Likierman, A. (1988) *Public Expenditure: The Public Spending Process*. Harmondsworth: Penguin.

Lindblom, C.E. (1979) 'Still muddling, not yet through'. *Public Administration Review* 39(6): 517–526.

Lindblom, C.E. (1982) 'Still muddling, not yet through', in McGrew, A. and Wilson, M.J. (eds), *Decision Making: Approaches and Analysis*. Manchester: Manchester University Press.

Ling, T. (1994) 'The new managerialism and social security', in Clarke, J., Cochrane, A. and McLaughlin, E. (eds), *Managing Social Policy*. London: Sage.

Ling, T. (2000) 'Unpacking partnership: health care', in Clarke, J., Gewirtz, S. and McLaughlin, E. (eds), *New Managerialism, New Welfare?* London: Sage.

Linneman, P.D. and Megbolugbe, I.F. (1994) 'Privatisation and housing policy'. *Urban Studies* 31(4/5): 635–651.

Lipsky, M. (1980) *Street-level Bureaucracy*. New York: Russell Sage.

Lister, R. (1994) 'The family and women', in Kavanagh, D. and Seldon, A. (eds), *The Major Effect*. London: Macmillan.

Lister, R. (1998) *Citizenship: Feminist Perspectives*. Basingstoke: Macmillan.

Lovelock, J. (2006) *The Revenge of Gaia*. London: Penguin and Allen Lane.

Lowe, R. (1993) *The Welfare State in Britain since 1945*. Basingstoke: Macmillan.

Lowe, R. (2005) *The Welfare State in Britain since 1945* (3rd edn). Basingstoke: Palgrave Macmillan.

Lukes, S. (1985) *Marxism and Morality*. Oxford: Oxford University Press.

Lukes, S. (2005) *Power: A Radical View* (2nd edn). Basingstoke: Palgrave.

Lund, B. (1996) *Housing Problems and Housing Policy*. London: Longman.

Lund, B. (2006) *Understanding Housing Policy*. Bristol: Policy Press.

Lynes, T. (1984) 'William Beveridge', in Barker, P. (ed.), *Founders of the Welfare State*. London: Heinemann.

Lyon, D. (1994) *Postmodernity*. Buckingham: Open University Press.

MacCallum, G.C. (1967) 'Negative and positive freedom'. *Philosophical Review* 76(3): 312–334.

MacCallum, G.C. (1991) 'Negative and positive freedom', in Miller, D. (ed.), *Liberty*. Oxford: Oxford University Press.

MacInnes, J. (1987) *Thatcherism at Work: Industrial Relations and Economic Change*. Milton Keynes: Open University Press.

Mack, J. and Lansley, S. (1985) *Poor Britain*. London: Allen & Unwin.

Macnicol, J. (1998) *The Politics of Retirement in Britain 1878–1948*. Cambridge: Cambridge University Press.

Macnicol, J. (2006) 'Age discrimination in history', in Bauld, L., Clarke, K. and Maltby, T. (eds), *Social Policy Review 18*. Bristol: Policy Press.

Macpherson, W. (1999) *The Stephen Lawrence Inquiry: Report of an Inquiry by Sir William Macpherson* (Cm 4262-1). London: The Stationery Office.

Majone, G. (1989) *Evidence, Argument and Persuasion in the Policy Process*. New Haven, CT: Yale University Press.

Malpass, P. (1996) 'The unravelling of housing policy in Britain'. *Housing Studies* 11(3): 459–470.

Malpass, P. (2003) 'The wobbly pillar? Housing and the British postwar welfare state'. *Journal of Social Policy* 32(4): 589–606.

Malpass, P. (2005) *Housing and the Welfare State*. Basingstoke: Palgrave.

Malpass, P. and Cairncross, L. (2006) 'Introduction', in Malpass, P. and Cairncross, L. (eds), *Building on the Past: Visions of Housing Futures*. Bristol: Policy Press.

Malpass, P. and Means, R. (1993) *Implementing Housing Policy*. Buckingham: Open University Press.

Malpass, P. and Murie, A. (1999) *Housing Policy and Practice* (5th edn). Basingstoke: Palgrave Macmillan.

Mansell, W. (2004) 'Provisional scores distort GCSE picture'. *Times Educational Supplement*, 21 October.

Mansell, W., Luck, A. and Paton, G. (2005) 'Ministers "misled" public on academies'. *Times Educational Supplement*, 7 October.

Marmot, M. (2004) *Status Syndrome*. London: Bloomsbury.

Marquand, D. (1988) *The Unprincipled Society*. London: Jonathan Cape.

Marquand, D. (1996) 'Moralists and hedonists', in Marquand, D. and Seldon, A. (eds), *The Ideas that Shaped Post-War Britain*. London: Fontana.

Marquand, D. (2004) *Decline of the Public*. Cambridge: Polity.

Marquand, D. and Seldon, A. (eds) (1996) *The Ideas that Shaped Post-War Britain*. London: Fontana.

Marr, A. (1996) *Ruling Britannia: The Failure and Future of British Democracy*. London: Penguin.

Marshall, J.D. (1985) *The Old Poor Law 1795–1834*. London: Macmillan.

Marshall, T.H. (1950) *Citizenship and Social Class*. Cambridge: Cambridge University Press.

Marshall, T.H. (1963) 'Citizenship and social class', in Marshall, T.H. (ed.), *Sociology at the Crossroads and Other Essays*. London: Heinemann.

Marshall, T.H. (1964) *Class, Citizenship and Social Development*. Chicago: University of Chicago Press.

Martin, J. and White, A. (1988) *The Prevalence of Disability among Adults. OPCS Surveys of Disability in Great Britain. Report 1*. OPCS Social Survey Division. London: HMSO.

Martinson, R. (1974) 'What works? Questions and answers about prison reform'. *Public Interest* 35 (Spring): 22–54.

Martinson, R. (1979) 'New findings, new views: a note of caution regarding sentencing reform'. *Hofstra Law Review* 7: 243–258.

Marx, K. and Engels, F. (1968) 'Manifesto of the Communist Party', in Marx, K. and Engels, F., *Selected Works in One Volume*. London: Lawrence & Wishart.

Mason, D. (2000a) *Race and Ethnicity in Modern Britain* (2nd edn). Oxford: Oxford University Press.

Mason, D. (2000b) 'Ethnicity', in Payne, G. (ed.), *Social Divisions*. Basingstoke: Palgrave.

Mason, D. (ed.) (2003) *Explaining Ethnic Differences: Changing Patterns of Disadvantage in Britain*. Bristol: Policy Press.

Matthews, R., Easton, H., Briggs, D. and Pease, K. (2007) *Assessing the Use and Impact of Anti-Social Behaviour Orders*. Bristol: Policy Press.

McBarnet, D. (1983) *Conviction*. London: Macmillan.

McKibbin, R. (1990) *The Ideologies of Class: Social Relations in Britain 1880–1950*. Oxford: Oxford University Press.

McKnight, A. (2005) 'Employment: tackling poverty through "work for those who can"', in Hills, J. and Stewart, K. (eds), *A More Equal Society? New Labour, Poverty, Inequality and Exclusion*. Bristol: Policy Press.

McLaughlin, E. (2005) 'Governance and social policy in Northern Ireland (1999–2004): the devolution years and postscript', in Powell, M., Bauld, L. and Clarke, K. (eds), *Social Policy Review 17*. Bristol: Policy Press.

McNally, S. and Vaitilingam, R. (2007) *Policy Analysis: Has Labour Delivered on the Policy Priorities of 'Education, Education, Education'? The Evidence on School Standards, Parental Choice and Staying On*. London: Centre for Economic Performance, LSE.

Mead, L. (1986) *Beyond Entitlement: The Social Obligations of Citizenship*. New York: Free Press.

Mead, L.M. (1997) 'From welfare to work: lessons from America', in Deacon, A. (ed.), *From Welfare to Work: Lessons from America*. London: Institute of Economic Affairs.

Means, R. (1995) 'Older people and the personal social services', in Gladstone, D. (ed.), *British Social Welfare: Past, Present and Future*. London: UCL Press.

Means, R. and Smith, R. (1998) *From Poor Law to Community Care: The Development of Welfare Services for Elderly People 1939–1971*. Bristol: Policy Press.

Means, R., Morbey, H. and Smith, R. (2002) *From Community Care to Market Care? The Development of Welfare Services for Older People*. Bristol: Policy Press.

Meikle, J. (2007) 'Cameron faces Tory revolt after retreat on grammar schools'. *The Guardian*, 17 May.

Middlemass, K. (1979) *Politics in Industrial Society*. London: André Deutsch.

Middlemass, K. (1986) *Power, Competition and the State. Vol. 1: Britain in Search of Balance*. London: Macmillan.

Miles, D. (2002) 'Is there a pensions crisis?' *Prospect*, December, pp. 46–50.

Mill, J.S. (1859) *On Liberty*. London: John W. Parker & Son.

Millar, J. (2003) 'Social policy and family policy', in Alcock, P., Erskine, A. and May, M. (eds), *The Student's Companion to Social Policy*. Oxford: Blackwell.

Millar, J. and Ridge, T. (2002) 'Parents, children, families and New Labour: developing family policy?', in Powell, M. (ed.), *Evaluating New Labour's Welfare Reforms*. Bristol: Policy Press.

Miller, D. (1976) *Social Justice*. Oxford: Clarendon Press.

Miller, D. (1990) 'Equality', in Hunt, G.M.K. (ed.), *Philosophy and Politics*. Cambridge: Cambridge University Press.

Miller, D. (1991) 'Introduction', in Miller, D., *Liberty*. Oxford: Oxford University Press.

Miller, D. (2000) *Citizenship and National Identity*. Cambridge: Polity.

Miller, D. (2003) *Political Philosophy: A Very Short Introduction*. Oxford: Oxford University Press.

Mills, W.C. (1970) *The Sociological Imagination* (3rd edn). New York: Oxford University Press.

Mishra, R. (1981) *Society and Social Policy*. London: Macmillan.

Mishra, R. (1984) *The Welfare State in Crisis*. Brighton: Wheatsheaf.

Mishra, R. (1990) *The Welfare State in Capitalist Society*. Hemel Hempstead: Harvester Wheatsheaf.

Mishra, R. (1999) *Globalization and the Welfare State*. Cheltenham: Edward Elgar.

Modood, T. (1997) 'Employment', in Modood, T., Berthoud, R., Lakey, J., Nazroo, J., Smith, P., Virdee, S. and Beishon, P. (eds), *Ethnic Minorities in Britain*. London: Policy Studies Institute.

Moggridge, D.E. (1976) *Keynes*. Glasgow: Fontana.

Mooney, G. and Scott, G. (2005) *Exploring Social Policy in the 'New' Scotland*. Bristol: Policy Press.

Morgan, K.O. (1990) *The People's Peace*. London: Oxford University Press.

Morgan, P. (1998) 'An endangered species?', in David, M.E. (ed.), *The Fragmenting Family: Does It Matter?* London: IEA Health and Welfare Unit.

Morris, J. (1991) *Pride Against Prejudice: Transforming Attitudes to Disability*. London: The Women's Press.

Morris, J. (1992) '"Us" and "Them"? Feminist research, community care and disability'. *Critical Social Policy*, 33 (Winter): 22–38.

Moss, P. (2000) 'Uncertain start: a critical look at some of New Labour's "early years" policies', in Dean, H., Sykes, R. and Woods, R. (eds), *Social Policy Review 12*. Newcastle: Social Policy Association/University of Northumbria.

Mount, F. (1982) *The Subversive Family: An Alternative History of Love and Marriage*. London: Jonathan Cape.

Mulhall, S. and Swift, A. (1996) *Liberals and Communitarians* (2nd edn). Oxford: Blackwell.

Mullard, M. (ed.) (1995) *Policy-Making in Britain: An Introduction*. London: Routledge.

Mullins, D. and Murie, A. (2006) *Housing Policy in the UK*. Basingstoke: Palgrave Macmillan.

Muncie, J. (1990) 'Failure never matters: detention centres and the politics of deterrence'. *Critical Social Policy* 28: 53–66.

Munn, M. (2006) 'Through the glass ceiling: equalities in the 21st century'. DCLG (www.communities.gov.uk), 23 October.

Murie, A. (2007) 'Housing policy, housing tenure and the housing market', in Clarke, K., Maltby, T. and Kennett, K. (eds), *Social Policy Review 19*. Bristol: Policy Press.

Murray, C. (1990) *The Emerging British Underclass*. London: IEA Health and Welfare Unit.

Murray, C. (1997) *Does Prison Work?* London: Institute of Economic Affairs.

Myers, N. and Kent, J. (1995) *Environmental Exodus. An Emergent Crisis in the Global Arena*. Washington, DC: The Climate Institute.

Myles, J. and Pierson, P. (2001) 'The comparative political economy of pension reform', in Pierson, P. (ed.), *The New Politics of the Welfare State*. Oxford: Oxford University Press.

National Audit Office (NAO) (2002) *The New Deal for Young People*. London: The Stationery Office.

National Audit Office (NAO) (2005) *More Than a Roof: Progress in Tackling Homelessness*. London: The Stationery Office.

National Offender Management Service (2007) *Population in Custody. Monthly Tables, June 2007, England and Wales*. http://www.justice.gov.uk/docs/population-in-custody-june07.pdf

Neilson, J. (1998) 'Equal opportunities for women in the European Union: success or failure?' *Journal of European Social Policy* 8(1): 64–79.

Nelken, D. (2002) 'White-collar crime', in Maguire, M., Morgan, R. and Reiner, R. (eds), *The Oxford Handbook of Criminology*. Oxford: Oxford University Press.

Netten, A. (2005) 'Personal social services', in Powell, M., Bauld, L. and Clarke, K. (eds), *Social Policy Review 17*. Bristol: Policy Press.

Nettleton, S. (1995) *The Sociology of Health and Illness*. Cambridge: Polity.

Newman, J. (2001) *Modernising Governance: New Labour, Policy and Society*. London: Sage.

Newman, J. and Clarke, J. (1994) 'Going about our business? The managerialisation of public services', in Clarke, J., Cochrane, A. and McLaughlin, E. (eds), *Managing Social Policy*. London: Sage.

Norman, A. (1985) *Triple Jeopardy: Growing Old in a Second Homeland*. London: Centre for Policy on Ageing.

Nozick, R. (1974) *Anarchy, State, and Utopia*. New York: Basic Books.

Nugent, N. (2006) *The Government and Politics of the European Union* (6th edn). Basingstoke: Palgrave Macmillan.

O'Connor, J. (1973) *The Fiscal Crisis of the State*. New York: St Martin's Press.

ODDC (2003) *Triple Jeopardy: African American Women with Disabilities*. Columbus, OH: Report by the Ohio Developmental Disabilities Council.

OECD (1981) *The Welfare State in Crisis*. Paris: Organisation for Economic Co-operation and Development.

OECD (1985) *Social Expenditure 1960–1990*. Paris: Organisation for Economic Co-operation and Development.

OECD (2004) *Balancing Work and Family Life: Helping Parents into Paid Employment*. Paris: Organisation for Economic Co-operation and Development.

OECD (2005) *Pensions at a Glance: Public Policies across OECD Countries*. Paris: Organisation for Economic Co-operation and Development.

Offe, C. (1984) *Contradictions of the Welfare State*. London: Hutchinson.

Office for National Statistics (ONS) (2004) *Social Trends No. 34*. London: ONS.

Office for National Statistics (ONS) (2005a) *Social Trends No. 35*. London: ONS.

Office for National Statistics (ONS) (2005b) *Children Looked After by Local Authorities, Year Ending 31 March 2001*. London: ONS.

Office for National Statistics (ONS) (2006a) *Social Trends No. 36*. London: ONS.

Office for National Statistics (ONS) (2006b) *Labour Force Survey*. London: ONS.

Office for National Statistics (ONS) (2007) *Social Trends No. 37*. London: ONS.

Office of the Deputy Prime Minister (ODPM) (2003) *Sustainable Communities: Building for the Future*. London: ODPM.

Office of the Deputy Prime Minister (ODPM) (2005a) *Sustainable Communities: Homes for All. A Five Year Plan from the Office of the Deputy Prime Minister*. London: ODPM.

Office of the Deputy Prime Minister (ODPM) (2005b) *Housing Statistics*. London: ODPM.

O'Higgins, M. (1985) 'Welfare, redistribution and inequality: disillusion, illusion and reality', in Bean, P., Ferris, J. and Whynes, D. (eds), *In Defence of Welfare*. London: Tavistock.

Oliver, M. (1990) *The Politics of Disablement*. Basingstoke: Macmillan.

Oliver, M. and Barnes, C. (1998) *Disabled People and Social Policy: From Exclusion to Inclusion*. Harlow: Longman.

Ormerod, D. (2005) *Smith and Hogan: Criminal Law*. Oxford: Oxford University Press.

Osbourne, D. and Gaebler, T. (1992) *Reinventing Government*. Reading, MA: Addison-Wesley.

Packer, H. (1968) *The Limits of the Criminal Sanction*. Stanford, CA: Stanford University Press.

Padfield, N. (2000) *Criminal Law*. London: Butterworth.

Pahl, J. (2003) 'The family and welfare', in Baldock, J., Manning, N. and Vickerstaff, S. (eds), *Social Policy* (2nd edn). Oxford: Oxford University Press.

Parker, G. (2006) 'Europe faces growth threat from ageing population'. *Financial Times*, 13 February.

Parker, J. (1972) *Social Policy and Citizenship*. Oxford: Martin Robertson.

Parkin, J. (2005) 'Academies' glitter may be fool's gold'. *Times Educational Supplement*, 7 October.

Parry, R. (1998) 'The view from Scotland', in Jones, H. and MacGregor, S. (eds), *Social Issues and Party Politics*. London: Routledge.

Parry, R. (2002) 'Delivery structure and policy development in post-devolution Scotland'. *Social Policy and Society* 1(4): 315–324.

Parry, R. (2008) 'Social policy and devolution', in Alcock, P., Erskine, A. and May, M. (eds), *The Student's Companion to Social Policy* (3rd edn). Oxford: Blackwell.

Pascall, G. (1986) *Social Policy: A Feminist Analysis*. London: Tavistock.

Pascall, G. (1997) *Social Policy: A New Feminist Analysis*. London: Routledge.

Pascall, G. (1999) *Social Policy: A Feminist Analysis* (2nd edn). London: Routledge.

Pateman, C. (1988) 'The patriarchal welfare state', in Gutmann, A. (ed.), *Democracy and the Welfare State*. Princeton, NJ: Princeton University Press.

Paton, G. (2005) 'Academies hit rock bottom'. *Times Educational Supplement*, 18 March.

Patsios, D. (2006) 'Pensioners, poverty and social exclusion', in Pantazis, C., Gordon, D. and Levitas, R. (eds), *Poverty and Social Exclusion in Britain: The Millennium Survey*. Bristol: Policy Press.

Paxman, J. (2003) *The Political Animal: An Anatomy*. London: Penguin.

Payne, G. (2006) *Social Divisions* (2nd edn). Basingstoke: Palgrave.

Peacock, A.T. and Wiseman, J. (1967) *The Growth of Public Expenditure in the United Kingdom*. London: Allen & Unwin.

Pearson, R. and Williams, G.L. (1984) *Political Thought and Public Policy in the Nineteenth Century: An Introduction*. London: Longman.

Peckham, S. (2007) 'One, or four? The National Health Service in 2006', in Clarke, K., Maltby, T. and Kennett, P. (eds), *Social Policy Review 19*. Bristol: Policy Press.

Pedersen, S. (1993) *Family, Dependence, and the Origins of the Welfare State: Britain and France 1914–1945*. Cambridge: Cambridge University Press.

Pelling, H. (1968) *Popular Politics and Society in Late Victorian Britain*. London: Macmillan.

Pelling, H. (1984) *The Labour Governments 1945–51*. London: Macmillan.

Pemberton, H. (2006) 'Politics and pensions in post-war Britain', in Pemberton, H., Thane, P. and Whiteside, N. (eds), *Britain's Pensions Crisis: History and Policy*. Oxford: British Academy/Oxford University Press.

Pemberton, H., Thane, P. and Whiteside, N. (eds) (2006a) *Britain's Pensions Crisis, ibid*.

Pemberton, H., Thane, P. and Whiteside, N. (2006b) 'Epilogue', in *Britain's Pensions Crisis, ibid*.

Pemberton, H., Thane, P. and Whiteside, N. (2006c) 'Introduction', in *Britain's Pensions Crisis, ibid*.

Penna, S. and O'Brien, M. (1996) 'Postmodernism and social policy: a small step forwards?' *Journal of Social Policy* 25(1): 39–61.

Pensions Commission (2004) *Pensions: Challenges and Choices. The First Report of the Pensions Commission*. London: The Stationery Office. www.pensionscommission.org.uk

Pensions Commission (2005) *A New Pension Settlement for the Twenty-First Century. The Second Report of the Pensions Commission*. London: The Stationery Office.

Pensions Commission (2006) *Implementing an Integrated Package of Pension Reforms. The Final Report of the Pensions Commission*. London: The Stationery Office.

Phelps, E.S. (ed.) (1973) *Economic Justice*. Harmondsworth: Penguin.

Phillips, A. (1999) *Which Equalities Matter?* Cambridge: Polity.

Phillips, T. (2005) 'Clement Attlee Lecture'. Commission for Racial Equality, http://www.cre.gov.uk/Default.aspx.LocID-0hgnew06b.RefLocID-0hg00900c002.Lang-EN.htm, accessed 5 June 2005.

Phillips, T. and Reid, J. (2004) *The Best Intentions: Race, Equity and Delivering Today's NHS*. London: Fabian Society.

Phillipson, C. (2006) 'Extending working life: problems and prospects for social and public policy', in Bauld, L., Clarke, K. and Maltby T. (eds), *Social Policy Review 18*. Bristol: Policy Press.

Pierre, J. and Peters, B.G. (2000) *Governance, Politics and State*. Basingstoke: Macmillan.

Pierson, C. (1996) 'Social policy', in Marquand, D. and Seldon, A. (eds), *The Ideas that Shaped Post-War Britain*. London: Fontana.

Pierson, C. (1998) *Beyond the Welfare State?* (2nd edn). Cambridge: Polity.

Pierson, C. (2006) *Beyond the Welfare State?* (3rd edn). Cambridge: Polity.

Pierson, C. and Castles, F.G. (eds) (2000) *The Welfare State Reader*. Cambridge: Polity.

Pierson, P. (1994) *Dismantling the Welfare State? Reagan, Thatcher, and the Politics of Retrenchment*. Cambridge: Cambridge University Press.

Pimlott, B. (1988) 'The myth of consensus', in Smith, L.M. (ed.), *The Making of Britain: Echoes of Greatness*. London: Macmillan and London Weekend Television.

Pimlott, B. (1993) *Harold Wilson*. London: HarperCollins.

Pimlott, B. (1994) *Frustrate their Knavish Tricks: Writings on Biography, History and Politics*. London: HarperCollins.

Pinder, J. (2001) *The European Union: A Very Short Introduction*. Oxford: Oxford University Press.

Pitts, J. and Smith, P. (1995) *Preventing School Bullying*. London: Police Research Group.

Plant, R. (1991) *Modern Political Thought*. Oxford: Blackwell.

Plant, R. (1996) 'Social democracy', in Marquand, D. and Seldon, A. (eds), *The Ideas that Shaped Post-War Britain*. London: Fontana.

Plant, R. (2001) 'Blair and ideology', in Seldon, A. (ed.), *The Blair Effect: The Blair Government 1997–2001*. London: Little, Brown.

Pliatzky, L. (1984) *Getting and Spending*. Oxford: Blackwell.

Pollard, M. (1984) *The Hardest Work under Heaven: The Life and Death of the British Coal Miner*. London: Hutchinson.

Pollitt, C. (1993) *Managerialism and Public Services*. Oxford: Blackwell.

Pollock, A.M. (2005) *NHS plc: The Privatisation of our Health Care*. London: Verso.

Porter, R. (1997) *The Greatest Benefit to Mankind: A Medical History of Humanity from Antiquity to the Present*. London: HarperCollins.

Powell, M. (1995) 'The strategy of equality revisited'. *Journal of Social Policy* **24**(2): 163–185.

Powell, M. (1997) *Evaluating the National Health Service*. Buckingham: Open University Press.

Powell, M. (ed.) (1999) *New Labour, New Welfare State?* Bristol: Policy Press.

Powell, M. (ed.) (2002) *Evaluating New Labour's Welfare Reforms*. Bristol: Policy Press.

Powell, M. and Hewitt, M. (2002) *Welfare State and Welfare Change*. Buckingham: Open University Press.

Power, M. (1993) *The Audit Explosion*. London: Demos.

Power, M. (1997) *The Audit Society*. Oxford: Oxford University Press.

Pratchett, L. (1999) 'Introduction: defining democratic renewal', *Local Government Studies* 25(4): 1–18.

Putnam, R. (2000) *Bowling Alone*. New York: Touchstone.

Race for Racial Justice (2005) http://www.r4rj.org.uk/immigrationlegislation.htm, accessed 6 June 2005.

Rae, D.W. (1981) *Equalities*. Cambridge: Harvard University Press.

Rake, K. (2001) 'Gender and New Labour's social policies'. *Journal of Social Policy* 30(2): 209–231.

Raphael, D.D. (1990) *Problems of Political Philosophy*. Basingstoke: Macmillan.

Ratcliffe, P. (2004) *'Race', Ethnicity and Difference: Imagining the Inclusive Society*. Maidenhead: Open University Press.

Rawls, J. (1972) *A Theory of Justice*. London: Oxford University Press.

Reay, D., Davies, J., David, M. and Ball, S. (2001) 'Choices of degree or degrees of choice? Class, 'race' and the higher education choice process'. *Sociology* 35(4): 855–874.

Rehnberg, C. (1997) 'Sweden', in Ham, C. (ed.), *Health Care Reform: Learning from International Experience*. Buckingham: Open University Press.

Reynolds, D. and Sullivan, M. (1987) *The Comprehensive Experiment*. Brighton: Falmer Press.

Rhodes, R. (1996) 'The new governance: governing without government'. *Political Studies* 44: 652–667.

Rhodes, R. (1997) *Understanding Governance: Policy Networks, Governance, Reflexivity and Accountability*. Buckingham: Open University Press.

Rhodes, R. (2000) 'Governance and public administration', in Pierre, J. (ed.), *Debating Governance*. Oxford: Oxford University Press.

Rhodes, R.A.W. (1988) *Beyond Westminster and Whitehall*. London: Unwin Hyman.

Rhodes, R.A.W. (1999) 'Foreword', in Stoker, G. (ed.), *The New Politics of British Local Governance*. London: Macmillan.

Richards, D. and Smith, M.J. (2003) *Governance and Public Policy in the UK*. Oxford: Oxford University Press.

Riley, K. (1998) *Whose School is it Anyway?* London: Routledge.

Ringen, S. (1987) *The Possibility of Politics: A Study in the Political Economy of the Welfare State*. Oxford: Clarendon Press.

Robbins, Lord (1963) *Report on Higher Education*. London: HMSO.

Roberts, J. (1984) 'T.H. Green', in Pelczynski, Z. and Gray, J. (eds), *Conceptions of Liberty in Political Philosophy*. London: Athlone Press.

Robinson, R. and Le Grand, J. (eds) (1994) *Evaluating the NHS Reforms*. London: King's Fund Institute.

Robson, W.A. and Crick, B. (eds) (1970) *The Future of the Social Services*. Harmondsworth: Penguin.

Rock, P. (1973) *Deviant Behaviour*. London: Hutchinson.

Rowntree, B.S. (1901) *Poverty: A Study of Town Life*. London: Macmillan.

Rummery, K. (2007) 'Modernising services, empowering users? Adult social care in 2006', in Clarke, K., Maltby, T. and Kennett, P. (eds), *Social Policy Review 19*. Bristol: Policy Press.

Rummery, K. and Glendinning, C. (1999) 'Negotiating needs, access and gate-keeping: developments in health and community care policies in the UK and the rights of disabled and older citizens'. *Critical Social Policy* **19**(3): 335–351.

Rummery, K. and Glendinning, C. (2000) 'Access to services as a civil and social rights issue: the role of welfare professionals in regulating access to and commissioning services for disabled and older people under New Labour'. *Social Policy and Administration* **34**(5): 529–550.

Sainsbury, D. (1996) *Gender, Equality and Welfare States*. Cambridge: Cambridge University Press.

Saraga, E. (ed.) (1998) *Embodying the Social: Constructions of Difference*. London: Routledge.

Sassi, F. (2005) 'Tackling health inequalities', in Hills, J. and Stewart, K. (eds), *A More Equal Society? New Labour, Poverty, Inequality and Exclusion*. Bristol: Policy Press.

Saville, J. (1957–58) 'The welfare state, an historical approach'. *New Reasoner* **1**(3): 5–25.

Schwartz, B. (2004) *The Paradox of Choice: Why Less is More*. London: HarperCollins.

Scott, P. (2002) 'The future of general education in mass higher education systems'. *Higher Education Policy* **15**: 61–75.

Scott, S. and Jackson, S. (2000) *Gender: A Sociological Reader*. London: Routledge.

Scruton, R. (1980) *The Meaning of Conservatism*. Harmondsworth: Penguin.

Sedlack, G. and Stanley, J. (1992) *Social Research: Theory and Methods*. Boston, MA: Allyn and Bacon.

Seebohm, F. (1968) *Report of the Committee on Local Authority and Allied Personal Social Services*. London: HMSO.

Seldon, A. (1994) 'Policy-making and Cabinet', in Kavanagh, D. and Seldon, A. (eds), *The Major Effect*. Basingstoke: Macmillan.

Sellin, T. (1938) *Culture Conflict and Crime*. New York: Social Science Research Council.

Sen, A. (1980) 'Equality of what?', in McMurrin, S.M. (ed.), *Liberty, Equality and Law*. Cambridge: Cambridge University Press.

Sen, A. (1987) *The Standard of Living*. Cambridge: Cambridge University Press.

Shakespeare, T. (1996) 'Disability, identity and difference', in Barnes, C. and Mercer, G. (eds), *Exploring the Divide: Illness and Disability*. Leeds: The Disability Press.

Shakespeare, T. (1998) 'Choices and rights, eugenics, genetics and disability equality'. *Disability and Society* **14**(5): 643–657.

Shakespeare, T. (2000) 'The social relations of care', in Lewis, G., Gewirtz, S. and Clarke, J. (eds), *Rethinking Social Policy*. London: The Open University in association with Sage.

Sharkey, P. (2006) *Essentials of Community Care* (2nd edn). Basingstoke: Palgrave Macmillan.

Sharp, K. and Earle, S. (2002) 'Feminism, abortion and disability: irreconcilable differences?' *Disability and Society* **17**(2): 137–145.

Sherry, M. (2004) 'Overlaps and contradictions between queer theory and disability studies'. *Disability and Society* **19**(17): 769–783.

Sieghart, P. (1985) *The Lawful Rights of Mankind*. Oxford: Oxford University Press.

Sked, A. and Cook, C. (1979) *Post-War Britain: A Political History*. Harmondsworth: Penguin.

Skidelsky, R. (ed.) (1988) *Thatcherism*. Oxford: Blackwell.

Skidelsky, R. (1996) *Keynes*. Oxford: Oxford University Press.

Skidelsky, R. (1997) *Beyond the Welfare State*. London: Social Market Foundation.

Slack, P. (1995) *The English Poor Law 1531–1782*. Cambridge: Cambridge University Press.

Smaje, C. (1995) *Health, 'Race' and Ethnicity: Making Sense of the Evidence*. London: King's Fund Institute.

Smart, C. (1990) 'Feminist approaches to criminology, or postmodern woman meets atavistic man', in Gelsthorpe, L. and Morris, A. (eds), *Feminist Perspectives in Criminology*. London: Routledge.

Smith, D. (1987) *The Rise and Fall of Monetarism: The Theory and Politics of an Economic Experiment*. Harmondsworth: Penguin.

Smith, D. (1993) *From Boom to Bust: Trial and Error in British Economic Policy*. Harmondsworth: Penguin.

Smith, D. (2005) 'The Treasury and economic policy', in Seldon, A. and Kavanagh, D. (eds), *The Blair Effect 2001–5*. Cambridge: Cambridge University Press.

Smith, K. (1989) *The British Economic Crisis: Its Past and Future*. Harmondsworth: Penguin.

Smith, M. (1999) *The Core Executive in Britain*. Basingstoke: Macmillan.

Smith, T. and Babbington, E. (2006) 'Devolution: a map of divergence in the NHS', in British Medical Association, *Health Policy Review – Issue 2: Different Approaches to Reforming Health Services*. London: BMA.

Social Exclusion Unit (SEU) (1998) *Bringing Britain Together: A National Strategy for Neighbourhood Renewal*. London: The Stationery Office.

Soil Association, http://www.soilassociation.org/web/sa/saweb.nsf

Spicker, P. (1995) *Social Policy: Themes and Approaches*. Hemel Hempstead: Prentice Hall / Harvester Wheatsheaf.

Stanko, E. (2001) 'The day to count: reflections on a methodology to raise awareness about the impact of domestic violence in the UK'. *Criminal Justice* 1(2): 215–226.

Stanley, L. and Wise, S. (1993) *Breaking Out Again: Feminist Consciousness and Feminist Research*. London: Routledge.

Statistics Commission (2005) *Measuring Standards in English Primary Schools*. Report no. 23. London: Statistics Commission.

Steger, M.B. (2003) *Globalization: A Very Short Introduction*. Oxford: Oxford University Press.

Stephens, M. and Quilgars, D. (2006) 'Strategic pragmatism? The state of housing policy', in Bauld, L., Clarke, K. and Maltby, T. (eds), *Social Policy Review 18*. Bristol: Policy Press.

Stephens, P. (1997) *Politics and the Pound: The Tories, the Economy and Europe*. London: Macmillan.

Stephens, P. (2001) 'The Treasury under Labour', in Seldon, A. (ed.), *The Blair Effect: The Blair Government 1997–2001*. London: Little, Brown.

Stewart, J. (2004) '"Scottish solutions to Scottish problems"? Social welfare in Scotland since devolution', in Ellison, N., Bauld, L. and Powell, M. (eds), *Social Policy Review 16*. Bristol: Policy Press.

Stewart, J. and Stoker, G. (1988) *The Future of Local Government*. Basingstoke: Macmillan.

Stewart, K. (2005a) 'Equality and social justice', in Seldon, A. and Kavanagh, D. (eds), *The Blair Effect 2001–5*. Cambridge: Cambridge University Press.

Stewart, W. (2005b) 'Doubts cast on academies'. *Times Educational Supplement*, 18 February.

Stoker, G. (1999) 'Introduction: the unintended costs and benefits of new management reform for British local government', in Stoker, G. (ed.), *The New Management of British Local Governance*. Basingstoke: Macmillan.

Stoker, G. and Mossberger, K. (1995) 'The post-Fordist local state: the dynamics of its development', in Stewart, J. and Stoker, G. (eds), *Local Government in the 1990s*. Basingstoke: Macmillan.

Sullivan, M. (1989) *The Social Politics of Thatcherism: New Conservatism and the Welfare State*. Swansea: University of Wales.

Sullivan, M. (1992) *The Politics of Social Policy*. London: Harvester Wheatsheaf.

Sullivan, M. (1996) *The Development of the British Welfare State*. London: Prentice Hall / Harvester Wheatsheaf.

Summers, D. (2007) 'Brown outlines legislative programme'. *The Guardian*, 11 July.

Sutherland, E. and Cressey, D. (1970) *Principles of Criminology* (6th edn). Philadelphia, PA: Lippincott.

Sutherland, S. (1999) *With Respect to Old Age: The Royal Commission on Long-Term Care* (the Sutherland Report). London: The Stationery Office.

Swann, D. (1988) *The Retreat of the State: Deregulation and Privatisation in the UK and US*. London: Harvester Wheatsheaf.

Swift, A. (2001) *Political Philosophy: A Beginners' Guide for Students and Politicians*. Cambridge: Cambridge University Press.

Sykes, R. and Alcock, P. (eds) (1998) *Developments in European Social Policy: Convergence and Diversity*. Bristol: Policy Press.

Sykes, R., Bochel, C. and Ellison, N. (2001a) 'The year in social policy', in Sykes, R., Bochel, C. and Ellison, N. (eds), *Social Policy Review 13: Developments and Debates 2000–2001*. Bristol: Policy Press.

Sykes, R., Palier, B. and Prior, P.M. (eds) (2001b) *Globalization and European Welfare States: Challenges and Change*. Basingstoke: Palgrave.

Tait, N. (2006a) 'Cancer sufferer loses drug fight'. *Financial Times*, 16 February.

Tait, N. (2006b) 'Breast cancer patient wins drug case'. *Financial Times*, 13 April.

Tappan, P. (2001) 'Who is the criminal?', in Henry, S. and Lanier, M. (eds), *What is Crime? Controversies over the Nature of Crime and What to Do About It*. Lanham, MD: Rowman and Littlefield.

Tarling, R. (1993) *Analysing Offending: Data Models and Interpretations*. London: HMSO.

Tawney, R.H. (1952) *Equality* (4th edn). London: Allen & Unwin.

Tawney, R.H. (1964) *Equality* (paperback edn). London: Allen & Unwin.

Taylor, A. (2006) 'Raise minimum wage, says TUC'. *Financial Times*, 9 September.

Taylor, A. (2007) 'CBI backs 3.2% rise in minimum wage'. *Financial Times*, 8 March.

Taylor, C. (1979) 'What's wrong with negative liberty?', in Ryan, A. (ed.), *The Idea of Freedom*. Oxford: Oxford University Press.

Taylor, I., Walton, P. and Young, J. (1973) *The New Criminology*. London: Routledge & Kegan Paul.

Taylor, R. (1994) 'Employment and industrial relations policy', in Kavanagh, D. and Seldon, A. (eds), *The Major Effect*. London: Macmillan.

Taylor, R. (2001) 'Employment relations policy', in Seldon, A. (ed.), *The Blair Effect: The Blair Government 1997–2001*. London: Little, Brown.

Taylor, R. (2005) 'Mr Blair's British business model – capital and labour in flexible markets', in Kavanagh, D. and Seldon, A. (eds), *The Blair Effect 2001–5*. Cambridge: Cambridge University Press.

Taylor, S. and Field, D. (eds) (2007) *Sociology of Health and Health Care*. Oxford: Blackwell.

Taylor-Gooby, P. (1985) *Public Opinion, Ideology and State Welfare*. London: Routledge.

Taylor-Gooby, P. (1991) *Social Change, Social Welfare and Social Science*. Hemel Hempstead: Harvester Wheatsheaf.

Taylor-Gooby, P. (1994) 'Postmodernism and social policy: a great leap backwards?' *Journal of Social Policy* 23(3): 385–404.

Teather, D. (2006) 'Glass ceiling still blocks women from executive floor'. *The Guardian*, 2 October.

Terrill, R. (1974) *R.H. Tawney and his Times*. London: André Deutsch.

Thane, P. (1996) *Foundations of the Welfare State*. London: Longman.

Thane, P. (2000) *Old Age in English History*. Oxford: Oxford University Press.

Thane, P. (2006a) 'Blair must not repeat Attlee's pensions mistake'. *Financial Times*, 24 May.

Thane, P. (2006b) 'The "scandal" of women's pensions in Britain: how did it come about?', in Pemberton, H., Thane, P. and Whiteside, N. (eds), *Britain's Pensions Crisis: History and Policy*. Oxford: British Academy/Oxford University Press.

Thatcher, M. (1987) Interview in *Woman's Own*, 31 October.

Thatcher, M. (1993) *The Downing Street Years*. London: HarperCollins.

The Information Centre (2007) *Community Care Statistics 2006: Home Help/Care Services for Adults, England*. London: The Information Centre.

Therborn, G. (2004) *Between Sex and Power: Family in the World, 1900–2000*. Abingdon: Routledge.

Therborn, G. and Roebroek, J. (1986) 'The irreversible welfare state: its recent maturation, its encounter with economic crisis, and its future prospects'. *International Journal of Health Services* 16(3): 319–338.

Threlfall, M. (2002) 'The European Union's social policy focus: from labour to welfare and constitutionalised rights?', in Sykes, R., Bochel, C. and Ellison, N. (eds), *Social Policy Review 14: Developments and Debates 2001–2002*. Lavenham, Suffolk: Social Policy Association.

Timmermans, S. and Gabe, J. (2004) *Partners in Health, Partners in Crime*. Oxford: Blackwell.

Timmins, N. (1995) *The Five Giants: A Biography of the Welfare State*. London: Fontana.

Timmins, N. (2005a) 'Doubts on funding NHS "monuments"'. *Financial Times*, 10 June.

Timmins, N. (2005b) 'Hewitt warns that failing hospitals will be closed'. *Financial Times*, 14 May.

Timmins, N. (2005c) 'NHS drugs regulator to withdraw approval of Alzheimer's treatment'. *Financial Times*, 2 March.

Timmins, N. (2005d) 'NHS plans for £200m overspend despite record funding'. *Financial Times*, 2 December.

Timmins, N. (2006a) 'Drip, drip of bad news drowns the good'. *Financial Times*, 2 March.

Timmins, N. (2006b) 'Financial mayhem exposes structural problems that beset the NHS'. *Financial Times*, 9 February.

Timmins, N. (ed.) (2006c) *Designing the 'New' NHS*. London: King's Fund.

Timmins, N. (2006d) 'Open for business: how private provision is bringing an agony of choice in the NHS'. *Financial Times*, 23 January.

Timmins, N. (2006e) 'Pension reform put at heart of welfare changes'. *Financial Times*, 16 November.

Timmins, N. (2006f) 'Pensions industry outlines rival scheme'. *Financial Times*, 10 February.

Timmins, N. (2006g) 'Pensions plan defers crucial decisions'. *Financial Times*, 13 December.

Timmins, N. (2006h) 'Protection needed for savings, says NAPF'. *Financial Times*, 9 September.

Timmins, N. (2006i) 'Turner attacks critics for "thoroughly bad arguments and red herrings"'. *Financial Times*, 10 February.

Timmins, N. (2007a) 'NHS spending rise beats expectations'. *Financial Times*, 10 October.

Timmins, N. (2007b) 'Hospital chief casts doubt on links with NHS'. *Financial Times*, 13 September.

Timmins, N. (2007c) 'Hain begins "crusade" for full employment'. *Financial Times*, 31 July.

Timmins, N. (2007d) 'Work is the route claimants must take, says Murphy'. *Financial Times*, 28 March.

Timmins, N. (2007e) 'Business "uncertain" about jobs plan role'. *Financial Times*, 19 July.

Timmins, N. (2007f) 'Call to revamp "woeful" New Deal'. *Financial Times*, 14 May.

Timmins, N. and Hall, B. (2006) 'Pensions revamp in jeopardy'. *Financial Times*, 22 March.

Titmuss, R.M. (1950) *Problems of Social Policy*. London: HMSO and Longmans Green & Co.

Titmuss, R.M. (1958) *Essays on 'The Welfare State'*. London: Allen & Unwin.

Titmuss, R.M. (1968) *Commitment to Welfare*. London: Allen & Unwin.

Titmuss, R.M. (1970) *The Gift Relationship*. London: Allen & Unwin.

Titmuss, R.M. (1974) *Social Policy*. London: Allen & Unwin.

Titmuss, R.M. (1987) 'Social welfare and the art of giving', in Abel-Smith, B. and Titmuss, K. (eds), *The Philosophy of Welfare*. London: Allen & Unwin.

Tobin, J. (1970) 'On limiting the domain of inequality'. *Journal of Law and Economics* 13 (2): 263–277.

Tomlinson, S. (2001) *Education in a Post-Welfare Society*. Milton Keynes: Open University Press.

Tomlinson, S. (2003) 'Globalization, race and education: continuity and change'. *Journal of Education and Change* 4(3): 213–230.

Tomlinson, S. (2004) 'The rise of the meritocracy', in Ellison, N., Bauld, L. and Powell, M. (eds), *Social Policy Review 16*. Bristol: Policy Press.

Tomlinson, S. (2005) *Education in a Post-Welfare Society* (2nd edn). Milton Keynes: Open University Press.

Townsend, P. (1979) *Poverty in the United Kingdom*. London: Allen Lane and Penguin.

Townsend, P. and Davidson, N. (1982) *Inequalities in Health*. Harmondsworth: Penguin.

Toynbee, P. (2006) 'Our children deserve the best, so we must be prepared to pay up'. *The Guardian*, 7 April.

Toynbee, P. and Walker, D. (2005) *Better or Worse? Has Labour Delivered?* London: Bloomsbury.

Tudor Hart, J. (1971) 'The inverse care law'. *Lancet*, i: 405–412.

Tymms, P. (2004) 'Are standards rising in English primary schools?' *British Educational Research Journal* 30(4): 477–494.

United Kingdom Parliament (2005) http://www.parliament.uk/directories/hci-olists/gender.cfm, accessed 24 May 2005.

Van Parijs, P. (ed.) (1992) *Arguing for Basic Income*. London: Verso.

Van Parijs, P. (1995) *Real Freedom for All*. Oxford: Oxford University Press.

Vincent, A. (1992) *Modern Political Ideologies*. Oxford: Blackwell.

Vincent, J. (2000) 'Age and old age', in Payne, G. (ed.), *Social Divisions*. Basingstoke: Palgrave.

Von Hirsch, A. (1976) *Doing Justice: The Choice of Punishments*. New York: Hill and Wang.

Waddell, G. and Burton, A.K. (2006) *Is Work Good for Your Health and Well-being?* London: The Stationery Office.

Waldegrave, W. (1993) *The Reality of Reform and Accountability in Today's Public Service*. London: Public Finance Foundation.

Walker, A. and Maltby, T. (1997) *Ageing Europe*. Buckingham: Open University Press.

Walker, N. (1991) *Why Punish?* Oxford: Oxford University Press.

Wanless, D. (2004) *Securing Good Health for the Whole Population: Final Report*. London: The Stationery Office.

Wanless, D. (2007) *Our Future Health Secured? A Review of NHS Funding and Performance*. London: King's Fund.

Weale, A. (1978a) 'Paternalism and social policy'. *Journal of Social Policy* 7(2): 157–172.

Weale, A. (1978b) *Equality and Social Policy*. London: Routledge.

Weale, A. (1985) 'The welfare state and two conflicting ideals of equality'. *Government and Opposition* 20(3): 315–327.

Weber, M. (1949) *Max Weber on the Methodology of the Social Sciences* (translated by E.A. Shils and H.A. Finch). Glencoe, IL: Free Press.

Webster, C. (ed.) (1993) *Caring for Health: History and Diversity*. Buckingham: Open University Press.

Webster, C. (1994) 'Conservatives and consensus: the politics of the National Health Service, 1951–64', in Oakley, A. and Williams, A.S. (eds), *The Politics of the Welfare State*. London: UCL Press.

Webster, C. (1998) *The National Health Service: A Political History*. Oxford: Oxford University Press.

Wedderburn, D. (1965) 'Facts and theories of the welfare state', in Miliband, R. and Saville, J. (eds), *The Socialist Register 1965*. London: Merlin Press.

Weeks, A. (1986) *Comprehensive Schools: Past, Present and Future*. London: Methuen.

Weller, P. (2000) 'In search of governance', in Davis, G. and Keating, M. (eds), *The Future of Governance*. St Leonards, NSW: Allen & Unwin.

West, D. (1982) *Delinquency: Its Roots, Careers and Prospects*. London: Heinemann.

White, M. and Wintour, P. (2005) 'Choice is a "tidal wave" that Labour must not ignore'. *The Guardian*, 11 February.

White, S. (2007) *Equality*. Cambridge: Polity.

Whitehead, C.M.E. (1993) 'Privatising housing: an assessment of UK experience'. *Housing Policy Debate* 4(1): 101–139.

Whitehead, M. (1987) *The Health Divide*. London: Health Education Council.

Whiteside, N. (1991) *Bad Times: Unemployment in British Social and Political History*. London: Faber.

Whiteside, N. (1998) 'Employment policy', in Ellison, N. and Pierson, C. (eds), *Developments in British Social Policy*. Basingstoke: Macmillan.

Wiggins, D. (1985) 'The claims of need' in Honderich, T. (ed.), *Morality and Objectivity*. London: Routledge.

Wilding, P. (1982) *Professional Power and Social Welfare*. London: Routledge.

Wilkinson, R.G. (1996) *Unhealthy Societies: The Afflictions of Inequality*. London: Routledge.

Willetts, D. (1989) 'The family', in Kavanagh, D. and Seldon, A. (eds), *The Thatcher Effect: A Decade of Change*. Oxford: Oxford University Press.

Willetts, D. (1992) *Modern Conservatism*. Harmondsworth: Penguin.

Willetts, D. (1994) *Civic Conservatism*. London: Social Market Foundation.

Williams, F. (1989) *Social Policy: A Critical Introduction*. Cambridge: Polity.

Williams, F. (2005) 'New Labour's family policy', in Powell, M., Bauld, L. and Clarke, K. (eds), *Social Policy Review 17*. Bristol: Policy Press.

Wilson, D. and Ashton, J. (2001) *What Everyone in Britain Should Know about Crime and Punishment*. Oxford: Oxford University Press.

Wilson, E. (1974) *Women and the Welfare State*. London: Red Rag Collective.

Wilson, J.Q. (1975) *Thinking about Crime*. New York: Basic Books.

Wilson, T. and Wilson, D. (eds) (1991) *The State and Social Welfare: The Objectives of Policy*. London: Longman.

Winter, J.M. (1984) 'R.H. Tawney', in Barker, P. (ed.), *Founders of the Welfare State*. London: Heinemann.

Wistow, G., Knapp, M., Hardy, B. and Allen, C. (1994) *Social Care in a Mixed Economy*. Buckingham: Open University Press.

Wolff, J. (1996) *An Introduction to Political Philosophy*. Oxford: Oxford University Press.

Women and Equality Unit (WEU) (2005) *Individual Income 1996/97 – 2003/04*. London: Department of Trade and Industry.

Woolmington v *DPP* (1935) AC 462 at 481.

World Bank (1994) *Averting the Old Age Crisis: Policies to Protect the Old and Promote Growth*. Oxford: Oxford University Press.

Wright, T. (1997) *Why Vote Labour?* Harmondsworth: Penguin.

Yeates, N. (2001) *Globalization and Social Policy*. London: Sage.

Yeates, N. (2002) 'The "antiglobalisation" movement and its implications for social policy', in Sykes, R., Bochel, C. and Ellison, N. (eds), *Social Policy Review 14: Development and Debates 2001–2002*. Lavenham, Suffolk: Social Policy Association.

Young, H. and Sloman, A. (1984) *But, Chancellor: An Inquiry into the Treasury*. London: BBC.

Glossary of terms

Acts of Settlement   Name given to a number of Acts of Parliament passed from the sixteenth century that defined who was eligible for parish relief. In order to try to keep Poor Law costs down, the parish was only responsible for paupers who were born within a parish or who had some other connection, for example through marriage.

Actus reus   The type of offence committed.

Adversarial   Description of the British legal system in which participants are pitted against one another either as plaintiff and respondent in civil law or prosecution and defendant in criminal law.

Altruism   Unselfish concern for others. The basis of a moral, or other-regarding, outlook, as opposed to a selfish or egoistic one. The question of how far social policies and welfare states depend on such altruistic concern for others has been much debated; some writers, such as Richard Titmuss in his book *The Gift Relationship* (1970) argued that it was an important underpinning for the welfare state.

'Basic Income' or 'Citizen's Income'   An idea which in various forms has been around for a long time. It involves a critique of existing social security systems, based on social insurance or social assistance principles, as exclusionary, and proposes their replacement by a universal tax-financed cash grant, payable to all individuals regardless of labour market position, marital status, etc. It involves removing the link between work and entitlement which is so important in most contemporary social security systems.

Beveridge   Sir William Beveridge, a civil servant/academic responsible for the publication of the Social Insurance and Allied Services Report of 1942 – the Beveridge Report – often considered the blueprint for much of the development of the post-war British welfare state.

Bretton Woods   Refers to the Bretton Woods system of monetary management regulations for the western capitalist states. A series of Bretton Woods agreements were signed in 1944 at Bretton Woods, New Hampshire, USA, and created the World Bank and the IMF.

Classical liberalism   Descriptive of a political doctrine usually associated with the nineteenth century and with early formulations of social policy. An interventionist role for the state may be justified where other social structures (markets) are seen to be failing and wherein state activity is minimal or residual.

Communitarianism   Range of ideas expressing the desire to re-establish or rediscover 'civil society', in which collective welfare is expressed through the agency of the active community and active citizen rather than that of a centralised state machinery.

Comprehensive schools   Schools offering education without attempting to differentiate between abilities of pupils along arbitrary academic or technical lines. Developed as the preferred method of state schooling during the 1960s and 1970s.

Consensus/welfare consensus   Term applied to the post-war political settlement characterised by the similarities exhibited in the economic policies of successive Labour (Gaitskell) and Conservative (Butler) Chancellors of the Exchequer. In particular, the consensus was said to be built upon the acceptance of the role of the state in the pursuit of welfare and greater equality together with the pursuit of full employment as an economic principle.

Consumerism   Neo-liberal doctrine which stresses the role of the individual as consumer of welfare services within a market or quasi-market oriented welfare state. It regards consumers as having sovereignty within markets which individuals lack in any state-dominated system of welfare provision.

Crime control   Model of criminal justice policy that is concerned with attempts to suppress crime and criminal activity, often without regard to the consequences for civil rights.

Crown Prosecution Service (CPS)   Government agency given responsibility for deciding whether to instigate, and pursue, criminal proceedings through the courts.

'Decline', 'declinism'   An influential view, mood or feeling held by opinion-formers, journalists and to some extent by politicians and the public about the state of the UK from the 1950s to the 1980s, namely that it was 'in decline'. The UK appeared to be relatively economically unsuccessful compared with, for example, many European countries and Japan. Growth rates were low by comparison with other countries, and there were endemic industrial relations problems and balance of payments crises. (In fact the UK's economic growth performance was quite respectable in comparison with its own past history.) This pessimistic mood or feeling was enhanced by two things: the UK's having 'won the war' in 1945 but now appearing much less successful than its defeated rivals; and the disappearance of the Empire between the 1940s and 1960s. 'Declinism' was in fact widely shared by left and right, but can be seen as underpinning the views particularly of the Thatcher Governments in the 1980s, which went on to claim that they had solved the problem of the UK's decline.

Democracy Movement   This is a non-party pressure group, set up to prevent the British Government from adopting the Euro as its currency, thereby replacing the pound sterling. The organisation is against an EU constitution, viewing the EU as an undemocratic superstate.

Democratic deficit   Term describing the lack or weakness of traditional democratic forms of control and scrutiny of the Executive arm of European policy making.

Deserving poor   Term applied to paupers thought to be more genuine and therefore deserving of parish relief. This might include those people who find themselves in poverty by virtue of illness, disability or old age.

Discrimination   The act of making distinctions – usually in reference to particular social groups, for example based on race or ethnicity, gender, class, sexual orientation – and treating differently (and less or more favourably) because of such distinctions; direct discrimination is where an individual or group is treated differently (and less favourably) directly, for example, because of their ethnicity, gender or sexual orientation; indirect discrimination is where an individual or group is treated differently (and less favourably) as an indirect consequence of a policy or practice.

Due process   Model of criminal justice policy that is concerned with the pursuit of justice within the criminal legal system.

Enabling Authority   The job of a local authority, for example, its adult social care department, is increasingly to co-ordinate and monitor the quality of social care provision within its locale rather than to act as a provider of such services. The Enabling Authority was to be key in the development of an internal market in social care following the passage of the NHS and Community Care Act 1990.

Enlightenment   This term describes the historical period at the end of the middle ages during which rational and scientific methods of thought and investigation were developed.

Equal opportunities policies   A range of policies designed to narrow gender or other inequalities within society, either by equalising outcomes of policy initiatives or equalising the environment within which policy operates.

Ethnocentrism   Term describing attitudes and the development of policies that explicitly or implicitly discriminate against minority ethnic groups.

European Community/European Union (EC/EU)   The economic association developed among European countries following the Second World War which aims to create a single market on the continent of Europe and to guarantee economic progress.

European Free Trade Association   Alternative form of economic association to the EU designed around bilateral agreement between member states rather than common agreements across all member states.

Exchange Rate Mechanism   Monetary system established within the EU designed to tie the rate of currency exchange of its member nations more closely and to minimise rapid and wild currency fluctuation.

Fabianism   A range of political ideas associated with the rise of the Labour Party in Britain which promotes an active and redistributive role for the state. Often described as the 'Parliamentary road'.

Five giants   The most pressing social problems – Want, Ignorance, Disease, Idleness and Squalor – as defined by the Beveridge Report.

Full employment   Unwritten government goal throughout much of the post-war era which sought to maintain consistently low levels of (male manufacturing) unemployment.

Grant Maintained Status Also known as 'opted out' schools, such schools are managed independently of their local authority and financed directly by the Education Department.

Health promotion Describes a set of policies designed to induce personal and individual responsibility for health issues. Usually involves a programme of health education to promote healthier lifestyles, for example by discouraging health-damaging behaviour such as smoking, heavy drinking or poor diet or by promoting particular health issues such as more careful sexual behaviour.

Historical Materialism Marx's theory of social development in which he suggested that all human societies were governed, in their development, by immutable historical laws.

Inter alia Literally meaning 'amongst other things'.

Invisible Hand Term coined by the economist Adam Smith to describe the 'natural' operation of the free market and its tendency to self-regulation.

'Keynesian social democracy', 'Keynesian welfare state' These are shorthand terms used to describe or refer to, typically, European welfare systems and states such as that of the UK from the 1940s until the 1970s, underpinned by a combination of economic policy and social policy in order to promote social goals. 'Keynesian' (which refers to the economist John Maynard Keynes, who developed a new theory about unemployment and economic policy in the 1930s) in this context refers to the commitment to use economic policy tools to maintain high or 'full' employment and to the belief that governments can effectively manage the economy to achieve this and other economic policy goals, including low inflation, balance of payments stability and a reasonable rate of economic growth. This is complemented by the development of a comprehensive range of high-quality universalist welfare services. The Keynesian welfare state concept is also typically associated with the concept of the post-war 'consensus'.

Laissez-faire Economic and political principle which argues for freedom of action for individuals, especially in commerce and economics, and is, therefore, against extensive government activity or intervention.

Laissez-faire capitalism Seen as a pure form of capitalism, it implies that governments should not intervene in the workings of the economy (laisser faire: to leave alone), and leave all to the workings of the 'market'. This school of thought believes business operations should be unimpeded.

Legitimacy, legitimation This involves a reference to states, governments, social orders and institutions (such as welfare institutions) and the degree to which they command the loyalty and support of the population and their authority is accepted.

Less eligibility Principle of the Poor Law that suggested that the relief given to the poor should be at a level below that of the lowest paid of labourers to ensure that the poor would choose work rather than relief.

Life expectancy The average period a person, of a given age, may expect to live.

Local management of schools A system of management in schools in which much decision making is devolved to head teachers and boards of governors rather than LEAs.

Means-test   Test of income or wealth which determines entitlements to welfare benefits. Not all benefits, however, are subject to a means-test.

Mens rea   Intention to commit a criminal act.

Micro-economic, macro-economic   Micro-economics refers to the sphere of economic activity, markets and market exchanges in particular sectors of the economy, to, for example, the behaviour of firms and enterprises in innovating, setting prices, determining output and production, to the labour market and the processes of determining wages and labour supply, and to families and households in making decisions about consuming, working and so on. Macro-economics is concerned with the level of the whole economy, rather than particular sectors or markets. It is concerned with such issues as price stability and inflation and the balance of payments. It is typically associated with such issues as monetary policy, e.g. whether the central bank should pursue price stability through inflation targeting, and with fiscal balance and fiscal policy – the appropriate level of taxes and the volume of public spending.

'Mixed economy of welfare' or 'welfare pluralism'   As descriptive terms, these refer to the fact that welfare in any society is a product of a variety of agencies and institutions, including voluntary, commercial and informal ones (such as the family), as well as statutory (public) agencies. The terms may also have a programmatic aspect to them, namely, that policy should seek to develop a plurality of welfare-providing institutions and try to move away from an exclusive reliance on one, such as statutory agencies.

Mode of production   Marx's term describing the organisation within a society of resources (forces of production) – capital, labour, land and raw materials.

Monetarism   Economic theory which emphasises the control of the money supply as a method of managing the economy and in particular of controlling inflation.

Morbidity   Measure of the rate of disease or illness in a society within a given period.

Mortality   Measure of the rate of death in a society within a given period.

National assistance   A system of welfare (mostly cash) benefits to which entitlement is most usually determined by the administration of a means-test. This system has operated under various guises over the past 50 years, developed as Supplementary Benefits and latterly Income Support.

National Curriculum   A standardised curriculum approved by the Department for Education which stresses the development of literacy and numeracy and allows for comparisons of achievement between schools.

National Insurance   A system of welfare (cash) benefits to which entitlement is determined by a National Insurance Contributions record.

National Minimum Wage (NMW)   Introduced from April 1999, the NMW is to be a key element of Labour's Welfare to Work strategy by, they hope, making low paid employment more attractive.

Negative equity   A term coined after the slump in the private housing market in the early 1990s. Describes a situation wherein the market value of a property is less than the outstanding mortgage liability.

Non-contributory benefits Range of cash benefits to which entitlement is determined by criteria other than National Insurance contributions.

People's Budget Lloyd-George's redistributive Budget of 1909 which imposed higher levels of taxation on the rich in order to finance spending on social policies, including pensions and contributions to the National Insurance fund.

Polytechnic A type of higher education institution developed in the 1960s offering degree-level study but specialising in the teaching of technical and vocational subjects. Polytechnics ceased to exist in Britain in 1991 as they were granted full university status.

Poor Law A system of pauper relief developed in Britain between the sixteenth and nineteenth centuries. In its earlier form, the parish was charged with responsibility for the poor living within its boundaries who would be helped with either outdoor relief – money or food and goods – which allowed the poor to carry on living and working within the parish. Alternatively the parish could provide indoor relief through workhouses, which would put the poor to work in return for assistance. The New Poor Law, which operated from 1834, did away with most outdoor relief and depended much more on the provision of help within the workhouse. The workhouse was intended to act as a deterrent and to encourage the poor to find work rather than rely on the help granted by the local Board of Guardians of the Poor who administered the new system.

Post-Fordism A term used in industrial sociology and political economy. 'Fordism' – the reference is to Henry Ford, the American creator of a mass-production car industry – refers to industrial processes – the mass-production of standardised products and components in large-scale manufacturing firms and enterprises which developed in the twentieth century for a mass market with supposedly uniform and standardised tastes. 'Post-Fordism' refers to an alleged decline of such standardised mass production and its replacement by a diversified model of smaller-scale production for a much more diversified market, perhaps involving a decline in the giant manufacturing firm, 'lean' production processes and outsourcing.

Power (dominance) and new criminology Model of criminal justice that sees crime as a 'social construct' such that neither individuals nor their behaviour should be regarded as inherently criminal.

Pre-fabrication Method of rapid housing construction in which house components were constructed in factories and assembled on site.

Pre-Sentence Reports (PSRs) Documents prepared for a criminal trial which provide the court with background information about the accused person.

Primary Health Care Health services provided often as the first point of treatment. Examples include General Practice, dentistry, health visiting services and locally based health clinics. Primary care has been identified as the cornerstone of 'New Labour' health policy, which intends to focus on the development of locality planning of health services.

Qualified Majority Voting (QMV) Refers to the new simplified system of voting in the European Union. Under this new system of Council decision-making, a qualified majority is achieved only if a decision is supported by 55% of Member States, including at least 15 of them, representing at least 65% of the Union's population. Unanimity is not required.

'Quasi-market' or 'internal market'   A kind of market associated with reforms of UK welfare agencies in the 1990s. It depends on the idea that there are two important elements in the organisation and delivery of welfare services – financing the service and providing or delivering it – and that these two elements can be separated to some extent. The agency remains part of the public sector, but an element of competition is injected into their operations by separating the function of purchasing the service from that of providing it. Henceforth, two different agencies are involved – a purchasing (or 'commissioning') agency (such as, in the NHS, a Primary Care Trust or PCT) and a providing agency (such as, in the NHS, a Foundation Hospital). The purchasing/commissioning agency, working on behalf of their local resident population, may select any provider on grounds of quality, cost, accessibility and so on. Versions of the idea have been applied to health, social care, housing and education in an attempt to improve quality, efficiency and responsiveness.

Queen's Counsel (QC)   Senior barristers who usually work in the higher levels of the court system – High Court, Court of Appeal, House of Lords.

Rational choice theory (also known as **public choice theory**)   An application of economic concepts and methodology to other areas of social life. It involves the idea that social life and social institutions, including the state and politics, can be understood as the outcome of behaviour by rationally-choosing individuals seeking to maximise advantage.

Relative deprivation   A term, made famous by the work of Peter Townsend, used in poverty research and policy. Above the level of destitution or absolute subsistence, poverty is only meaningful if defined in terms of a relationship, between a norm of an average or generally acceptable or 'decent' standard of living in a particular society, shared by most people, and groups unable, because of lack of income, to share in this. Such groups may be described as 'relatively deprived'. The concept acknowledges the constantly-evolving nature of poverty and of the societal norm of decency.

Reserve army of labour   Groups of workers maintained in capitalist societies who are available to work when the economic system enters one of its periodic boom cycles.

Restructuring   This can refer to one of two things: 1. A general process of economic and industrial change, such as that accompanying the decline of manufacturing industry and rise of service industries, as in the UK from the 1970s to the 1990s, or with 'post-Fordist' transformations of the industrial sphere; 2. Changes in public sector organisations, such as welfare delivery agencies, particularly associated with the decline of the traditional post-war rational-bureaucratic public administration model and development of so-called 'new public management', involving new forms of management, 'quasi'-markets and purchaser-provider separation.

Serious Fraud Office   State-sponsored organisation responsible for the investigation of commercial malpractice such as insider trading.

Skills shortage/skills mismatch Two terms used to describe shortfalls in education and training policy. Skills shortage is a term particularly related to school leavers, who lack education in the skills relevant to and required by industry and the economy generally. Skills mismatch is a term referring to the type of skills possessed by workers and their inapplicability to the needs of the economy. An example would be where there have been redundancies in traditional industries, say engineering, and a rise in new technologies, computing and telecommunications, and the skills of the traditional industry are not readily transferred to the new.

Social Chapter Annex to the Maastricht Treaty which lays down proposals to widen the concept of European social policy, initially without British participation.

Social Charter More correctly called the Community Charter of the Fundamental Rights of Workers, this represents a key stage in the widening of the concept of European social policy beyond simply the rights attributed to those in employment.

Social control A sociological concept which refers to the achievement of social order through the regulation of society and social life by various means, including, in complex, differentiated, modern societies, the exercise of state power, behaviour-regulating law and legislation, agencies of coercion such as armed forces and police, and also such means as religion and education.

Standard Attainment Tests (SATs) A system of assessing school children at ages 7, 11 and 14 which is used to measure a child's progress and upon which School League Tables have been based.

Stigma A term made famous by the American sociologist Erving Goffman in his book of that title (1963). Stigma involves the idea of 'spoiled identity'. It involves loss of status or dignity in some sense. Students of social policy in the 1960s and 1970s such as Richard Titmuss were particularly concerned with the issue of how and to what extent social policies and services might engender stigma among service users. The issue was perhaps most serious for long-term recipients of services in the social care sector and some parts of means-tested social security, but was important wherever distinctions were made between service beneficiaries or users on, for example, income grounds. Examples could include school children receiving free school meals who were identified as such. The Poor Law was an example of a social policy that was, to some extent, deliberately designed to stigmatise.

Sub-regional governance Refers to the regional groupings of national states engaged in applying supranational economic and political policies and regulation, such as the European Union (EU), the North American Free Trade Association (NAFTA) and the Organisation of African Unity (OAU).

Subsidiarity Doctrine of policy making in the European Union which holds that policy decisions should be taken at the lowest appropriate level and that national governments should take precedence over the European Commission.

Tenure Set of legal rights to occupy property whether as rented, leased or owner-occupied property.

Tripartism A term denoting the 'three-way' organisation and management of compulsory and secondary education in Britain after the Second World War. Secondary schooling was split between the grammar, modern and technical schools, entry for which would be determined by assessment – the eleven-plus examination. Management in the education system was divided between the Ministry for Education, Local Education Authorities and teachers in schools.

United Kingdom Independence Party (UKIP)   A libertarian political party, founded in 1993, whose main goal is the UK's withdrawal from the EU, on the basis that the latter has destroyed the country's political sovereignty.

Undeserving or indolent poor   Term applied to paupers thought to be less genuine and therefore not deserving of parish relief. This might include those simply unemployed and regarded as indolent or lazy, beggars and 'tramps' who moved about the country in search of work.

Underclass   A term describing a stratum of the poor within a population which is said to be living outside and detached from established social norms and is both reliant upon and encouraged by a generous welfare benefits system.

Universal, universalism   These terms refer to welfare services and programmes which are in some sense available to all, not just some section of the population. Child Benefit is, for example, available to all mothers with dependent children, regardless of income level. Universal may be contrasted with 'selective' social services or benefits, but the distinction is a difficult one. Means-tested social security benefits (Income Support, Jobseekers' Allowance) might be regarded as 'selective' benefits (by contrast with Child Benefit), but in reality anyone meeting the eligibility criteria is entitled. Perhaps the distinction is better thought of in terms of a distinction between benefits and services which are only available on the basis of a means-test (selective) and those which are not, such as Child Benefit, the State Retirement Pension and NHS care (universal). Universalism and universal benefits are often associated with an equality-promoting, 'institutional' model of the welfare state, in the sense of one that promotes universal equal citizenship, selectivism and selective benefits in comparison with a welfare system merely focused on relieving poverty, but the reality is more complex.

Utilitarianism   Philosophy expounded by (particularly) Jeremy Bentham which argued that all human decisions were a choice between pleasure and pain and that rational individuals would usually satisfy (short-term) pleasure. In turn, Bentham argued that the correct role for the (welfare) state was to maximise human pleasure.

Welfare and rehabilitation   Model of criminal justice that seeks to rehabilitate the 'criminal' back into wider society.

Welfare to Work   Programme of employment assistance, more widely available than earlier targeted schemes, which employs a system of subsidy for employers who create permanent jobs for the unemployed. Initially targeted at the younger unemployed, it was later extended to include the long-term unemployed, single parents and the disabled.

Winter of discontent   Period of industrial unrest, particularly in the public sector, between the autumn of 1978 and spring of 1979, which marked the end of the Labour government's policy of wages control in order to control the economy.

Index